FAMILY VIOLENCE AND NURSING PRACTICE

2nd Edition

Janice Humphreys, PhD, RN, NP, FAAN, is Associate Professor and Vice Chair for Faculty Practice in the Department of Family Health Care Nursing at the University of California at San Francisco. Previous to her position at UCSF, Dr. Humphreys taught at the University of Michigan and Wayne State University Schools of Nursing. She is a Pediatric Nursing Practitioner and actively serves several professional organizations, including elected offices for the Nursing Network on Violence Against Women (Pres. 2003–2005); the American Academy of Nursing Co-Chair Expert Panel on Violence (2006–present); and Board Member for the Academy on Violence and Abuse (2008–present). She is an ad hoc referee for numerous professional journals, including the *Journal of Family Nursing*; the *Journal of Midwifery/Women's Health*; *Nursing Research*; *Clinical Child and Family Psychology*; the *Journal of Interpersonal Violence*; the *Journal of Pediatrics*; and *Nursing Outlook*. She is a Fellow in the American Academy of Nursing (invited 2006).

Jacquelyn C. Campbell, PhD, RN, FAAN, is Professor and Anna D. Wolf Chair at the Johns Hopkins University School of Nursing, and the National Program Director for the Robert Wood Johnson Foundation Nurse Faculty Scholars Program. She is the recipient of multiple honors and awards, including the Pathfinder Award for Nursing Research of the Friends of the National Institute of Nursing Research (2006), and three honorary doctorates (the University of Goteberg, Sweden; the University of Massachusetts; and Grand Valley State University, Michigan). Her >200 publications include peer-reviewed research, book chapters, and seven books. She has served as consultant on violence against women globally, health disparities, and research training on violence. She has been Principal Investigator of seven major research grants, from NIH, NIJ, CDC, and DoD, on a variety of abuse topics including: Abuse Status/Health Consequences for African American and Afro-Caribbean Women; Domestic Violence Enhanced Home Visitation; Health/Employment Outcomes of Workplace Violence for Nursing Personnel; and Risk Assessment Validation. Dr. Campbell is a Fellow in the American Academy of Nursing (1988), an elected member of the Institute of Medicine (2000), and President of the Board of Directors of the Family Violence Prevention Fund.

FAMILY VIOLENCE AND NURSING PRACTICE

2nd Edition

Janice Humphreys, PhD, RN, NP, FAAN
Jacquelyn C. Campbell, PhD, RN, FAAN

EDITORS

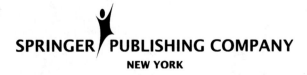

SPRINGER PUBLISHING COMPANY
NEW YORK

Springer Publishing Company, LLC
11 West 42nd Street
New York, NY 10036
www.springerpub.com

Acquisitions Editor: Margaret Zuccarini
Project Editor: Peter Rocheleau
Project Manager: Amor Nanas
Cover Design: TG Design
Composition: The Manila Typesetting Company

ISBN: 978-0-8261-1828-8

E-book ISBN: 978-0-8261-1829-5

14/ 5 4 3

The author and the publisher of this work have made every effort to use sources believed to be reliable to provide information that is accurate and compatible with the standards generally accepted at the time of publication. Because medical science is continually advancing, our knowledge base continues to expand. Therefore, as new information becomes available, changes in procedures become necessary. We recommend that the reader always consult current research and specific institutional policies before performing any clinical procedure. The author and publisher shall not be liable for any special, consequential, or exemplary damages resulting, in whole or in part, from the readers' use of, or reliance on, the information contained in this book. The publisher has no responsibility for the persistence or accuracy of URLs for external or third-party Internet Web sites referred to in this publication and does not guarantee that any content on such Web sites is, or will remain, accurate or appropriate.

Library of Congress Cataloging-in-Publication Data

Family violence and nursing practice / [edited by] Janice Humphreys, Jacquelyn C. Campbell. — 2nd ed.
    p. ; cm.
Includes bibliographical references and index.
ISBN 978-0-8261-1828-8 — ISBN 978-0-8261-1829-5 (e-book)
    1. Family violence. 2. Nursing.
I. Humphreys, Janice. II. Campbell, Jacquelyn.
[DNLM: 1. Domestic Violence. 2. Nursing Care. 3. Nurse's Role.
WY 150 F1987 2010]
RC569.5.F3F37 2010
362.82'92–dc22

                                                                        2010024115

Printed in the United States of America by Gasch Printing

To Rick and Jack, with love

—Janice

With love to Christy and Brad and Nik,
Grace, Sophie, Nadia, Nathan, and Leila

and for always, Reg

and in tribute to
Dorothy and Joe Bowman
and
Constance Morrow

—Jackie

Contents

vii

Contributors

Angela Frederick Amar, PhD, RN
Assistant Professor, William F. Connell School of Nursing
Boston College
Chestnut Hill, MA

Sarah Anderson, PhD, RN, CEN, SANE-A
Research Assistant Professor, University of Virginia School of Nursing
Charlottesville, VA

Sandra L. Annan, PhD, RN
Professor, James Madison University College of Integrated Science and
    Technology
Department of Nursing
Harrisonburg, VA

Helene Berman, PhD, RN
Professor, School of Nursing
Scotiabank Research Chair, Centre for Research & Education on Violence Against Women
    and Children, The University of Western Ontario
London, Ontario, Canada

Shreya Bhandari, PhD, MSW
Post Doctoral Research Fellow, Sinclair School of Nursing
University of Missouri
Columbia, MO

Jamie Blankenship, BSN, RN
Research Assistant, NYU College of Nursing
New York, NY

Tina Bloom, PhD, MPH, RN
University of Missouri Sinclair School of Nursing
Columbia, MO

Linda F. C. Bullock, PhD, RN, FAAN
Professor, University of Missouri Sinclair School of Nursing
Columbia, MO

Candace Burton, PhD(c), RN
School of Nursing, University of California—San Francisco
San Francisco, CA

Billy Caceres, BSN, RN
Research Assistant, NYU College of Nursing
New York, NY

Angela Chandracomar, BSN, RN
Research Assistant, NYU College of Nursing
New York, NY

Mary Ann Curry, DNSc, RN
Professor Emeritus, Oregon Health and Science University School of Nursing
Sherwood, OR

Jessica E. Draughon, PhD(c), RN
Doctoral Candidate, Johns Hopkins University School of Nursing
Santa Rosa, CA

Rochelle Einboden, MN, RN
Lecturer, University of British Columbia School of Nursing
Vancouver, British Columbia, Canada

Nancy Fishwick, PhD, RN, FNP
Director and Associate Professor
University of Maine School of Nursing
Orono, ME

Marilyn Ford-Gilboe, RN, PhD
Professor and Faculty Scholar, Arthur Labatt Family School of Nursing
The University of Western Ontario
London, Ontario, Canada

Nina M. Fredland, PhD, RN, FNP
Assistant Professor, The University of Texas at Austin School of Nursing
Austin, TX

Terry Fulmer, PhD, RN, FAAN
Erline Perkins McGriff Professor and Dean
New York University College of Nursing
New York, NY

Jessica M. Gill, RN, PhD
Assistant Clinical Investigator, National Institute of Nursing Research
Bethesda, MD

Nancy Glass, PhD, MPH, RN, FAAN
Associate Professor, Johns Hopkins University School of Nursing
Baltimore, MD

Rosa M. Gonzalez-Guarda, PhD, MPH, RN
Assistant Professor
M. Christine Schwartz Center for Nursing and Health Studies
University of Miami School of Nursing and Health Studies
Coral Gables, FL

Sepali Guruge, PhD, RN
Associate Professor, Daphne Cockwell School of Nursing
Ryerson University
Toronto, Ontario, Canada

Jennifer L. Hardesty, PhD
Assistant Professor, University of Illinois at Urbana-Champaign
Urbana, IL

Dena Hassouneh, PhD, RN
Associate Professor, Oregon Health Sciences University School of Nursing
Portland, OR

Susan J. Kelley, PhD, RN, FAAN
Dean and Professor, College of Health and Human Sciences
Atlanta, GA

Ursula A. Kelly, PhD, RN, ANP-BC, PMHNP-BC
Visiting Scholar, Nell Hodgson Woodruff School of Nursing, Emory University
Nurse Scientist, Atlanta VA Medical Center
Atlanta, GA

Kathryn Laughon, PhD, RN
Associate Professor, University of Virginia School of Nursing
Charlottesville, VA

Annie Lewis-O'Connor, NP-BC, MPH, PhD
Program Director of Nursing Practice, Center for Women and Newborns
Brigham and Women's Hospital Instructor, Harvard Medical School
Boston, MA

Marguerite B. Lucea, PhD, MSN, MPH, RN
Doctoral Candidate, Johns Hopkins University School of Nursing
Washington, DC

Marilyn Merritt-Gray, MN, RN
Professor, Faculty of Nursing, University of New Brunswick
Fredericton, New Brunswick, Canada

Nina Ng, BSN, RN
Research Assistant, NYU College of Nursing
New York, NY

Barbara J. Parker, RN, PhD, FAAN
Theresa A. Thomas Professor of Nursing
Claude Moore Nursing Education Building
Charlottesville, VA

Mary C. Sengstock, PhD, CCS
Professor of Sociology, Wayne State University
Detroit, MI

Phyllis W. Sharps, PhD, RN, CNE, FAAN
Professor and Chair, Dept. of Community Public Health Nursing
Johns Hopkins University School of Nursing
Baltimore, MD

Daniel J. Sheridan, PhD, RN, FNE-A, FAAN
Associate Professor, Johns Hopkins University School of Nursing
Baltimore, MD

Janette Y. Taylor, PhD, RN, WHCNP-BC
Associate Professor, University of Iowa College of Nursing
Iowa City, IA

Agnes Tiwari, PhD, RN
Associate Professor, Department of Nursing Studies
The University of Hong Kong, Pokfulam, Hong Kong

Joan C. Urbancic, PhD, RN
Professor Emeritus, University of Detroit Mercy
Detroit, MI

Colleen Varcoe, RN, PhD
Professor, Associate Director, Research
University of British Columbia School of Nursing
Vancouver, BC

Stephanie J. Woods, PhD, RN
Professor, College of Nursing, The University of Akron
Akron, OH

Heather Wopat, BSN, RN
Research Assistant, NYU College of Nursing
New York, NY

Judith Wuest, RN, PhD
Professor, Faculty of Nursing, University of New Brunswick
Fredericton, New Brunswick, Canada

Preface

A woman enters the emergency department with facial bruises and severe abdominal pain. She is asked how her injuries occurred, and she mumbles that she fell down a flight of stairs. Her male companion glowers in the doorway of the cubicle. The nurse firmly asks him to wait outside and gently proceeds with obtaining a detailed history from the woman including assessment for family violence.

In another part of the hospital, a newly postpartum battered mother in the obstetrical unit fears going home and does not know where to go. Her nurse-midwife helps arrange her discharge directly to an abused woman shelter.

A 14-year-old daughter of a woman who has five other children is being seen in an outpatient clinic with her mother. The mother voices the concern, "I don't want to have to 'do time' for what I might do to her." Mother and daughter are counseled by the nurse who begins the process of connecting this family with resources that can help them.

These are just three illustrations of the multitude of possible practice situations where nurses are encountering family violence. Family violence is widespread and a global concern that has both immediate and lifelong health consequences. Nursing has an important role to play in the prevention, identification, treatment, and scholarly investigation of family violence.

The second edition of *Family Violence and Nursing Practice* continues to be a landmark resource that provides uniquely comprehensive, nursing-focused coverage of family violence and offers both practicing nurses and nursing students of every level a clear view of the essential theories, interventions, and issues surrounding family violence. Written by recognized nursing experts, this easy to comprehend, yet detailed, overview of family violence includes coverage of: intimate partner violence (IPV) (including abuse during pregnancy, same sex IPV, intimate partner homicide, stalking, violence against women with disabilities, and dating violence), child abuse, children witnessing violence, sexual assault (child and adult), and elder abuse. *Family Violence and Nursing Practice* includes evidence-based practice guidelines for multiple health care settings, gives in-depth attention to cultural issues and culturally relevant practice, and provides abundant displays and tables that offer quick access to essential standards for care. With this edition practice assessment forms are included along with model interventions that give practical strategies for addressing family violence, as well as appendices that provide handy forms for abuse assessment. Also included are chapters on legal and forensic issues addressing the nurse's role and responsibilities when confronting family violence and a unique chapter on international work in family violence.

Violence is a common health problem of tremendous magnitude. Violence occurs against all family members and is an indicator of complex family needs and issues. Nursing is in an excellent position to be actively involved with other professionals by initiating, coordinating, and evaluating the multidisciplinary approach to violence families.

There is growing recognition of nursing's contribution to the needs of those experiencing family violence. Although we recognize that nursing research and practice are and must be interdisciplinary in nature, we maintain that nursing has a unique role to play and discipline-specific knowledge to contribute. Since the first version of this text was published in 1982, thousands of nurses have become involved in a variety of ways in the care of survivors of family violence. Nurses provide direct care to survivors in shelters, homes, hospitals, and community settings. Nurses are frequently members of boards of directors at shelters and other agencies assisting survivors. Nursing research on family violence has evolved rapidly and is reported in the literature with ever greater frequency. One of the most visible outcomes is Nursing Network on Violence Against Women International (www.NNVAWI.org). This grassroots organization was a direct outgrowth of the 1985 Surgeon General's Workshop on Violence and Public Health. Immediately following that meeting and every 2 years since, the NNVAWI has held a conference where participants exchange practice ideas, research findings, theory, and policy initiatives related to all forms of violence against women. Over time, the group has become truly international. Since the first edition of the book, forensic nursing and the International Association of Forensic Nursing (www.iafn.org) have grown in importance, with the forensic nursing role in family violence having become increasingly recognized. The American Nurses' Association has a long-standing (1991) resolution addressing the nursing role in violence against women, as has the Emergency Nurses' Association, the National Black Nurses' Association, the Hispanic Nurses' Association, the Association on Women's Health and Obstetrical Nursing, and the College of Nurse Midwives. The American Academy of Nursing has a policy task force (Expert Panel) on violence. Nurses have increasingly contributed to health care policy addressing family violence. Exciting developments—yet much more can be done in terms of policy formation, nursing research, practice and education.

Family Violence and Nursing Practice conveys nursing interventions based on existing theories and research on families and all forms of family violence, and emphasizes the strengths and health potential of survivors and families—an approach that empowers nursing to contribute to the prevention of this worldwide health concern.

Janice Humphreys
Jacquelyn C. Campbell

This book evolved from our professional interest in research on and commitment to those who experience family violence. For the existence of this text, we owe a great many thanks:

To our many friends and colleagues who provided support and indulgence.

To our expert contributing authors who share our concern about family violence.

To our invaluable funding sources, including the National Institute of Nursing Research, the National Institute of Justice, the Centers for Disease Control and Prevention, the National Institutes of Child Health and Development, Mental Health, and Drug Abuse, and the National Center for Minority Health and Health Disparities.

To Margaret Zuccarini, Executive Acquisitions Editor of Springer Publishing Company for her advice, counsel, and patience.

To our students, who have challenged us to grow.

To the abused women and children who freely shared their problems and concerns, took part in our research, and showed us over and over again what courage and strength really means.

To the profession of nursing for providing an opportunity to care about the needs of other human beings.

To each other for continuing friendship, and the sharing of ideas.

Janice Humphreys
Jacquelyn C. Campbell

1

Theories of Aggression and Family Violence

Marguerite B. Lucea, PhD, MSN, MPH, RN
Nancy Glass, PhD, MPH, RN, FAAN
Kathryn Laughon, PhD, RN

INTRODUCTION

Violence in the family cannot be fully understood without analysis of the broader picture of violence, in general. This chapter provides a background of the major theoretical frameworks found in the current literature and used to explain violence in our society. A concept analysis and a summary of the perspectives on violence from domain-specific theories as well as integrated theories are presented as a basis for nursing conceptualization of violence as a health problem. The chapter concludes with special considerations, including the influence of the existing structural violence in society, cultural attitudes, and social organization on behaviors.

One way to estimate the magnitude of the health concern that violence represents is to examine homicide statistics. Among established market (or industrialized) economies, the rate of homicide in the United States was 5.6 per 100,000 in 2005 (Bureau of Justice Statistics, 2007), a much higher rate than countries such as Canada (1.95), England (1.62), France (1.64), and Germany (0.98) (United Nations Office on Drugs and Crime, 2006). In the United States, males are 77% of the victims and almost 90% of the offenders. Homicide is the second leading cause of death among Americans aged 15–24, with rates in 2005 being 3.7 times higher for men compared to women, and 6.2 times higher for African Americans compared to Whites including both men and women (Bureau of Justice Statistics, 2007; Centers for Disease Control and Prevention (CDC), 2008). Further, the rate of violent victimization other than homicide was 23.3 per 1,000 persons older than 12 years in 2006 (U.S. Department of Justice, 2007).

If nursing identifies prevention of health problems as a major area of concern, an examination of causes of violence is mandated. When we understand more about the complex causal picture of violence, we can work to prevent the problem by eliminating or reducing those causal or risk factors. To approach the research literature on the causes of violence, we must begin with an examination of the concepts involved.

CONCEPT ANALYSIS

Concepts that initially appear to be relatively simple and are used frequently in common language should be carefully scrutinized before the field, based on this concept, can be understood. This process is known as concept analysis (Walker & Avant, 1995). When violence literature is studied, there is striking disagreement among authors about definitions of even the most frequently used terms and, more importantly, their attached values and connotations. Is aggression always bad? Can violence and aggression be used to achieve moral human aspirations or should nonviolence always be the method? An abbreviated concept analysis is presented of the two most important ideas in understanding this field-aggression and violence.

Aggression

Aggression is defined as "any offensive action, attach or procedure and overt or suppressed hostility, ether innate or resulting from continued frustration and directed outward or against oneself." The root is Latin from the word *aggressio*, which means attack (Webster's, 1996). From these beginnings, there is a variety of definitions used in the literature and in common usage. The synonyms listed for the adjective form, *aggressive*, reflect two different perspectives. Synonyms include *hostile, belligerent, assailant, pugnacious, vicious, contentious*; the second group includes *self-assertive, forceful, bold, enterprising, energetic*, and *zealous*. The disparate synonyms reflect the ambivalence about aggression in American society. Connotations of aggression as negative or positive are also grounded in the sex–role stereotypes held about male and female behavior. The most commonly held perspectives allow for healthy expressions of aggression as drives for accomplishment and mastery.

Yet this meaning of aggression has typically applied only to men. Aggressive men are often described as bold, forceful, enterprising, energetic, zealous, and/or self-assertive. For women, aggression is usually not viewed as positively because, even today, aggression in women violates gender norms. These norms are the standards for appropriate male and female behavior within a society. When a woman acts in an aggressive manner, her behavior is often judged as hostile, belligerent, or contentious because it does not reflect assumptions about female nature as kind and nurturing. These opposing interpretations of the term *aggression* suggest that perceptions of this concept are grounded in the social context of the behavior. Views of aggressive behavior are derived from how males and females are expected to act in society.

Over the past 30 years, there has been a shift from regarding aggression as innate or as a basic personality characteristic to studying aggression as a behavior that is a deliberate attempt to harm others, regardless of gender. Anderson and Carnegay (2004) cite a frequently used definition of aggression as being "a behavior directed toward another individual and carried out with the intent to harm" (p. 170). Scholars now include psychological injury as one of the possible results of aggression. Nursing literature also has addressed aggression, distinguishing assertiveness from aggression. Herman (1979) describes aggression as getting what is wanted at the expense of others. Aggressive behavior is seen as dominating, deprecating, humiliating, and embarrassing to others, whereas "assertion is the direct, honest, and appropriate expression of one's thoughts, feelings, opinions and beliefs . . . without infringing on the right of others" (Herman, 1979). This distinction seems useful and is accepted as a basic premise of this book. Aggression, therefore, is seen as destructive in intent either physically or psychologically and as infringing on the rights of others.

Violence

Aggression can be seen on a continuum with violence at the extreme end, encompassing destructive results as well as aggressive intent. Webster defines *violence* as the "exertion of any physical force so as to injure or abuse." The word originates from the Latin *violare*, to violate or dishonor. Consistent with the official definition and its Latin root, common associations with violence are much more negative than those associated with aggression. Yet much violence is socially tolerated as in police violence, war, and self-defense. The appropriateness of violence depends on the agent, the circumstances, the status of the victim, and the degree of harm inflicted. Some authors have insisted that violence is a reflection of conflicting groups and interests in any society. Yet entire cultures, such as the Semai in Malaysia, are totally nonviolent wherein any kind of violence is absolutely disallowed (Robarchek & Robarchek, 1998).

American culture officially condemns violence, but it is covertly sanctioned in many ways. Violent characters are glorified on television, in books, and in music; threats to hurt and kill each other are made in jest as a constant part of common language. In addition, violent video games, such as *Mortal Kombat* and *Grand Theft Auto*, encourage the use of violence through an interactive and engrossing medium in which the player must be the aggressor. The teaching of U.S. history is hinged on the different wars in which the country has engaged. In addition, American society is undecided whether hitting a child is legitimate punishment. In fact, corporal punishment of children in the home is legal in the United States, even though it has been outlawed in 24 countries around the world (Global Initiative, 2006). This societal ambivalence toward violence is reflected in the rates of violent crime and in violence in families.

THEORETICAL FRAMEWORKS EXPLAINING VIOLENCE

The complexity of etiology of violence is reflected in the many theories as to its causes (see Table 1.1). The theoretical frameworks that attempt to illuminate the causative factors of violence can be divided in a variety of ways. For the purposes of this chapter, the two major groupings are "domain-specific" and "integrated" theories. Domain-specific theories refer to those in the areas of biology, psychology, and sociology that focus on one aspect of violence causation. Integrative theories incorporate several of the aforementioned domains in their presentation of the theoretical basis of violent behaviors.

This review of theoretical frameworks cannot be considered exhaustive. It indicates the problems with determining causality of problems of violence and points out some of the inconsistencies, gaps, and difficulties in the traditional theoretical field. It also serves to underpin the theoretical information concerned with specific aspects of violence in the family. Note there are multiple explanations for violent behavior, and various theories are not mutually exclusive.

TABLE 1.1 Overview of Theories of Violence and Aggression

Theory	Level of Research Support	Strengths	Limitations
DOMAIN-SPECIFIC THEORIES			
Biological perspective			
Neurotransmitters (NE, 5-HT, dopamine), enzymes (MOA), specific genes	Limited but growing	Examines neurochemical relationships as foundational to behavior manifestations	Preliminary research thus far limited to associations, not causal relationships. Not able to account entirely for behaviors
Sex hormones (testosterone) and hormone-binding globulin	Limited with mixed results	Strong evidence for link between anabolic androgenic steroid use and violence	Inconclusive evidence regarding naturally occurring hormones and hormone-binding globulins
Brain areas	Moderate overall	Good evidence for link between abnormalities in prefrontal, medial temporal, and amygdala regions and aggression	Limited in identifying underlying causes of abnormalities
Alcohol and drugs	Weak for psychopharmacological basis Moderate as supplement to other theories	Research supports influence of executive functioning and personality on relationship between alcohol and aggression Link between stimulant drugs and aggression has been demonstrated	Insufficient as stand-alone theory/cause Relationship may be confounded by social factors—research is unclear
Psychological perspective			
Frustration–aggression	Weak	Could be considered relevant to family violence, as individual goals may be thwarted by others in family	Lacks specifics regarding stimuli of aggression and personality influences
Cognitive (cognitive neoassociation, script, and social information processing)	Moderate	Incorporates biological foundations. Has been applied to both violent victimization and perpetration	Limited ethnic diversity and small sample sizes limit generalizability to population

Sociocultural perspective

Structural violence	Limited to moderate	Encompasses societal structures that allow inequities; allows for influence of society on individual behaviors	Very broad, difficult to explain all behaviors
Intrafamilial resource	Limited to moderate	Specifically addresses sociological underpinnings of family violence	Focuses primarily on who holds resource power, not other factors present in families
Cultural consistency	Limited to moderate	Several aspects of culture seen as influential on individual behavior; helps in understanding violence causation within cultures	Does not account for individual characteristics (biological, psychological, etc.) of aggressors

INTEGRATED THEORIES

Social cognitive	Moderate to strong	Incorporates biological, psychological and sociological factors to causation of violence	Further research required to assess role of mediating and moderating influences
General aggression model	Limited due to relative newness of theory	Allows violence to be related to several motives. May be good for developing multisystem interventions	New theory requires testing of components
Ecological	Strong	Use of nested "systems" accounts for complexity of violent behaviors	Many studies examine role of some systems on violent behaviors, but few examine all systems in one study
Adolescent-limited (AL) versus life-course persistent (LCP)	Strong	Unique in that it has been applied in several longitudinal studies	Limited research on how child abuse (sexual or physical) influences whether a child follows LCP or AL path

Domain-Specific Theories

The Biological Perspective

Early theories on violence in the 1960s and 1970s favored the evolutionary and instinctivist basis, purporting that aggression is normal and serves to preserve species through the favoring of genes that promoted strength (Lorenz, 1966). Dominance and subordination was seen as inevitable (Ardrey, 1966). However, these theories have long fallen out of favor and offer little to the field. Instead, theories that emphasize the neurochemical underpinnings of violent behavior have taken precedence when examining the role of biology in violence. It should be noted that while biologic factors play a significant role in the development of aggressive behaviors, scientists exploring this singular dimension of violence do not purport that biology explains all aspects of violent behavior. Experts in this field recognize that biology and genetics must be considered in tandem with environmental and learning factors (Bernet, Vnencak-Jones, Farahany, & Montgomery, 2007; Reif et al., 2007).

Violence, as defined earlier in the chapter, is aggression that has harm as the outcome (e.g., death). The environmental and psychological roots of aggressive behavior have been studied for centuries, but it is only in the past 40 years that scientists have systematically explored biological links to aggressive behavior (see Table 1.2). Recent studies using both animal and human models suggest a role of enzymatic and neurotransmitter systems as inhibitors and facilitators of aggressive behavior (Alia-Klein et al., 2008; Francesco Ferrari, Palanza, Parmigiani, de Almeida, & Miczek, 2005; Mejia, Ervin, Baker, & Palmour, 2002; Nelson & Trainor, 2007). Evidence also points to androgens such as testosterone and their binding globulins as having a role in aggressive behavior (Aluja & Garcia, 2007; Brooks & Reddon, 1996). In addition, some recent studies have worked on isolating specific candidate genes linked to increased aggressiveness (Burt & Mikolajewski, 2008; Guo, Roettger, & Shih, 2007).

NEUROTRANSMITTERS, ENZYMES, AND ASSOCIATED GENES. During recent decades, the roles that monoamine neurotransmitters of norepinephrine (NE), serotonin (5-HT), and dopamine and the enzyme monoamine oxidase A play in aggressive and violent behaviors has been the subject of several recent studies. Abnormal serotonin levels have demonstrated association with impulsive and aggressive behaviors. Most often, 5-HT_{1A} and 5-HT_{2A} levels in the brain were inversely correlated with aggressive acts, including self-aggression, such that low extracellular levels were associated with increased aggression (Meyer et al., 2008; Ryding, Lindström, & Träskman-Bendz, 2008; Witte et al., 2009). Researchers have also shown that the major metobolite of serotonin, 5-hydroxyindolacetic acid (5-HIAA), is reduced in the cerebrospinal fluid (CSF) of subjects with a history of aggression (Dolan, Anderson, & Deakin, 2001).

The brain's dopaminergic system appears to play a role in aggressive behavior. Animal studies suggest that an increase in brain dopamine activity creates a state in which animals are more prepared to respond impulsively and aggressively to stimuli in the environment (Blackburn, Pfaus, & Phillips, 1992). Linked to both the dopaminergic and serotonergic findings, preliminary evidence supports a genetic disturbance in neurotransmitter function that might predispose individuals to aggressive behaviors (Alia-Klein et al., 2008; Reif et al., 2007). Interruption of and lowering of the normal activity of monoamine oxidase A (MAO-A), the enzyme responsible for metabolizing monoamine neurotransmitters, has been linked to violent behaviors in both humans and animals

TABLE 1.2 *Biological Factors and Irregularities Related to Increased Aggression*

Biological Factor	Purpose as Applicable to Aggression (Not Exhaustive)	Irregularities Associated With Increased Aggression or Violence
Neurotransmitter		
Norepinephrine (NE)	Integral for attentiveness, emotions, learning Also can be released in blood to cause increase in heart rate and contraction of blood vessels	Elevated levels in the brain
Serotonin (5-HT)	Contributes to regulation of mood, pain, sleep	Low extracellular 5-HT_{1A} and 5-HT_{2A} in brain Low 5-HIAA (metabolite) in CSF
Dopamine	Modulates mood	Increased dopaminergic activity Genetic disruption of dopamine D2 receptor (DRD2) or dopamine transporter (DAT1)
Enzyme		
Monoamine oxidase A	Metabolizes brain neurotransmitters NE, 5-HT, dopamine	Deficient levels or gene mutations
Sex hormone		
Anabolic androgenic steroid (AAS)	Externally supplemented; used as "performance-enhancing" drug	Lifetime and past year use
Testosterone (naturally occurring)	Steroid hormone for development of male reproductive system and maintenance of secondary sex characteristics. Also effects memory and attention	Elevated levels (although research findings are inconsistent)
Sex hormone-binding globulin (SHGB)	Glycoprotein active in regulating distribution of sex hormones between free and protein-bound states	Elevated levels (suggested to have mediating role between testosterone and aggression)

(Alia-Klein et al., 2008; Mejia et al., 2002). In addition, variations in the dopamine D2 receptor (DRD2) and the dopamine transporter (DAT1) genotypes have been linked to violent delinquency in young adults (Guo et al., 2007).

Even with the growing body of research in this area, however, the findings are still preliminary. The studies have been conducted on limited samples, and most have looked only at associations. The exact role of the neurotransmitters on regulating aggression is still not entirely clear and subject to further study.

SEX HORMONES. In human beings, androgens (male hormones naturally produced in the body) have often been associated with the regulation of aggressive behavior, although the nature of the role remains unclear. Testosterone, including anabolic androgenic steroid (AAS) use, has been studied extensively in relationship to human assertiveness, dominance, and aggression. A clear link has been made between AAS use (both past year and lifetime use) and increased aggression among adolescents (Beaver, Vaughn, Delisi, & Wright, 2008; Ricci, Schwartzer, & Melloni Jr., 2009; Schwartzer, Ricci, & Melloni Jr., 2009). One interesting finding in recent research on naturally occurring testosterone has been that the relationship between testosterone and violence is not limited to men, but was found to be higher in women (Cashdan, 1995; von der Ahlen, Lindman, Sarkola,

Makisalo, & Eriksson, 2002). Another is that the level of sex hormone-binding globulin (SHGB) is more associated with increased aggressiveness among a sample of inmates than their serum testosterone (Aluja & Garcia, 2007).

However, increased levels of naturally occurring testosterone are not always predictive of increased aggression. Archer (2006) reviewed the literature available on testosterone and violence, and determined there were conflicting results. Boys going through puberty experienced a surge in systemic testosterone levels, yet they do not necessarily demonstrate more violent behaviors. In addition, in reviewing the extant literature, Archer concludes that there is a great deal of variation in the relationship between testosterone and aggression. It is most pronounced in samples consisting of offenders and young adults, although these can be confounded.

BRAIN AREAS AND LESIONS. Brain imaging and neurological studies have converged on the conclusion that certain areas of the brain are more closely linked to aggression and violence than others. Functional and structural deficits in the prefrontal cortex, medial temporal lobe, and the amygdala have been consistently linked to antisocial and aggressive acts (Bufkin & Luttrell, 2005; Raine, 2002). Damage to these areas affects a person's ability to make decisions, comprehend consequences of their actions, accurately interpret social cues, and regulate negative emotions. Brain imaging research, however, is unable to determine the underlying cause of the structural and functional brain abnormalities identified, and it is unclear when in a person's life difficulties first occur.

With this in mind, however, the study of patients who suffer brain injuries can provide important evidence to the neurobiology of aggressive behavior. Older studies found that a history of head trauma was significantly more common in male batterers than in nonviolent men (Rosenbaum et al., 1994). In one meta-analysis of traumatic brain injury (TBI) and violence, persons with histories of TBIs were 66% more likely to be at risk for violence than the non-TBI controls (fixed-estimate odds ratio = 1.66, 95% CI 1.12–2.31) (Fazel, Philipson, Gardiner, Merritt, & Grann, 2009). However, there is indication that it may not be the matter of having a TBI history, but the extent of that TBI. A recent study (Turkstra, Jones, & Toler, 2003) used a sample of convicted domestic violence perpetrators and noncriminal controls, matched for race, age, and socioeconomic status. The actual frequency of TBI was not significantly different, although the causes for TBI in the convicted offenders were more likely interpersonal in nature and the TBIs were more severe than the controls. The offenders also reported significantly more problems with aggression and anger than their nonviolent controls.

ROLE OF ALCOHOL AND DRUGS. There has also been extensive research on the role of substances such as alcohol and drugs on the neural mechanisms for aggression (Giancola, 2002). It is important to note, however, that the effects of alcohol alone on an individual's behavior are not a stand-alone theory. The general population and researchers have long associated substance abuse with violence, but the relationships are extremely complex. Violent crime and alcohol are associated in research, but as first pointed out by Moyer (1987), neither are most criminals alcoholics nor the majority of alcoholics violent criminals. Laboratory experiments have shown increased aggression with alcohol ingestion, but there is variability in the studies, and not all subjects react the same. Research has not substantiated a "direct cause paradigm," the theory that alcohol directly causes aggression. Rather, alcohol detrimentally affects certain psychological and physiological processes that then may lead to the expression of aggressive behavior (Giancola, 2002).

Previous research examined the cognitive effects of alcohol on inhibitions and instigation perceptions. Cognitive models of violence postulate that aggressive behavior is determined by the relative balance of a combination of both instigative (e.g., threats, insults) and inhibitory (e.g., anxiety, norms of reciprocity) cues present in hostile interpersonal situations. The instigative cues increase the probability of an aggressive act, whereas inhibitory cues decrease the probability of an aggressive act (Giancola, 2002).

"Blaming the booze" for decreasing inhibitions and allowing misperceptions of situations may oversimplify the relationship. Researchers recently found that the effect of cognitive expectations on actions following alcohol ingestion was negated when baseline temperament was incorporated into the model, such that those with more aggressive baseline personalities were more likely to be aggressive when alcohol was introduced (Giancola, Godlaski, & Parrott, 2005). Other recent studies have examined the role of "general" trait anger and dispositional aggressivity in the interplay between alcohol and aggressive behavior and had similar results (Giancola, Saucier, & Gussler-Burkhardt, 2003; Giancola, 2004a; Parrott & Zeichner, 2002). Behavioral anger was the strongest risk factor for alcohol-related aggression (Giancola et al., 2003).

In addition, men with higher scores in both behavioral and cognitive anger had an increase in aggression when ingesting alcohol, while women with only high behavioral anger scores showed a higher level of aggression in the same study. Similarly, using a sample of social drinkers, researchers found that a person with a difficult temperament, regardless of gender, was more likely to be aggressive. Yet, with the introduction of alcohol, only the men with difficult temperaments showed an increase in aggression over their baseline (Giancola, 2004a).

The extent to which this relationship between alcohol and increased aggression is affected by executive functioning (EF) of an individual's brain has been subject of recent research. EF is considered a "higher-order cognitive construct involved in the planning, initiation, and regulation of goal-oriented behaviors," and this includes a person's ability to maintain attention, problem solve, reason abstractly, and organize information contained in the working memory and utilize it appropriately (Giancola, 2007). It may also play a role in temperament regulation. EF activities have been linked to the prefrontal cortex in the brain, an area also strongly influenced by levels of serotonin, dopamine, and MAO-A, which have been previously discussed.

EF has been examined as a moderator of the relationship between alcohol and aggression, similarly to the role of difficult temperament. Men with higher EF demonstrated lower aggressive behavior, whether or not they had ingested alcohol, and only those men with lower EF scores showed an increase in aggression with the ingestion of alcohol (Giancola, 2004b). Of the women in the same study, simply the belief that they had ingested alcohol (regardless of alcohol or placebo group) suppressed aggressive actions, but this did not hold true for men. Giancola, Parrott, and Roth (2006) re-examined the positive relationship between difficult temperament and alcohol-related aggression by assessing the role of EF. They found that, among men, EF mediated this relationship by reducing the effect of difficult temperament on alcohol-related aggression by 20%.

Whether alcohol has an effect on serotonin, and how this is related to aggression, has just begun to be studied in humans and only to a limited extent. Heinz et al. (2000) found that there may be a genetic susceptibility of certain individuals to neurotoxic effects of chronic alcohol that result in decreased 5-HT transporter availability. A decrease in 5-HTT functioning effects the normal serotonin levels in the brain, and may be related to increased aggression (see previous section on neurotransmitters). When examining acute alcohol consumption, McCloskey, Berman, Echevarria, and Coccaro (2009) found that higher levels of 5-HT lowered aggression, while acute alcohol consumption increased aggressive acts. However, the two occurred independently of one another, and no overlapping influence was discovered.

The extent to which offender and victim alcohol consumption impacts the violence suggests that, while offender drinking is associated with increased negative outcomes, victim drinking does not play as significant of a role. Using the data from the National Violence Against Women Survey (NVAWS), Thompson and Kingree (2006) examined the reports of 1,756 women who reported experiencing physical assault by their partners. Women with partners who had been drinking were more likely to be injured than those whose partners had not been drinking.

However, a woman's alcohol consumption was not significantly related to outcomes (Thompson & Kingree, 2006). Although a review of studies among college students found links between both offender and victim alcohol ingestion and the likelihood of sexual assault (Abbey, 2002), recent work has found stronger support for the connection between offender drinking and sexual assault than victim ingestion. Brecklin and Ullman (2002) recently analyzed the data from 859 female sexual assault victims identified through the National Violence against Women Survey. The analysis showed that offender behavior (e.g., drinking and aggression), not victim behavior, is an important determinant of sexual assault outcomes for women (Brecklin & Ullman, 2002). Offenders who were drinking were 80% more likely to complete the rape, and high levels of offender aggression increased the risk of victim injury by nearly nine times (OR 8.91, $p < 0.001$) and medical care outcomes by 3.5 times (OR3.52, $p < 0.05$) in multivariate analysis, controlling for demographic, drinking, and assault characteristics (Brecklin & Ullman, 2002).

The literature on illicit drug use and crime often find strong associations between illicit drug use and both violent and property offending (Martin & Bryant, 2001). Goldstein's (1985) conceptual framework for the relationship of drugs and violence identified three factors through which they may be linked; these include the specific drugs' psychopharmacological effects, the user's economic needs, and the violence associated with the distribution and control of illicit drugs (Goldstein, 1985). These factors do not take into account, however, the effect of experiencing child sexual, emotional, and physical abuse as a precursor to drug use in adulthood, which has been demonstrated in several studies (Kennedy, 2008; Miller, 2002).

Research on substance abuse and violence has shown that stimulant drugs such as crack cocaine are the strongest predictors of violence (Fals-Stewart, Golden, & Schumacher, 2003); this is not true with opiates such as heroin (Moore et al., 2008). As with alcohol, effects of drugs on violent behavior appear to be associated with social, individual, and situational factors rather than neurophysiological causes for the majority of drugs. The majority of studies have found little evidence of a psychopharmacological basis for an illicit drug-violence association (Martin & Bryant, 2001). Potential exceptions are stimulants such as cocaine and amphetamines. In studies completed with primates, stump-tail macaques (monkeys) were given amphetamines. After receiving the drug, it was noted that the monkeys' aggressive behaviors increased significantly. Although more research has been done on linking human amphetamine use and violence using longitudinal data (Fals-Stewart et al., 2003), the support of a direct causal link between the two remains weak. Investigators are challenged to disentangle the relationships among alcohol, illicit drug use, and violence. Often the studies fail to distinguish between the many different substances used by the individuals and the combined effects of multiple drugs on aggression (Martin & Bryant, 2001).

LIMITATIONS OF THE BIOLOGICAL PERSPECTIVE. All human beings experience anger and may behave aggressively with enough provocation such that sorting out the interactions of psychological and environmental factors with basic genetics and physiology is extremely complex. As the empirical evidence suggests, there is considerable credence to the position that neurobiologic systems do influence aggressive behavior. However, a direct casual link is difficult to establish with the existing evidence.

In addition, the majority of research examining the relationship between neurobiology and aggression has been conducted with men, although there are an increasing number of studies that are examining both men and women. Unfortunately, the majority of the research also has been conducted with limited sample sizes, and therefore generalizability, to broader populations is restricted. Neurophysiologists still lack evidence that explains the complete difference between males and females in their aggressive or non-aggressive behavior when responding to stimuli, as testosterone only partially explains the difference.

The Psychological Perspective

Also considered domain-specific theories are the theories generated from the field of psychology. These explanations of violence vary greatly. A few psychologists echo Freud's theories that aggression is a basic instinct or drive (Freud, 1932). Others de-emphasize or refute that view and identify other psychological traits that characterize the violent person. Psychoanalytic frameworks, whose basic premise is that some basic need has been thwarted in the violent individual, usually by some form of faulty child rearing (Warren & Hindelang, 1979) have not been substantiated empirically and therefore will not be addressed here. The following psychological theories will be addressed below: frustration–aggression theory, cognitive neoassociation theory, script theory, and social information processing theory. The first two will only be mentioned in a cursory manner, as their influence in the field of violence has greatly decreased in recent years.

FRUSTRATION–AGGRESSION THEORY. This theory was first proposed by Dollard, Doob, Miller, Mowrer, and Sears (1939). They postulated that if an obstacle to achieving a desired goal is presented, this results in frustration, which in turn is the cause of all aggression. This theory is based on the belief that aggression is innate to humans. One could imagine that this concept of aggression resulting from frustration is relevant to family violence, where conflict often arises when an individual's goals may be thwarted by another individual within the family unit or by the family as an organism in itself. However, it lacks specifics regarding which frustrating events will results in aggression, why some people respond to frustration by withdrawing, and what determined differing aspects of aggression (i.e., physical, emotional, etc.) (Gelles & Straus, 1979) and has not been supported by evidence.

COGNITIVE THEORIES. Three interrelated theories use cognition and response as the basis for violent behaviors. According to the Cognitive neoassociation theory, stress related to noxious stimuli triggers memories, emotions and behaviors lead to fight (anger) or flight (fear) responses. Thoughts, affect, and behavior are linked in memory and are triggered by unpleasant and stressful conditions or feelings (Berkowitz, 1990). Whether the ultimate response to a given trigger is fight or flight depends on prior conditioning, genetic predisposition, and an appraisal of the best course of action for the situation. Aggressiveness and the associated thoughts, emotions, and behaviors are linked inextricably in memory. Berkowitz suggests that a wide range of stressors such as physical pain, excessive heat, economic uncertainty, and political unrest can all lead to an increase in aggressive behaviors in humans (Berkowitz, 1998).

Closely related to this is the Script theory that suggests that as humans develop, they learn certain scripts for given situations, which both explain and guide behavior (Abelson, 1981; Shanck & Abelson, 1977). Scripts are both learned by observation and reinforced by conditioning. Thus, society's response to an individual's use of a particular script will influence if and how that script is used in the future. Huesmann (1998) stated that "more aggressive people are presumed to have encoded a larger number of aggressive scripts" (p. 87). The longer scripts persist as a response, the more refined and resistant to modification they become. Huesmann also postulates that negative emotional arousal (such as feeling angry) will "prime" individuals to retrieve more aggressive scripts and result in the individual retrieving the most well-learned scripts, and evaluating the scripts less carefully.

The Social information processing (SIP) theory blends the two aforementioned cognitive theories, holding that human behavior, including aggression, is influenced by several domains but is mediated by cognitive processes (Dodge & Coie, 1987; Milner, 2000). Behavior is modeled within a hierarchical system, with biological and neurochemical processes at the lowest level, while higher-order information retrieval and cognitive processing are required for more complex behaviors. SIP theory postulates that human behaviors include the following four steps: behavioral cues are recognized and interpreted, scripts are retrieved (and enacted), the script is evaluated, and the environmental response is evaluated.

SIP has been used explain the link between early experience or witnessing of violence and later aggressive behavior in several studies. An examination of incarcerated juveniles found that both violent victimization and exposure to severe violence resulted in more approval of aggression as an effective approach, more hostile perceptions of others' behaviors, and more aggressive behaviors (Shahinfar, Kupersmidt, & Matza, 2001). A study of elementary school children found that both violent victimization and witnessing violence was associated with aggressive behavior and mediated through social information processing rather than emotional factors (Schwartz & Proctor, 2000).

Other research has explored how SIP may influence a parent's likelihood to physically abuse their children. Cognitive schemas, such as empathetic perspective-taking, internal locus of control, and accurate developmental expectations, put parents at less risk for physical abuse, beyond certain contextual variables, such as stress and anger expression (Rodriguez & Richardson, 2007). In particular, external locus of control was highly predictive of potentiality to abuse, overreaction in discipline, and demonstration of physical aggression toward the child. In another study comparing mothers who had been identified as neglectful to those who were not, the neglectful mothers were less able to interpret their infant's signals accurately and were less likely to identify when the child was in distress (Hildyard & Wolfe, 2007). These studies, however, used limited sample sizes and were not all ethnically diverse, which indicates the need for further research in this area with larger, more diverse sample sizes.

The Sociocultural Perspective

Another domain in which researchers have developed theories explaining the basis of violent behavior is the social–cultural domain. The sociocultural theories of violence generally consider some of the biological and psychological aspects of causation, but their basic proposition is that social structure and conditions are more important (West, 1979). For several decades, they have vehemently rejected the notion that aggression is an instinct or a drive and postulate that most violent offenders do not generally act destructively (Chatterton, 1976). Except for these areas of agreement, there is a great variation in approaches. There are theorists who emphasize any one of the following aspects: the structural violence inherent in our society, cultural attitudes fostering violence, and the role of resources.

STRUCTURAL VIOLENCE THEORY. The theory of structural violence contends that there are certain mechanisms in place in a society that incur violence upon certain individuals and give way to the endorsement of violence between individuals. First put forth by Galtung (1969) and (1996), structural violence is embedded within a society, much less overt than direct violence between individuals, but much more influential. Of particular note is the vertical violence that takes place through the structure of society through political, legal, economic, or other mechanisms, which promotes unequal access to various basic needs as well as those needed for advancement. This structural violence can lead to interpersonal violence, which has direct impact on the health of those individuals as well as the health of the larger society. Structural violence theorists would point out issues in the United States such as health disparities, poor urban schooling, homicide rates, and several other areas which could be seen as indications of structural violence. In addition, globally, conflict between ethnicities such as those that occurred and are occurring in the Rwandan genocide, the conflict in Darfur, the Sri Lankan civil war, the conflict in Bosnia, and several others could also be considered results of structural violence.

One illustration where structural violence can play a part in interpersonal violence is that of poverty. Berkowitz (1998), in his review of literature, noted that poverty, or a more complex variable of economic deprivation, was a good predictor of aggressive behavior in adolescents (Berkowitz, 1998). Anderson and Anderson's (1998) model testing found that socioeconomic status was positively related to violent crime independent of other factors. Jewkes' (2002) review of the relationship between intimate partner violence (IPV) and poverty found that there is a strong positive correlation between poverty and rates of violence, and that this relationship may be mediated through stress or a crisis in male role identity. The analysis of risk factors for intimate partner femicide of Campbell et al. (2003) found that the male partner's unemployment significantly increased the risk of lethal violence among battered women.

INTRAFAMILIAL RESOURCE THEORY. The resource theory is one of the only theories that specifically applies to family violence, and for that reason, we include it for discussion. Originally described by Goode (1971), this theory rests on the assumption that systems, including familial systems, rely on some extent of violence or a threat of violence. The theory posits that persons with the most resources hold the most power and therefore can command a certain level of force over the others. These resources can be economic, material, social, personal, or familial among others, but the person with the most resources often does not feel the need to use force. Rather, when other resources are constrained or limited, violence becomes a resource used to gain control or additional force. Violence is also used by someone who lacks sufficient resources to hold the most power.

This could be construed as being related to structural violence, although it is most often applied to the familial level. Tang (1999), in her study on Hong Kong Chinese couples, found that couples who had an egalitarian distribution of power demonstrated less interpersonal violence than those couples with unequal marital power in either direction (Tang, 1999). Similar results were found in a nationally representative sample of Korean couples (Kim & Emery, 2003) and among Filipino couples (Ansara & Hindin, 2009).

CULTURAL CONSISTENCY THEORY. Elements of a culture tend to be interdependent. Knowledge of the interdependent factors within a culture and their relationship to violence can ultimately provide a framework of cultural norms. This knowledge not only provides a greater understanding of what leads to abuse, but it can also help influence the development of cultures that are free of violence (Levinson, 1989).

The cultural consistency theory explains that even cultural norms that are not directly related to violence can have an effect on violence that occurs within the culture. For example, according to Carroll's seminal work, Mexican American boys may be so afraid of their father's punishment that there is little communication between the two. Because of the poor communication, the boys unwittingly act in such a way that they offend their fathers and are punished severely (Carroll, 1980). Family structure that contains stress and physical abuse models violence, which is then acted out by the next generation. In the cultural consistency theory, the norms of this family behavior reflect the values of the society as a whole. The norms are tied to the structure of the systemic aspects of the culture, and in this way, violence tends to be consistent with the norms and values of the society (Carroll, 1980). This explanation, thus, helps in understanding the causation of violence within a culture. Cultural consistency theory explains why societies that are known for warfare are also associated with high rates of individual violence.

According to the cultural spillover hypothesis of the cultural consistency framework, the more a society tends to use physical force toward socially approved ends, the greater the likelihood that this legitimization of force will be generalized to other areas of life (Baron, Straus, & Jaffee, 1988). Examples of the use of force in a society are in maintaining order in schools, controlling crime, or dominating international events for the country's self-interest. Evidence exists that in states where there is a strong emphasis on physical punishment of children, strict or corporal punishment in schools, and high levels of incarceration, there is more, rather than less, interpersonal violence (Baron et al., 1988).

Integrated Theories

Social Cognitive Theory

Social cognitive theory incorporates biological, psychological, and sociological factors of causation of violence, although it emphasizes the sociological aspects more than the others. Bandura is the originator and best-known proponent of the social cognitive theory as an explanation for aggression. He calls the theory psychological because it grows out of the school of behavioral psychology, yet it obviously contains aspects of several different frameworks. Bandura originally named the theory "social learning theory" (Bandura, 1973). He reformulated the theory, however, to include more cognitive processes to account for observational learning and renamed the theory accordingly (Bandura, 1986).

Individuals begin life, according to this theory, with a blank slate, and violence is learned. Bandura defines aggression as "behavior that results in personal injury and in destruction of property" including that the injury "may be psychological." He also notes that the behavior must be labeled as aggressive by society, this labeling determined by the action's intensity, the intentions attributed to the performer by others, and the characteristics of the labeler. Bandura believes that aggressive behavior may be considered adaptive or destructive depending on the situation in which it is used. He acknowledges the role of biological subcortical structures in producing destructive behavior, but believes that the social situation is most important in determining the frequency, form, circumstances, and target of the action.

Bandura postulates that rather than arising from instinct or frustration, aversive experiences result in emotional arousal, which an individual perceives as fear, anger, sorrow, or even euphoria, depending on prior learning, cognitive interpretation, and other people's reactions to the same experience. Moreover, "frustration or anger arousal is a facilitative but not a necessary condition for aggression" (Bandura, 1973). Bandura concludes that the majority of events that stimulate aggression (such as insults, status threats, or unjust treatment) do so through learned experience. As an illustration, not all people who have experienced divorce, parental rejection, poverty, mental illness, or brain damage ever become violent. He perceives the motivation for aggression as reinforcement based, not biologically determined.

The acquisition of aggressive behavior can be learned through modeling or observational learning or by direct experience or practice. Performance is determined by both internal (biological and cognitive) and external instigators (Bandura, 1973; Bandura, 1979). Bandura showed this through experiments with children. He notes also that observation of other's behavior also provides clues as to whether an action will be rewarded or punished when it occurs. If a child sees a parent or peer gain status, dominance, resources, or power using violence, he or she will be more likely to use it (Bandura, 1973). It has often been noticed that violent men are more likely to have been abused as children, and these ideas also help to explain why some peer groups (such as gangs) and subcultures are known for violence (Bandura, 1973). Bandura (1973) found that the parents of aggressive boys from middle class homes, although they neither abused their children nor displayed antisocial violence, "repeatedly modeled and reinforced combative attitudes and behavior."

Bandura later explains that behavior learned from models is reinforced if the imitative actions are perceived as useful to the person (Bandura, 1979). If aggression is successful and dominance is achieved by it, then the aggression is reinforced (Laborit, 1978). A year-long study of school children showed that children who demonstrated aggression-encouraging cognitions in the fall and perceived more support in the environment for these cognitions were more likely to demonstrate aggressive behavior through the school year (Egan, Monson, & Perry, 1998).

Various applications of the full social–cognitive model have been tested as explanations of aggression and have generally been supported. A test of applying the social–cognitive model to men who physical abuse their intimate partners found support for the model (Copenhaver, 2000). These men did not have fewer coping skills than nonviolent men, but the abusive men tended to interpret ambiguous situations negatively and thus respond with violence. Empirical evidence supports the theoretical propositions that aggressive behavior is learned, at least in many cases, and growing research seeks to explain the mediating and moderating variables through which this may occur.

GENERAL AGGRESSION MODEL. Synthesizing elements from the above models, as well as several others, Anderson and Bushman (2002) proposed the General Aggression Model (GAM). Previously, aggressive acts had been classified into dichotomous pairs:

either hostile or instrumental, impulsive or premeditated, proactive or reactive. However, these pairings did not permit understanding of the interplay between cognition and decision-making processes. In addition, the pairings had potential to be confounded by other pairings. For instance, an act of instrumental aggression (being aggressive to obtain something beyond the "rewards" of the aggressive act) could not be entirely independent of impulsivity or premeditation (Anderson & Carnagey, 2004). Therefore, Anderson and colleagues (2002, 2004) developed GAM as a more integrated theory blending social cognition and development, where situational, individual, and biological variables are considered in the larger schema of violent acts. In this model, inputs from the person (traits, sex, beliefs, attitudes, values, and scripts) and the situation (aggressive cues, provocation, frustration, discomfort, drugs, and incentives) both influence the person's internal state (affect, cognition, and arousal) and thereby determine the outcomes (appraisal and decision processes that lead to either thoughtful or impulsive action).

This model's strengths lie in several areas (Anderson & Bushman, 2002). It has streamlined several domain-specific theories into a more parsimonious one. It also allows violence to be related to several motives, rather than the isolated dichotomies discussed in the preceding paragraph. The authors also believe that this model can serve as the basis for creating multisystem violence interventions, targeting chronic aggression instead of focusing on only one type of behavior. However, the newness of the theory precludes the existence of a body of research testing the components of the theory.

ECOLOGICAL THEORY. One of the most integrated theories concerning violence in societies as well as in families is the Ecological theory, first proposed by Bronfenbrenner (1977). He proposed that a person's behavior and development resulted from interactions among several systems: microsystems, mesosystems, exosystems, and macrosystems. This model, as applied to violence, attends to the interactions among the system levels. The microsystem pertains to individual factors (biology, history of witnessing or experiencing abuse, general demographics such as age, sex, education, mental health status, and substance use). The mesosystem refers to the interactions between the individuals and their close relationships (such as with partners, peers, and families). The exosystem refers to the community contexts for the individual (such as schools, places of work, neighborhoods), while macrosystems are considered the societal structures (norms and beliefs about violence, masculinity factors, gender roles, racisim, etc.) (see Figure 1.1). The goal behind applying this model to examining violence and aggression among individuals is to identify multilevel preventions strategies.

The ecological approach has been widely applied in violence research, particularly in the areas of adolescent violence, violence against women, revictimization experiences of female partners, and to some extent, elder abuse. Strong family functioning has been shown to be an important influence in decreasing youth violence, just as community violence has been a strong influence on increased individual violence (Brook, Brook, & Whiteman, 2007; Gorman-Smith, Henry, & Tolan, 2004; Tolan, Gorman-Smith, & Henry, 2003a). Among high-poverty African American youth, exposure to violence in the community strongly predicted individual violent behavior so much so that violence exposure even limited the effect of healthy parenting processes on violent behavior (Spano, Vazsonyi, & Bolland, 2009). At the same time, high levels of collective efficacy within a community (exosystem) have a protective effect against the occurrence of violent victimization and homicide (Sampson, Raudenbush, & Earls, 1997). In a longitudinal study of urban youth, strong community structures (exosystem) positively influenced parenting

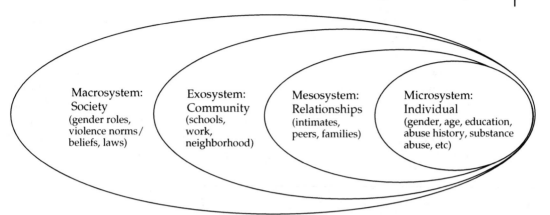

FIGURE 1.1   The ecological model as it relates to violence. *Source:* Dahlberg, L. L., & Krug, E. G. (2002). *Violence—A Global Public Health Problem. World Report on Violence and Health.* Geneva, Switzerland: World Health Organization. Adapted with permission from the World Health Organization.

practices (mesosystem), which in turn meant the youth were less likely to be involved in gangs (mesosystem) (Tolan, Gorman-Smith, & Henry, 2003b). Not entirely surprisingly, gang membership (mesosystem) positively influenced violent behaviors of the youth (microsystem). In a similar study of male youths in inner city Chicago, researchers found that family types characterized by strong interpersonal relationships and effective parenting had a direct negative effect on youth violence as well as an indirect effect mediated through decreased gang membership and peer violence (Henry, Tolan, & Gorman-Smith, 2001).

The role of the community can play a substantial role in violence revictimization as well. Child abuse (microsystem) has identified as a risk factor for intimate partner abuse (mesosystem) in adult life (see subsequent chapters). High community cohesiveness has been shown to significantly decrease the effect of childhood emotional abuse on whether an individual experiences physical IPV as an adult (Obasaju, Palin, Jacobs, Anderson, & Kaslow, 2009; Sampson et al., 1997). At the same time, neighborhood disorder, poverty, and structural inequality expressed by racism has an additive effect on the same relationship (Cunradi, Caetano, Clark, & Schafer, 2000; Sampson, Morenoff, & Raudenbush, 2005).

The ecological theory has also been applied to elder abuse, in an effort to better understand the risk and protective factors related to this kind of family violence. Parra-Cardona, Meyer, Schiamberg, and Post (2007) present the theory framed in a culturally relevant manner for Latino families with elders at risk for abuse. Risk factors at the microsystem level of the elder included being female, having a high level of dependency, having mental health issues, being foreign-born, and limited English proficiency. Other risk factors within families included a discrepancy in cultural identities and lack of recognition of those differences. Systemically, risk factors included lack of connection with resources, health care barriers, anti-immigration barriers, and traditional gender roles. Schiamberg and Gans (2000) applied another overarching system in their model of elder abuse, and that is the chronosystem—how change and continuity over time influence the relationship in question (Schiamberg & Gans, 2000). This is perhaps of particular importance when thinking of elder abuse because the elder's status (physical and mental) may worsen over time, and attitudes toward the elderly can change, thereby increasing caregiver strain and increasing the risk for abuse.

ADOLESCENT-LIMITED VERSUS LIFE-COURSE PERSISTENT MODEL. The last integrated theory that will be discussed in this chapter is that of the adolescent-limited versus life-persistent model of antisocial (and violent) behaviors (Moffitt, 1993). According to Moffitt, there is a larger group of youth who engage in antisocial behaviors in adolescence, but that these behaviors are limited to this period of development. These behaviors are more often internally focused, such as withdrawing from interactions and isolating oneself from others, although they can be externally expressed through violence as well. Conversely, there is a small group of individuals who exhibit continued antisocial behaviors throughout their lifetimes, and the majority of these antisocial behaviors are externally directed (i.e., violence and aggression). For those who exhibit life-course persistent antisocial tendencies, their interpersonal problems work together with their environments throughout their development, and this culminates in a personality that is pathological.

According to this theory, persons who are in the life-course persistent group have lower cognitive functioning (Raine et al., 2005), insufficient parental guidance, temperament and behavior problems as children than those in the adolescent-limited group (Moffitt & Caspi, 2001). A longitudinal study over 20 years used a large sample of young, male criminal offenders to examine the cognitive functioning portion of the theory, finding that it held for Whites and Latinos, but not for African Americans (Donnellan, Ge, & Wenk, 2000). Those with life-course persistent behavioral problems also have more difficulty in partnerships as young adults and report more IPV (both victimization and perpetration) than their adolescent-limited counterparts. Those at least risk for such violence in partnerships are those who experience no antisocial behaviors throughout their childhoods (Woodward, Fergusson, & Horwood, 2002).

This theory is becoming more widely applied in recent years. Scientists are more closely examining these groupings in terms of the influence of genetics (Burt & Mikolajewski, 2008). In addition, it is one of the only theories that has been examined through several longitudinal studies, all of which lend support to lower social functioning and more dysfunctional personal relationships over time for those in the life-course persistent group (Bergman & Andershed, 2009; Huesmann, Dubow, & Boxer, 2009).

SPECIAL CONSIDERATIONS

Certain considerations must be made when reflecting on the pervasiveness in so many societies of violence on a macro level of society as well as a micro level of the interpersonal and family. These have been alluded to in some of the theories discussed above, but they are important to make special note of here.

Cultural Positioning

In this discussion, culture refers to homogeneous nations, political subdivisions within nations, ethnic groups, or small-scale societies (Levinson, 1989). The culture of an individual is one's "social heredity." The role of culture in relationship to violence must be understood. The problem of understanding culture as a causative influence is a complex one, however, because there is likely to be a multiplicity of mingled antecedents associated with violence.

For instance, there are many different cultures in the United States. All of the theories presented may at least partially explain the effect of culture on violence, yet studies of differences among ethnic groups within the United States indicate the complexity of the influences. In order to be useful, variables that are implicated in abuse must have explanatory power both within and between cultures. It is also important to not assume that members of ethnic groups can be characterized similarly in terms of characteristics that are related to abuse.

One of the variables that have been shown important to consider is the level of acculturation of the family or couple into the United States in conjunction with socioeconomic status. An extensive review of literature on acculturation and violence among minority adolescents found several investigations demonstrating that increased acculturation is associated with an increase in youth violence among Latinos and Asian Pacific Islanders, while ethnic group identity and involvement in culture-of-origin activities were found to be protective (Smokowski, David-Ferdon, & Stroupe, 2009). By the same token, however, low acculturation was a risk factor for increased victimization, except in the realm of dating violence for Latino youth. In their study of Chinese, Cambodian, Laotian/Mien, and Vietnamese adolescents and the influence of acculturation on violence, Le and Stockdale found enough differences between the groups to warrant further cross-cultural comparisons before definitive conclusions could be made (Le & Stockdale, 2008).

To this end, an interactional approach is needed to understand the effect of cultural differences on ethnic groups (Gelfand & Fandetti, 1986; Sorenson, 1996). Assessment should be made of the ethnic groups for (1) language, generation of the immigrant, cultural homogeneity of the neighborhood, degrees of activity in traditional religions, socioeconomic status, attitudes about violence and (2) the interaction of these factors with the institutions of work, school, social services, medical services, and community. Ethnic identity and levels of oppression have also been found to be important variables in relationship to violence, but there has yet to be sufficient study to specify their exact roles and the interactions of these variables with other factors. Several studies have shown that socioeconomic status accounts for differences in prevalence in husband to wife abuse U.S. ethnic groups, and when socioeconomic class is controlled for, the differences in violence between ethnicities often disappears (Dearwater et al., 1998; DeMaris, 1990; Lockhart, 1987; Schafer, Caetano, & Clark, 1998; Torres, 1991; Walton-Moss, Manganello, Frye, & Campbell, 2005).

Furthermore, the extent to which violence is "accepted" in a society is also related to how it is positioned. For instance, if aggression is seen as a normative behavior in a culture, attitudes concerning the use of violence are more relaxed. An excellent example of this is in the United States, one of the most violent of market economies. The United States has a long history of violence used as a means to achieve socially approved ends. American culture reflects at least a covert acceptance of violence in the media, in attitudinal surveys, and in choice of heroes. In the 1990s, Senator Moynihan suggested that aggression and other deviant behavior have become so pervasive in American society that rather than address the behaviors, the boundaries of deviancy have been refined so that previously stigmatized behavior is now considered normal (Moynihan, 1993). Farrell (2000) notes that there is a tendency toward excess in American culture, including excessive violence (what he terms "berserk" behavior) that is encouraged through the spectrum of entertainment and news media, which has now become the norm in and the selling point of the reality television shows of the 2000s. Successful interventions must take this context into consideration when developing programs and planning for sustainable change in individuals as well as society.

Meaning of Violence Cross-Culturally

The meaning of the term *violence* within a culture varies through time as well as from culture to culture. Historically in the United States, the *Journal of Marriage and the Family* first mentioned "family violence" after 1970, and not until after 1973 were there references to "wife abuse" in *The New York Times*. The first official declaration of violence as a health problem was by former Surgeon General Dr. C. Everett Koop in 1985 (DHHS, 1986). Behaviors generally understood as abuse in one culture may be considered legitimate in another. Torres' (1991) comparison of Mexican Americans and Anglo-Americans demonstrated differences in behaviors that were considered abusive. Although there was no difference in the severity and frequency of violence between the two groups, Mexican Americans labeled their experience of being hit as abuse less frequently. Whether the differences were related to ethnicity or to sociocultural factors such as religion, education, and economic factors that are characteristic of each group, it is apparent that abuse occurs within a context that influences interpretation (Counts, Brown, & Campbell, 1999; Torres, 1991).

The absence of reports of abuse in a culture does not mean it does not exist. An unstated assumption in much of the anthropological literature is that if the persons interviewed or observed did not know, acknowledge, or admit there was abuse, it was not classified as abuse (Korbin, 1991). If abuse is a function of a person's perception of being victimized, the culture's beliefs and norms become important in understanding the influence of culture on recognition of violence as well as the culture's definition of violence. Because of different cultures' perceptions of what constitutes abuse and the complexity of different cultural systems, it may not be possible to attain a universal definition of family violence that is culturally specific (Korbin, 1991).

Yet, certain societies are totally nonviolent both interpersonally and in warfare, according to many different anthropologists and other reporters. The existence of such cultures provides powerful evidence that cultural forces and learning are at least as important as biology in explaining the occurrence of violence. The characteristics of such societies assist in identifying possible primary prevention approaches. Nonviolent societies tend to be more egalitarian than hierarchical in sex roles and ethnic groups' arrangements, treat children with kindness and without corporal punishment, value cooperation over competition, and are not tied to violence and control of women (Counts et al., 1999; Levinson, 1989; Paddock, 1975; Whiting, 1965).

With this in mind, violence and abuse cannot be understood outside of cultural context. The complexity of violence is magnified by varied cultural systems. For instance, complicating factors within the United States are that members of the various cultures and ethnic groups differ in their level of acculturation and oppression. There will be important differences between one person's beliefs and those of persons from other cultures or ethnic groups. Yet, membership in a culture or ethnic group cannot forecast the person's perception or reaction to violence. The influence of spiritual, moral, somatic, psychological, and metaphysical as well as the economic, kinship, and territoriality issues need to be taken into account to discern the individual and family's views of violence and abuse. Only then can nurses and other health practitioners structure their approaches to ethnic groups for perception and management of the problem (Flaskerud, 1984).

Social Organization

Social organization is defined in sociology as the pattern of relationships between and among individuals and social groups and how the individuals are related to each other and the whole group (Straus, 1974). Proponents of the influence of social organization on family violence posit that violence can be found in the structure of the society, and it affects how the family members relate to each other. One of the aspects of social organization is gender relationships and gender inequalities.

Gender Inequality

Traditionally patriarchal societies have viewed violence toward wives as a male prerogative, stemming from the idea that a woman is the property of men (Dobash & Dobash, 1998; Heise, Ellsberg, & Gottemoeller, 1999). There is inconsistent evidence about any direct correlation between the status of women and violence against women cross-culturally (Counts et al., 1999). Issues that complicate research in this realm are (1) the many spheres and indicators of women's status (Whiting, 1965), (2) failure to measure women's status at the cultural or ethnic group level rather than in individual couples, and (3) the possibility of a curvilinear relationship between violence and women's status (Campbell, 1999, 2001). In other words, in cultures where women are totally subjugated, women may not be beaten often because there are other societal mechanisms in place that keep women's status low. In societies where there is equality between males and females, wife beating is limited. It is where women's status is changing rapidly or disputed that domestic violence is highly prevalent. In Bangladesh, for instance, microfinance programs targeting women's economic empowerment have shown that initial involvement of the women is associated with an increase in partner violence, perhaps from the challenging of very traditional gender norms, but longitudinal involvement beyond 5 years demonstrates a dramatic reduction in violence (Kabeer, 2001; Schuler, Hashemi, Riley, & Akhter, 1996). In the Philippines, both male- and female-dominated household decision-making patterns were associated with increased risk for IPV, while joint decision making was protective (Hindin & Adair, 2002).

As previously mentioned, the concept of women's status is complex and cannot be described by only one factor. Status may differ between the public and private spheres of culture, as well as among dimensions of power, prestige, and rewards, which are indicators of status in the United States. Cross-cultural indicators related to women's status that have been associated with wife beating are matrilocality, virtue as honor, male sexual jealousy, strong association of women with nature, cultural sanctions allowing wife beating, other violence against women, female entrapment in marriage (divorce restrictions), male control of production, and male domestic decision making (Counts et al., 1999; Levinson, 1989).

The effect of gender inequality can also be seen culturally in the maltreatment of female children. Female infants and small children are more likely to be malnourished and receive inadequate medical care than their brothers in societies where there is male gender preference (Heise et al., 1999; Korbin, 1991). In India and the People's Republic of China, amniocentesis has been used for sex determination and then followed by abortion of female fetuses. Understanding these complex relationships and the underlying motivations is important to prevention of violence.

SUMMARY

Studying the interactions among biological, social, environmental and psychological factors in the expression of aggression is the most promising approach in violence research. The causes of violence are multifactorial and somewhat elusive, and therefore, the theories that provide the best framework for understanding are those that take several levels of human interaction into account. No one theory has surfaced as the absolute explanation, although the integrated theories hold a great deal of promise. As nurses, we must be aware of the multifaceted roots of violent behavior. Interventions for our clients who have either been victimized or who are perpetrating violence must be developed with an understanding of this, and we must continually be aware of our own experiences and perceptions of violence, in order to serve our clients in a therapeutic and effective manner.

REFERENCES

Abbey, A. (2002). Alcohol-related sexual assault: A common problem among college students. *Journal of Studies on Alcohol. Supplement, 3*(14), 118–128.

Abelson, R. P. (1981). Psychological status of the script concept. *American Psychologist, 36,* 715–729.

Alia-Klein, N., Goldstein, R. Z., Kriplani, A., Logan, J., Tomasi, D., Williams, B., et al. (2008). Brain monamine oxidase-A activity predicts trait aggression. *Journal of Neuroscience, 28*(19), 5099–5104.

Aluja, A., & Garcia, L. F. (2007). Role of sex hormone-binding globulin in the relationship between sex hormones and antisocial and aggressive personality in inmates. *Psychiatry Research, 152*(2–3), 189–196.

Anderson, C. A., & Anderson, K. B. (1998). Temperature and aggression: Paradox, controversy, and a fairly clear picture. In R. G. Geen & E. Donnerstein (Eds.), *Human aggression: Theories, research and implications for practice* (pp. 247–298). San Diego, CA: Academic Press.

Anderson, C. A., & Bushman, B. J. (2002). Human aggression. *Annual Review of Psychology, 53,* 27–51.

Anderson, C. A., & Carnagey, N. L. (2004). Violent evil and the general aggression model. In A. Miller (Ed.), *The social psychology of good and evil* (pp. 168–192). New York: Guilford.

Ansara, D. L., & Hindin, M. J. (2009). Perpetration of intimate partner aggression by men and women in the Philippines: Prevalence and associated factors. *Journal of Interpersonal Violence, 24*(9), 1579–1590.

Archer, J. (2006). Testosterone and human aggression: An evaluation of the challenge hypothesis. *Neuroscience & Biobehavioral Reviews, 30*(3), 319–345.

Ardrey, R. (1966). *The territorial imperative.* New York: Antheneum.

Bandura, A. (1973). *Aggression: A social learning analysis.* New York: General Learning Press.

Bandura, A. (1979). The social learning perspective. In H. Toch (Ed.), *Psychology of crime and criminal justice* (pp. 198–236). New York: Holt, Rinehart, and Winston.

Bandura, A. (1986). *Social foundations of thought and action: A social cognitive theory.* Englewood Cliffs, NJ: Prentice-Hall.

Baron, L., Straus, M., & Jaffee, D. (1988). A test of the cultural spillover theory. *Annals of the New York Academy of Sciences, 528,* 79–110.

Beaver, K. M., Vaughn, M. G., Delisi, M., & Wright, J. P. (2008). Anabolic–androgenic steroid use and involvement in violent behavior in a nationally representative sample of young adult males in the united states. *American Journal of Public Health, 98*(12), 2185–2187.

Bergman, L. R., & Andershed, A. K. (2009). Predictors and outcomes of persistent or age-limited registered criminal behavior: A 30-year longitudinal study of a Swedish urban population. *Aggressive Behavior, 35*(2), 164–178.

Berkowitz, L. (1998). Affective aggression: The role of stress, pain, and negative affect. In R. G. Geen & E. Donnerstein (Eds.), *Human aggression: Theories, research and implications for practice* (pp. 49–72). San Diego, CA: Academic Press.

Berkowitz, L. (1990). On the formation and regulation of anger and aggression: A cognitive–neoassociationistic analysis. *American Psychologist, 45*, 494–503.

Bernet, W., Vnencak-Jones, C. L., Farahany, N., & Montgomery, S. A. (2007). Bad nature, bad nurture, and testimony regarding MAOA and SLC6A4 genotyping at murder trials. *Journal of Forensic Science, 52*(6), 1362–1371.

Blackburn, J. R., Pfaus, J. G., & Phillips, A. G. (1992). Dopamine functions in appetitive and defensive behaviours. *Progress in Neurobiology, 39*(3), 247–279.

Brecklin, L. R., & Ullman, S. E. (2002). The roles of victim and offender alcohol use in sexual assaults: Results from the national violence against women survey. *Journal of Studies on Alcohol, 63*(1), 57–63.

Bronfenbrenner, U. (1977). Toward an experimental ecology of human development. *American Psychologist, 32*, 513–531.

Brook, J. S., Brook, D. W., & Whiteman, M. (2007). Growing up in a violent society: Longitudinal predictors of violence in Columbian adolescents. *American Journal of Community Psychology, 40*(1–2), 82–95.

Brooks, J. H., & Reddon, J. R. (1996). Serum testosterone in violent and nonviolent young offenders. *Journal of Clinical Psychology, 52*(4), 475–483.

Bufkin, J. L., & Luttrell, V. R. (2005). Neuroimaging studies of aggressive and violent behavior: Current findings and implications for criminology and criminal justice. *Trauma, Violence, & Abuse, 6*(2), 176–191.

Bureau of Justice Statistics. (2007). *Homicide trends in the U.S.* Retrieved May 15, 2009, from http://www.ojp.usdoj.gov/bjs/homicide/homtrnd.htm#contents

Burt, S. A., & Mikolajewski, A. J. (2008). Preliminary evidence that specific candidate genes are associated with adolescent-onset antisocial behavior. *Aggressive Behavior, 34*, 437–445.

Campbell, J. C. (1999). Sanctions and sanctuaries: Wife beating within culture contexts. In D. A. Counts, J. K. Brown & J. C. Campbell (Eds.), *To have and to hit: Anthropological perspectives on wife beating* (pp. 219–232). Chicago, IL: University of Illinois Press.

Campbell, J. C. (2001). Global perspectives on wife beating and health care. In M. Martinez (Ed.), *Prevention and control of aggression and its impact on victims* (pp. 215–228). New York: Kluwer.

Campbell, J. C., Webster, D., Koziol-McLain, J., Block, C., Campbell, D., Curry, M. A., et al. (2003). Risk factors for femicide in abusive relationships: Results from a multisite case control study. *American Journal of Public Health, 93*(7), 1089–1097.

Carroll, J. C. (1980). A cultural-consistency theory of family violence in Mexican-American and Jewish-ethic groups. In M. A. Strauss & G. T. Hotaling (Eds.), *The social causes of husband–wife violence* (pp. 68–85). Minneapolis, MN: University of Minnesota Press.

Cashdan, E. (1995). Hormones, sex, and status in women. *Hormones and Behavior, 29*(3), 354–366.

Centers for Disease Control and Prevention (CDC). (2008). *Death rates by age and age-adjusted death rates for the 15 leading causes of death in 2005: United states.* Retrieved May 15, 2009, from http://www.disastercenter.com/cdc/Leading%20Cause%20of%20Death%201999-2005.html

Chatterton, M. R. (1976). The social contexts of violence. In M. Borland (Ed.), *Violence in the family* (pp. 15–36). Atlantic Highlands, NJ: Humanities Press.

Copenhaver, M. M. (2000). Testing a social-cognitive model of intimate abusiveness among substance-dependent males. *American Journal of Drug and Alcohol Abuse, 24*(4), 603.

Counts, D., Brown, J., & Campbell, J. C. (1999). *To have and to hit: Cultural perspectives on wife beating.* Chicago: University of Illinois Press.

Cunradi, C. B., Caetano, R., Clark, C. L., & Schafer, J. (2000). Neighborhood poverty as a predictor of intimate partner violence among white, black, and Hispanic couples in the United States: A multi-level analysis. *Annals of Epidemiology, 10*(5), 297–308.

Dearwater, S. R., Coben, J. H., Campbell, J. C., Nah, G., Glass, N. E., McLoughlin, E., et al. (1998). Prevalence of intimate partner abuse in women treated at community hospital emergency departments. *Journal of the American Medical Association, 280*(5), 433–438.

DeMaris, A. (1990). The dynamics of generational transfer in courtship violence: A biracial exploration. *Journal of Marriage and the Family, 52*, 219–231.

DHHS. (1986). Surgeon general's workshop on violence and public health. Washington, DC.

Dobash, R. E., & Dobash, R. P. (1998). *Rethinking violence against women.* Thousand Oaks, CA: Sage.

Dodge, K. A., & Coie, J. D. (1987). Social information-processing factors in reactive and proactive aggression in children's peer groups. *Journal of Personal and Social Psychology, 53*, 1146–1158.

Dolan, M., Anderson, I. M., & Deakin, J. F. W. (2001). Relationship between 5-HT function and impulsivity and aggression in male offenders with personality disorders. *British Journal of Psychiatry, 178*(4), 352–359.

Dollard, J., Doob, L. W., Miller, N. E., Mowrer, O. H., & Sears, R. R. (1939). *Frustration and aggression.* New Haven, CT: Yale University Press.

Donnellan, M. B., Ge, X., & Wenk, E. (2000). Cognitive abilities in adolescent-limited and life-course-persistent criminal offenders. *Journal of Abnormal Psychology, 109*(3), 396–402.

Egan, S. K., Monson, T. C., & Perry, D. G. (1998). Social-cognitive influences on change in aggression over time. *Developmental Psychology, 34*(6), 1155.

Fals-Stewart, W., Golden, J., & Schumacher, J. A. (2003). Intimate partner violence and substance use: A longitudinal day-to-day examination. *Addictive Behaviors, 28*(9), 1555–1574.

Farrell, K. (2000). The berserk style in American culture. *Cultural Critique, 46,* 179–209.

Fazel, S., Philipson, J., Gardiner, L., Merritt, R., & Grann, M. (2009). Neurological disorders and violence: A systematic review and meta-analysis wit a focus on epilepsy and traumatic brain injury. *Journal of Neurology, epub ahead of print.*

Flaskerud, J. H. (1984). A comparison of perceptions of problematic behavior by six minority groups and mental health professionals. *Nursing Research, 33*(4), 190–197.

Francesco Ferrari, P., Palanza, P., Parmigiani, S., de Almeida, R. M. M., & Miczek, K. A. (2005). Serotonin and aggressive behavior in rodents and nonhuman primates: Predispositions and plasticity. *European Journal of Pharmacology, 526*(1–3), 259–273.

Freud, S. (1932). Why war? In R. Maple & D. R. Matheson (Eds.), *Aggression, hostility, and violence* (pp. 118–132). New York: Holt, Rinehart, Winston.

Galtung, J. (1969). Violence, peace and peace research. *Journal of Peace Research, 6*(3), 167–191.

Galtung, J. (1996). *Peace by peaceful means: Peace and conflict development and civilization.* London, UK: Sage.

Gelfand, D. E., & Fandetti, D. V. (1986). The emergent nature of ethnicity: Dilemmas in assessment. *Social Casework: The Journal of Contemporary Social Work,* (542), 550.

Gelles, R. J., & Straus, M. A. (1979). Determinants of violence in the family: Toward theoretical integration. In W. R. Burr, R. Hill, F. I. Nye & I. L. Reiss (Eds.), *Contemporary theories about the family* (pp. 549–581). New York: Free Press.

Giancola, P. R. (2002). Alcohol-related aggression during the college years: Theories, risk factors and policy implications. *Journal of Studies on Alcohol. Supplement, Mar*(14), 129–139.

Giancola, P. R., Godlaski, A. J., & Parrott, D. J. (2005). "So I can't blame the booze?": Dispositional aggressivity negates the moderating effects of expectancies on alcohol-related aggression. *Journal of Studies on Alcohol, 66*(6), 815–824.

Giancola, P. R., Saucier, D. A., & Gussler-Burkhardt, N. L. (2003). The effects of affective, behavioral, and cognitive components of trait anger on the alcohol-aggression relation. *Alcoholism, Clinical and Experimental Research, 27*(12), 1944–1954.

Giancola, P. R. (2004a). Difficult temperament, acute alcohol intoxication, and aggressive behavior. *Drug and Alcohol Dependence, 74*(2), 135–145.

Giancola, P. R. (2004b). Executive functioning and alcohol-related aggression. *Journal of Abnormal Psychology, 113*(4), 541–555.

Giancola, P. R. (2007). The underlying role of aggressivity in the relation between executive functioning and alcohol consumption. *Addictive Behaviors, 32*(4), 765–783.

Giancola, P. R., Parrott, D. J., & Roth, R. M. (2006). The influence of difficult temperament on alcohol-related aggression: Better accounted for by executive functioning? *Addictive Behaviors, 31*(12), 2169–2187.

Global Initiative. (2006). *Global summary of the legal status of corporal punishment of children.* Retrieved May 9, 2009, from http://www.violencestudy.org/IMG/pdf/140705-02.pdf

Goldstein, P. J. (1985). The drugs/violence nexus: A tripartite conceptual framework. *Journal of Drug Issues,* (15), 493–506.

Goode, W. J. (1971). Force and violence in the family. *Journal of Marriage and the Family, 33,* 624–636.

Gorman-Smith, D., Henry, D. B., & Tolan, P. H. (2004). Exposure to community violence and violence perpetration: The protective effects of family functioning. *Journal of Clinical and Child Adolescent Psychology, 33*(3), 439–449.

Guo, G., Roettger, M. E., & Shih, J. C. (2007). Contributions of the DAT1 and DRD2 genes to serious and violent delinquency among adolescents and young adults. *Human Genetics, 121,* 125–136.

Heinz, A., Jones, D. W., Mazzanti, C., Goldman, D., Ragan, P., Hommer, D., et al. (2000). A relationship between serotonin transporter genotype and in vivo protein expression and alcohol neurotoxicity. *Biological Psychiatry, 47(7)*, 643–649.

Heise, L., Ellsberg, M., & Gottemoeller, M. (1999). *Ending violence against women*. Baltimore, MD: Johns Hopkins University Population Reports.

Henry, D. B., Tolan, P. H., & Gorman-Smith, D. (2001). Longitudinal family and peer group effects on violence and nonviolent delinquency. *Journal of Clinical Child Psychology, 30(2)*, 172–186.

Herman, S. J. (1979). Assertive nurses breathe! *Journal of the New York State Nurses Association, 10(3)*, 6–8.

Hildyard, K., & Wolfe, D. (2007). Cognitive processes associated with child neglect. *Child Abuse & Neglect, 31(8)*, 895–907.

Hindin, M. J., & Adair, L. S. (2002). Who's at risk? factors associated with intimate partner violence in the Philippines. *Social Science & Medicine, 55(8)*, 1385–1399.

Huesmann, L. R. (1998). The role of information processing and cognitive schema in the acquisition and maintenance of habitual aggressive behavior. In R. G. Geen & E. Donnerstein (Eds.), *Human aggression: Theories, research, and implications for social policy* (pp. 73–109). New York: Academic Press.

Huesmann, L. R., Dubow, E. F., & Boxer, P. (2009). Continuity of aggression from childhood to early adulthood as a predictor of life outcomes: Implications for he adolescent-limited and life-course-persistent models. *Aggressive Behavior, 35(2)*, 136–149.

Jewkes, R. K. (2002). Intimate partner violence: Causes and prevention. *Lancet, 359(9315)*, 1423–1429.

Kabeer, N. (2001). Conflicts over credit: Re-evaluating the empowerment potential of loans to women in rural Bangladesh. *World Development, 29*, 63–84.

Kennedy, S. (2008). Childhood abuse related to nicotine, illicit and prescription drug use by women: Pilot study. *Psychological Reports, 103(2)*, 459–466.

Kim, J., & Emery, C. (2003). Marital power, conflict, norm consensus, and marital violence in a nationally representative sample of Korean couples. *Journal of Interpersonal Violence, 18(2)*, 197–219.

Korbin, J. E. (1991). Cross-cultural perspectives and research directions for the 21st century. *Child Abuse and Neglect, 15*, 67–77.

Krug, E. G., L. L. Dahlberg, J. A. Mercy, A. B. Zwi, & R. Lozano, eds. (2002). World report on violence and health. World Health Organization: Geneva R

Laborit, H. (1978). Biological and sociological mechanisms of aggression. *International Social Science Journal, 30*, 738–745.

Le, T. N., & Stockdale, G. (2008). Acculturative dissonance, ethnic identity, and youth violence. *Cultural Diversity and Ethnic Minority Psychology, 14(1)*, 1–9.

Levinson, D. (1989). *Family violence in cross cultural perspective*. Newbury Park, CA: Sage.

Lockhart, L. L. (1987). A reexamination of the effects of race and social class on the incidence of marital violence: A search for reliable differences. *Journal of Marriage and the Family, 49*, 603–610.

Lorenz, K. (1966). *On aggression*. New York: Bantam Books.

Martin, S. E., & Bryant, K. (2001). Gender differences in the association of alcohol intoxication and illicit drug abuse among persons arrested for violent and property offenses. *Journal of Substance Abuse, 13*, 563–581.

McCloskey, M. S., Berman, M. E., Echevarria, D. J., & Coccaro, E. F. (2009). Effects of acute alcohol intoxication and paroxetine on aggression in men. *Alcoholism, Clinical and Experimental Research, 33(4)*, 581–590.

Mejia, J. M., Ervin, F. R., Baker, G. B., & Palmour, R. M. (2002). Monoamine oxidase inhibition during brain development induces pathological aggressive behavior in mice. *Biological Psychiatry, 52*, 811–822.

Meyer, J. H., Wilson, A. A., Rusjan, P., Clark, M., Houle, S., Woodside, S., et al. (2008). Serotonin receptor binding potential in people with aggressive and violent behavior. *Journal of Psychiatry & Neuroscience, 33(6)*, 499–508.

Miller, W. R. (2002). Concomitance between childhood sexual and physical abuse and substance use problems. A review. *Clinical Psychology Review, 22(1)*, 22–77.

Milner, J. S. (2000). Social information processing and child physical abuse: Theory and research. In D. J. Hansen (Ed.), *Nebraska symposium on motivation, vol. 46, 1998: Motivation and child maltreatment* (pp. 39–84). Lincoln, NE: University of Nebraska Press.

Moffitt, T. E. (1993). Adolescence-limited and life-course-persistent antisocial behavior: A developmental taxonomy. *Psychological Review, 100(4)*, 674–701.

Moffitt, T. E., & Caspi, A. (2001). Childhood predictors differentiate life-course persistent and adolescence-limited antisocial pathways among males and females. *Development and Psychopathology, 13*(2), 355–375.

Moore, T. M., Stuart, G. L., Meehan, J. C., Rhatigan, D. L., Hellmuth, J. C., & Keen, S. M. (2008). Drug abuse and aggression between intimate partners: A meta-analytic review. *Clinical Psychology Review, 28*(2), 247–274.

Moyer, K. E. (1987). *Violence and aggression.* New York: Paragon House.

Moynihan, D. P. (1993). Defining deviancy down. *American Scholar, 62,* 17–30.

Nelson, R. J., & Trainor, B. C. (2007). Neural mechanisms of aggression. *Nature Reviews Neuroscience, 8,* 536–546.

Obasaju, M. A., Palin, F. L., Jacobs, C., Anderson, P., & Kaslow, N. J. (2009). Won't you be my neighbor?: Using an ecological approach to examine the impact of community on revictimization. *Journal of Interpersonal Violence, 24*(1), 38–53.

Paddock, J. (1975). Studies on antiviolent and "normal" communities. *Aggressive Behavior, 1,* 217–233.

Parra-Cardona, J. R., Meyer, E., Schiamberg, L., & Post, L. (2007). Elder abuse and neglect in Latino families: An ecological and culturally relevant theoretical framework for clinical practice. *Family Process, 46*(4), 451–470.

Parrott, D. J., & Zeichner, A. (2002). Effects of alcohol and trait anger on physical aggression in men. *Journal of Studies on Alcohol, 63,* 196–204.

Raine, A. (2002). The role of prefrontal deficits, low autonomic arousal, and early health factors in the development of antisocial and aggressive behavior in children. *Journal of Child Psychology and Psychiatry, 43*(4), 417–434.

Raine, A., Moffitt, T. E., Caspi, A., Loeber, R., Stouthamer-Loeber, M., & Lynam, D. (2005). Neurocognitive impairments in boys on the life-course persistent antisocial path. *Journal of Abnormal Psychology, 114*(1), 38–49.

Reif, A., Rosler, M., Freitag, C. M., Schneider, M., Eujen, A., Kissling, C., et al. (2007). Nature and nurture predispose to violent behavior: Serotonergic genes and adverse childhood environment. *Neuropsychopharmacology, 32,* 2375–2383.

Ricci, L. A., Schwartzer, J. J., & Melloni Jr., R. H. (2009). Alterations in the anterior hypothalamic dopamine system in aggressive adolescent AAS-treated hamsters. *Hormones and Behavior, 55*(2), 348–355.

Robarchek, C. A., & Robarchek, C. J. (1998). Reciprocities and realities: World views, peacefulness, and violence among Semai and Waorani. *Aggressive Behavior, 24,* 123–133.

Rodriguez, C. M., & Richardson, M. J. (2007). Stress and anger as contextual factors and preexisting cognitive schemas: Predicting parental child maltreatment risk. *Child Maltreatment, 12*(4), 325–337.

Rosenbaum, A., Hoge, S. K., Adelman, S. A., Warnken, W. J., Fletcher, K. E., & Kane, R. L. (1994). Head injury in partner-abusive men. *Journal of Consulting and Clinical Psychology, 62*(6), 1187–1193.

Ryding, E., Lindström, M., & Träskman-Bendz, L. (2008). The role of dopamine and serotonin in suicidal behaviour and aggression. In Giuseppe Di Giovann, Vincenzo Di Matteo and Ennio Esposito (Ed.), *Progress in brain research* (pp. 307–315). Elsevier.

Sampson, R. J., Morenoff, J. D., & Raudenbush, S. (2005). Social anatomy of racial and ethnic disparities in violence. *American Journal of Public Health, 95*(2), 224–232.

Sampson, R. J., Raudenbush, S. W., & Earls, F. J. (1997). Neighborhoods and violent crime: A multilevel study of collective efficacy. *Science, 277*(5328), 918–924.

Schafer, J., Caetano, R., & Clark, C. L. (1998). Rates of intimate partner violence in the united states. *American Journal of Public Health, 88*(11), 1702–1704.

Schiamberg, L. B., & Gans, D. (2000). Elder abuse by adult children: An applied framework for understanding contextual risk factors and the intergenerational character of quality of life. *International Journal of Aging & Human Development, 50*(4), 329–359.

Schuler, S. R., Hashemi, S. M., Riley, A. P., & Akhter, S. (1996). Credit programs, patriarchy and men's violence against women in rural Bangladesh. *Social Science and Medicine, 43,* 1729–1742.

Schwartz, D., & Proctor, L. J. (2000). Community violence exposure and children's social adjustment in the school peer group: The mediating roles of emotion regulation and social cognition. *Journal of Consulting and Clinical Psychology, 68*(4), 670–683.

Schwartzer, J. J., Ricci, L. A., & Melloni Jr., R. H. (2009). Interactions between the dopaminergic and GABAergic neural systems in the lateral anterior hypothalamus of aggressive AAS-treated hamsters. *Behavioural Brain Research, 203*(1), 15–22.

Shahinfar, A., Kupersmidt, J. B., & Matza, L. S. (2001). The relation between exposure to violence and social information processing among incarcerated adolescents. *Journal of Abnormal Psychology, 110*(1), 136–141.

Shanck, R. C., & Abelson, R. P. (1977). *Scripts, plans, goals and understanding: An inquiry into human knowledge structures.* Hillsdale, NJ: Erlbaum.

Smokowski, P. R., David-Ferdon, C., & Stroupe, N. (2009). Acculturation and violence in minority adolescents: A review of the empirical literature. *Journal of Primary Prevention, epub ahead of print*

Sorenson, S. (1996). Violence against women: Examining ethnic differences and commonalities. *Evaluation Review, 20*(2), 123–145.

Spano, R., Vazsonyi, A. T., & Bolland, J. (2009). Does parenting mediate the effects of exposure to violence on violent behavior? An ecological–transactional model of community violence. *Journal of Adolescence, 32*(5), 1321–1341.

Straus, M. (1974). Leveling, civility, and violence in the family. *Journal of Marriage and the Family, 36,* 18–25.

Tang, C. S. (1999). Marital power and aggression in a community sample of Hong Kong Chinese families. *Journal of Interpersonal Violence, 14*(6), 586–602.

Thompson, M. P., & Kingree, J. B. (2006). The roles of victim and perpetrator alcohol use in intimate partner violence outcomes. *Journal of Interpersonal Violence, 21*(2), 163–177.

Tolan, P. H., Gorman-Smith, D., & Henry, D. B. (2003a). The developmental ecology of urban males' youth violence. *Developmental Psychology, 39*(2), 274–291.

Tolan, P. H., Gorman-Smith, D., & Henry, D. B. (2003b). The developmental ecology of urban males' youth violence. *Developmental Psychology, 39*(2), 274–291.

Torres, S. (1991). A comparison of wife abuse between two cultures: Perceptions, attitudes, nature and extent. *Issues in Mental Health Nursing, 12*(1), 20–21.

Turkstra, I., Jones, D., & Toler, L. (2003). Brain injury and violent crime. *Brain Injury, 17*(1), 39–47.

U.S. Department of Justice. (2007). Criminal victimization, 2006. *OJP Factsheet,*

United Nations Office on Drugs and Crime. (2006). *Ninth united nations survey of crime trends and operations of criminal justice systems.* Retrieved May 15, 2009, from http://www.unodc.org/pdf/research/9th_survey/CTS9ByIndicatorExtract.pdf

von der Ahlen, B., Lindman, R., Sarkola, T., Makisalo, H., & Eriksson, C. J. P. (2002). An exploratory study on self-evaluated aggression and androgens in women. *Aggressive Behavior, 28*(4), 273–280.

Walker, L. O., & Avant, K. C. (1995). *Strategies for theory construction in nursing* (3rd ed.). Norwalk: Appleton & Lange.

Walton-Moss, B. J., Manganello, J., Frye, V., & Campbell, J. C. (2005). Risk factors for intimate partner violence and associated injury among urban women. *Journal of Community Health, 30,* 377–389.

Warren, M. Q., & Hindelang, M. J. (1979). Current explanation of offender behavior. In H. Toch (Ed.), *Psychology of crime and criminal justice* (pp. 62–80). New York: Hale, Rinehardt, Winston.

Webster's. (1996). *Webster's Encyclopedic Unabridged Dictionary of the English Language.* New York: Random House.

West, D. J. (1979). The response to violence. *Journal of Medical Ethics, 5,* 128–136.

Whiting, B. B. (1965). Sex identify conflict and physical violence: A comparative study, part 2. *American Anthropology, 67,* 128–135.

Witte, A. V., Floel, A., Stein, P., Savli, M., Mein, L., Wadsak, W., et al. (2009). Aggression is related to frontal serotonin-1A receptor distribution as revealed by PET in healthy subjects. *Human Brain Mapping, epub ahead of print*

Woodward, L. J., Fergusson, D. M., & Horwood, L. J. (2002). Romantic relationships of young people with childhood and adolescent onset antisocial behavior problems. *Journal of Abnormal Child Psychology, 30*(3), 231–243.

2

Family Violence: Long-Term Health Consequences of Trauma

Stephanie J. Woods, PhD, RN
Jessica Gill, RN, PhD

INTRODUCTION

The effects of family violence are far-reaching, resulting in physical, emotional, mental, social, and spiritual deficits in women and children who experience it. Intimate partner violence (IPV) also impacts families, communities, and society as a whole. The acute, repetitive acts of violence, stress, and injury, coupled with the ongoing, chronic stress states that are associated with IPV and other forms of abuse adversely affect women's physiologic balance and well-being, which in turn influences short- and long-term health. These declines in health are likely a result of changes in biopsychophysiological function further supporting nursing's conceptualization of the holistic definition of health. Research over the past decade in women who experience IPV and other forms of trauma shows that the experience of IPV and, in many cases, childhood sexual abuse alters neuroendocrine and immune function, and that posttraumatic stress disorder symptomatology exerts an additional effect (Gill, Vythilingam, & Page, 2008; Woods, Page, Hall, & Alexander, 2008a; Woods, Page, & Alexander, 2003; Woods, Page, O'Campo, Pugh, Ford, & Campbell, 2005a; Woods, Wineman, Page, Hall, Alexander, & Campbell, 2005b).

In this chapter, the physical and mental health consequences of family violence in women are outlined first. Next, there is a section devoted to a brief discussion of the stress response, as well as several theories that may explain the mechanisms of altered functioning of the neuroendocrine and inflammatory/immune systems in persons who have experienced violence and trauma. Lastly, empirical findings related to neuroendocrine and inflammatory/immune activities in abused women and children and their contributions to declines in health are presented.

Family Violence as Trauma and Health Consequences

Epidemiological surveys have shown that one in three American women will experience physical, emotional, or sexual abuse by a family member or intimate partner at some point during their lifetime (The Commonwealth Fund, 1999; Tjaden & Thoennes, 2000).

Intimate partner violence (IPV), also known as domestic violence and spousal abuse, takes a variety of forms, including physical violence, emotional abuse, sexual violence, threats of violence, and risk of homicide (Parker, McFarlane, Soeken, Silva, & Reel, 1999; Woods et al., 2005b). A woman involved in an ongoing intimately abusive relationship is subject to acute and chronic threats, injuries, and harm, which result from the frequent and/or intense intentional violent acts. Although persons exposed to repeated trauma have some opportunity to anticipate and develop strategies for managing the trauma and stress associated with it, they also face periods of prolonged fear, uncertainty, and hyperarousal (Connor, Davidson, & Lee, 2003; McFarlane & Yehuda, 1996).

Effects of IPV and Other Forms of Family Violence for Women

Women exposed to violence and trauma experience a wide range of long-term health problems, as do men (Breiding, Black, & Ryan, 2008), although the prevalence of IPV and IPV-related injury is significantly less for men, and effects have been studied less often. IPV is a significant risk factor for psychological and emotional health problems for women, including depression (Dienemann, Boyle, Baker, Resnick, Weiderhorn, & Campbell, 2000), substance abuse (Curry, 1998; Walton-Moss, Morrison, Yeo, et al., 2003), and post-traumatic stress disorder (PTSD) (Bennice, Resick, Mechanic, & Astin, 2003; Woods, Hall, Campbell, & Angott, 2008b). Following a meta-analysis of 11 studies, Golding (1999) reported a prevalence rate of almost 64% for PTSD in women in a violent intimate relationship. Rates of PTSD are as high as 92% in women seeking help at crisis shelters and domestic violence agencies (Woods et al., 2008b). There is also evidence that PTSD is often comorbid with other mental health problems. Women with PTSD often have comorbid depression (Breslau, Kessler, Chilcoat, Schultz, Davis, & Andreski, 1998; Kessler, Sonnega, Bromet, Hughes, & Nelson, 1995; O'Campo et al., 2006). PTSD symptoms also have been found to increase the risk for illicit drug and alcohol abuse in women experiencing IPV, with each symptom cluster of PTSD uniquely contributing to this risk (Sullivan & Holt, 2008).

Women who are abused by their male partner suffer acute physical injuries as well as negative effects on their long-term physical health (see Figure 2.1) (Campbell, 2002; Coker, Davis, Arias, Desai, Sanderson, & Brandt, 2002; Garcia-Moreno, Watts, Jansen, Ellsberg, & Heise, 2003; Woods et al., 2008b). Women who experience intimate abuse rate their health as lower than nonabused women (Lown & Vega, 2001; Wittenberg et al., 2007). Women experiencing IPV have stress-related health problems, including neuromuscular pain, headaches, seizures, sleep problems, hypertension, and increased susceptibility to viral and bacterial infections (Campbell et al., 2002; Coker et al., 2002; Garcia-Moreno et al., 2003; Woods et al., 2008b). IPV increases the risk of contracting a sexually transmitted disease (Silverman, Decker, Saggurti, Balaiah, & Raj, 2008; Alvarez, Pavao, Mack, Chow, Baumrind, & Kimerling, 2009) and significantly increases the risk of cervical cancer by 2.7 times (Coker, Hopenhayn, DeSimone, Bush, & Clifford, 2009). Gastrointestinal problems are also associated with experiences of IPV. For example, 71% of women with IPV have at least one functional gastrointestinal disease (FGID), and in two-thirds of these women, the onset of FGID symptoms occurred simultaneously or soon after the beginning of an IPV relationship (Perona et al., 2005).

Even when women leave the violent relationship, their health is at risk. Women who have been out of an abusive relationship an average of 20 months or longer continue

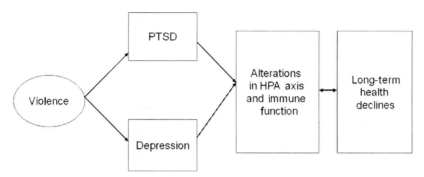

FIGURE 2.1 Psychiatric and physical health declines following violence.

to experience chronic pain, including back and neck pain, headaches, pelvic pain, and swollen and painful joints (Woods & Wineman, 2004; Wuest, Merritt-Gray, Ford-Gilboe, Lent, Varcoe, & Campbell, 2008). In a sample of abused women, PTSD symptom severity mediated the symptoms of chronic pain (Wuest et al., 2009). Empirical evidence has consistently shown that trauma-exposed women with PTSD, with or without accompanying depression, have significantly more self-reported physical and mental health complaints, physician-diagnosed illnesses, and chronic health problems compared with women who have not been exposed to trauma (Calhoun, Wiley, Dennis, & Beckham, 2009; Laffaye, Kennedy, & Stein, 2003). Researchers tracking health care costs of battered women over an 11-year period found that women who experienced ongoing physical violence from a male partner spent 42% more on health care than nonabused women (Bonomi, Anderson, Rivara, & Thompson, 2009). In addition, women experiencing emotional abuse, but no physical violence, by a male intimate partner had annual health care costs that were 33% higher than nonabused women.

Research has also shown a relationship between different types of maltreatment experienced as a child and long-term physical health problems (Dube, Felitti, Dong, Giles, & Anda, 2003; Felitti et al., 1998; Frances, Caldji, Champange, Plotsky, & Meaney, 1999; Goodwin & Stein, 2004). Women abused as children, but not as adults, had significantly more physical health symptoms compared with women who never experienced abuse (McCauley et al., 1997). In addition, adults (male and female) abused as children have different biological responses to stressors, which are linked to vulnerability to depression and anxiety symptoms when they get older (Lupien, McEwen, Gunnar, & Heim, 2009). Adding to the evidence, women who have experienced childhood abuse or have witnessed IPV between their parents are more likely to experience IPV as adults through complex interactions with PTSD, substance abuse, and risk behaviors (Dube, Anda, Felitti, Edwards, & Williamson, 2002; Fargo, 2009). Therefore, trauma leads to long-term vulnerabilities that underlie health declines in adulthood; however, a better understanding of how to prevent these declines is required.

The evidence that health consequences of intimate partner and other forms of family violence for women are long-lasting is strong and persuasive. The physiological effects of trauma and the relation to health declines may be explained through four main theoretical frameworks. These frameworks illustrate how the physiological effects of chronic stress result in excessive demands on the body, which can result in long-term health declines.

THE STRESS RESPONSE

It is important to understand the dynamic interplay between the physiologic, immunologic, and psychological responses to stress, particularly in persons experiencing the repeated acute and ongoing chronic stress situations associated with family violence. These biological changes can underlie risk for psychological and physical health declines; however, a full understanding of these complex processes is lacking, in part because of the paucity of prospective studies. There may also be adaptations that contribute to a more resilient response to IPV and child abuse; but again, factors that promote resilience are not well understood. Several theories have been posited to explain the alterations in neuroendocrine and inflammatory/immune activity in persons who have experienced trauma: allostasis, psychoneuroimmunology, risky early family environment, and psychobiological resilience. A brief description of the stress response and the four potential frameworks is described in the following section.

Autonomic and Neuroendocrine Systems

During an acute stress or threat situation, the body has a physiologic "fight-or-flight" response, which activates the hypothalamic–pituitary–adrenal (HPA) axis and the sympathetic nervous system (SNS). These activations result in the release of the glucocorticoid cortisol and the catecholamines epinephrine and norepinephrine; the release and interactions of these mediators are well orchestrated and are adaptive as a short-term response to stress (McEwen & Wingfield, 2003). Glucocorticoids help to promote survival by mobilizing and replenishing energy stores and reducing nonessential activity in other body systems, including the immune system (McEwen & Seeman, 1999). Cortisol also turns off the acute stress response via a negative feedback loop on all components of the HPA axis. In the short-term, the acute stress response is protective; however, repeated and prolonged stress states can result in serious physical and psychiatric health declines (see Figure 2.2). Repeated or prolonged stress results in upregulation of the HPA axis, in part, through central and peripheral increases in the numbers and sensitivity of glucocorticoid receptors (Stam, 2007). In chronically stressed animals, this process results in a reduction in the volume of the hippocampus, a neuronal structure required for the processing of new information and memory recall.

Immune System

The HPA axis and their mediators have an interrelated, integrative role with inflammatory and immune activities (Black, 1995; McEwen, 1998; McEwen & Stellar, 1993; van der Kolk & Saporta, 1993), which may be disrupted following exposure to extreme or chronic stress like intimate partner and family violence (see Figure 2.3). Cortisol's role in the inflammatory/immune response is one of immunosuppression. Cortisol exerts its immunosuppressive effects by inhibiting lymphocyte function and cytokine production, T-cell proliferation, killer cell and macrophage activity, and depressing immunoglobulin synthesis through activation of glucocorticoid receptors that reduce the NFK-b inflammatory pathway (Chrousos, 1995; Raison and Miller, 2003). Persistent low cortisol levels

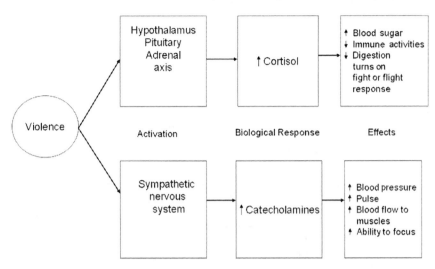

FIGURE 2.2   The acute stress response.

in chronically stressed or traumatized persons may cause tissue damage, suppress cellular immunity, and increase vulnerability for chronic pain syndromes, cardiovascular pathology, and onset of autoimmune disorder (Heim, Ehlert, & Hellhammer, 2000; Heim, Ehlert, Hanker, & Hellhammer, 1998; McEwen, 1998). Low cortisol levels may also result in an inability to contain the acute stress response (Yehuda, 2000).

Cytokines are proteins that facilitate communication and link the immune, nervous, and neuroendocrine systems (Coe & Laudenslager, 2007; Rabin, 1999). The HPA axis and immune system exert well-described, bidirectional effects. While IL-6 and TNF-α stimulate the HPA axis to produce cortisol, cortisol, in turn, suppresses the production and activity of inflammatory cytokines and immune cells including macrophages, thereby protecting against excessive proinflammatory consequences (Kunz-Ebrecht, Mohamed-Ali, Feldman, Kirschbaum, & Steptoe, 2003; Raison & Miller, 2003; Fries et al., 2005). Cortisol also serves to restrain excessive cytokine and inflammatory immune cell activity (Kunz-Ebrecht et al., 2003; Raison & Miller, 2003). Yet, IL-6 can interact with all components of the HPA axis and directly stimulate production of cortisol (Artz, Pereda, Castro, Pagotto, Renner, & Stalla, 1999). Therefore, glucocorticoids and inflammatory cytokines are synergistic, in that they function to protect the individual from the pathological consequences of each other (Chrousos, 1995).

Not only may cytokines contribute to risk for medical conditions, but an excess of inflammatory cytokines results in "sickness behavior," which includes symptoms of malaise, fatigue, reduced appetite, and altered sleep patterns (Elenkov, Iezzoni, Daly, Harris, & Chrousos, 2005). In support of this, administration of virus antigens to humans increased levels of proinflammatory cytokines (IL-1b and IL-6), and these elevations were also positively correlated with symptoms of "sickness behavior" (Vollmer-Conna et al., 2004). In addition, depressive symptoms and major depression are a known side effect of immune cytokines in patients undergoing treatment for cancer (Maes, Capuron, et al., 2001b; Capuron, Ravaud, Miller, & Dantzer, 2004) or hepatitis C (Maes, Bonaccorso, et al., 2001a; Beratis et al., 2005; Wichers, Kenis, Koek, Robaeys, Nicolson, & Maes, 2007).

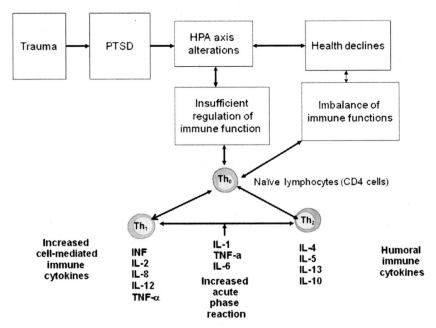

FIGURE 2.3 Biological alterations in PTSD.

There is a consistent association between long-term exposure to stress and altered immune function (Herbert & Cohen, 1993; Kang & Fox, 2001). Segerstrom and Miller (2004), in a meta-analysis of psychoneuroimmunology research, reported that chronic stress and the severity of stressors were key factors in moderating both the nature and intensity of alterations in immune function. Moreover, while prolonged stress can suppress some immune activities, it also appears to induce a chronic, systemic state of inflammation (Kiecolt-Glaser, Preacher, MacCallum, Atkinson, Malarkey, & Glaser, 2003) as evidenced by increased circulating concentrations of the inflammatory biomarkers C-reactive protein (CRP) and IL-6 and an increased immune response to placed antigens and wound recovery (Christian, Graham, Padgett, Glaser, & Kiecolt-Glaser, 2006). Repeated and sustained activation of the stress response along with altered immune function and chronic, low-grade, systemic inflammation, without any time for rest and recovery, increases the risk for physical health problems including hypertension, cardiovascular disease, metabolic syndrome, altered immune function, and diabetes (Black, 2006; Lundberg, 2005).

Neuronal Response

The perception of stress results in activation of brain areas that both initiate the stress response as well as moderate it so that is it not excessive. Chronic activation of these areas, which often occurs in persons who have experienced violence and trauma, can change the function, structure, and communication pathways (Bremner, 2006). In women experiencing IPV and PTSD, there is increased activation of the bilateral anterior insula in anticipation of negative images (Simmons, Paulus, Thorp, Matthews, Norman, & Stein, 2008). The anterior insula is a component of the amygdala, which is responsible for initiating the stress response when an individual perceives fear. In a meta-analysis of studies in adults abused as children, researchers Woon and Hedges (2008) found a significant reduction in the volume of the hippocampus, a structure needed to form and recall memories, and an initiator and regulator of the stress response. In both men and women, more trauma experiences resulted in greater amygdala re-activity and less responsive suppression of the amygdala by the medial prefrontal cortex, the structure responsible for modulating responses to the environment (Ganzel, Kim, Glover, & Temple, 2008).

Framework of Allostasis

Allostasis is the active process of adapting to change and maintaining homeostasis through interactions among the autonomic, neuroendocrine, and immune systems (McEwen, 1998). Stress begins in the brain and affects the brain as well as the rest of the body through the initiation of the stress response. Stress, within the allostatic framework, is described by McEwen and Wingfield (2003) as "*events* that are threatening to an individual and which elicit physiological and behavioral responses as part of allostasis in addition to that imposed by the normal cycle [of daily activity]" (p. 4). Additionally, responses often experienced by persons during times of acute stress, including anxiety, worry, and increased vigilance, may intensify the release and actions of physiological mediators (McEwen & Wingfield, 2003).

Allostatic load refers to the cumulative wear and tear on the body as it tries to adapt to adverse and repeated psychosocial and physical stressors and includes interpersonal relationships, lifestyle, and environmental factors (McEwen, 2000a). There are several ways in which allostatic load may accumulate (McEwen, 2000b; Stewart, 2006), including repeated surges of the physiologic mediators due to frequent stress or violence, or repeated stress over prolonged periods of time. Allostatic load can occur if the stress response continues to respond to stressors and is no longer sufficiently shutting down the stress response. Lastly, load may result if others systems need to compensate due to an insufficient initial allostatic response. Allostatic load can be sustained for a limited time; however, chronic stress can lead to excess exposure to autonomic, neuroendocrine, and immune mediators resulting in changes in the chemistry, structure, and function of the body over time (McEwen, 2000a). These changes put persons at risk for health declines. Allostasis has been proposed and/or used as a guiding framework for research with women experiencing intimate partner violence (Woods, 2008b) and female war veterans (Groer & Burns, 2009), as it provides a comprehensive physiological explanation of the chronic stress of trauma and violence and links these to observed health declines.

Psychoneuroimmunology

A second possible and related framework that links psychological well-being and distress with neuroendocrine and immune system activity and health is the psychoneuroimmunological model (PNI). The basic concepts of the PNI model are that physical and psychological stress and trauma result in activation of the SNS and increased release of catecholamines, decreased cortisol levels over time, and alterations in immune activity including proinflammatory cytokine production (Coe & Laudenslager, 2007; Figley et al., 2009). Both the allostasis/allostatic load framework and the PNI model include mechanisms for cumulative wear and tear of lifetime trauma and prolonged or chronic stress situations. However, the PNI model emphasizes immune competence and the link between proinflammatory cytokines and inflammatory/immune activities and behavioral influences and their relationships with PTSD, depression, and other psychological and physical health problems. Coe and Laudenslager (2007), in an analysis of two decades of research published in *Brain, Behavior, and Immunity*, concluded that studies using a PNI framework have extended knowledge about inflammation and inflammation physiology, and the many types of psychological, behavioral, and environmental factors that can affect immune function and health. The PNI model has been proposed and used to guide research and interventions in several populations, including those exposed to chronic violence (Figley, Hall, Nash, & Temoshok, 2009; Laudenslager et al., 1998) and persons with HIV, cancer, and pain (Carlson, Speca, Faris, & Patel, 2007; Maier, 2003; McCain et al., 2003).

Risky Early Family Environment

A third potential framework to explain alterations in stress systems and their relationships with physical and mental health outcomes in adulthood is the risky early family environment. Building on, in part, the framework of allostasis, Taylor, Lerner, Sage, Lehman, and Seeman (2004) have posited a theoretical perspective that exposure to risky early environments "creates a cascade of risks that exacerbate or lead to vulnerabilities" (p. 1368). This cascade of risk may result in disturbances in the neuroendocrine response to stress which may lead to a broad array of physical and psychological outcomes. Anda et al. (2006) stated that extreme and repetitive childhood stressors are often kept secret and that the accompanying changes resulting from frequent acute stress responses is not always visible. However, both the chronic trauma and repeated stress responses have detrimental effects on the developing neural networks and the neuroendocrine systems of children. Repetti, Taylor, and Seeman (2002), in an integrative biobehavioral literature review, noted that the repeated stress of a risky early environment may result in chronic activation of the HPA axis and sympathetic nervous system in children. This can lead to increased cardiovascular reactivity with possible long-term effects in adulthood including hypertension and cardiovascular disease.

Emotional regulation, including recognizing emotions of self and others, managing emotional states, and difficulties with social relationships can also be challenging for those exposed to early risky environments, further contributing to increased vulnerability (Repetti et al., 2002). Adult children from risky family environments have been found to have little amygdala activation when observing fearful/angry faces and increased activation when labeling the emotional character of those faces compared to adult children from nonrisky environments who showed the expected patterns of amygdala reactivity (Taylor, Eisenberg, Saxbe, Lehman, & Lieberman, 2006a). Taylor and associates speculated that children who experience a risky early family environment may not be able to detect threats or have the emotional regulation skills to cope with threats.

Psychobiological Resilience

A fourth potential framework for explaining responses to violence and trauma is psychobiological resilience. Although most people are exposed to at least one trauma during their lives, the majority do not develop posttraumatic stress disorder or depression or a stress-related physical health condition (Kessler et al., 1995; Breslau et al., 1998; Kimmerling, 2004). One possible explanation for this is resilience, a common, yet less understood contributor to physical and mental health. Resilience was first identified as an anomaly based on exceptional coping in studies of children raised under severely adverse circumstances who, despite their environment, excelled in education, health, and interpersonal relationships (Rutter, 1979). More recently, epidemiological studies (Breslau & Kessler, 2001; Kessler et al., 1995) and research of survivors of the World Trade Center Attack (Bonanno, Galea, Bucciarelli, & Vlahov, 2007) and the Oklahoma City Bombing (North, Pfefferbaum, Tivis, Kawasaki, Reddy, & Spitznagel, 2004) have confirmed that resilience is a common response to trauma and has been termed as "ordinary magic" (Masten, 2001). Bonanno and Mancini (2009) state that resilience is "the maintenance of relatively stable levels of psychological and physical functioning" (p. 371). This conceptualization shifts the focus from individual limitations to individual strengths, competencies, and capacities and is a critical step to understanding how resilience can be fostered in those exposed to trauma.

There are multiple psychosocial factors associated with resilience. These include positive emotions and optimism, humor, cognitive flexibility, cognitive explanatory style and reappraisal, acceptance, religion/spirituality, altruism, social support, role models, coping style, exercise, capacity to recover from negative events, and stress inoculation (Southwick, Vythilingam, & Charney, 2005). Psychological factors are dependent on physiologic and genetic factors to mitigate stress, and include genetic predisposition and epigenetic and neural mechanisms, which mediate adaptive changes in the neural circuits that involve neurotransmitter and molecular pathways (Feder, Nestler, & Charney, 2009). These changes shape the functioning of the neural circuits that regulate fear, emotion reactivity, reward, and social behavior, which together are thought to mediate resilience and successful coping with stress.

NEUROENDOCRINE AND IMMUNE CHANGES IN WOMEN EXPOSED TO VIOLENCE

Research examining physiologic and immunologic changes in women experiencing the acute and chronic stress of intimate partner violence is in its infancy. In this section, known empirical findings related to altered neuroendocrine and immune activity, risky early environments, and epigenetic changes in women and children experiencing intimate partner and family violence are highlighted. Findings in other samples of trauma-exposed individuals are also discussed. The physical health problems associated with such changes are discussed.

Alterations in Neuroendocrine Activity in Women Experiencing IPV

Cortisol is the most studied biological measure in persons with PTSD. One of the first findings in PTSD research was a reduction in the level of cortisol, which was counterintuitive as these patients were known to exhibit chronically high stress levels. Decreased cortisol levels have been associated with chronic PTSD in persons who have experienced a broad array of trauma, in both women and men, from children to Holocaust survivors and the children of Holocaust survivors, when compared to those with similar trauma experiences, those with no PTSD, and healthy comparison groups (Gill, Vythilingam, & Page, 2008; Goenjian, Yehuda, Pynoos, Steinberg, Tashjian, Yang et al., 1996; Olff, Guzelcan, de Vries, Assies, & Gersons, 2006; Yehuda, Bierer, Schmeidler, Aferiat, Breslau, & Dolan, 2000; Yehuda, Schmeidler, Wainberg, Binder-Brynes, & Duvdevani, 1998; Yehuda,

Kahana, Binder-Brynes, Southwick, Mason, & Giller, 1995). In a recent meta-analysis, cortisol was found to be lower only in studies that used serum or plasma, samples of persons with chronic PTSD and primarily women, and those with high levels of depression (Meewisse, Reitsma, de Vries, Gerson, & Olff, 2007). Research has also shown an association between depression and comorbid PTSD (PTSD + MDD), with higher salivary cortisol levels in PTSD + MDD, but not in PTSD – MDD compared to control groups (Young & Breslau, 2004). However, lower levels of plasma cortisol have been observed in PTSD + MDD in community samples of men and women (Vythilingam et al., in press), and in PTSD + MDD compared to healthy control groups and to depressed groups (Oquendo et al., 2003).

Altered cortisol patterns have been reported in women who are experiencing intimate partner violence. Inslicht et al. (2006) found that women survivors of IPV with lifetime PTSD ($n = 29$) had significantly higher cortisol levels at four time points throughout the day compared to women exposed to IPV without PTSD even after controlling for age, depression, and abuse characteristics. Higher evening cortisol levels have also been reported in crisis sheltered abused women compared to nonabused women (Pico-Alfonso, Garcia-Linares, Celda-Navarro, Herbert, & Martinez, 2004). However, these investigators did not find an association between cortisol levels and PTSD symptoms.

In contrast, approximately half of 116 battered women in a cross-sectional study of women seeking help for IPV, with most reporting moderate to severe PTSD symptoms, exhibited altered levels of diurnal cortisol, and an altered cortisol pattern, including blunted, flat, or reversed diurnal patterns (Woods et al., 2003). In a follow-up study, almost 65% of 142 women, primarily from crisis shelters, and who were demonstrating high levels of PTSD symptomatology, had altered diurnal cortisol patterns; approximately 55% of the women exhibited a blunt or flat diurnal pattern (Woods et al., 2008a).

Studies that have examined the function of the HPA axis through responses to administration of stimulators have generally demonstrated "supersensitivity." Excessive suppression of cortisol and adernocorticotrophin (ACTH) in response to dexamethasone has been reported in samples of combat veterans, women who were abused as children, and in women who experienced domestic violence (Griffin, Resick, & Yehuda, 2005; Newport, Heim, Bonsall, Miller, & Nemeroff, 2004; Stein, Yehuda, Keverola, & Hanna, 1997; Yehuda, Boisoneau, Lowy, Giller, 1995; Yehuda, Boisoneau, Mason, & Giller, 1993). Hydrocotisone easily crosses the blood–brain barrier and acts on both glucocorticoid and mineralocorticoid receptors in the hippocampus and hypothalamus. One study with combat veterans with PTSD has shown a graded "central" sensitivity to glucocorticoids (Yehuda, Yang, Buchsbaum, & Golier, 2006). In addition, preliminary evidence supports distinct differences in glucocorticoid sensitivity between patients with PTSD + MDD and PTSD – MDD. Compared to PTSD + MDD, those with PTSD – MDD had greater suppression of plasma cortisol following a standard dexamethasone suppression test (DST) (Kudler, Davidson, Meador, Lipper, & Ely, 1987) and a low-dose DST (Golier Schmeidler, Legge, & Yehuda, 2006; Griffin et al., 2005). Cortisol and ACTH response to the dexamethasone-/corticotrophin-releasing hormone test was also significantly different between individuals with PTSD + MDD and PTSD – MDD (de Kloet et al., 2008).

In summary, even though the empirical evidence is limited, and the direction of neuroendocrine changes is not consistent, it is clear that women who have been abused by an intimate partner, particularly those who also experienced PTSD and/or depression, have altered HPA axis activity. Findings of a blunted or flat diurnal cortisol pattern are particularly important in light of the results from Sephton, Sapolsky, Kraemer, and Spiegel

(2000) and Abercrombie, Giese-Davis, Sephton, Epel, Turner-Cobb, and Spiegel (2004) who reported that a relatively flat or abnormal diurnal cortisol variation was predictive of early mortality in women with metastatic breast cancer. Moreover, a relatively flat diurnal cortisol pattern was associated with both low circulating counts of natural killer (NK) cells and suppressed NK activity in women with metastatic breast cancer (Sephton et al., 2000). These results underscore the importance of evaluating cortisol at multiple time points and of determining the role of altered circadian patterns to health of women. Accordingly, additional research is needed in women abused by intimate partners to determine the role of PTSD and depression, HPA axis functioning, and the associated implications for physical and psychological health.

Altered Inflammatory/Immune Activity

In a review of empirical literature, Gill, Woods, and Page (2009) suggested that excessive activity of the inflammatory/immune response is associated with chronic PTSD. This excessive activity may contribute to the early and increased morbidity often seen in persons who have experienced trauma and PTSD symptoms, including women and children experiencing family violence.

Empirical evidence has shown alterations in both immune cell enumeration and efficacy in some persons with PTSD. Abused women experiencing PTSD have a significantly higher number of leukocytes and absolute lymphocyte subset counts than comparison women and controlling for smoking and body mass index (Woods et al., 2003). Yet, despite having higher levels of circulating lymphocytes compared to nonabused women, the cytotoxic potential of the T and NK (natural killer) cells in abused women was decreased, indicating reduced functional efficacy of these immune cells (Woods et al., 2005b). In a recent study, participants with PTSD had more memory T cells, but fewer naïve T cells that would be used to fight off new antigens, and also less regulatory T cells that would regulate the immune response to an antigen (Sommershof et al., 2009). This finding extends those of Altemus, Dhabhar, and Yang's. (2006), which consistently showed an excessive response to placed antigens in abused women, indicating an insufficiently regulated immune response. These findings also suggest that abused women with PTSD may have compromised immune responsiveness.

Women who have experienced trauma, including interpersonal violence as an adult or child, and are suffering from PTSD symptoms, have been found to have higher levels of stimulated proinflammatory cytokines IL-6 and TNF-α production compared to both trauma and nontrauma control groups (Gill et al., 2008). In the same study, those with comorbid MDD had higher stimulated IL-6 levels compared to those women with PTSD alone (Gill et al., 2008). In addition, PTSD was a mediator of the relationship between IFN-γ and IPV. Women currently experiencing IPV have been found to have high mean levels of IL-6 (Woods, Hall, Foster, & Page, 2009), values that were consistent with those found in patients with mild congestive heart failure (Tsutamoto et al., 1998) and women 2 to 3 decades older who were participating in the Framingham Offspring Study (Loucks, Sullivan, D'Agostino, Larson, Berkman, & Benjamin, 2006). Women experiencing IPV have also been found to have higher levels of stimulated proinflammatory cytokine interferon-γ (IFN-γ) compared to nonabused women (Woods et al., 2005a). High levels of inflammatory cytokines are a biological predictor of symptoms of metabolic syndrome in young adults, which resulted in increased risk for coronary artery disease (Jacobs et al., 2009) and also symptoms of pain following surgery (Wang, Hamza, Wu, & Dionne, 2009).

The role of inflammation in the development of serious health problems has also come under study. C-reactive protein (CRP) is a protein biomarker of the inflammatory process, and as such, is widely recognized as a clinically useful marker for chronic inflammation. Inflammation occurs locally, through recruitment and activation of immune cells, and systemically, via increased secretion of C-reactive protein (CRP) and other complement components (Janeway, 2005). These higher levels of inflammation damage the vascular endothelium, a prerequisite for plaque and clot formation (Andersen & Pedersen, 2008), which could result in unstable angina, myocardial infarction, ischemic arrhythmias, sudden cardiac death, or stroke (Gokce, Keaney, Hunter, Watkins, Menzoian, & Vita, 2002). Chronic inflammation is also an independent risk factor for cardiovascular disease, cancer, hypertension, diabetes, and autoimmune disease. Growing empirical evidence has suggested that depression, history of childhood maltreatment, and cumulative exposure to stress are associated with chronic inflammation (Danese, Moffitt, Pariante, Ambler, Poulton, & Caspi, 2008; Kling et al., 2007; Taylor, Lehman, Kiefe, & Seeman, 2006b) and may explain findings of subsequent cardiac mortality in adults experiencing childhood maltreatment (Felitti et al., 1998).

Little research has examined CRP levels in abused women. One exception is a study with 152 women currently experiencing intimate abuse and an average age of approximately 34 years. Almost 40% of the participants had CRP values over 3 mg/l; almost 16% had CRP levels over 10 (Woods et al., 2009). According to the American Heart Association, CRP values of 3 or higher put the person at high risk for cardiovascular disease. Thirty-eight percent of the women in the Framingham Offspring Study (Dhingra et al., 2007) had CRP values greater than 3, but the women in the Framingham sample were, on average, 20–30 years older than the participants in the study by Woods study. This suggests that women experiencing IPV may be experiencing chronic inflammation, which may, over more extended periods of time, contribute to early morbidity. Dhingra and colleagues also reported increased odds of having at least one common inflammatory condition, such as cancer or pulmonary disease, with rising CRP values.

These findings, taken together, indicate an association between increased inflammatory and immune activity and violence and trauma in women. Increased inflammation has been associated with cardiovascular disease, hypertension, chronic pain, and diabetes (Andersen & Pedersen, 2008; Campbell et al., 2002; Dhingra et al., 2007; Dobie, Kivlahan, Maynard, Bush, Davis, & Bradley, 2004; Jacobs et al., 2009; Kimerling, 2004; Wang et al., 2009). Thus, interventions that lower markers of inflammation may be of great benefit in reducing the health consequences for women experiencing violence. Psychological interventions, including meditation (Pace et al., 2009) and relaxation (Koh, Lee, Beyn, Chu, & Kim, 2008), lower IL-6 levels and could be of benefit. Hydrocortisone administered orally for 1 month reduced PTSD symptoms in three patients in a double-blind placebo-controlled cross-over study; however, information regarding changes in immune function was not provided (Aerni et al., 2004; de Quervain, 2006). In a prospective study, hydrocortisone reduced the risk of developing PTSD symptoms, lowered IL-6 levels, and improved health outcomes in patients undergoing a cardiac surgery (Weis et al., 2006). Novel drugs that lower IL-6 levels (Woo et al. 2005) and nonsteroidal anti-inflammatory drugs (NSAIDS) should be evaluated as putative or adjunctive treatments for PTSD.

Risky Early Family Environments

Risky early family environment is a multifaceted concept and has been measured using a variety of factors, including childhood abuse, harsh discipline, maternal rejection, chaotic or neglectful parenting, family conflict, disorganized households, and lack of nurturance and physical affection (Danese 2007; Felitti et al., 1998; Repetti et al., 2002; Taylor et al., 2006b). Risky early family environment and low socioeconomic status (SES) in childhood have been related to higher levels of anxiety and depression (Repetti et al., 2002), altered metabolic functioning (Lehman, Taylor, Kiefe, & Seeman, 2005), changes in neuroendocrine responses to stress (Anda et al., 2006; Taylor et al., 2004), and major physical health problems (Felitti et al., 1998).

Taylor and colleagues (2006b), using Year 15 CARDIA study data, reported that low childhood SES and risky early family environment were associated with increased levels of C-reactive protein in adulthood via higher body mass index and psychosocial factors such as depression and social support. Danese and associates (2007), in a longitudinal-prospective study of 972 participants, reported that exposure to maltreatment during childhood was significantly associated with increased risk of clinically relevant CRP levels 20 years later in adulthood. This relationship existed even after controlling for other risk factors such as smoking, physical activity, and diet.

Further, research has shown that the effects of early life stressors are cumulative and contribute to a wide array of physical and mental health deficits throughout the life span (Allen, Matthews, & Sherman, 1997; Danese et al., 2007; Felitti et al., 1998; McEwen, 1998; Repetti et al., 2002; Taylor et al., 2006b). Empirical evidence has shown that exposure to trauma during childhood may increase vulnerability to future stress and results in long-term neurobiological changes in the individual's stress response (Bremner, Southwick, Johnson, Yehuda, & Charney, 1993; Heim, Newport, Bonsall, Miller, & Nemeroff, 2001; Follette, Polusny, Bechtle, & Naugle, 1996; Friedman, Jalowiec, McHugo, Wang, & McDonagh, 2007; Resnick, Yehuda, Pitman, and Foy, 1995; Yehuda & Flory, 2007) and increases the risk for PTSD onset (DeBellis, 1997; DeBellis & Putnam, 1994; Heim & Nemeroff, 2001). Moreover, adult children of Holocaust survivors with PTSD were three times more likely to develop PTSD (Yehuda et al., 1998) and to have lower cortisol levels when compared to demographically matched comparison group (Yehuda, Bierer, Schmeidler, Aferiat, Breslau, & Dolan, 2000).

There is a paucity of research that examines the relationship between risky early environments, and how those experiences may contribute to risk for neuroendocrine and immune function alterations in abused women, and contribute to risk for psychological and physical health declines. Women abused as children were found to be at six times the risk for chronic fatigue syndrome and to have a lower wakening cortisol response, which were significantly associated (Heim, Nater, Maloney, Boneva, Jones, & Reeves, 2009). An initial study found that childhood physical, emotional, and sexual abuse and childhood emotional neglect predicted higher B cell counts in abused women, suggesting that childhood maltreatment altered immune function (Woods et al., 2005b). In addition, childhood physical and emotional neglect was related to an increased CD8 (suppressor/cytotoxic) cell count. Although these immune findings need to be viewed with caution, they suggest the need for additional research to disentangle the complex pathways among the neuroendocrine and immune systems and risky early environments.

Epigenetic Changes in Abused Children and Risk for Psychiatric Symptoms

The relationship between early life stress and psychological and physical health may relate to epigenetic changes. Epigenetics refers to changes in phenotype or gene expression that are caused by environmental factors and not from changes in the underlying DNA sequence. Epigenetic changes may underlie the risk for behavioral changes and psychiatric symptoms in those who experience childhood abuse (Hohoff, 2009). In a recent study, hippocampal neurons retrieved from suicide completers with a history of childhood abuse had increased cytosine methylation of NR3C1, which is a glucocorticoid receptor, a change that would result in blunted HPA axis functioning (McGowan et al., 2009). In rats exposed to abusive caretaking during infancy, there was an increased methylation of the gene for brain-deprived neurotrophic factor (BDNF), a neurotrophin linked to regulation of mood, learning, and appetite (Roth, Lubin, Funk, & Sweatt, 2009). Therefore, there is evidence for a link between epigenetic changes and the negative consequences of trauma; however, additional studies are needed in humans to understand these complex relationships.

SUMMARY

There are long-term health consequences of violence for women and children. Several potential frameworks integrating physiological pathways and psychological responses to trauma and violence have been posited. By developing a better understanding of how IPV may alter neuroendocrine and immune functioning, and how these changes may underlie health declines, more effective treatments can be developed. Even when women and children are no longer exposed to family violence, they are at risk for long-term health declines. In addition, few individuals experience only one trauma during their lifetimes (Breslau et al., 1998). To date, there is little evidence regarding the effect of multiple traumas on the health of the individual.

Prevention of family violence is foremost. Interventions that include traditional cognitive and psychological therapy, mind–body-based interventions, and medications that ease psychological distress and reduce inflammation may assist in re-balancing the effects of chronic stress and help to offset the health risk that family violence exerts. Many interventions for women and children who have experienced violence are described in others chapters of this book. There has been little prospective research or research that combines study of both biological measures and interventions in persons experiencing chronic stress due to violence and trauma. Such research would enhance understanding of the underlying physiologic and immunologic changes that occur in persons in chronic stress situations. Further, this type of research would improve interventions. Nurses are in a key place to initiate such research as well as comprehensive interventions that will have the power to change the lifelong biological imprint that violence and trauma have on women and children.

REFERENCES

Abercrombie, H. C., Giese-Davis, J., Sephton, S., Epel, E. S., Turner-Cobb, J. M., & Spiegel, D. (2004). Flattened cortisol rhythms in metastatic breast cancer patients. *Psychoneuroendocrinology, 29,* 1082–1092.

Aerni, A., Traber, R., Hock, C., Roozendaal, B., Schelling, G., Papassotiropoulos, A., et al. (2004). Low-dose cortisol for symptoms of posttraumatic stress disorder. *American Journal of Psychiatry, 161*(8), 1488–1490.

Allen, M. T., Matthews, K. A., & Sherman, F. S. (1997). Cardiovascular reactivity to stress and left ventricular mass in youth. *Hypertension, 30,* 782–787.

Altemus, M., Dhabhar, F. S., & Yang, R. (2006). Immune function in PTSD. *Annals of the New York Academy of Science, 1071,* 167–183.

Alvarez, J., Pavao, J., Mack, K. P., Chow, J. M., Baumrind, N., & Kimerling, R. (2009). Lifetime interpersonal violence and self-reported *Chlamydia trachomatis* diagnosis among California women. *Journal of Women's Health (Larchmt), 18*(1), 57–63.

Anda, R. F., Felitti, V. J., Bremner, J. D., Walker, J. D., Whitfield, C., Perry, B. D., et al. (2006). The enduring effects of abuse and related adverse experiences in childhood: A convergence of evidence from neurobiology and epidemiology. *European Archives of Psychiatry and Clinical Neuroscience, 256,* 174–186.

Andersen, K., & Pedersen, B. K. (2008). The role of inflammation in vascular insulin resistance with focus on IL-6. *Hormones and Metabolism Research, 40*(9), 635–639.

Artz, E., Pereda, M. P., Castro, C. P., Pagotto, U., Renner, U., & Stalla, G. K. (1999). Pathophysiological role of the cytokine network in the anterior pituitary gland. *Frontiers in Neuroendocrinology, 20,* 71–95.

Bennice, J. A., Resick, P. A., Mechanic, M., & Astin. M. (2003). The relative effects of intimate partner physical and sexual violence on post-traumatic stress disorder symptomatology. *Violence and Victims, 18*(1), 87–94.

Beratis, S., Katrivanou, A., Georgiou, S., Monastirili, A., Pasmatzi, P., Gourzis, P., et al. (2005). Major depression and risk of depressive symptomatology associated with short-term and low-dose interferon-alpha treatment. *Journal of Psychosomatic Research, 58*(1), 15–18.

Black, P. H. (1995). Psychoneuroimmunology: Brain and immunity. *Science and Medicine, 2*(6), 16–25.

Bonanno, G. A., Galea, S., Bucciarelli, A., & Vlahov, D. (2007). What predicts psychological resilience after disaster? The role of demographics, resources, and life stress. *Journal of Consulting and Clinical Psychology, 75*(5), 671–682.

Bonomi, A. E., Anderson, M. L., Rivara, F. P., & Thompson, R. S. (2009). Health care utilization and costs associated with physical and nonphysical-only intimate partner violence. *Health Services Research, 44*(3), 1052–1067.

Breiding, M. J., Black, M. C., & Ryan, G. W. (2008). Chronic diseases and health risk behaviors associated with intimate partner violence—18 U.S. states/territories, 2005. *Annals of Epidemiology, 18*(7), 538–544.

Bremner, J. D. (2006). Traumatic stress: effects on the brain. *Dialogues of Clinical Neuroscience, 8*(4), 445–461.

Bremner, J. D., Southwick, S. M., Johnson, D. R., Yehuda, R., & Charney, D. S. (1993). Childhood physical abuse and combat-related posttraumatic stress disorder in Vietnam veterans. *American Journal of Psychiatry, 150,* 235–239.

Breslau, N., & Kessler, R. C. (2001). The stressor criterion in DSM-IV posttraumatic stress disorder: an empirical investigation. *Biological Psychiatry, 50*(9), 699–704.

Breslau, N., Kessler, R. C., Chilcoat, H, D., Schultz, L. R., Davis, G. C., & Andreski, P. (1998). Trauma and posttraumatic stress disorder in the community: the 1996 Detroit Area Survey of Trauma. *Archives of General Psychiatry, 55*(7), 626–632.

Calhoun, P. S., Wiley, M., Dennis, M. F., & Beckham, J. C. (2009). Self-reported health and physician diagnosed illnesses in women with posttraumatic stress disorder and major depressive disorder. *Journal of Traumatic Stress, 22*(2), 122–130.

Campbell, J. C. (2002). Health consequences of intimate partner violence. *Lancet, 359,* 1331–1336.

Campbell, J., Jones, A. S., Dienemann, J., Kub, J., Schollenberger, J., O'Campo, P., et al. (2002). Intimate partner violence and physical health consequences. *Archives of Internal Medicine, 162*(10), 1157–1163.

Capuron, L., Ravaud, A., Miller, A. H., & Dantzer, R. (2004). Baseline mood and psychosocial characteristics of patients developing depressive symptoms during interleukin-2 and/or interferon-alpha cancer therapy. *Brain, Behavior, and Immunity, 18*(3), 205–213.

Carlson, L. E., Speca, M., Faris, P., & Patel, K. D. (2007). One year pre-post intervention follow-up of psychological, immune, endocrine and blood pressure outcomes of mindfulness-based stress reduction (MBSR) in breast and prostate cancer outpatients. *Brain, Behavior, and Immunity, 21,* 1038–1049.

Christian, L. M., Graham, J. E., Padgett, D. A., Glaser, R., & Kiecolt-Glaser, J. K. (2006). Stress and wound healing. *Neuroimmunomodulation, 13*(5–6), 337–346.

Chrousos, G. P. (1995). The hypothalamic–pituitary–adrenal axis and immune-mediated inflammation. *The New England Journal of Medicine, 332*(20), 1351–1362.

Coe, C. L., & Laudenslager, M. L. (2007). Psychosocial influences on immunity, including effects on immune maturation and senescence. *Brain, Behavior, & Immunity, 21*, 1000–1008.

Coker, A. L., Davis, K. E., Arias, I., Desai, S., Sanderson, M., & Brandt, H. M. (2002). Physical and mental health effects of intimate partner violence for men and women. *American Journal Preventive Medicine, 23*(4), 260–268.

Coker, A. L., Hopenhayn, C., DeSimone, C. P., Bush, H. M., & Clifford, L. (2009). Violence against women raises risk of cervical cancer. *Journal of Women's Health (Larchmt), 18*(8), 1179–1185.

The Commonwealth Fund. (1999). *Violence and abuse.* New York: The Commonwealth Fund.

Connor, K. M., Davidson, J. R. T., & Lee, L. (2003). Spirituality, resilience, and anger in survivors of violent trauma: A community survey. *Journal of Traumatic Stress, 16*(5), 487–494.

Curry, M. A. (1998). The interrelationships between abuse, substance use, and psychosocial stress during pregnancy. *JOGNN, 27*, 692–699.

Danese, A., Moffitt, T. E., Pariante, C. M., Ambler, A., Poulton, R., & Caspi, A. (2008). Elevated inflammation levels in depressed adults with a history of childhood maltreatment. *Archives of General Psychiatry, 65*(4), 409–416.

Danese, A., Pariante, C. M., Caspi, A., Taylor, A., & Poulton, R. (2007). Childhood maltreatment predicts adult inflammation in a life-course study. *Proceedings of The National Academy of Science (PNAS), 104*(4), 1319–1324.

DeBellis, M. D. (1997). Posttraumatic stress disorder and acute stress disorder. In R. T. Ammerman & M. Hersen (Eds.), *Handbook of Prevention and Treatment with Children and Adolescents* (pp. 455–494). New York: John Wiley & Sons, Inc.

DeBellis, M. D., & Putnam, F. W. (1994). The psychobiology of childhood maltreatment. *Child and Adolescent Psychiatric Clinics of North America, 3*, 663–677.

de Kloet, C., Vermetten, E., Lentjes, E., Geuze, E., van Pelt, J., Manuel, R., et al. (2008). Differences in the response to the combined DEX-CRH test between PTSD patients with and without co-morbid depressive disorder. *Psychoneuroendocrinology, 33*(3), 313–320.

de Quervain, D. J. (2006). Glucocorticoid-induced inhibition of memory retrieval: implications for posttraumatic stress disorder. *Annals of the New York Academy of Science, 1071*, 216–220.

Dienemann, J., Boyle, E., Baker, D., Resnick, W., Weiderhorn, N., & Campbell, J. (2000). Intimate partner abuse among women diagnosed with depression. *Issues in Mental Health Nursing, 21*, 499–513.

Dhingra, R., Gona, P., Nam, B. H., D'Agostino, R. B., Sr, Wilson, P. W., Benjamin E. J., O'Donnell C. J. (2007). C-reactive protein, inflammatory conditions, and cardiovascular disease risk. *American Journal of Medicine, 120*, 1054–1062.

Dobie, D. J., Kivlahan, D. R., Maynard, C., Bush, K. R., Davis, T. M., & Bradley, K. A. (2004). Posttraumatic stress disorder in women veterans: Associations with self-reported health problems and functional impairment. *Archives of Internal Medicine, 164*, 394–400.

Dube, S. R., Anda, R. F., Felitti, V. J., Edwards, V. J., & Williamson, D. F. (2002). Exposure to abuse, neglect, and household dysfunction among adults who witnessed intimate partner violence as children: Implications for health and social services. *Violence & Victims, 17*(1), 3–17.

Dube, S. R., Felitti, V. J., Dong, M., Giles, W. H., & Anda, R. F. (2003). The impact of adverse childhood experiences on health problems: Evidence from four birth cohorts dating back to 1900. *Preventive Medicine, 37*, 268–277.

Elenkov, I. J., Iezzoni, D. G., Daly, A., Harris, A. G., & Chrousos, G. P. (2005). Cytokine dysregulation, inflammation and well-being. *Neuroimmunomodulation, 12*(5), 255–269.

Fargo, J. D. (2009). Pathways to adult sexual revictimization: Direct and indirect behavioral risk factors across the lifespan. *Journal of Interpersonal Violence, 24*(11), 1771–1791.

Feder, A., Nestler, E. J., & Charney, D. S. (2009). Psychobiology and molecular genetics of resilience. *Nature Reviews Neuroscience, 10*(6), 446–457.

Felitti, V. J., Anda, R. F., Nordenberg, D., Williamson, D. F., Apitz, A. M., Edwards, V., et al. (1998). Relationship of childhood abuse and household dysfunction to many of the leading causes of death in adults. *American Journal of Preventive Medicine, 14*, 245–258.

Figley, C. R., Hall, N., Nash, W. P., & Temoshok, L. (2009). *Combat stress injuries: Towards a psychoneuro-immunological model for research, treatment, and prevention.* Poster presented at the Psychoneuroimmunology Research Conference, Breckenridge, CO.

Follette, V. M., Polusny, M. A., Bechtle, A. E., & Naugle, A. E. (1996). Cumulative trauma: The impact of child sexual abuse, adult sexual assault and spouse abuse. *Journal of Traumatic Stress, 9,* 25–35.

Frances, D. D., Caldji, C., Champagne, F., Plotsky, P. M., & Meaney, M. J. (1999). The role of corticotropin-releasing factor–norepinephrine systems in mediating the effects of early experience on the development of behavioral and endocrine responses to stress. *Biological Psychiatry, 46,* 1153–1166.

Friedman, M. J., Jalowiec, J., McHugo, G., Wang, S., & McDonagh, A. (2007). Adult sexual abuse is associated with elevated neurohormone levels among women with PTSD due to childhood sexual abuse. *Journal of Traumatic Stress, 20,* 611–617.

Fries, E., Hesse, J., Hesse, J., Hellhammer, J., Hellhammer, D. L. (2005). A new view on hypocortisolism. *Psychoneuroendocrinology, 30*(10), 1010–1016.

Ganzel, B. L., Kim, P., Glover, G. H., & Temple, E. (2008). Resilience after 9/11: multimodal neuroimaging evidence for stress-related change in the healthy adult brain. *Neuroimage, 40*(2), 788–795.

Garcia-Moreno, C., Watts, C., Jansen, H., Ellsberg, M. C., & Heise, L. (2003). Responding to violence against women: WHO's Multicountry study on women's health and domestic violence. *Health & Human Rights, 6,* 113–129.

Gill, J., Woods, S. J., & Page, G. G. (2009). PTSD is associated with an excess of inflammatory/immune activities. *Perspectives in Psychiatric Care, 45*(4), 262–277.

Gill, J., Vythilingam, M., & Page. GG. (2008). Low cortisol, high DHEA, and high levels of stimulated TNF-α and IL-6 in women with PTSD. *Journal of Traumatic Stress, 21*(6), 530–539.

Goenjian, A. K., Yehuda, R., Pynoos, R. S., Steinberg, A. M., Tashjian, M., Yang, R. K., et al. (1996). Basal cortisol and dexamethasone suppression of cortisol and MHPG among adolescents after the earthquake in Armenia. *American Journal of Psychiatry, 153,* 929–934.

Gokce, N., Keaney, J. F., Hunter, L. M., Watkins, M. T. Menzoian, J. O., & Vita, J. A. (2002). Risk stratification for postoperative cardiovascular events via noninvasive assessment of endothelial function: a prospective study. *Circulation, 105*(13), 1567–1572.

Golier, J. A., Schmeidler, J., Legge, J., & Yehuda, R. (2006). Enhanced cortisol suppression to dexamethasone associated with Gulf War deployment. *Psychoneuroendocrinology, 31*(10), 1181–1189.

Golding, J. M. (1999). Intimate partner violence as a risk factor for mental disorders: A meta-analysis. *Journal of Family Violence, 14*(2), 99–132.

Goodwin, R. D., & Stein, M. B. (2004). Association between childhood trauma and physical disorders among adults in the United States. *Psychological Medicine, 34,* 509–520.

Griffin, M. G., Resick, P. A., & Yehuda, R. (2005). Enhanced cortisol suppression following dexamethasone administration in domestic violence survivors. *American Journal of Psychiatry, 162*(6), 1192–1199.

Groer, M. W., & Burns, C. (2009). Stress response in female veterans: An allostatic perspective. *Rehabilitation Nursing, 34*(3), 96–104.

Heim, C., Nater, U. M., Maloney, E., Boneva, R., Jones, J. F., & Reeves, W. C. (2009). Childhood trauma and risk for chronic fatigue syndrome: Association with neuroendocrine dysfunction. *Archives of General Psychiatry, 66*(1), 72–80.

Heim, C., & Nemeroff, C. B. (2001). The role of childhood trauma in the neurobiology of mood and anxiety disorders: Preclinical and clinical studies. *Biological Psychiatry, 49,* 1023–1039.

Heim, C., Newport, D. J., Bonsall, R., Miller, A. H., & Nemeroff, C. B. (2001). Altered pituitary–adrenal axis responses to provocative challenge tests in adult survivors of childhood abuse. *American Journal of Psychiatry, 158,* 575–581.

Heim, C., Ehlert, U., & Hellhammer, D. H. (2000). The potential role of hypocortisolism in the pathophysiology of stress-related bodily disorders. *Psychoneuroendocrinology, 25*(1), 1–35.

Heim, C., Ehlert, U., Hanker, J. P., & Hellhammer, D. H. (1998). Abuse-related posttraumatic stress disorder and alterations of the hypothalamic–pituitary–adrenal axis in women with chronic pelvic pain. *Psychosomatic Medicine, 60,* 309–318.

Herbert, T. B., & Cohen, S. (1993). Stress and immunity in humans: A meta-analytic review. *Psychosomatic Medicine, 55,* 364–379.

Hohoff, C. (2009). Anxiety in mice and men: a comparison. *Journal of Neural Transmission, 116*(6), 679–87.

Inslicht, S. S., Marmar, C. R., Neylan, T. C., Metzler, T. J., Hart, S. L., Otte, C., et al. (2006). Increased cortisol in women with intimate partner violence-related posttraumatic stress disorder. *Psychoneuroendocrinology, 31*, 825–838.

Jacobs, M., van Greevenbroek, M. M., van der Kallen, C. J., Ferreira, I., Blake, E. E., Feskens, E. J., et al. (2009). Low-grade inflammation can partly explain the association between the metabolic syndrome and either coronary artery disease or severity of peripheral arterial disease: the CODAM study. *European Journal of Clinical Investigation, 39*, 437–444.

Janeway, C. (2005). *Immunobiology.* New York: Garland Science Publishing.

Kang, D. H., & Fox, C. (2001). Th1 and Th2 cytokine responses to academic stress. *Research in Nursing & Health, 24*, 245–257.

Kessler, R. C., Sonnega, A., Bromet, E., Hughes, M., & Nelson, C. B. (1995). Posttraumatic stress disorder in the National Comorbidity Survey. *Archives of General Psychiatry, 52*(12), 1048–1060.

Kiecolt-Glaser, J. K., Preacher, K. J., MacCallum, R. C., Atkinson, C., Malarkey, W. B., & Glaser, R. (2003). Chronic stress and age-related increases in the proinflammatory cytokine IL-6. *Proceedings of the National Academy of Sciences, 100*, 9090–9095.

Kimerling, R. (2004). An investigation of sex differences in nonpsychiatric morbidity associated with posttraumatic stress disorder. *Journal of the American Medical Women's Association, 59*, 43–47.

Kling, M. A., Alesci, S., Csako, G., Costello, R., Luckenbaugh, D. A., Bonne, O., et al. (2007). Sustained low-grade pro-inflammatory state in unmedicated, remitted women with major depressive disorder as evidenced by elevated serum levels of the acute phase proteins C-reactive protein and serum amyloid A. *Biological Psychiatry, 62*(4), 309–313.

Koh, K. B., Lee, Y. J., Beyn, K. M., Chu, S. H., & Kim, D. M. (2008). Counter-stress effects of relaxation on proinflammatory and anti-inflammatory cytokines. *Brain Behavior and Immunity, 22*, 1130–1137.

Kudler, H., Davidson, J., Meador, K., Lipper, S., & Ely, T. (1987). The DST and posttraumatic stress disorder. *American Journal of Psychiatry, 144*(8), 1068–1071.

Kunz-Ebrecht, S. R., Mohamed-Ali, V., Feldman, P. J., Kirschbaum, C., & Steptoe, A. (2003). Cortisol responses to mild psychological stress are inversely associated with proinflammatory cytokines. *Brain Behavior and Immunity, 17*(5), 373–383.

Laffaye, C., Kennedy, C., & Stein, M. B. (2003). Post-traumatic stress disorder and health-related quality of life in female victims of intimate partner violence. *Violence & Victims, 18*(2), 227–238.

Laudenslager, M. L., Aasal, R., Adler, L., Berger, C. L., Montgomery, P. T., Sandberg, E., et al. (1998). Elevated cytotoxicity in combat veterans with long-term post-traumatic stress disorder: Preliminary observations. *Brain, Behavior, & Immunity, 12*(1), 74–79.

Lehman, B. J., Taylor, S. E., Kiefe, C. I., & Seeman, T. E. (2005). Relation of childhood socioeconomic status and family environment to adult metabolic functioning in the CARDIA study. *Psychosomatic Medicine, 67*, 846–854.

Lown, E. A., & Vega, W. A. (2001). Intimate partner violence and health: Self-assessed health, chronic health, and somatic symptoms among Mexican American women. *Psychosomatic Medicine, 63*(3), 352–360.

Loucks, E. B., Sullivan, L. M., D'Agostino, R. B., Larson, M. G., Berkman, L. F., & Benjamin, E. J. (2006). Social networks and inflammatory markers in the Framingham Heart Study. *Journal of Biosocial Science, 38*, 835–842.

Lundberg, U. (2005). Stress hormones in health and illness: The roles of work and gender. *Psychoneuroendocrinology, 30*, 1017–1021.

Lupien, S. J., et al. (2009). *Effects of stress throughout the lifespan on the brain, behavior and cognition.* Nat Rev Neurosci, 10(6), 434–445.

Maes, M., Bonaccorso, S., Marino, V., Puzella, A., Pasquini, M., Biondi, M., et al. (2001a). Treatment with interferon-alpha (IFN alpha) of hepatitis C patients induces lower serum dipeptidyl peptidase IV activity, which is related to IFN alpha-induced depressive and anxiety symptoms and immune activation. *Molecular Psychiatry, 6*(4), 475–480.

Maes, M., Capuron, L., Rayaud, A., Gualde, N., Bosmans, E., Egyed, B., et al. (2001b). Lowered serum dipeptidyl peptidase IV activity is associated with depressive symptoms and cytokine production in cancer patients receiving interleukin-2-based immunotherapy. *Neuropsychopharmacology, 24*(2), 130–40.

Maier, S. (2003). Bidirectional immune–brain communication: Implications for understanding stress, pain, and cognition. *Brain, Behavior, & Immunity, 17*(2), 69–85.

Masten, A. S. (2001). Ordinary magic. Resilience processes in development. *American Psychology, 56*(3), 227–238.

McCain, N. L., Munjas, B. A., Munro, C. L., Elswick, R. K., Wheeler-Robins, J. L., Ferreira-Gonzalez, A., et al. (2003). Effects of stress-management on PNI-based outcomes in persons with HIV disease. *Research in Nursing & Health, 26,* 102–117.

McCauley, J., Kern, D. E., Kolodner, K., Dill, L., Schroeder, A. F., DeChant, H. K., et al. (1997). Clinical characteristics of women with a history of childhood abuse: Unhealed wounds. *JAMA, 277*(17), 1362–1368.

McEwen, B. S. (1998). Protective and damaging effects of stress mediators. *The New England Journal of Medicine, 338,* 171–179.

McEwen, B. S. (2000a). Allostasis and allostatic load: Implications for neuropyschopharmacology. *Neuropyschopharmacology, 22,* 108–124.

McEwen, B. S. (2000b). The neurobiology of stress: From serendipity to clinical relevance. *Brain Research, 886,* 172–189.

McEwen, B. S., & Stellar, E. (1993). Stress and the individual: Mechanisms leading to disease. *Archives of Internal Medicine, 153,* 2093–2101.

McEwen, B. S., & Seeman, T. (1999). Protective and damaging effects of mediators of stress: Elaborating and testing the concepts of allostasis and allostatic load. *Annals of the New York Academy of Sciences, 896,* 30–47.

McEwen, B. S., & Wingfield, J. C. (2003). The concept of allostasis in biology and biomedicine. *Hormones and Behavior, 43,* 2–15.

Meewisse, M. L., Reitsma, J. B., de Vries, G. J., Gerson, B. P., & Olff, M. (2007).Cortisol and posttraumatic stress disorder in adults: systematic review and meta-analysis. *British Journal of Psychiatry, 191,* 387–392.

McFarlane, A. C., & Yehuda, R. (1996). Resilience, vulnerability, and the course of posttraumatic reactions. In B. A. van der Kolk, A. C. McFarlane, & L. Weisaeth (Eds.), *Traumatic stress: The effects of overwhelming experience on mind, body, and society* (pp 155–181). New York: The Guilford Press.

McGowan, P. O., Sasaki, A., D'Alessio, A. C., Dymov, S., Labonté, B., Szyf, M., et al. (2009). Epigenetic regulation of the glucocorticoid receptor in human brain associates with childhood abuse. *Nature Neuroscience, 12*(3), 342–348.

Newport, D. J., Heim, C., Bonsall, R., Miller, A. H., & Nemeroff, C. B. (2004). Pituitary–adrenal responses to standard and low-dose dexamethasone suppression tests in adult survivors of child abuse. *Biological Psychiatry, 55*(1), 10–20.

North, C. S., Pfefferbaum, B., Tivis, L., Kawasaki, A., Reddy, C., & Spitznagel, E. L. (2004). The course of posttraumatic stress disorder in a follow-up study of survivors of the Oklahoma City bombing. *Annals of Clinical Psychiatry, 16*(4), 209–215.

O'Campo, P., Kub, J., Woods, A., Garza, M., Snow Jones, A., Gielen, et al. (2006). Depression, PTSD and co-morbidity related to intimate partner violence in civilian and military women. *Brief Treatment and Crisis Intervention Journal, 6*(2), 99–110.

Olff, M., Guzelcan, Y., de Vries, G., Assies, J., & Gersons, B. P. R. (2006). HPA- and HPT-axis alterations in chronic posttraumatic stress disorder. *Psychoneuroimmunology, 31,* 1220–1230.

Oquendo, M. A., Echavarria, G., Galfalvy, H. C., Grunebaum, M. F., Burke, A., Barrera, A., et al. (2003). Lower cortisol levels in depressed patients with comorbid post-traumatic stress disorder. *Neuropsychopharmacology, 28*(3), 591–598.

Pace, T. W., Negi, L. T., Adame, D. D., Cole, S. P., Sivilli, T. I., Brown, T. D., et al. (2009). Effect of compassion meditation on neuroendocrine, innate immune and behavioral responses to psychosocial stress. *Psychoneuroendocrinology, 34*(1), 87–98.

Parker, B., McFarlane, J., Soeken, K., Silva, C., & Reel, S. (1999). Testing an intervention to prevent further abuse to pregnant women. *Research in Nursing and Health, 22,* 59–66.

Perona, M., Benasayag, R., Perolló, A., Santos, J., Zárate, N., Zárate, P., et al. (2005). Prevalence of functional gastrointestinal disorders in women who report domestic violence to the police. *Clinical Gastroenterology and Hepatology, 3*(5), 436–41.

Pico-Alfonso, M. A., Garcia-Linares, M. I., Celda-Navarro, N., Herbert, J., & Martinez, M. (2004). Changes in cortisol and dehydroepiandrosterone in women victims of physical and psychological intimate partner violence, *Biological Psychiatry, 56,* 233–240.

Rabin, B. S. (1999). *Stress, immune function, and health: The connection.* New York: Wiley-Liss.

Raison, C. L., & Miller, A. H. (2003). When not enough is too much: the role of insufficient glucocorticoid signaling in the pathophysiology of stress-related disorders. *American Journal of Psychiatry, 160*(9), 1554–65.

Repetti, R. L., Taylor, S. E., & Seeman, T. E. (2002). Risky families: Family social environments and the mental and physical health of offspring. *Psychological Bulletin, 128,* 330–366.

Resnick, H. S., Yehuda, R., Pitman, R. K., & Foy, D. W. (1995). Effect of previous trauma on acute plasma cortisol level following rape. *American Journal of Psychiatry, 152,* 1675–1677.

Roth, T. L., Lubin, F. D., Funk, A. J., & Sweatt, J. D. (2009). Lasting epigenetic influence of early-life adversity on the BDNF gene. *Biological Psychiatry, 65*(9), 760–769.

Rutter, M. (1979). Protective factors in children's responses to stress and disadvantage. *Annals of the Academy of Medicine of Singapore, 8*(3), 324–338.

Segerstrom, S. C., & Miller, G. E. (2004). Psychological stress and the human immune system: A meta-analytic study of 30 years of inquiry. *Psychological Bulletin, 130*(4), 601–630.

Sephton, S. E., Sapolsky, R. M., Kraemer, H. C., & Spiegel, D. (2000). Diurnal cortisol rhythm as a predictor of breast cancer survival. *Journal of the National Cancer Institute, 92*(12), 994–1000.

Silverman, J. G., Decker, M. R., Saggurti, N., Balaiah, D., & Raj, A. (2008). Intimate partner violence and HIV infection among married Indian women. *JAMA, 300*(6), 703–710.

Simmons, A. N., Paulus, M. P., Thorp, S. R., Matthews, S. C., Norman, S. B., & Stein, M. B. (2008). Functional activation and neural networks in women with posttraumatic stress disorder related to intimate partner violence. *Biological Psychiatry, 64*(8), 681–690.

Sommershof, A., Aichinger, H., Engler, H., Adenauser, H., Catini, C. Boneberg, E. M., et al. (2009). Substantial reduction of naive and regulatory T cells following traumatic stress. *Brain Behavior and Immunity, 23*(8), 1117–1124.

Southwick, S. M., Vythilingam, M., & Charney, D. S. (2005). The psychobiology of depression and resilience to stress: Implications for prevention and treatment. *Annual Review of Clinical Psychology, 1,* 255–291.

Stam, R. (2007). PTSD and stress sensitisation: a tale of brain and body Part 2: animal models. *Neuroscience and Biobehavioral Reviews, 31*(4), 558–584.

Stein, M. B., Yehuda, R., Keverola, C., & Hanna, C. (1997). Enhanced dexamethasone suppression of plasma cortisol in adult women traumatized by childhood sexual abuse. *Biological Psychiatry, 42*(8), 680–686.

Stewart, J. A. (2006). The detrimental effects of allostasis: Allostatic load as a measure of cumulative stress. *Journal of Physiological Anthropology, 25,* 133–145.

Sullivan, T. P., & Holt, L. J. (2008). PTSD symptom clusters are differentially related to substance use among community women exposed to intimate partner violence. *Journal of Trauma Stress, 21*(2), 173–180.

Taylor, S. E., Eisenberger, N., Saxbe, D., Lehman, B. J., & Lieberman, M. D. (2006a). Neural responses to emotional stimuli are associated with childhood family stress. *Biological Psychiatry, 60,* 296–301.

Taylor, S. E., Lehman, B. J., Kiefe, C. I., & Seeman, T. E. (2006b). Relationship of early life stress and psychological functioning to adult C-reactive protein in the coronary artery risk development in young adults study. *Biological Psychiatry, 60,* 819–824.

Taylor, S. E., Lerner, J. S., Sage, R. M, Lehman, B. J., & Seeman, T. E. (2004). Early environment, emotions, responses to stress and health. *Journal of Personality, 72,* 1365–1393.

Tjaden, P., & Thoennes, N. (2000). *Extent, nature, and consequences of intimate partner violence.* Findings from the National Violence Against Women Survey No. NCJ 1818671. Washington, DC: US Department of Justice.

Tsutamoto, T., Hisanaga, T., Wada, A., Maeda, K., Ohnishi, M., Fukai, D., et al. (1998). Interleukin-6 spillover in the peripheral circulation increases with the severity of heart failure, and the high plasma level of interleukin-6 is an important prognostic predictor in patients with congestive heart failure. *Journal of American College of Cardiology, 31*(2), 391–398.

van der Kolk, B. A., & Saporta, J. (1993). Biologic response to psychic trauma. In J. P. Wilson & B. Raphael (Eds.), *International handbook of traumatic stress syndromes* (pp. 25–33). New York: Plenum Press.

Vollmer-Conna, U., Fazou, C., Cameron, B., Li, H., Brennan, C., Luck, L., et al. (2004). Production of pro-inflammatory cytokines correlates with the symptoms of acute sickness behaviour in humans. *Psychological Medicine, 34*(7), 1289–97.

Vythilingam M, Gill, J., Luckenbaugh DA, Gold PW, Collin C, Bonne O, et al. (in press). Low early morning plasma cortisol in post-traumatic stress disorder is associated with comorbid depression but not with enhanced glucocorticoid feedback inhibition. *Psychoneuroendocrinology* Apr; 35(3), 442–450.

Walton-Moss, B., Morrison, C., Yeo, R., Woodruff, K., Woods, A., Campbell, J. C., et al. (2003). Interrelationships of violence and psychiatric symptoms in women with substance use disorders. *Journal of Addictions Nursing, 14,* 193–200.

Wang, X. M., Hamza, M., Wu, T. X., & Dionne, R. A. (2009). Upregulation of IL-6, IL-8 and CCL2 gene expression after acute inflammation: Correlation to clinical pain. *Pain, 142*(3), 275–283.

Weis, F., Kilger, E., Roozendaal, B., de Quervain, D. L., Lamm, P., Schmidt, M., et al. (2006). Stress doses of hydrocortisone reduce chronic stress symptoms and improve health-related quality of life in high-risk patients after cardiac surgery: a randomized study. *Journal of Thoracic and Cardiovascular Surgery, 131*(2), 277–282.

Wichers, M. C., Kenis, G., Koek, G. H., Robaeys, G., Nicolson, N. A., & Maes, M. (2007). Interferon-alpha-induced depressive symptoms are related to changes in the cytokine network but not to cortisol. *Journal of Psychosomatic Research, 62*(2), 207–214.

Wittenberg, E., Joshi, M., Thomas, K. A., & McCloskey, L. A. (2007). Measuring the effect of intimate partner violence on health-related quality of life: a qualitative focus group study. *Health and Quality of Life Outcomes, 5,* 67.

Woo, P., Wilkinson, N., Prier, A. M., Southwood, T., Leone, V., Livermore, P., et al. (2005). Open label phase II trial of single, ascending doses of MRA in Caucasian children with severe systemic juvenile idiopathic arthritis: Proof of principle of the efficacy of IL-6 receptor blockade in this type of arthritis and demonstration of prolonged clinical improvement. *Arthritis Research & Therapy, 7*(6), R1281–R1288.

Woods, A. B., Page, G. G., O'Campo, P., Pugh, L. C., Ford, D., & Campbell, J. C. (2005a). The mediation effect of posttraumatic stress disorder symptoms on the relationship of intimate partner violence and IFN-γ levels. *American Journal of Community Psychology, 36*(1/2), 159–175.

Woods, S. J., Page, G. G., & Alexander, T. S. (2003). *Symptoms of PTSD, WBC counts, and diurnal cortisol circadian patterns in intimately abused women.* Poster presented at the Psychoneuroimmunology Research Society 10th International Annual Meeting. Amelia Island, FL.

Woods, S. J., & Wineman, N. M. (2004). Trauma, posttraumatic stress disorder symptom clusters, and physical health symptoms in postabused women. *Archives of Psychiatric Nursing, 18*(1), 26–34.

Woods, S. J., Wineman, N. M., Page, G. G., Hall, R. J., Alexander, T. S., & Campbell, J. C. (2005b). Predicting immune status in women with PTSD and childhood and adult violence. *Advances in Nursing Science, 28*(4), 332–345.

Woods, S. J., Page, G. G., Hall, R. J., & Alexander, T. S. (2008a). *Physical health symptoms and discomfort, diurnal cortisol patterns, and immune function in currently abused women.* Paper presented as part of the symposium The Complexities of Health and Resource Access for Women Who Have Experienced Intimate Partner Violence at The State of the Science Congress, Washington, DC.

Woods, S. J., Hall, R. J., Campbell, J. C., & Angott, D. M. (2008b). Physical health and posttraumatic stress disorder symptoms in women experiencing intimate partner. *Journal of Midwifery and Women's Health, 53,* 538–546.

Woods, S. J., Hall, R. J., Foster, K. E., & Page, G. G. (2009). *Predicting CRP levels in young- and middle-aged women experiencing intimate partner violence.* Poster presented at the Psychoneuroimmunology Research Society 16th International Annual Meeting. Breckenridge, CO.

Woon, F. L., & Hedges, D. W. (2008). Hippocampal and amygdala volumes in children and adults with childhood maltreatment-related posttraumatic stress disorder: a meta-analysis. *Hippocampus, 18*(8), 729–736.

Wuest, J., Ford-Gilboe, M., Merrit-Gray, M., Varcoe, C., Lent, B., Wilk, P., et al. (2009). Abuse-related injury and symptoms of posttraumatic stress disorder as mechanisms of chronic pain in survivors of intimate partner violence. *Pain Medicine, 10*(4), 739–747.

Wuest, J., Merritt-Gray, M., Ford-Gilboe, M., Lent, B., Varcoe, C., & Campbell, J. C. (2008). Chronic pain in women survivors of intimate partner violence. *The Journal of Pain, 9*(11), 1049–1057.

Yehuda, R. (2000). Biology of post-traumatic stress disorder. *Journal of Clinical Psychiatry, 61*(suppl 7), 14–21.

Yehuda, R. D., Boisoneau, D., Lowy, M. T., & Giller, E. L., Jr. (1995). Dose–response changes in plasma cortisol and lymphocyte glucocorticoid receptors following dexamethasone administration in combat veterans with and without posttraumatic stress disorder. *Archives of General Psychiatry, 52*(7), 583–593.

Yehuda, R. D., Boisoneau, D., Mason, J. W., & Giller, E. L. (1993). Glucocorticoid receptor number and cortisol excretion in mood, anxiety, and psychotic disorders. *Biological Psychiatry, 34*(1–2), 18–25.

Yehuda, R., Kahana, B., Binder-Brynes, K., Southwick, S. M., Mason, J. W., & Giller, E. L. (1995). Low urinary cortisol excretion in Holocaust survivors with posttraumatic stress disorder. *American Journal of Psychiatry, 152,* 982–986.

Yehuda, R., Schmeidler, J., Wainberg, M., Binder-Brynes, K., & Duvdevani, T. (1998). Vulnerability to posttraumatic stress disorder in adult offspring of Holocaust survivors. *American Journal of Psychiatry, 155*(9), 1163–1171.

Yehuda, R., Bierer, L. M., Schmeidler, J., Aferiat, D. H., Breslau, I., & Dolan, S. (2000). Low cortisol and risk for PTSD in adult offspring of Holocaust survivors. *American Journal of Psychiatry, 157*(8), 1252–1259.

Yehuda, R., & Flory, J. D. (2007). Differentiating biological correlates of risk, PTSD, and resilience following trauma exposure. *Journal of Traumatic Stress, 20,* 435–447.

Yehuda, R., Yang, R. K., Buchsbaum, M. S., & Golier, J. A. (2006). Alterations in cortisol negative feedback inhibition as examined using the ACTH response to cortisol administration in PTSD. *Psychoneuroendocrinology, 31*(4), 447–451.

Young, E. A., & Breslau, N. (2004). Cortisol and catecholamines in posttraumatic stress disorder: An epidemiologic community study. *Archives General Psychiatry, 61,* 394–401.

3

Theories of Intimate Partner Violence

Ursula A. Kelly, PhD, RN, ANP-BC, PMHNP-BC
Rosa M. Gonzalez-Guarda, PhD, MPH, RN
Janette Taylor, PhD, RN, WHCNP-BC

DEFINITIONS AND SCOPE

The issue of abuse and violence within intimate adult relationships began to receive public attention in the 1970s, largely through the efforts of grassroots women's groups (Shepard, 2005). Scholarly attention to this significant social and health problem has increased dramatically over the past 3 decades (Rhatigan, Moore, & Street, 2005). This chapter provides an overview of theoretical frameworks that attempt to explain the *causes* of abuse within intimate adult relationships and a brief review of frameworks explaining *women's responses* to abuse and violence over time (see chapter 5 for a complete explanation of these frameworks as the basis for nursing care). The historical roots and traditional and contemporary theoretical approaches to the phenomena are analyzed. The chapter concludes with suggestions for a theoretical base for nursing research and practice with women in abusive relationships.

Definition of Terms

We have adopted the term "intimate partner violence" (IPV) to encompass the diverse realities of abuse within the intimate relationships of adults. The Centers for Disease Control and Prevention's (CDC's) (Saltzman, Fanslow, McMahon, & Shelley, 2002) definition for IPV can be summarized as follows: threats or intentional use of physical and/or sexual violence with the potential to cause injury, disability, or death; or psychological/emotional abuse and/or coercive tactics when there has been prior physical and/or sexual violence perpetrated by a current or former spouse or nonmarital partner, for example, dating, boyfriend, or girlfriend. The World Health Organization's (WHO) definition does not necessitate the presence of physical or sexual violence in addition to psychological violence in its definition of IPV: "As well as acts of physical aggression such as hitting or kicking, violence by intimate partners includes forced intercourse and other forms of sexual coercion, psychological abuse such as intimidation and humiliation, and controlling behaviors such as isolating a person from family and friends or restricting access to information and assistance" (Krug, Dahlberg, Mercy, Zwi, & Lozano, 2002, p. 24).

IPV can occur in all kinds of intimate relationships, including marriage, committed relationships in opposite sex and same sex relationships, and dating relationships of adults and adolescents, and can continue even after a relationship has ended. Gender asymmetry is often the dynamics in IPV, though at times, IPV can be bilateral, meaning, both partners are violent. When IPV is bilateral, the use of severe violence and control, called "intimate terrorism," by men exceeds that of women (Johnson, 2006) and the injuries inflicted by men are far more severe than those they receive (Weston, Temple, & Marshall, 2005). Low-level violence between intimate partners is often more bilateral and less often includes forced sex and controlling behaviors. The kind of domestic violence that is seen in domestic violence shelters, the criminal justice system, among women with mental health problems from IPV, and in emergency departments is primarily directed toward women and is characterized by coercive control. In these relationships, women may, indeed, use physical violence, but it is almost always in self-defense (Babcock, Miller, & Siard, 2003; Swan & Snow, 2003). We will use the term "battering of female partners" to characterize these relationships and to make clear the severity of this abuse and its gender specificity.

Battering has been defined as deliberate and repeated physical aggression and/or sexual assault inflicted on a woman by a man with whom she has or has had an intimate relationship within a context of coercive control (Campbell, 1989; Campbell & Humphreys, 1993). Battering is thus a pattern, not a single incident, and the underlying dynamic is power and control of the (almost always) female victim. Although it is true that, in some small proportion of cases, a woman may be the primary perpetrator of battering against a male partner, the preponderance of evidence suggests that the incidence is very low. The consensus of most experts on IPV is that the kind of repetitive, prolonged, serious assault involving severe injury, done intentionally with minimal provocation, and in the interest of coercive control, or battering, is almost exclusively reserved for women (Johnson & Leone, 2005).

The context of coercive control refers to the variety of strategies in which the abusive partner keeps the woman fearful of future harm to herself and her children, and, in fact, even doubtful of her own reality. Examples of controlling strategies include emotional and verbal abuse, restriction of her contact with others (social isolation), controlling her personal and household finances (economic abuse), and using intimidating and threatening behavior. These controlling behaviors are depicted in the "Power and Control Wheel" developed by the Duluth, Minnesota, Domestic Abuse Intervention Project. The "Power and Control Wheel" is widely used in public and professional education literature (see, for example, Warshaw & Ganley, 1998).

IPV and battering are not restricted to heterosexual relationships. Battering in lesbian and gay male relationships has been described in the literature, but relatively little data-based research on the subject has been conducted, particularly among racial and ethnic minority populations (Feldman, Diaz, Ream, & Ei-Bassel, 2007; Owen & Burke, 2004; Renzetti, 1992; Turell, 2000). Similar to research reports of the prevalence of IPV in heterosexual relationships, reports of IPV in lesbian and gay male relationships have a wide range, from less than 10% to more than 50% (Eaton et al., 2008; Waldner-Haugrud, Gratch, & Magruder, 1997; West, 2002). Turell (2000) reported similar rates of physical violence but an 83% prevalence of emotional abuse among lesbians and gay men. Overall, available data suggest that the rates of IPV among heterosexual and same-sex couples are roughly equal (Stanley, Bartholomew, Taylor, Oram, & Landolt, 2006). However, results from one study that included a random sample of same-sex couples indicated that the prevalence of IPV among same-sex male couples was significantly higher than the level among same-sex female couples (Tjaden & Thoennes, 1999). Evidence from an early qualitative study suggested that the fundamental IPV dynamics of power and control among intimate partners are often similar in heterosexual and same-sex relationships (Renzetti, 1992). However, several researchers have challenged a reliance on heterosexually gendered theoretical and empirical analyses of IPV power dynamics in research with same-sex couples, particularly lesbian couples, arguing instead for analyses that consider the power dynamics of intersecting identities (race, socioeconomic status, age, disability, and sexual orientation) (Brown, 2008) and minority stress (Balsam & Szymanski, 2005; Brown, 2008). Certainly, much more research is needed in this area.

Scope of the Problem

When considering descriptions of the extent of IPV, it is important to note: (1) how IPV is defined and measured, that is, psychological, physical, and/or sexual violence; (2) within what timeframe, typically past year or adult lifetime occurrence; and (3) in what population or setting, for example, national survey, community sample, or clinical setting. Most reported IPV prevalence rates include physical and sexual violence only (Garcia-Moreno, Jansen, Ellsberg, Heise, & Watts, 2006; Tjaden & Thoennes, 2000). However, more recently, psychological abuse has been included in prevalence reports, as researchers recognize its pervasive nature, severity, and harmful effects (Basile, Arias, Desai, & Thompson, 2004; Bonomi, Anderson, Cannon, Slesnick, & Rodriguez, 2009; Coker et al., 2002; Hazen, Connelly, Soriano, & Landsverk, 2008; Thompson et al., 2006).

In the United States, most population-based estimates of lifetime physical and sexual IPV prevalence range from 25% to 50% , with the most usual range between 25% and 35% (Coker et al., 2002; Garcia-Moreno et al., 2006; Tjaden & Thoennes, 2000). Worldwide, these same rates range from 15% to 71%, with most results ranging from 30% to 60% (Garcia-Moreno et al., 2006). Rates of past year IPV range from 1.8% to 14% in population-based studies and up to 44% in health care settings (Bonomi et al., 2009; Coker et al., 2002; Thompson et al., 2006), although the more usual prevalence in health care settings is between 10% and 23%. Women are two times more likely to be physically or sexually assaulted by a current or former intimate partner than an acquaintance, family member, friend, or stranger (Tjaden & Thoennes, 2000). As high as these figures are, it is commonly accepted that reported data represent underestimates of the true incidence and prevalence of IPV. For nurses, it is important to remember that at least 1 in every 10 women in health care settings is in a violent relationship (Sampselle, 1991). Poor women and young women are particularly at risk (Tjaden & Thoennes, 2000). Women who are separated and divorced are also at increased risk, but since these data are from cross-sectional surveys, it is not clear if the marital dissolution occurred before or after the violence.

ABUSE OF FEMALE PARTNERS AND HOMICIDE

One of the most frightening aspects of abuse of female partners is its connection with homicide of women, particularly in the United States, which has the highest level of intimate partner homicide of any industrialized country (Krug et al., 2002). The level of danger for women in abusive relationships is illustrated by U.S. Crime Report data that in the past decade, 33% of all female homicide victims were murdered by a husband, ex-husband, or boyfriend (Rennison, 2003). The percentage is even higher (40% to 50%) when ex-boyfriends are included among perpetrators (Campbell et al., 2003). In contrast, less than 4% of U.S. male homicide victims are killed by an intimate partner (Rennison, 2003). IPV is clearly the most important risk factor for intimate partner femicide. In a nursing study of risk factors for intimate partner femicide, Campbell et al. (2003) reported that 70% of the total sample and 79% of the women killed between the ages of 18 and 50 were physically abused by their murderer before they were killed.

Battered women themselves are acutely aware that they are in danger of being killed. One of the strongest risk factors for femicide in battering relationships is when women take deliberate action to sever a dangerously abusive relationship (Campbell et al., 2003). Women frequently remain in dangerous relationships because of the realistic fear of life-threatening consequences, but their fears have not always been treated as valid. Often, the explicit or implicit question of "Why does she stay?" still lingers in the public's mind. Battering men feel that an intimate partner leaving the relationship is the ultimate loss of control. Many batterers have been heard to say something like "If I can't have you, no one can." Approximately one-third of femicides by intimate partners are followed by suicide of the male partner. This phenomenon almost never happens when a woman kills a man.

Homicide of the Abuser

Women do not usually kill people. In fact, they perpetrate about 12% of the homicides in the United States (Fox & Zawitz, 2007). When women do kill, it often involves a male partner and is done in self-defense. Historically, women who killed their batterers were charged with first- or second-degree murder or a reduced charge of manslaughter, or they had to plead temporary insanity (Gillespie, 1989). Because the battered woman's lethal act is not always at the same point in time as the assaults directed at her, she usually could not claim self-defense as the motive for her action because a self-defense legal defense requires the reasonable belief of imminent danger of death or serious injury. Fortunately, many courts have broadened the definition of self-defense to take into account the circumstances of battered women. In the 1980s and early 1990s, governors in several states granted clemency to battered women serving prison sentences because their actions are now considered justifiable (Grossfeld, 1991).

There have been few studies of women who killed their batterers. In a classic early study, Browne (1987) interviewed 42 women facing murder or attempted murder charges in the death or serious injury of their mates. In comparison to men who abused their wives but had not been killed, the men who had been killed had a history of frequent drug and alcohol abuse, extensive police records for a variety of criminal offenses, had often threatened to kill someone, and had abused their own children significantly more than the men in the nonhomicide group. Furthermore, women who were charged with murder sustained significantly more severe injury and had been injured more often, including forced sex from their partners, than women whose abusive partner was still living. These women made many attempts to obtain outside intervention for the violence directed at them, but the responses they received from the criminal justice system were ineffective. Browne (1987) concluded that women who murder their abusers have become trapped in a seemingly inescapable spiral of escalating violence against them, desperately fear for their lives and the lives of their children, and therefore take lethal action for survival. A similar nursing study of 12 women incarcerated for killing their batterers supported most of Browne's conclusions with the exception that these women did not note an escalation in the frequency or severity of the physical or sexual abuse directed at them prior to murdering the batterer (Foster, Veale, & Fogel, 1989). In Campbell's (1981) early study of intimate partner homicide, as in Foster and colleagues' and Browne's studies, the majority (75%) of women who killed an intimate partner had been physically assaulted before the homicide occurred.

The rates of women killing their male intimate partners have decreased by 75% since 1976, from 1,304 victims in 1976 to 329 in 2005. In 1976, approximately equal numbers of U.S. men were killed by an intimate partner as killed their spouse or ex-partner. In 2005, the ratio was 4:1, with four women killed by an intimate partner for every male killed (Fox & Zawitz, 2007). The decrease in men being killed is associated with states where there are strong laws that protect battered women and provide substantial resources and services, including shelters (Browne, Williams, & Dutton, 1998). It seems that in states where there are resources and laws that protect battered women, battered women feel less like their only recourse is to kill their abuser.

HISTORICAL PERSPECTIVE

IPV and violence against women in general have deep historical roots and continue to be condoned and even legally sanctioned in many societies. In their classic early study of wife beating, Dobash and Dobash (1979) placed such abuse in its historical context as a form of behavior which:

> has existed for centuries as an acceptable, and, indeed, a desirable part of a patriarchal family system within a patriarchal society, and much of the ideology and many of the institutional arrangements which supported the patriarchy through the subordination, domination and control of women are still reflected in our culture and our social institutions. (p. 31)

A fundamental aspect of current cultural support for abusing women is embedded in the historical and contemporary context of the many forms of violence against women that operate to maintain the patriarchal structure of most societies. Patriarchy can be defined as "any kind of group organization in which males hold dominant power and determine what part females shall and shall not play" (Rich, 1979, p. 78). Speaking about the United States, hooks (1984) extended the definition of patriarchy and located it within the dynamics of violence when she observed that domestic violence:

> is inextricably linked to all acts of violence in this society that occur between the powerful and the powerless, the dominant and the dominated. While male supremacy encourages the use of abusive force to maintain male domination of women, it is the Western philosophical notion of hierarchical rule and coercive authority that is the root cause of violence against women, of adult violence against children, of all violence between those who dominate and those who are dominated. (p. 118)

This analysis of power dynamics allows us to better see the foundations upon which oppression is grounded. Isolated acts of female intimate partner abuse do not keep our society sexist, but when the acts are multiplied and coupled with the frightening incidence of rape, homicide of women, and genital mutilation and joined with the historical precedents of suttee, witch burning, foot binding, mutilating surgery, and female infanticide, the power of patriarchy can be seen as based ultimately upon violence.

Violence Against Women Historically and Internationally

The Bible provides an early written prescription for the physical punishment of wives. Deuteronomy 22:13-21 lists a law condemning brides to death by stoning if unable to prove virginity (Davidson, 1978). In early Rome, husbands and fathers could legally beat or put women to death for many reasons, but especially for adultery or suspected infidelity, reflecting "not so much thwarted love but loss of control and damage to a possession" (Dobash & Dobash, 1979, p. 37). Constantine, the emperor and religious leader of the Byzantium branch of Christianity, set the example for treatment of wives by putting his own young wife to death by scalding (Davidson, 1978). By medieval times, the widespread nature of wife beating had been documented in several ways. In Spanish law, a woman who committed adultery could be killed with impunity. Female sexual infidelity was punishable by beating, as was disobedience in France. Italian men punished unfaithful women with severe flogging and exile for 3 years (Dobash & Dobash, 1979). A medieval theological manual refers to the necessity of men beating their wives "for correction" according to church doctrine. The medieval "age of chivalry" promoted the ideal of female chastity before marriage and fidelity after marriage, which was an important aspect of male property rights and outward sign of the master maintaining control (Dobash & Dobash, 1979). This glorification and objectification of women as asexual, weak adornments contributed to their subjugation. The close of the Middle Ages saw the rise of the nuclear family along with the development of modern states and the beginning of capitalism, all of which eroded the position of women and strengthened the authority of men. In sixteenth-century England, allegiance to fathers and husbands was equated with loyalty to the king and God (Dobash & Dobash, 1979).

The "witch-hunts" in Western Europe from the 1500s to the 1700s represent one of the best documented forms of systematic violence against women. Though the actual number can never be known, authoritative estimates range from two hundred thousand to nine million women murdered, often by hanging or burning, as punishment for their perceived healing abilities, assumed to have been acquired through "consorting with Satan" (Achterberg, 1991). Feminist analysis of this practice is that the main crime of the women involved was a lack of submission to the stereotyped role of the subservient medieval woman.

The Effects of Capitalism and Protestantism

Capitalism and Protestantism developed simultaneously. The basic unit of production moved outside of the family, and for the first time, wages were paid for work on a regular basis. Domestic work received no wages and therefore became devalued.

The Protestant religion idealized marriage and equated wifely obedience with moral duty. The head of the household gained much of the power that formerly belonged to priests (Dobash & Dobash, 1979). John Knox insisted that the "natural" subordination of women was ordained by God. Wife beating was discouraged by the Protestant theologians, but the husband's right to do so was acknowledged, and the practice was widespread (Dobash & Dobash, 1979). As May explained, "children, property, earnings, and even the wife's conscience belonged to the husband" (May, 1978, p. 38). During the seventeenth, eighteenth, and nineteenth centuries in the Western world, there was little objection to the husband using force, as long as it did not exceed certain limits. A wife could be beaten if she "caused jealousy, was lazy, unwilling to work in the fields, became drunk, spent too much money, or neglected the house" (May, 1978, p. 138). While the Reformation set the tone in the rest of Europe, Napoleon influenced France, Holland, Italy, and sections of Switzerland and Germany. He thought of wives as "fickle, defenseless, mindless beings, tending toward Eve-like evil" and deserving of punishment for misdeeds such as "causing" bankruptcy or criminality in her husband (Davidson, 1978, pp. 14–16). He is quoted as saying to the Council of State:

> The husband must possess the absolute power and right to say to his wife: "Madam, you shall not go out, you shall not go to the theatre, you shall not receive such and such a person; for the children you bear shall be mine." (Davidson, 1978, p. 15)

The common saying of the times was, "Women, like walnut trees, should be beaten every day" (Davidson, 1978, p. 14). There are many forms of violence against women throughout the world. During the same time period as the witch burnings in Europe, the practice of suttee, or inclusion of the widow and concubines in the male's funeral pyre, was being carried out in India. Women were often drugged or coerced to the pyre. Even when she was not forced, the widow knew that her alternatives to death on the pyre consisted of prostitution or a life of servitude and starvation with her husband's relatives. Cultural beliefs held the widow to blame for the man's death, if not during her present life, then in her past ones. The Chinese custom of foot binding was forced by male insistence that women were not attractive unless their feet were tiny stumps caused by years of excruciatingly painful breaking of the bones and binding. As a result, women were forced to be absolutely dependent on men, since they could take only a few tottering steps without assistance. The practice of female genital cutting began prior to colonialization in several countries of Africa and the Middle East (Boddy, 1998).

In similar practices, Western medicine in the late nineteenth century used the surgical procedures of clitoridectomy, oophorectomy, and hysterectomy to "cure" masturbation, insanity, deviation from the "proper" female role, heightened sexual appetites, and rebellion against husband or father (Daly, 1978). Radical feminists have argued that the medical practices of superfluous hysterectomies, unnecessarily mutilating surgery for breast cancer, and the use of IUDs and coercive sterilization of impoverished or mentally retarded women in the 1960s and 1970s were evidence of continued violence against women by male-dominated medicine. Control of reproductive rights and the development and use of particularly risky and permanent methods of contraception, for example, Norplant and antifertility "vaccines," have come into question as part of an ongoing discrimination against women, especially poor women and women of color (Roberts, 1997; Shapiro, 1985; Silliman & King, 1999).

Legalization of Violence Against Women

Lest we think that the practices of violence against women are confined to other countries and other times, we need to remember that the United States of America was founded on the equal rights of white men, not of women (and not of persons of color). John Adams rejected his wife's plea for better treatment of women in the new government. Sir William Blackstone's interpretation of English law that upheld the husband's right to employ moderate chastisement in response to improper wifely behavior was used as a model for American law. In 1824, the state of Mississippi legalized wife beating, and in 1886, a proposed law for punishment of husbands who beat their wives was defeated in Pennsylvania. North Carolina passed the first law against wife beating, but the court pronounced that it did not intend to hear cases unless there was permanent damage or danger to life (Davidson, 1978). British common law in the eighteenth century also established the legal right of a man to use force with his wife to insure that she fulfilled her wifely obligations, "the consummation of marriage, cohabitation, conjugal rights, sexual fidelity and general obedience and respect for his wishes" (Dobash & Dobash, 1979, pp. 14, 74). When John Stuart Mill petitioned Parliament to end the brutal treatment of British wives in 1869, the legal changes that followed were directed not toward eliminating the practice of wife beating but toward limiting the amount of damage that was being done. The nineteenth century in England was also marked by more tolerance of conjugal violence in the lower classes while more chivalry was expected by the upper classes (May, 1978).

As late as 1915, a London police magistrate reaffirmed that wives could be beaten at home legally as long as the stick used was no bigger than the man's thumb ("the rule of thumb" from a 1782 judge's proclamation) (Dobash & Dobash, 1979; May, 1978). It was legal for men to rape their wives in every state in the United States until the early 1970s. Laws preserving the legality of marital rape were common in the United States until the late 1980s and early 1990s (Russell, 1990). It continues to be difficult for women to prosecute their husbands for rape (Kirkwood & Cecil, 2001). Clearly, the law has been condoning violence toward wives for centuries. Dobash and Dobash (1979) summarized this relationship, "The ideologies and institutions that made such treatment both possible and justifiable have survived, albeit somewhat altered from century to century, and have been woven in to the fabric of our culture and are thriving today" (p. 31).

Widespread cultural tolerance for violence against women, and IPV in particular, continued through the 1980s (Carmody & Williams, 1987). There was clearly a cultural shift in the late 1980s and early 1990s with far fewer Americans believing that domestic violence is a private matter and far more believing that the police should intervene, at least if there is injury to the victim (Klein, Campbell, Soler, & Ghez, 1997). However, men are still less convinced than women that domestic violence is a serious problem that needs attention, not only in the United States, but all over the world.

Contemporary Forms of Violence Against Women Internationally

Female infanticide, homicide of women, and genital mutilation are three forms of violence directed at females that are rooted in history and continue today. They are found in their most blatant forms in societies that rigidly adhere to male dominance. Because of the higher life expectancy of females, the proportion of women in the population should be higher than men; however, world population statistics show that the male population exceeds that of females. The worldwide male to female ratio is 102:100, with 105 male births for every 100 female births (United Nations, 2009). This imbalance is highest in Arab and Islamic countries and India, with the United Arab Emirates having the highest male/female ratio of 205:100 (United Nations, 2009). The population of India has had a steadily increasing male to female ratio, as sex selection through abortion of female fetuses continues in order to avoid the high costs of dowries (Center for Social Research, 2008).

India and Arabic and Islamic nations also practice the killing of adult women with frightening regularity. "Honor crimes" are acts of violence, usually murder, committed by male family members against female family members who are perceived to have brought dishonor upon the family, either through "dishonorable acts," including divorce, premarital sex, or herself being the victim of a sexual assault or rape, or even because of rumor of impropriety (Hussain, 2006). While data on honor killings are difficult to obtain, it is estimated that worldwide 5,000 women are killed each year for "honor." For example, in 2008 in Afghanistan alone, there were 96 cases of so-called honor killings (Human Rights Watch, 2009).

Female genital mutilation, also called "cutting" and abbreviated as "FGM" or "FGM/C" is defined by the WHO (2008) as all procedures involving partial or total removal of the external female genitalia or other injury to the female genital organs for nonmedical reasons and is considered a human rights violation. FGM/C is widespread in much of East, West, and Central Africa, in parts of the Middle East, and in certain immigrant communities in North America and Europe. The mutilation can take the form of removal of the tip of the clitoris, complete clitoridectomy, or excision of some or all of the external genitalia and may be accompanied by infibulation—the narrowing or closure of the vaginal opening by sewing with catgut or using thorns, leaving a small opening for urination and menstrual flow. Infibulation involves opening the aperture further for intercourse and childbirth and resewing at the husband's command (WHO, 2008). FGM is traumatic and painful; girls are often held down during the procedure and then incapacitated for several days or weeks (Talle, 2007). The serious health consequences are both immediate and long term (WHO, 2008).

Between 100 and 140 million girls and women in the world have undergone FGM/C, and 3 million girls in Africa are considered at risk for FGM/C annually (WHO, 2008). In Somalia, more than 90% of girls undergo FGM/C by the age of 12, and the practice is still very much in favor (WHO, 2008). In Ethiopia, the practice is widespread and deep rooted, although there is a slowly growing rejection of the practice among younger women (Rahlenbeck & Mekonnen, 2009). FGM/C is deeply entrenched in inequitable social and political structures. In areas where FGM/C is widely practiced, it is supported by both men and women, reflecting the extreme social pressure to conform or risk ostracism and other social disadvantages (WHO, 2008). International political and grassroots efforts, in addition to the work of the WHO and other nongovernmental organizations over the past few decades, are gradually increasing support for the abolition of FGM/C.

A form of violence against women more in the realm of public awareness is rape. In her classic work, Dworkin (1976) states: "Rape is no excess, no aberration, no accident, no mistake—it embodies sexuality as the culture defines it," (p. 46). Rape takes many forms: sexual abuse of children, gang rape, forced intercourse with wives, sexual torture of female prisoners, intercourse with therapists, forced sexual initiation, bride capture, and group rape as a puberty rite, as well as the more identified form as sexual assault on a female by an unknown male (Brownmiller, 1975; Krug et al., 2002). Rape is "an exercise of domination and the infliction of degradation upon the victim" and serves to restrict the independence of women and remind them of their vulnerability, thereby keeping them subjugated across all patriarchal societies (Schram, 1978, p. 78). Rape and forced sex across a continuum of relationships and contexts continues to be common in the United States as well as in developing countries (Tjaden & Thoennes, 2000) (see also chapter 16). In the United States, more than half of women who are raped are younger than 18 years old; more than two-thirds of female rape victims are raped by someone they know (Tjaden & Thoennes, 2000). Rape is a crime of violence, not sex, and has long been used as systematic weapon of war (Diken & Laustsen, 2005; Power, 2002; Krug et al., 2002). Recent systematic uses of rape as a war strategy and a form of genocide were in the former Yugoslavia (mainly in Bosnia and Kosovo) and in civil wars in Rwanda, Liberia, and Uganda. The United Nations estimated that a quarter of a million women were raped as part of the 1994 Rawandan genocide, in a campaign that lead to unimaginable suffering with devastating long-term personal, familial, and societal consequences, including HIV/AIDS (Amnesty International, 2004; Mukamana & Brysiewicz, 2008). Estimates of the same extent of rape in 2007–2010 in the Democratic Republic of the Congo have been documented.

Sex trafficking of women and children has existed for centuries, but has garnered public attention recently. Sex trafficking, or human trafficking for the purposes of sexual exploitation, occurs internationally, as well as into and within the United States. The U.S. government estimates that 50,000 women are trafficked into the United States every year, primarily from Southeast Asia, the former Soviet Union, and Latin America (Raymond & Hughes, 2001). According to the United Nations, exploitation rather than coercion is the operative dynamic in sex trafficking, meaning that exploitation can occur with or without an individual's consent, for example, prostitution or voluntary migration (Hughes, 2001). Like other forms of sexual violence against women, the physical and mental health consequences of sex trafficking are profound and long lasting.

THEORETICAL FRAMEWORKS

IPV has been recognized as a serious threat to the safety, health, and well-being of women, children, and families by social reform groups at various times. For example, concern for the plight of abused women and children was intertwined with the primary goals of the suffragists in Great Britain and the United States, by those who promoted temperance in the late 1800s, and by those who promoted family planning and women's reproductive rights in the early and mid-1900s (Pleck, 1987). Abuse was blamed on poverty, drunkenness, and "brutish" men. The second wave of the women's movement in the 1960s raised awareness that violence against women was more prevalent than had been realized, and that attributions to poverty and alcohol could not account for the abuse experienced by women from all walks of life.

Scholarly attention to the problem has increased exponentially in the past three decades, as public and private funds have been allocated for research, education, treatment services, and prevention programs. Many theories have been offered to explain the social structures, cultural traditions, and personal behaviors that create and perpetuate abuse and violence. Feminist critiques remind us that focusing exclusively on individual and couple dynamics fails to explain why so many women are abused by their intimate partners. Additional important critiques of existing theoretical frameworks have come from those who point out their questionable relevancy to persons of racial and ethnic minority groups and those exposed to other systems of oppression such as heterosexism, classism, ageism, ableism, and religion/spirituality (Barnes, 1999; Chavis & Hill, 2009; Phillips, 1998; West, 1998). Only recently have researchers and policy makers begun to explore the adequacy of theories with persons of color and varied ethnicities. Race and ethnicity shape the experience and interpretation of IPV in myriad ways, including culturally based family structures and subordinate roles for women. The poverty experienced by persons of racial and ethnic minorities in the United States clearly complicates women's experiences, particularly in terms of unequal access to social resources and financial independence (West, 1998). Recent efforts that integrate research findings and theoretical explanations from many disciplines hold promise in our search for theories that help us explain, predict, ameliorate, and ultimately prevent IPV.

Theories of Causation

Contemporary theories of causation are those that attempt to explain and predict the motivations, circumstances, and other factors that characterize individuals who perpetrate abuse and violence within intimate partner relationships. In general, traditional frameworks for understanding the causes of IPV have fallen into one of several categories: (a) biological theories of criminal behavior, (b) theories of psychopathology of individual perpetrators, (c) family systems theories, or (d) social learning theories (Cunningham et al., 1998). A summary of these traditional theories can be found in Exhibit 3.1.

As can be noted through the criticisms highlighted in Exhibit 3.1, none of the traditional theories completely explain why an individual may perpetrate IPV. For example, although social learning theory posits that aggression toward an intimate partner is a learned behavior that can be transmitted from generation to generation, not all children exposed to aggressive parents become perpetrators. The need to integrate research findings from various perspectives and disciplines has led to the development of more comprehensive and contemporary explanations for IPV, such as theories that describe gender-based inequities, oppression and power, sociocultural models that draw from various traditional theories, and ecological frameworks that describe various levels of influence (e.g., individual, relationship, community, and societal). These comprehensive approaches are the primary focus of this section.

Theories/Models of Gender-Based Inequities, Systems of Oppression and Power

Masculinity or Male Socialization as a Synthesizing Framework

One of the most widely adopted synthesizing frameworks for understanding violence against women is masculinity and male socialization. Discussions of male socialization and masculinity often include generalizations; however, these processes often differ across cultural groups and communities. Induction into male roles may vary within families. Still, psychological, sociological, and anthropological literature (Archer, 1994; Connell, 1995; Gilmore, 1990; Miedzian, 1991), and more recently feminist scholarship and

EXHIBIT 3.1 | *Traditional Theories for Understanding Causes of IPV: Level of Focus, Explanations for IPV, and Criticisms*

Psychological Perspectives
- *Focus*: Individual psychopathology of both the perpetrator and the victim
- *Explanations*:
  - Abuse is deliberately provoked by women who required this behavior to meet their need for suffering (female masochism).
  - Perpetrator abusive behavior results from mood disorders, personality disorders, psychoneurological effects from head injury and posttraumatic stress disorder (PTSD).
  - Extreme jealousy of the intimate female partner and subsequent violence of abusive men dates back to evolutionary forces to reproduce and pass along genes for survival of the species (genetic or heritable predisposition).
- *Criticisms*: Female masochism leads to victim blaming; psychoneurological explanations may be associated with aggression but do not cause IPV and do not explain how perpetrators usually target their aggression toward intimate partners; does not consider important sociocultural factors (Cunningham et al., 1998; Wilson & Daly, 1993)

Alcohol and Drugs as Causes of IPV
- *Focus*: Individual use of alcohol or drugs by the perpetrator and social norms regarding these behaviors.
- *Explanation*:
  - Alcohol and/or drug use leads to a biochemical "disinhibiting effect," whereby a person's usual voluntary behavior constraints are temporarily removed, resulting in aggressive behaviors.
  - Drinking provides a period of time during which one may behave in ways that would be socially unacceptable if sober (e.g., aggression toward female partner).
  - Alcohol and/or drugs alter cognitive processes so that individuals interpret individual cues as threatening.
  - Alcohol and/or drugs serve as a risk factor for IPV occurrence, more severe IPV, perpetrator reassault after intervention, and intimate partner femicide.
- *Criticisms*: Partners are not always drunk when abusive or abusive when they are drunk; appears to potentiate abuse tendencies among batterers but not cause abuse (Gondolf, 1997a; Kantor, 1993; Kantor & Straus, 1987; Kub, Campbell, Rose & Soeken, 1999; Sharps et al., 2001; Testa & Leonard, 2001)

Family Systems Theories and Family Stress Theory
- *Focus*: Family members and their interaction with social systems
- *Explanation*:
  - The manner in which the family functions, such as role expectations, communication patterns and power status of family members, are affected by the response and feedback of family members.
  - Family violence is the result of the behaviors of both the perpetrator and the victim and is often the fault of all those involved.
- *Criticisms*: Minimizes the responsibility of the perpetrator and exaggerates the responsibility of the victim (Cunningham et al., 1998)

Social Learning Theory
- *Focus*: Individual learning through the interactions and norms established within families, groups, and society
- *Explanation:*
  - Abusive behaviors are learned by children during childhood; children observe and imitate the behaviors adults model for them.
  - As children grow, these behaviors are reinforced by society (e.g., boys are taught not to use aggression to cope with negative feelings).
- *Criticisms:* Not all children who are exposed to abuse during childhood become abusive as adults, and not all perpetrators wore abused as children; does not incorporate other factors that may serve as risk or protective factors for the perpetration of IPV (Cunningham et al., 1998; Maxfield & Widom, 2001; Strauss & Gelles, 1990)

studies of masculinities (Diamond, 2006; Levant & Pollack, 1995; Phillips, 2006; Schrock & Schwalbe, 2009), have influenced current thinking about gendered roles in general. This section will briefly examine explanations for male socialization, delineate characteristics associated with it, and explain the association of patriarchal attitudes with gender inequity and violence against women.

Patriarchy and Socialization for Masculinity

There are wide ranges of unequal relationships and social systems among groups. Such inequalities exist in the United States and globally. In the United States, patriarchy, which addresses the dynamics of inequality, domination, and control, is a key concept in critical theory and feminist studies. The literal meaning of patriarchy is "rule of the father"; however, it is routinely used in U.S. feminist studies to mean "male domination" (Macey, 2001; Pilcher & Wheelan, 2004). In the family social system, the father is the head of the household and has virtually unchallenged authority over women and children who are viewed as subordinates. Patriarchy also refers to the dominance of men in social or cultural systems such as government. Patriarchy is a learned process; training for the male role starts early and consists of a range of complex social and psychological processes geared toward indoctrination into patriarchy (Sherriff, 2007; Swain, 2003). Patriarchal systems hold multiple advantages for many men and numerous disadvantages for women and children. Gender violence and overall threats to women's rights are frequent disadvantages for women living within patriarchal systems.

The origins of patriarchy, masculinity, and gender violence are difficult to trace. The concept of machismo or compulsive masculinity can be found in psychological, sociological, and anthropological literature and is also discussed in much of the domestic violence research. In more contemporary scholarship, it is addressed within the study of masculinities (for examples, see Archer, 1994; Connell, 1995; Gilmore, 1990; Miedzian, 1991).

SOCIALIZATION FOR MASCULINITY. The training for the male role starts early. More stringent demands are made and enforced more harshly on boys than on girls at an early age. Around the world, even preschool boys are more aggressive than girls, yet the amount of that aggression is culturally dependent. Male school and peer group activities are explicitly organized around struggle, boys are encouraged to restrict their activities to masculine pursuits even in kindergarten, and boys are encouraged to hunt, fight, participate in sports, and play violent video games in all-male company (Miedzian, 1991). Violence can be viewed "as a clandestine masculine ideal in Western culture" (Toby, 1966, p. 19). The ideal male wields authority, especially over women, has unlimited sexual prowess, is invulnerable, has competition as his guiding principle, never discloses emotion, is tough and brave, has great power, is adept at one-upsmanship, can always fight victoriously if he needs to and does not really need anyone. A popular contemporary concept that represents socialization for masculinity in Latino culture is "machismo." Machismo has been defined by Latino women and men as being a cultural inheritance that promotes negative ideals among males that are associated with aggression toward partners, substance abuse, and promiscuity (Fiorentino, Berger, & Ramirez, 2007; Gonzalez-Guarda, Ortega, Vasquez, & DeSantis, 2009). On the other hand, the concept of caballerismo (male chivalry), such as protecting and providing for the family, encompasses the positive aspects associated with the male role in Latino culture that can counterbalance the negative behaviors associated with machismo (Arciniega, Anderson, Tovar-Blank, & Tracey, 2008). All-male groups in any culture, such as gangs in our inner cities today, or fraternities in universities, or all male sports, sports fans, or drinking groups tend to facilitate the expression of aggression and provide group standards for maleness and masculinity such as bravery and toughness (Malamuth et al., 1991; Miedzian, 1991; Smith, 1987; Tiger, 1969). These standards have been nearly universal around the world and almost impossible to achieve (Gilmore, 1990). Although the tough, macho man ideal has lessened in its hold on middle class American and European cultures, it is still present in many subcultures and in much of the world.

Feminist Theory and Feminist Intersectionality

Articulated most eloquently by Dobash and Dobash (1979; 1993; 1998), Pence, Paymar, Ritmeester, and Shepard (1993), and Stark (2007), feminist theories of IPV emphasize the underlying premises of the need for power and control on the part of batterers and the societal arrangements of patriarchy and tolerance (not support for) of violence against women that support individual abusers in seeing this behavior as tolerable. These theories also incorporate aspects of social learning theory, with the premise that perpetrating abusive behavior is a choice to use a set of learned behaviors. Although it is difficult to prove individual abuser's beliefs in these abstract premises, the continuing gender differences in perceptions about IPV (Klein et al., 1997), historical and international records of violence against women associated with cultural norms of male ownership of women, and lack of equal power relationships within homes are evidence in support of this theoretical framework (e.g., Counts, Brown, & Campbell, 1999; Levinson, 1989). Several international studies from South Africa, India, and China associate male justification for men hitting women and beliefs in male domination of household affairs associated with reported wife beating (Abrahams, 2002; Martin, Tsui, Maitra, & Marinshaw, 1999; Wood & Jewkes, 2001; Xu, Campbell, & Zhu, 2001).

Feminist theory has evolved to account for additional factors and complexities that intersect with gender to place women and other vulnerable groups at a disadvantage in establishing equitable power relationships with their partners and society in general. Much of this theoretical development has been led by social scientists, domestic violence advocates, and minority women who have conceptualized violence against women as much more than just a gender issue. For example, Black feminist theory emerged in response to the predominately white women's movement and predominately male black civil rights movement, neither of which completely represented the experience of both being black and a woman. In Black feminist theory, the interaction between gender, race, and class are conceptualized as being part of an overarching structure of domination (Collins, 2000; Crenshaw, 1991). Similarly, Chicanas and Latinas felt that their concerns were not being adequately represented by either the Chicano movement or the women's movement. Chicana feminist theory describes the dynamics between race/ethnicity, social class, linguistics, and nationalism. Chicana feminists also focused on approaches they felt were unique to their culture, such as the need to challenge traditional and exaggerated gender roles that were present in Latino households, while still preserving strong family structures and the important role of women in the home (Anzaldua, 1990; Ortega, 2006; Roth, 2004). Native American and other indigenous feminists find that postcolonial frameworks that emphasize the role of historical trauma, as well as the many different tribal traditions in male–female relationships are important in understanding the often high rates of IPV among aboriginal peoples worldwide (Bohn, 1993; Hamby, 2006).

Feminist theorists and other social scientists have recommended the use of feminist intersectionality as a means of not only obtaining a more comprehensive understanding of the multiplicative effects of social inequalities experienced by vulnerable and marginalized groups, but also of conducting research and developing interventions that address health disparities (Kelly, 2009a). Feminist intersectionality is a body of knowledge that is driven by the pursuit of social justice and seeks to explain the processes in which various social positions, such as gender, race, ethnicity, class, age, sexual orientation, disability status, and religion, shape the health of individuals, families, communities, and society as a whole (Chavis & Hill, 2009; Weber, 2006). Feminist intersectionality is built upon the assumptions that every social group has unique qualities and can therefore not be considered homogenous to one another; that individuals are positioned within social structures that influence power relationships; and that there are interactions between different social identities, for example, race, gender, and immigrant status, that have multiplicative effects on health and well-being.

Power and Control/The Duluth Model

Most gender-based theories describing IPV, as well as more comprehensive approaches that have evolved from these, describe the lack of power and control women and other marginalized groups encounter within their intimate relationships. The Power and Control Wheel is a tool developed by the Domestic Abuse Intervention Program (DAIP) in Duluth, Minnesota in the early 1980s. Also known as the Duluth Model, the Power and Control Wheel has been used as part of a curriculum for batterers and victims of domestic violence (Pence et al., 1993). Recently, the Power and Control Wheel has been adapted to describe how various systems of oppression, for example, racism, classism, and sexism, influence the experience of victims of IPV (Chavis & Hill, 2009) (see Figure 3.1). In the original Power and Control Wheel, battering is characterized by a pattern of abusive behaviors that are used to control and dominate an intimate partner. This is depicted by placing the words "power and control" at the core of the wheel. Tactics that are commonly used to control an intimate partner and make them vulnerable to physical and sexual violence are the spokes of the wheel (www.theduluthmodel.org). The eight tactics that are specified include (a) intimidation, for example, making the partner afraid by using looks, gestures, and actions, such as smashing things; (b) emotional abuse, for

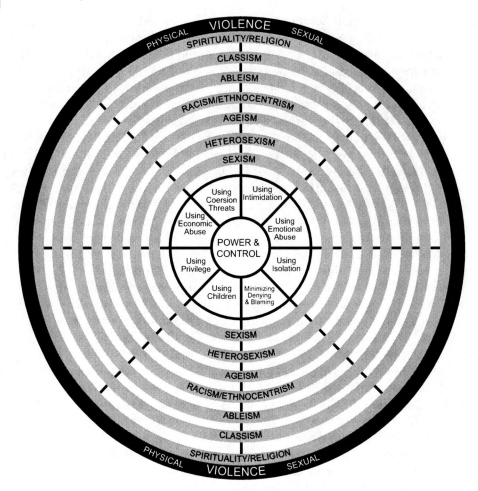

FIGURE 3.1 The multicultural power and control wheel.

example, putting a partner down and making her feel guilty; (c) isolation, for example, controlling a partner's interactions with family and friends; (d) minimizing, denying, and blaming, for example, saying that the abuse was nothing of significance, did not happen or was a partner's responsibility; (e) using children, for example, having children relay messages to a partner, threatening to take custody of children; (f) using privilege, for example, treating partners as servants; (g) economic abuse, for example, interfering with a partner getting a job; and (h) using coercion and threats, for example, threatening to hurt a partner or commit suicide. Chavis and Hill (2009) added seven distinct rings surrounding these tactics on the wheel to represent multiple forms of oppression that are interconnected. These include (a) sexism, (b) heterosexism, (c) ageism, (d) racism/ethnocentrism, (e) disability/ableism, (f) classism and (g) spirituality/religion. The tactics can manifest themselves differently through these oppressive systems. For example, for an immigrant, racial/ethnic minority woman who is undocumented, economic abuse can be represented through having her partner threaten to report her to the authorities for work that she does "under the table."

Critical Theory

Critical theory, also known as critical theory of society or critical social theory (CST), has several meanings across philosophy and the social sciences. Critical theory is described as "a whole range of theories which take a critical view of society and the human sciences or which seek to explain the emergence of their objects of knowledge" (Macey, 2001, p. 74). The intellectual underpinnings of the theory are often credited to the works of Horkheimer (1972, 1982, 1987, 1993) and Habermas (1971, 1973, 1975, 1979, 1984, 1985, 1987) as well as several others. Today, CST continues to emerge and is expressed by a variety of domestic and international/transnational scholars. In particular, social theories articulated by diverse groups of women demonstrate the complexity of life experiences within intersecting oppressions that include (but are not limited to) race, class, gender, sexuality, ethnicity, nation, and religion (see, e.g., Collins, 2000; Denzin, Lincoln, & Smith, 2008; Mohanty, 2003; Riley, Mohanty, & Pratt, 2008). One of the many organizing principles of CST is the idea that individuals and groups have different political, social, and historic contexts, which are characterized by injustice. Although people seek to alter their social and economic situations, often they are constrained by multiple forms of social, cultural, and political domination. A second principle is that social critique of the status quo is essential so that constraining conditions can be exposed. Additionally, critical social theorists advocate for empowerment, liberation, and emancipation from alienation and domination. Collins (2000) succinctly summarized the goal of CST when she stated, "What makes critical social theory 'critical' is its commitment to justice, for one's own group and/or for that of other groups" (p. 298).

Social Cultural Models

A multifactorial model of IPV, which combines elements of family systems theory, social learning theory, social structures, and cultural factors, was first developed by Straus and Gelles (1990). This model recognizes the societal background of a high level of violence in our culture, the sexist organization of the society and its family system, and cultural norms legitimizing violence against family members. With this background of societal influences, the family is believed to be inherently at high risk for violent interaction by virtue of the great amount of time family members spend interacting; the broad range of activities over which conflict can occur; the intensity of emotional involvement of the members; the involuntary nature of family membership; the impingement of family members on each other's personal space, time, and lifestyles; and the assumption of family members that they have the right to try to change each other's behavior (Straus, 1980). Within these societal and family contexts, Straus and others believe that people can be socialized to use violence for conflict resolution. Children learn this by observing parental violence, experiencing physical punishment, seeing their parents tolerate sibling fighting, and, if boys, being taught to value violence. This socialization teaches the association of love with violence and justifies the use of physical force as a morally correct means of solving disputes.

Ecological Frameworks

More recently, an "ecological framework" has been proposed by the WHO to describe violence as a global, public health problem (see chapter 1). This framework integrates research findings from several disciplines, including feminist theory, into an explanatory framework of the origins of gender-based intimate partner violence (Heise, 1998).

The ecological approach views IPV as a multifaceted phenomenon that is the result of a dynamic interplay among individual, relationship, community, and societal factors that influence an individual's risk to perpetrate or become a victim of violence. These factors can be imagined as concentric circles nested within a larger circle (Centers for Disease Control & Prevention, 2009; Dahlberg & Krug, 2002) (see Figure 3.2). At the individual level, the person who perpetrates or is a victim of abuse and violence possesses a set of biological and personality traits and a personal history that shape his or her behaviors and interactions with other individuals (for example, with the intimate partner and with other family members) and with the broader community and society. Individual-level factors that are partially predictive of becoming abusive include (a) demographic factors such as age, education, and income; (b) witnessing domestic violence as a child; (c) experiencing physical or sexual abuse as a child and, to a lesser extent, having an absent or an emotionally abusive father; and (d) substance use.

The second level of influence includes close relationships with partners, family members, and peers that can influence the risk of the individual to perpetrate or become a victim of violence. Several aspects of the relationship level, especially in terms of family structure and functioning, have been identified as risk factors for the development of IPV. These include (a) male economic and decision-making authority in the family, (b) male control of wealth and resources in the family, and (c) marital conflict, especially in relationships with asymmetrical power structures. The third level of factors is the community, and includes settings such as neighborhoods, schools, and workplaces that serve as the context in which individuals and relationships exist. For example, research conducted at this level of influence has demonstrated that communi-

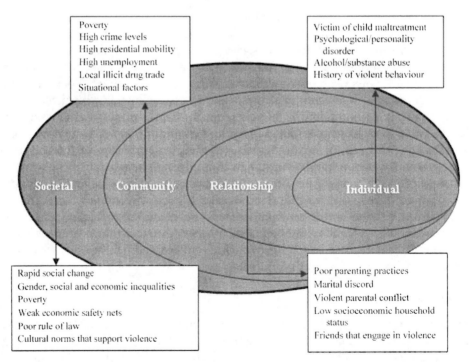

FIGURE 3.2 The ecological model for understanding violence with examples of risk factors (WHO, 2009).

ties with high residential mobility, that is, high flow of individuals moving in and out, high population densities, and lack of cohesion among residents, are associated with higher levels of violence. Local gun and drug trade and community poverty and unemployment rates have also been identified as risk factors for the perpetration of and/or victimization by violence.

For example, research has consistently demonstrated that, although violence against women occurs in all socioeconomic groups, IPV is more common in low-income families and in households in which the man is unemployed. The underlying cause of this increase in risk for IPV is unclear, but it is possible that poverty at the community level may underlie much stress and conflict within intimate couples, such that the influence of community poverty is manifested at the relationship level.

The fourth and last level of factors is the societal level. This includes broad societal factors that create a climate that encourages or discourages violence at the community, relationship, and individual levels, including the rules, norms, and social expectations that govern personal behavior and social inequities between groups, for example, poverty, sexism, health disparities. For example, a factor at the societal level that has been identified as being associated with violence is that of social isolation of women and other marginalized groups. Sources of support and assistance may not be readily available to women who have been socially and/or geographically cut off from their social network, thus making them vulnerable to IPV and its consequences. It is also at this level of analysis that the patriarchal roots of IPV and other systems of oppression that were examined earlier in this chapter can be illuminated. The WHO's ecological approach to understanding violence and other ecological models that identify risk and protective factors associated with the perpetration of IPV integrate research findings from various disciplines into a comprehensive framework that improves our understanding of the origins, or causes, of IPV.

The need for treatment and prevention strategies that move beyond the individual and relationship levels becomes clear based on ecological models that elucidate the influence of factors that are present across all levels of influence, that is, individual, relationship, community, and societal, and how these interact with one another to create the context in which violence occurs. The WHO ecological model for understanding violence provides some direction regarding what type of interventions can be developed to target the different levels of influence. For example, specific approaches that target the individual level may include strategies that promote healthy attitudes, beliefs, and practices regarding relationships and IPV, while approaches that target the broader community and societal level may focus on social marketing campaigns that change social norms and policies that address social and economic inequities between different groups (Dahlber & Krug, 2002). However, there is a broad recognition that in order to develop more effective interventions that aim to change behaviors such as violence and abuse, comprehensive strategies that target multiple levels of influence must be developed (Sallis, Owen, & Fisher, 2008).

TYPOLOGIES OF BATTERERS AND OF INTIMATE PARTNER VIOLENCE

An important conclusion reached by many who work with men who batter their female partners is that there is no single personality profile, social characteristic, or "type" of man who batters, and there may be at least two distinct types of IPV, two types of batterers, and three subtypes of batterers (Holtzworth-Munroe and Stuart, 1994; Jacobson & Gottman, 1998; Johnson, 1995; 2006). Variability among perpetrators has been described along several dimensions, including (a) motives for the abuse or violence; (b) the nature, severity, and frequency of the violence; (c) whether or not the perpetrator commits violence outside the family as well as within the family; and (d) whether or not the perpetrator is affected by a psychological or personality disorder (Holtzworth-Munroe, 2000; Johnson & Ferraro, 2000) (Exhibit 3.2). This insight is particularly important in the area of programs to reduce men's use of violence in their intimate relationships. Program developers and clinicians want to know "what works," "for whom," and "under what circumstances?" (Gondolf, 1997b).

Our understanding of the causes of men's violence against women in intimate relationships has significantly improved over the past three decades of research and theory development. Theoretical explanations have progressed from simplistic single-factor attributions (for example, men's witnessing abuse in childhood, or men's alcohol abuse), to (a) more nuanced explanations taking into account how factors interact, (b) more complicated typologies of batterers as a heterogeneous group, (c) integration of research findings and theoretical models from disparate fields of study into synthesizing explanatory frameworks, and finally, to (d) ongoing research that is making important distinctions among men who batter in order to enhance the efficacy of treatment approaches. Frameworks that better address the intersections of IPV, gender, race, and ethnicity are still clearly needed, as are frameworks that include the issues of same-sex partners who experience violence within their intimate relationships. It is important to remember that these three decades of scientific work were inspired by women telling their stories of abuse and violence at the hands of the person who claimed to love them most. It is equally important to keep future empirical and theoretical work grounded in women's realities, in which safety from further harm and empowerment for difficult decisions are integral to all work with women in abusive relationships.

EXHIBIT 3.2 | *Typologies Of Batterers And Of Intimate Partner Violence*

Two types of intimate partner violence

1. Terroristic battering (formerly patriarchal terrorism)
Defining characteristics
- Violence is almost entirely perpetrated toward females
- Increases in severity and frequency over time
- Motivated by desires for power and control
- Perpetrators are unrepentant
- Behavior is difficult to modify

2. Common couple violence
Defining characteristics
- More common
- More likely to have females as well as males as perpetrators
- Perpetrators more amenable to interventions (Johnson, 1995; 2006)

Two types of batterers

1. "Cobras"

Defining characteristics

* Display an overall internal calmness during verbally aggressive arguments
* A "cold physiology," with low heart rates and other measures
* Sociopaths with a high degree of criminal behavior and violence
* Resemble the "generally violent–antisocial batterers"

2. "Pit bulls"

Defining characteristics

* Display various measures of emotional distress
* Exhibit expected higher heart rates
* Deprive their partners of any independence and closely monitor their daily activities
* Suspect sexual betrayal in the most innocuous contexts, and eventually lose control of their emotions and erupt in violence
* Resemble "dysphoric–borderline batterers" (Jacobson & Gottman, 1998; Johnson & Ferraro, 2000)

Three subtypes of batterers

1. "Family-only batterer"

Defining characteristics

* Use the lowest levels of physical, psychological, and sexual abuse against their partners
* Least likely to be violent outside the home
* Do not show evidence of psychopathology

2. "Dysphoric-borderline batterer"

Defining characteristics

* Perpetrate a moderate or severe degree of physical abuse against their partners
* May also be violent outside the family
* Are likely to show characteristics of depression, anxiety, and/or borderline personality disorder

3. "Generally violent–antisocial batterer"

Defining characteristics

* Most violent type of batterer both to his intimate partner and to those outside the family
* Most likely to show evidence of antisocial personality disorder (Holtzworth-Munroe, 2000; Holtzworth-Munroe & Stuart, 1994)

THEORIES OF WOMEN'S RESPONSES TO INTIMATE PARTNER VIOLENCE

One of the most difficult dynamics of IPV for professionals and the general public to understand is why a woman would stay with an abusive partner, sometimes for many years. This question has been addressed from many perspectives, some of which have promoted victim-blaming attributions. The past three decades of research have resulted in a growing appreciation for the complexity and resourcefulness of women's strategic actions as they attempt to resolve the abuse in their relationship or, if needed, to break free of the abusive relationship, even in the face of ongoing danger and hardship. In fact, the majority of abused women do leave the abusive relationship or manage to make the violence end, but it may take many years for this to happen (Campbell et al., 1998). The important questions to be answered are not "Why does she stay?" but instead, "Why do so many men beat their partners?" and "What is preventing her from staying safe?"

This section of the chapter will review historical theoretical formulations of women's responses to IPV, which relied heavily on the field of psychology, and then discuss contemporary understandings of these responses, many of which are derived from ecological, sociological, and systems theories. A summary of these theories can be found in Exhibit 3.3. One important thing to remember, however, is that research has shown us

---

EXHIBIT 3.3 | HISTORICAL AND CONTEMPORARY THEORIES FOR UNDER-STANDING WOMEN'S RESPONSES TO IPV: LEVEL OF FOCUS, EXPLANATIONS, CRITIQUE, AND CHALLENGES

HISTORICAL
Psychological Theories
- *Focus*: Individual psychopathology of the victim
- Risk factors for being abused and remaining in the abusive relationship
  - *Explanation*: Women with low self-esteem and mental health problems, for example, symptoms of depression, anxiety, posttraumatic stress disorder, personality disorders, and substance abuse problems are more likely to remain in abusive relationships.
  - *Critique*: Research does not support low self-esteem or mental health problems as being risk factors for IPV. Rather, the low self-esteem and mental health problems seen in abused women are very likely the *result* of the violence rather than a precursor.
- Responses to IPV
  - *Explanations:*
    - *Learned Helplessness*: Repeated abuse leaves the victim unable to get out of the abusive relationship because of her depression, apathy, and poor problem solving.
    - *Traumatic Bonding*: Abused women develop strong emotional bonds to their abusers.
  - *Critique*: Women's responses to abuse are not passive. Coping with the abuse is an active process that involves creativity, problem solving, and strategizing. Typically, love precedes the abuse. The emotional bond may remain despite the abuse. Women want the abuse to end, not necessarily the relationship.

CONTEMPORARY
Psychological Theories
- *Focus*: Individual strengths and resiliency
- *Explanations*:
  - Women's responses to IPV are active processes, requiring creativity, perseverance, and inner strength.
  - These responses vary over time as women adapt to individual circumstances using multiple strategies.

* Women use various strategies to protect themselves and their children, seeking safety in whatever ways they can.
* Ongoing IPV can erode women's sense of inner strength and resiliency. Their self-efficacy can be negatively impacted by the abuse, making moving toward change very difficult.
* Social support, both perceived and tangible, is an important component of intervention for women who are experiencing IPV.
* *Challenges*:
  * Identifying and assisting women who are abused but who do not seek services requires effective screening and community outreach, both of which are difficult to implement universally.
  * Assisting women who are abused to recognize and tap into their inner strengths can be difficult.
  * Accessing resources to provide abused women with tangible support is difficult, particularly women who are marginalized or in socially oppressed groups.

Critical Social Theories
* *Focus*: Context of individuals' lives: political, social, economic, cultural, historical
* *Explanations*:
  * Women who are poor, from a minority ethnic group, or are immigrants face compounded barriers to leaving the abuser and to recovering from the abuse due to the socially unjust contexts in which they live.
  * Abused women face many external barriers to leaving or escaping an abusive intimate partner and to getting help from officials, including health care providers.
  * Official helping agencies can perpetuate the abuse, treat abused women in demeaning and punitive ways, and become "intrusive," even after a woman has left the relationship.
* *Critique*:
  * These theories do not take into account the roles women's inner emotional and psychological states also contribute to their responses to IPV.
* *Challenges*
  * Identifying points of immediate intervention is difficult when considering unjust systems at the societal level. Social action is a long-term intervention; effective short-term and immediate interventions need to be developed.
  * Changing the responses of helping agencies universally in order to make it "safe" for women to seek services is challenging. As nurses, we cannot guarantee that there will not be negative ramifications from systems if she seeks services.

that individuals respond to trauma and violence in individual ways within individual contexts. This has implications for development of effective prevention programs and clinical interventions.

An important caveat to bear in mind is that many women undoubtedly *do*, in fact, extricate themselves from relationships at the onset of abuse, or soon after, without seeking help outside of their own network, for example, at domestic violence shelters, calling the police, or involving the court system. Because most research on women's responses to IPV has relied on samples of women who have sought some type of formal assistance, for example, health care, social services, or use of the legal system, our knowledge of women who quickly break free without complications is very limited. Therefore, the theoretical and empirical work accomplished, thus far, is most useful in understanding the responses of women who endure abuse over a longer period of time and whose abuse becomes public by virtue of their help-seeking behaviors and involvement with official agencies.

Historical Perspectives

Psychological Perspectives

LOW SELF-ESTEEM. Research and theory from psychological perspectives have extensively explored personality and psychological factors related to women's responses to abusive relationships. Low self-esteem is often suggested in popular literature as a reason for women's continued involvement in abusive relationships. Women with low self-esteem are thought to be vulnerable to abuse, more tolerant in permitting the abuse to continue, and less likely to seek outside intervention. However, research has failed to support this persistent notion. The conclusion of most research in this area is twofold. First, as with most psychological attributes characteristic of battered women, the low self-esteem that many abused women experience is likely the consequence of the abuse and of the stigma associated with abuse rather than a preexisting condition. Second, women with low self-esteem are no more likely to become involved in an abusive relationship than are women with higher levels of self-esteem.

MENTAL HEALTH PROBLEMS. Similarly, various mental health problems, including symptoms of depression, posttraumatic stress disorder (PTSD), and alcohol and drug abuse, are consistently found to be more prevalent among abused women than women who have not been abused (Dienemann et al., 2000; Campbell, Kub, Belknap, & Templin, 1997; Golding, 1999). Again, most evidence supports our understanding that these symptoms are sequelae of trauma of IPV rather than precursors to it. The more trauma women have experienced in their lifetimes, such as abuse in childhood or sexual assault, in addition to IPV, the more symptoms they are likely to exhibit. Even though these symptoms are a consequence of the violence, they may interfere with a woman's problem solving and coping abilities. Therefore, interventions need to take these potential mental health problems into account (see chapter 5).

LEARNED HELPLESSNESS. Martin Seligman's theory of learned helplessness was promoted as a reasonable explanation of women's psychological and behavioral responses to abuse in the late 1980s (Walker, 1979, 1984). The original model stated that passivity, poor problem solving, and depression result when uncontrollable bad events occur, and future responses are expected to be futile, reflective of motivational, cognitive, and emotional deficits. Applied to women in abusive relationships, learned helplessness theory suggests that repeated abuse leads to the development of a cognitive perception by the victim that she is unable to resolve her current abusive situation and leads to depression and apathy, resulting in an inability to leave the relationship. Walker (1984) found some support for learned helplessness in a sample of battered women, especially in terms of depression. However, many did not perceive a loss of control of events in their lives, nor did they show low self-esteem. Rather than becoming passive and immobilized over time, as predicted by the learned helplessness model, women's help-seeking activities increased as the frequency and severity of violence increased.

TRAUMATIC BONDING. The theory of traumatic bonding (Dutton & Painter, 1981) has been used to explain the process wherein abused women develop strong emotional bonds or attachments to their abusers. This is similar to the Stockholm syndrome, in which abducted hostages develop loyalty to hostage takers, regardless of the risk or danger they face.

CYCLE THEORY OF VIOLENCE. Lenore Walker was one of the first researchers to describe a dynamic process in abusive relationships that she called the "cycle theory of violence" (Walker, 1979, 1984). From extensive interviews with battered women in which they described battering incidents, Walker described a three-phase cycle of violence. The first, the "tension-building phase," is characterized by an escalation of tension with verbal abuse and minor battering incidents. The woman engages in placating behavior, trying desperately to avoid serious incidents. This phase may last for weeks or years, until the tension has mounted to the breaking point. Phase two, "the acute battering incident," is the outbreak of serious violence that may last from 2 to 24 hours. The woman is powerless to affect the outcome of the second phase and can only try to protect herself and her children. In the third phase, the man becomes contrite, loving, and promises to reform, reinforcing the woman's hope that the beatings will end. Unfortunately, the cycle almost always repeats itself. Over time, the third phase occurs less often, leaving the woman trapped between the pre-outburst tension and battering episodes.

Empirical tests of Walker's cycle of violence theory lend inconsistent support for the three phases. Sixty-five percent of Walker's sample gave evidence of a tension-building phase prior to the battering, and 58% described loving contrition after the battering (Walker, 1984). Dobash and Dobash (1984) used similar research methods, but did not find support for Walker's third phase of the cycle of violence; only 14% of the batterers in their sample apologized after the worst incident of assault. Painter and Dutton (1985) found unpredictable behavior on the part of men after they violently attacked their female partner. Nevertheless, Walker's cycle of violence theory has been accepted by advocates and women themselves as a plausible explanation for the behavior of abused women. The three-phase cycle often appears in clinical protocols for professional education and in community education efforts by women's groups.

CONTEMPORARY THEORIES. Theorizing about women's responses to IPV has evolved with the application of two theories: critical social theory and resiliency, described by some as a strength-based approach. Together, these shifts in thinking offer a richer understanding of the processes involved in women's responses to IPV. Robust descriptive qualitative research has been reported about the emotional processes of being in, leaving, and recovering from abusive relationships and, more recently, adaptive responses and strategies used in these processes. More and more, analyses of these data reflect a strength-based theoretical approach and the application of critical social theory.

Most research on IPV in the past two decades has focused on individual components of women's responses, often operationalized in dichotomous ways, for example, decisions to stay or leave, to disclose the abuse or not, to seek outside help or not. Discussions of the influences on women's responses to abuse typically dichotomize them into internal versus external, that is, personal versus sociocultural. For example, Lazarus and Folkman (1984) described two types of coping: emotion-focused (internal) and problem-focused (external). Problem-focused coping is used to manage specific problems, for example, the abuse itself, getting childcare, etc., while emotion-focused coping is used to manage the distress that accompanies these problems. The two-part decision making model (Choice & Lamke, 1997) frames abused women's processes of evaluating whether to leave their relationships based on two questions. The first question, "Will I be better off?" reflects internal psychological processes. The second question, "Can I do it?" includes intrapsychic components, but also incorporates structural barriers, for example, lack of access to resources, such as employment and affordable childcare. The application of critical social theory to women's responses to IPV creates a shift from dichotomous to increasingly complex understandings.

CRITICAL SOCIAL THEORIES. Contemporary perspectives on women's responses to IPV are largely based on ecological systems theory and critical social theory, both described earlier, rather than purely psychological theories. Essentially, women's responses to IPV are no longer thought of as purely internal, mostly dysfunctional, psychological processes. The context of a woman's response is now considered more influential than her inner processes. The influence of social systems, such as children's protective services, the police, court systems, and health care providers on abused women's responses have been well-described. These formal systems may be barriers to or facilitators of assistance to abused women. For example, mothers' "external" or public responses to the violence may depend on their perceptions of or experiences with children's protective services. They might not disclose the abuse to anyone for fear of having their children removed from their custody (Kelly, 2006; Varcoe & Irwin, 2004), or they may be penalized for the abuser's behavior because of their (the women's) "failure to protect" (Kopels & Sheridan, 2002). Ineffective responses by police or court systems will prompt women to respond differently than if they received the legal assistance they were seeking, perhaps staying in the relationship and "managing" the abuse as best they can. Understanding the complex contexts of women's responses to the abuse is essential to understanding the complexity of their responses to it (see Moe, 2007). Contemporary theories articulate the context of women's responses to IPV more broadly than previous theories. Critical analyses of the influences of societal-level systems, for example, the political climate, the economy, health care systems, and culture now appear in IPV-related nursing and social sciences literature.

MARGINALIZATION. Marginalization is a concept used by nurses (Hall, Stevens, & Meleis, 1994) that describes difference, that is, deviation from the norm, as a negative characteristic. Living at the margins, which are defined as "the peripheral, boundary-determining aspects of persons, social networks, communities and environments," (Hall et al., 1994, pp. 24–25) negatively impacts health. Marginalization has come to be associated with vulnerability; marginalized and vulnerable populations have become topics for nursing research and scholarship. Victims and survivors of IPV have long been considered vulnerable, in part due to their marginalization that results from the violence.

FEMINIST INTERSECTIONALITY. Feminist intersectionality is a theory generated by Black feminist writers in the past three decades that recognizes that oppressed groups and individuals live at the margins of society with inequitable access to resources resulting in societal inequities and social injustice (Collins, 1986, 2000; Crenshaw, 1991; Hurtado, 1996; Mullings & Schulz, 2006; Zambrana, 1987). The negative effects on health from belonging to more than one oppressed group are multiplicative and unique. The application of intersectionality to IPV involves examining the multiplicative effects of structural inequalities in the lives of battered women. Add to this, each woman's social location and cultural background and the complexity of women's responses to IPV becomes clear (Sokoloff & Dupont, 2005).

Consider, for example, a woman who is being abused who is an immigrant with limited English proficiency and a grade school education, who is in the United States with her husband and three children without her own family, and is unemployed. She will have a limited spectrum of possible responses to IPV relative to a white woman who is a U.S. citizen, has a high level of education, is employed, and has a network of friends and family nearby. At the same time, if the white woman is in severe danger from the abuser, does not have access to household finances, and believes that she would lose custody of her children and her social network if she disclosed the abuse to anyone, she too will have a limited spectrum of responses available to her. Both women will also have their unique internal emotional and psychological responses to the violence. This example illustrates the importance of recognizing the impact of both the intersection of race, class, and gender and individuals' internal experiences on women's responses to IPV.

RESILIENCY. There has been a tremendous shift in perspective in the past 20 years from viewing abused women as helpless victims to resilient and resourceful survivors. Resilience is a construct that has been broadly defined as positive coping, adaptation, and persistence. It is most commonly referred to as the ability "to bounce back" successfully despite exposure to adverse circumstances, severe risk, or trauma (Greene, 2002). It is a biopsychosocial and spiritual phenomenon, which is best understood as a dynamic lifelong process, rather than a character trait. As circumstances change, with different risks, vulnerabilities, and protective factors, resilient or adaptive outcomes may change. This shift in perspective has been likened to moving from a deficiency model to a competence model (Hamby & Gray-Little, 1997), developing agency (Hage, 2006; Lempert, 1996), surviving (Davis, 2002; Taylor, 2004), and having strength (Irwin, Thorne, & Varcoe, 2002) (see Table 3.1). Strength-based approaches and interventions derive from the recognition of both the active role that abused women take in responding to and coping with IPV and the common patterns that can be seen in their responses.

SURVIVOR MODELS. Gondolf and Fisher (1988) first reframed battered women as active survivors rather than helpless victims. Survivor models are strongly supported by contemporary research (Campbell, Rose, Kub, & Nedd, 1998; Gondolf & Fisher, 1988;

TABLE 3.1 *Reformulations of Women's Responses to Intimate Partner Violence*

	Historical	Contemporary
Personal attributes	Weak	Strong
	Helpless	Resilient
	Victim	Survivor
Definition of response	Decision to stay or leave	Ongoing process of seeking safety for self and children
Mental and emotional reaction	Psychologically dysfunctional	Complex of internal and external factors
Coping style	Passive	Active
	Static	Adaptive

Hoff 1990). Data from 6,612 records from 50 battered women's shelters in Texas showed battered women persistently seeking help in ending the abuse directed at them (Gondolf & Fisher, 1988). Help-seeking efforts increased rather than decreased when the batterer's level of violence increased, particularly when he engaged in more antisocial or criminal behavior, in general. The inadequate response of social agencies to the needs of battered women was the most notable impediment to safety rather than internal characteristics of the women. The authors suggest that helping agencies must strengthen their advocacy role for women and remove the barriers that keep women trapped in abusive relationships rather than concentrate on "treating" victims.

The notion of women as "survivors" rather than victims has been further developed in contemporary research that has examined the process of women leaving an abusive relationship, often based on qualitative data from in-depth interviews. These studies have illuminated the complexity of women's experiences with, and responses to, IPV. An important unifying theme in this growing body of research is that women's responses to abuse reflect a dynamic process that evolves according to the nature of the abuse, their interpretations of the abuse and the relationship as a whole, as well as to their expectations of the pragmatic consequences of remaining in or severing the relationship, including the potential responses of systems that are intended to help them. Nurse researchers have made particularly important contributions to this body of knowledge.

PROCESSES OF EXPERIENCING, LEAVING, AND RECOVERING FROM ABUSIVE RELATIONSHIPS

Women's responses to IPV have been examined under three broad categories: processes of experiencing, getting out of, and recovering from abusive relationships. First, it is important to understand the various circumstances under which women get out of abusive relationships. At times, it is completely volitional, and a woman can leave the relationship or separate from her partner when she chooses without threat or danger. At times, the process of getting out is more emotionally and practically complicated, and a woman might have to use several strategies to extricate herself from the relationship or may return several times before ending the relationship for good. For some women, getting out of an abusive relationship requires escaping, literally, with its attendant risks and danger. Each of these words, leaving, separating, extricating, and escaping all have different connotations in terms of women's choices, as well as the relative dangers they face when getting out of abusive relationships. None of these words can capture the nuanced process for each woman of getting out of the abusive relationship, nor the level of risk involved at any one point in time. In this chapter, when we use the word leaving, it is in full recognition that leaving is not always a simple choice, nor a safe one. Further, leaving a relationship does not always equate with the end of violence, as we discuss later.

Several researchers have documented the experience of becoming embroiled in, coping with, and extricating oneself from an abusive relationship from the perspective of women who have lived through IPV. No longer is leaving the abusive relationship considered the only success in women's responses. Researchers have identified the strategies women use to seek safety for themselves and their children while they are still in the abusive relationship. Nurse researchers have also identified and described the ongoing violence that can continue after a woman has left the relationship, women's processes of

moving forward and recovering from the violence, and the broader context of these processes. The strengths and creative resistance strategies that women draw on in the face of
IPV are demonstrated in this research.

In a nursing investigation of women's experiences with IPV, Landenburger (1989,
1998) described a cumulative and multidimensional process that women go through in
abusive relationships that influences choices about staying in or leaving the relationship. Four phases of binding, enduring, disengaging, and recovering emerged from a
qualitative analysis of in-depth interviews with women who were in, or recently out of,
an abusive relationship. Women went through the four phases, but not necessarily in a
linear fashion, as they experienced changes in the meaning ascribed to the abuse, in interactions with the abusive partner, and in perceptions of themselves. In the first phase,
the "binding" phase, when the relationship is new and promising, women respond to
abuse with redoubled efforts to make the relationship work and to prevent future abuse
by appeasing the partner. In the second phase, or time of enduring, a woman tolerates
the abuse because of the positive aspects of the relationship, feels at least partially responsible for the abuse, and sets aside her own needs, desires, and goals in order to fully
attend to those of the abuser; also all in an effort to prevent or reduce further abuse.
Though a woman may tentatively seek outside help at this time, she does not openly
disclose her circumstances to others for fear of the consequences to her safety and to her
partner's social status. The phase of disengaging involves the woman labeling her situation as being abusive and herself as undeserving of abusive treatment. A breaking point
may be reached at which women are cognizant of the danger they or their children are in,
as well as the knowledge that they might attempt to kill the abuser. As women struggle
with independent living and safety concerns, they may leave and return to the abusive
relationship several times. After successfully dealing with the many barriers that could
trap them in the abusive relationship, some women enter a phase of recovery in which
they remain separated from the abuser. An important point for nurses and other helpers
to realize is that, from the woman's perspective, the abuse was just one aspect of a whole
relationship that may still have some positive elements in it—the woman wants the
abuse to stop, but may want to maintain the good aspects of the relationship (Campbell
et al., 1998).

Reclaiming self, regenerating family, strengthening capacity, and promoting health
serve as the explanatory core of women's responses to IPV in the nursing research program of Ford-Gilboe, Wuest, and Merritt-Gray (2005), Merritt-Gray and Wuest (1995),
Wuest, Ford-Gilboe, Merritt-Gray, and Berman (2003), Wuest and Merritt-Gray (1999),
(2001), and Wuest, Merritt-Gray, and Ford-Gilboe (2004). In these researchers' feminist
grounded-theory studies, women described the process of living in, and eventually leaving, an abusive relationship. A variety of strategies were employed in three stages of
reclaiming the self, "counteracting abuse" and, later, in "breaking free" and "not going
back" to the relationship. The strategic actions that women employed in resisting the
abuse contradict the view of battered women as passive victims.

Sustaining the separation from the abusive partner, or "not going back" is an important stage, since the process of leaving an abusive relationship can be so long and
arduous that, after leaving, women experience depleted reserves of emotional and
physical energy, ambivalence, and uncertainty (Wuest & Merritt-Gray, 1999). When
women move forward as single mothers, they "regenerate their family" by creating a
new family unit with open and safe interaction in contrast to the destructive environment they have left. This involves processes of mothers and children working as a team

and living together differently (Wuest et al., 2004). However, in the process of moving forward, women often face "intrusion" by social systems, as they search for employment, apply for financial assistance, and enlist the assistance of law enforcement and the court system in custody issues or ongoing stalking or harassment from the abusive partner. An important phase in the recovery process includes "strengthening their capacity" to limit this intrusion and to promote the health of their family. Taylor (2004) described a recovery process from IPV of "moving from surviving to thriving" in her ethnographic study of African American women. In this process, women moved from sharing secrets/shattering silences, the reclaiming the self, renewing the spirit, self-healing through forgiveness, finding inspiration in the future, to self-generativity by engaging in social activism (p. 35).

Several researchers have described the role of motherhood in women's experiences of and responses to IPV. Lutz, Curry, Robrecht, Libbus, and Bullock (2006) described the conflicting process of double binding that pregnant women engage in as they bind to the unborn child in preparation for being a mother and at the same time bind with their abusive partner. Women who are abused and are mothers strategize to protect their children's physical safety and emotional well-being (Ulrich et al., 2006). They make decisions about disclosing the abuse or seeking help in efforts to maintain custody of their children or co-parent with the abusers (Hardesty & Ganong, 2006; Varcoe & Irwin, 2004; Zink, Elder, & Jacobsen, 2003). In a study with battered Latina mothers, Kelly (2009b) found that realizing threats to the safety and well-being of their children was pivotal to these mothers' decisions to leave the abuser.

Cultural differences and nuances in women's responses to IPV are important to understand. Campbell (2008) analyzed the results of four studies conducted over 20 years with African American women who had experienced IPV. They reported that unique considerations of these women in any public responses they made to the abuse were concerns about bringing disgrace or more discrimination to the black community by disclosing the violence or risking racist intervention by police if they called them for assistance. In one study Campbell et al. (1998), found that the IPV was not always the women's biggest concern, in the face of poverty, unemployment, substance abuse, problems with their families or children, and mental health concerns.

Researchers who have investigated the responses of women from various cultures to IPV cite the resilience and resourcefulness of these women and the creative and adaptive strategies they use to respond to the violence (Shiu-Thornton, Senturia, & Sullivan, 2005), the extreme suffering and isolation of abused immigrant women, and the fatalistic role of religion and spirituality (Bhuyan, Mell, Senturia, Sullivan, & Shiu-Thornton, 2005).

Using a longitudinal design in which women were interviewed at three different time points over 3 years, Campbell and colleagues (1998) also described the resourcefulness of women's approaches to resolving the violence in their relationships. The majority of the sample was still in the abusive relationship at the beginning of the study; therefore, the results do not rely on women's reflections on an abusive relationship they left long ago. In contrast to other explications of women's responses to abuse, the overall goal of women in this study was to resolve the abuse (achieve nonviolence) rather than necessarily leave the intimate relationship. Women's stories revealed that the notion of "staying" or "leaving" an abusive relationship is a gross oversimplification of women's status in the relationship. For example, an "in/out" category was developed to describe women who were ambivalent about maintaining or leaving the relationship. These women may have left, or had him thrown out, more than once; however, they continued to have positive feelings for the partner and, though certain that they wanted the abuse to end, they were not convinced that the entire relationship had to be sacrificed to achieve nonviolence.

Another important insight gained from the study is that, in fact, leaving the intimate relationship and ending the violence were often independent outcomes. For some women, violence continues, and may even escalate, after they leave the abusive partner. The reality is that women are easily stalked by their ex-partner and can be harassed for years by virtue of legal proceedings, child custody and visitation rules, and other reasons for continued contact. It is essential for nurses and the public to understand that leaving or ending the abusive relationship does not necessarily end the violence for women and their children. Efforts to assist and support women must be made with full cognizance of this dangerous reality. Questions such as "Why don't you just leave?" need to be eliminated from our set of responses to women's disclosure of abuse. Although the complexity of women's stories over 3 years did not support description of a process with distinct phases or stages, women did describe various circumstances and events that played pivotal roles in their quest for nonviolence (Campbell et al., 1998). For example, achieving financial independence provided an important psychological and pragmatic boost that helped some women leave the relationship. For others, realization that their children's well-being was in jeopardy or that they themselves were becoming violent in response served as a catalyst for leaving the abusive partner.

In summary, theoretical frameworks of women's responses to IPV have evolved in complexity and explanatory power over the past 30 years. Contemporary research refutes the image of women as passive victims in abusive relationships. Rather, women actively respond to the abusive behaviors with creative and resourceful strategies, the goal being to be free of violence, perhaps while maintaining the relationship, but, more often, requiring dissolution of the relationship. Though this is a complicated process, a pattern of normative stages or phases have been described in qualitative research. Detailed knowledge of the process can be used to develop phase-specific nursing assessments and interventions with women who are experiencing IPV. The reality of ongoing danger and harassment from the perpetrator has been illustrated in women's narrative accounts and in review of homicide data. Those who are in positions to help women must remain aware that leaving an abusive relationship does not necessarily ensure the safety of women and their children; rather, the level of danger may increase for some time after leaving. Evaluation of danger and review of safety plans must be an integral component of work with women, even after they have left an abusive partner. Clearly, further research on the typologies of batterers, described earlier in this chapter, will improve the accuracy of danger assessments and appropriate safety plans for women and their children.

SUMMARY

IPV is clearly a public health problem of considerable magnitude in North America and around the world. Nurses have many roles to play in primary prevention efforts as well as in the application of appropriate interventions with those who have experienced abuse in intimate relationships. Although attention to the issue is fairly recent in the nursing and health care community, the problem itself is not a new phenomenon. Historical records reveal that "wife beating" has been socially sanctioned in patriarchal societies throughout history, and indeed, there continues to be cultural support, to varying degrees, for men to dominate and control their wives and partners through aggressive means (Dobash & Dobash, 1979, 1993; Heise, 1998; Krug et al., 2002). In this chapter, we reviewed the evolution of theoretical frameworks that explain the causes of IPV, including psychobiologic explanations, socialization theories, family system stressors, and an ecological framework for understanding gender-based violence against women. The concept of machismo was seen to be important in explaining the behavior of abusive men. Recent progress in understanding the types of men who batter, extremely important knowledge for those who work with men who batter and those who wish to improve the safety of women and children, was described. Theoretical frameworks that describe and explain women's responses to IPV were described chronologically, beginning with victim-blaming perspectives, followed by theories in which the victim is viewed as passive and helpless, and concluding with more recent frameworks that highlight the strength and creativity of women's resistance to, and resolution of, IPV. Though our knowledge remains imperfect, contemporary understanding of the causes of men's violence against women and women's responses to IPV provides an important base for the development of nursing assessment tools and interventions for primary prevention, early detection, and therapeutic approaches with those who experience IPV.

REFERENCES

Abrahams, N. (2002). *Men's use of violence against intimate partners: A study of working men in Cape Town.* Cape Town, SA: University of Cape Town.

Achterberg, J. (1991). *Woman as healer.* Boston: Shambhala.

Amnesty International. (2004). Rwanda:"Marked for Death": Rape survivors living with HIV/AIDS in Rwanda. http://www.amnesty.org/en/library/info/AFR47/007/2004/en.

Anderson, E. (1999). *Code of the streets.* NY: W. W. Norton.

Anzaldua, G. (1990). *Making face, making soul haciendo caras: Creative and critical perspectives by women of color.* San Francisco, CA: Aunt Lute Foundation Books.

Archer, J. (Ed.) (1994). *Male violence.* London & NY: Routledge.

Arciniega, G. M., Anderson, T. C., Tovar-Blank, Z. G., & Tracey, T. J. G. (2008). Toward a fuller conception of machismo: Development of a traditional machismo and caballerismo scale. *Journal of Counseling Psychology, 55*(1), 19–33.

Babcock, J. C., Miller, S. A., & Siard, C. (2003). Toward a typology of abusive women: Differences between partner-only and generally violent women in the use of violence. *Psychology of Women Quarterly, 27*(2), 153–161.

Balsam, K. F., & Szymanski, D. M. (2005). Relationship quality and domestic violence in women's same-sex relationships: The role of minority stress. *Psychology of Women Quarterly, 29*(3), 258–269.

Barnes, S. Y. (1999). Theories of spouse abuse: Relevance to African Americans. *Issues in Mental Health Nursing, 20,* 357–371.

Basile, K. C., Arias, I., Desai, S., & Thompson, M. P. (2004). The differential association of intimate partner physical, sexual, psychological, and stalking violence and posttraumatic stress symptoms in a nationally representative sample of women. *Journal of Traumatic Stress, 17*(5), 413–421.

Bhuyan, R., Mell, M., Senturia, K., Sullivan, M., & Shiu-Thornton, S. (2005). "Women must endure according to their karma": Cambodian immigrant women talk about domestic violence. *Journal of Interpersonal Violence, 20*(8), 902–921.

Boddy, J. (1998). Violence embodied? Circumcision, gender politics, and cultural aesthetics. In R. E. Dobash & R. E. Dobash (Eds.), *Rethinking violence against women* (pp. 77–110). Thousand Oaks, CA: Sage.

Bohn, D. (2003). Lifetime physical and sexual abuse, substance abuse, depression, and suicide attempts among Native American women. *Issues in Mental Health Nursing, 24,* 333–352.

Bonomi, A. E., Anderson, M. L., Cannon, E. A., Slesnick, N., & Rodriguez, M. A. (2009). Intimate partner violence in Latina and non-Latina women. *American Journal of Preventive Medicine, 36*(1), 43–48.

Bonomi, A. E., Anderson, M. L., Reid, R. J., Rivara, F. P., Carrell, D., & Thompson, R. S. (2009). Medical and psychosocial diagnoses in women with a history of intimate partner violence. *Archives of Internernal Medicine, 169*(18), 1692–1697.

Brown, C. (2008). Gender-role implications on same-sex intimate partner abuse. *Journal of Family Violence, 23,* 457–462.

Browne, A. (1987). *Battered women who kill.* New York: Free Press.

Browne, A., Williams, K. R., & Dutton, D. R. (1998). Homicide between intimate partners. In Smith, M. D. & Zahn, M. *Homicide: A sourcebook of social research* (pp. 149–164). Thousand Oaks, CA: Sage.

Brownmiller, S. (1975). *Against our will: Men, women, and rape.* NY: Bantam Books.

Campbell, J. C. (1981). Misogyny and homicide of women. *Advances in Nursing Science, 3*(2), 67–85.

Campbell, J. C. (1989). A test of two explanatory models of women's responses to battering. *Nursing Research, 38*(1), 18–24.

Campbell, J., Campbell, D. W., Gary, F., Nedd, D., Price-Lea, P., Sharps, P. W., et al. (2008). African American women's responses to intimate partner violence: an examination of cultural context. *Journal of Aggression, Maltreatment & Trauma, 16*(3), 277–295.

Campbell, J. C., & Humphreys, J. (1993). *Nursing care of survivors of family violence.* St. Louis: Mosby.

Campbell, J. C., Kub, J., Belknap, R. A., & Templin, T. (1997). Predictors of depression in battered women. *Violence Against Women, 3*(3), 276–293.

Campbell, J., Rose, L., Kub, J., & Nedd, D. (1998). Voices of strength and resistance: A contextual and longitudinal analysis of women's responses to battering. *Journal of Interpersonal Violence, 13*(6), 743–762.

Campbell, J, Webster, D, Koziol-McLain, J, Block, C. R., Campbell, D. W., et al. (2003). Risk factors for intimate partner femicide. *American Journal of Public Health, 93*(7), 1089–1097.

Carmody, D. C., & Williams, K. R. (1987). Wife assault and perceptions of sanctions. *Violence and Victims, 2*(1), 25–38.

Center for Social Research. (2008). Annual Report. New Dehli. [On-line] Available: http://www.csrindia.org/PDF/annualreport.pdf.

Centers for Disease Control & Prevention [CDC], (2009). Violence prevention—The social ecological model: A framework for prevention. Retrieved November 9, 2009, from http://www.cdc.gov/ViolencePrevention/overview/social-ecologicalmodel.html.

Chavis, A. Z., & Hill, M. S. (2009). Integrating multiple intersecting identities: A multicultural conceptualization of the power and control wheel. *Women & Therapy, 32,* 121–149.

Choice, P., & Lamke, L. K. (1997). A conceptual approach to understanding abused women's stay/leave decision. *Journal of Family Issues, 18,* 290–314.

Coker, A. L., Davis, K. E., Arias, I., Desai, S., Sanderson, M., Brandt, H. M., et al. (2002). Physical and mental health effects of intimate partner violence for men and women. *American Journal of Preventive Medicine, 23*(4), 260–268.

Collins, P. H. (1986). Learning from the outsider within: The sociological significance of Black feminist thought. *Social Problems, 33*(6), S14–S32.

Collins, P. H. (2000). *Black feminist thought: Knowledge, consciousness, and the politics of empowerment.* New York: Routledge.

Connell, R. (1995). *Masculinities.* Cambridge: Polity Press.

Counts, D. A., Brown, J. K., & Campbell, J. C. (1999). *To have and to hit: Cultural perspectives on wife beating.* Chicago: University of Illinois Press.

Crenshaw, K. (1991). Mapping the margins: Intersectionality, identity politics, and violence against women of color. *Stanford Law Review, 43*(6), 1241–1299.

Cunningham, A., Jaffe, P., Baker, L., Dick, T., Malla, S., Mazaheri, N., & Poisson, S. (1998). Theory-driven explanations of male violence against female partners: Literature update and related implications for treatment and evaluation. [Online]. Available: http://www.lfcc.on.ca/maleviolence.pdf.

Dahlberg, L. L., & Krug, E. G. (2002). Violence-a global public health problem. In E. Krug, L. L. Dahlberg, J. A. Mercy, A. B. Zwi, & R. Lozano R (Eds.), *World report on violence and health* (pp 1–56). Geneva, Switzerland: World Health Organization.

Daly, M. (1978). *Gyn/Ecology: The metaethics of radical feminism.* Boston: Beacon Press.

Davidson, T. (1978). *Conjugal crime: Understanding and changing the wifebeating problem.* NY: Hawthorne Books.

Davis, R. E. (2002). "The strongest women": Exploration of the inner resources of abused women. *Qualitative Health Research, 12*(9), 1248–1263.

Dearwater, S., Coben, J., Nah, G., Campbell, J., McLoughlin, E., & Glass, N. (1998). Prevalence of domestic violence in women treated at community hospital emergency departments. *JAMA, 280*(5), 433–438.

Denzin, N. K, Lincoln, Y. S., & Smith, L. T. (Eds.). (2008). *Handbook of critical and indigenous methodologies.* Thousand Oaks, CA: Sage.

Diamond, M. (2006). Masculinity unraveled: The roots of male gender identity and the shifting of male ego ideals throughout life. *Journal of the American Psychoanalytic Association, 54* (4), 1099–1130.

Dienemann, J., Boyle, E., Baker, D., Resnick, W., Wiederhorn, N., & Campbell, J. (2000). Intimate partner abuse among women diagnosed with depression. *Issues in Mental Health Nursing, 21,* 499–513.

Diken, B., & Laustsen, C. B. (2005). Becoming abject: Rape as a weapon of war. *Body Society, 11*(1), 111–128.

Dobash, R. E., & Dobash, R. P. (1998). *Rethinking violence against women.* Thousand Oaks, CA: Sage Publications.

Dobash, R. E., & Dobash, R. E. (1993). *Women, violence, and social change.* London: Routledge.

Dobash, R. E., & Dobash, R. P. (1984). The nature and antecedents of violent events. *British Journal of Criminology, 23,* 269–288.

Dobash, R. E., & Dobash, R. P. (1979). *Violence against wives.* NY: Free Press.

Dutton, D. G., & Painter, S. L. (1981). Traumatic bonding: The development of emotional attachments in battered women and other relationships of intermittent abuse. *Victimology, 6,* 139–155.

Dworkin, A. (1976). *Our blood: Prophecies and discourses on sexual politics.* NY: Harper & Row.

Eaton, L., Kaufman, M., Fuhrel, A., Cain, D., Cherry, C., Pope, H., et al. (2008). Examining factors coexisting with interpersonal violence in lesbian relationships. *Journal of Family Violence, 23*(8), 697–705.

Feldman, M. B., Diaz, R. M., Ream, G. L., & Ei-Bassel, N. (2007). Intimate partner violence and HIV sexual risk behavior among Latino gay and bisexual men. *Journal of LGBT Health Research, 3*(2), 9–19.

Fiorentino, D. D., Berger, D. E., & Ramirez, J. R. (2007). Drinking and driving among high-risk young Mexican-American men. *Accident Analysis and Prevention, 39,* 16–21.

Ford-Gilboe, M., Wuest, J., & Merritt-Gray, M. (2005). Strengthening capacity to limit intrusion: Theorizing family health promotion in the aftermath of woman abuse. *Qualitative Health Research, 15*(4), 477–501.

Foster, L. A., Veale, C. M., & Fogel, C. I. (1989). Factors present when battered women kill. *Issues in Mental Health Nursing, 10,* 273–284.

Fox, J. A. & Zawitz, M. W. (2007). *Homicide trends in the United States.* Washington, DC: Department of Justice. Bureau of Justice Statistics.

Garcia-Moreno, C., Jansen, H. A. F. M., Ellsberg, M., Heise, L., & Watts, C. H. (2006). Prevalence of intimate partner violence: findings from the WHO multi-country study on women's health and domestic violence. *Lancet, 368*(9543), 1260–1269.

Gillespie, C. K. (1989). *Justifiable homicide.* Columbus: Ohio State University Press.

Gilmore, D. D. (1990). *Manhood in the making: Cultural concepts of masculinity.* New Haven, CT: Yale University Press.

Golding, J. M. (1999). Intimate partner violence as a risk for mental disorders: A meta-analysis. *Journal of Family Violence, 14,* 99–132.

Gondolf, E. W. (1997a). Patterns of reassault in batterer programs. *Violence and Victims 12*(4), 373–387.

Gondolf, E. W. (1997b). Batterer programs: What we know and need to know. *Journal of Interpersonal Violence, 12*(1), 83–98.

Gondolf, E. W., & Fisher, E. R. (1988). *Battered women as survivors: An alternative to learned helplessness.* Lexington, MA: Lexington Books.

Gonzalez-Guarda, R. M., Ortega, J., Vasquez, E., & De Santis, J. (2009). La mancha negra: Substance abuse, violence and sexual risk among Hispanic males. *Western Journal of Nursing Research.* Online First, November 14, DOI:10.1177/0193945909343594.

Greene, R. R. (2002). *Resiliency: An integrated approach to practice, policy, and research.* Washington, DC: NASW Press.

Greenfield, L. A., Rand, M. R., Craven, D., Klaus, P. A., Perkins, C. A., Ringel, C., Warchol, G., & Matson, C. (1998). *Violence by intimates: Analysis of data on crimes by current or former spouses, boyfriends and, girlfriends*, Washington, DC: US Department of Justice.

Grossfeld, S. (1991, September 2). *"Safer" and in jail: Women who kill their batterers.* (pp. 1, 12, 13). Boston: Boston Globe.

Habermas, J. (1971). *Knowledge and human interests.* Boston: Beacon Press.

Habermas, J. (1973). *Theory and practice.* Boston: Beacon Press.

Habermas, J. (1975). *Legitimation crisis.* Boston: Beacon Press.

Habermas, J. (1979). *Communication and the evolution of society.* Boston: Beacon.

Habermas, J. (1984). *The theory of communicative action, Volume 1.* Boston: Beacon Press.

Habermas, J. (1987). *The theory of communicative action, Volume 2.* Boston: Beacon Press.

Habermas, J. (1985). *The philosophical discourse of modernity.* Cambridge: MIT Press.

Hage, S. M. (2006). Profiles of women as survivors: The development of agency in abusive relationships. *Journal of Counseling and Development, 84*(1), 83–94.

Hall, J. M., Stevens, P. E., & Meleis, A. I. (1994). Marginalization: A guiding concept for valuing diversity in nursing knowledge development. *Advances in Nursing Science, 16*(4), 23–41.

Hamby, S. L., & Gray-Little, B. (1997). Responses to partner violence: Moving away from deficit models. *Journal of Family Psychology, 11,* 339–350.

Hamby, S. L. (2006). The importance of community in a feminist analysis of domestic violence among Native Americans. In N. J. Sokoloff & C. Pratt (Eds.), *Domestic violence at the margins: Readings on race, class, gender and culture* (pp. 174–193). New Brunswick, NJ: Rutgers University Press.

Hardesty, J. L., & Ganong, L. H. (2006). How women make custody decisions and manage co-parenting with abusive former husbands. *Journal of Social and Personal Relationships, 23*(4), 543–563.

Hazen, A. L., Connelly, C. D., Soriano, F. I., & Landsverk, J. A. (2008). Intimate partner violence and psychological functioning in Latina women. *Health Care for Women International, 29*(3), 282–299.

Heise, L. (1998). Violence against women: An integrated, ecological framework. *Violence Against Women, 4,* 262–290.

Holtzworth-Munroe, A. (2000). A typology of men who are violent toward their female partners: Making sense of the heterogeneity of husband violence [Online serial]. *Current Directions in Psychological Science, 9*(4).

Holtzworth-Munroe, A., & Stuart, G. L. (1994). Typologies of male batterers: Three subtypes and the differences among them. *Psychological Bulletin, 116,* 476–497.

Hoff, L. A. (1990). *Battered women as survivors.* London: Routledge.

Hooks, B. (1984). *Feminist theory: From margin to center.* Boston, MA: South End Press.

Horkheimer, M. (1972). *Bemerkungen zur religion.* Frankfurt: Fisher Verlag.

Horkheimer, M. (1982). *Critical theory.* New York: Seabury Press.

Horkheimer, M. (1987). *Eclipse of reason.* Boston: Beacon Press.

Horkheimer, M. (1993). *Between philosophy and social science.* Cambridge: MIT Press.

Hughes, D. M. (2001). The 'Natasha' trade: The transnational shadow market of trafficking in women. *National Institute of Justice Journal,* 9–15.

Human Rights Watch. (2009). "We have the promises of the world".

Hurtado, A. (1996). Strategic suspensions: Feminists of color theorize the production of knowledge. In M. F. Belenky, N. R. Goldberger, J. M. Tarule, & B. M. Clinchy (Eds.), *Knowledge, difference, and power: Essays inspired by women's ways of knowing* (pp. 372–392). New York: Basic Books.

Hussain, M. (2006). Take my riches, give me justice: A contextual analysis of Pakistan's honor crimes legislation. *Harvard Journal of Law & Gender, 29,* 223–246.

Irwin, L. G., Thorne, S., & Varcoe, C. (2002). Strength in adversity: Motherhood for women who have been battered. *Canadian Journal of Nursing Research, 34*(4), 47–57.

Jacobson, N., & Gottman, J. (1998). *When men batter women: New insights into ending abusive relationships.* NY: Simon & Schuster.

Johnson, M. P., & Ferraro, K. J. (2000). Research on domestic violence in the 1990s: Making distinctions. *Journal of Marriage and the Family, 62,* 948-963.

Johnson, M. P. (1995). Patriarchal terrorism and common couple violence: Two forms of violence against women. *Journal of Marriage and the Family, 57,* 283–294.

Johnson, M. P. (2006). Conflict and control: Gender symmetry and asymmetry in domestic violence. *Violence against Women, 12*(11), 1003–1018.

Johnson, M. P., & Leone, J. M. (2005). The differential effects of intimate terrorism and situational couple violence: Findings from the National Violence Against Women Survey. *Journal of Family Issues, 26*(3), 322–349.

Kantor, G. K. (1993). Refining the brushstrokes in portraits on alcohol and wife assaults. In *APA, Alcohol and interpersonal violence: fostering multidisciplinary perspectives* (pp. 281–290). Washington, DC: National Institute on Alcohol Abuse and Alcoholism, NIH.

Kantor, G. K., & Straus, M. A. (1987). The "drunken bum" theory of wife beating. *Social Problems, 34*(3), 213–230.

Kelly, U. (2006). "What will happen if I tell you?" Battered Latina women's experiences of healthcare. *Canadian Journal of Nursing Research, 38*(4), 78–95.

Kelly, U. (2009a). Integrating intersectionality and biomedicine in health disparities research. *Advances in Nursing Science, 32*(2), E42–E56.

Kelly, U. (2009b). "I'm a mother first": The influence of mothering in the decision-making processes of battered immigrant Latino women. *Research in Nursing & Health, 32*(3), 286–297.

Kirkwood, M. K., & Cecil, D. K. (2001). Marital rape: A student assessment of rape laws and the marital exemption. *Violence Against Women, 7*(11), 1234–1253.

Klein, E., Campbell, J., Soler, E., & Ghez, M. (1997). *Ending domestic violence: Changing public perceptions.* Newbury Park: Sage.

Kopels, S., & Sheridan, M. C. (2002). Adding legal insult to injury: Battered women, their children, and the failure to protect. *Affilia, 17*(1), 9–29.

Krug, E. G., Dahlberg, L. L., Mercy, J. A., Zwi, A. B., & Lozano, R. (2002). *World report on violence and health.* Geneva: World Health Organization.

Kub, J., Campbell, J. C., Rose, L., & Soeken, K. (1999). Role of substance use in the battering relationship. *Journal of Addictions Nursing, 11*(4), 171–179.

Landenburger, K. M. (1998). Exploration of women's identity: Clinical approaches with abused women. In J. C. Campbell (Ed.), *Empowering survivors of abuse: Health care for battered women and their children* (pp. 61–69). Thousand Oaks, CA: Sage.

Landenburger, K. (1989). A process of entrapment in and recovery from an abusive relationship. *Issues in Mental Health Nursing, 3,* 209–227.

Lazarus, R. S., & Folkman, S. (1984). *Stress, appraisal, and coping.* New York: Springer.

Lempert, L. B. (1996). Women's strategies for survival: Developing agency in abusive relationships. *Journal of Family Violence, 11*(3), 269–289.

Levant, R. F., & Pollack, W. S. (Eds.). (1995). *A new psychology of men.* New York: Basic.

Levinson, D. (1989). *Family violence in cross cultural perspective.* Newbury Park: Sage.

Lutz, K. F., Curry, M. A., Robrecht, L. C., Libbus, M. K., & Bullock, L. (2006). Double binding: Abusive intimate partner relationships, and pregnancy. *Canadian Journal of Nursing Research, 38*(4), 118–134.

Macey, D. (2001). *The Penguin dictionary of critical theory.* New York: Penguin Books.

Malamuth, N., Sockloskie, R., Koss, M., & Tanaka, J. (1991). Characteristics of aggressors against women: Testing a model using a national sample of college students. *Journal of Consulting and Clinical Psychology, 59,* 670–681.

Martin, S. L., Tsui, A. O., Maitra, K., & Marinshaw, R. (1999). Domestic violence in Northern India. *American Journal of Epidemiology, 150,* 417–426.

Maxfield, M. G., & Widom, C. S. (2001). An update on the "cycle of violence" (pp. 1–7). Washington, DC: U.S. Department of Justice. National Institute of Justice Research in Brief.

May, M. (1978). Violence in the family: An historical perspective. In J. P. Martin (Ed.), *Violence and the family* (pp. 135–163). Chicester: John Wiley & Sons.

Merritt-Gray, M., & Wuest, J. (1995). Counteracting abuse and breaking free: The process of leaving revealed through women's voices. *Health Care for Women International, 16*(5), 399–412.

Miedzian, M. (1991). *Boys will be Boys: Breaking the links between masculinity and violence.* NY: Anchor Doubleday.

Moe, A. (2007). Silenced voices and structured survival: Battered women's help seeking. *Violence Against Women, 13*(7), 676–699.

Mohanty, C. T., (2003). *Feminism without borders: Decolonizing theory, practicing solidarity.* Durham, NC: Duke University Press.

Mukamana, D., & Brysiewicz, P. (2008). The lived experience of genocide rape survivors in Rwanda. *Journal of Nursing Scholarship, 40*(4), 379–384.

Mullings, L., & Schulz, A. (2006). Intersectionality and health: An introduction. In A. J. Schulz & L. Mullings (Eds.), *Gender, race, class, and health: Intersectional approaches* (pp. 3–17). San Francisco, CA: Jossey-Bass.

Ortega, M. (2006). Being lovingly, knowingly ignorant: White feminism and women of color. *Hypatia, 21*(3), 56–74.

Owen, S. S., & Burke, T. W. (2004). An exploration of prevalence of domestic violence in same-sex relationships. *Psychological Reports, 95,* 129–132.

Painter, S. L., & Dutton, D. (1985). Patterns of emotional bonding in women: Traumatic bonding. *International Journal of Women's Studies, 8,* 363–375.

Pence, E., Paymar, M., Ritmeester, T., & Shepard, M. (Eds.) (1993). *Education groups for men who batter. The Duluth Model.* NY: Springer.

Phillips, D. (1998). Culture and systems of oppression in abused women's lives. *JOGNN, 27,* 678–683.

Phillips, D. (2006). Masculinity, male development, gender, and identity: Modern and postmodern meanings. *Issues in Mental Health Nursing, 27* (4), 403–423.

Pilcher, J. & Wheelan, I. (2004). *50 Key Concepts in Gender Studies.* London: Sage Publications.

Pleck, E. (1987). *Domestic tyranny: The making of American social policy against family violence from Colonial times to the present.* NY: Oxford University Press.

Power, S. (2002). *A problem from hell.* New York: Basic Books.

Rahlenbeck, S. I., & Mekonnen, W. (2009). Growing rejection of female genital cutting among women of reproductive age in Amhara, Ethiopia. *Culture, Health & Sexuality: An International Journal for Research, Intervention and Care, 11*(4), 443–452.

Raymond, J. G., & Hughes, D. M. (2001). *Sex trafficking of women in the United States: International and domestic trends.* United States Department of Justice.

Relf, M. V. (2001). Battering and HIV in men who have sex with men: A critique and synthesis of the literature. *Journal of the Association of Nurses in AIDS Care, 12*(3), 41–48.

Rennison, C. M. (2000). *Violent victimization and race, 1993-98.* Washington, DC: Bureau of Justice Statistics, US Department of Justice.

Rennison, C. M. (2003). *Intimate partner violence, 1993–2001.* Washington, DC: Department of Justice. Bureau of Justice Statistics.

Renzetti, C. M. (1992). *Violent betrayal: Partner abuse in lesbian relationships.* Thousand Oaks, CA: Sage.

Rhatigan, D. L., Moore, T. M., & Street, A. E. (2005). Reflections on partner violence: 20 Years of research and beyond. *Journal of Interpersonal Violence, 20*(1), 82–88.

Rich, A. (1979). *On lies, secrets, and silence.* New York: W. W. Norton.

Riley, R. L., Mohanty, C. T., & Pratt, M. B. (Eds.). (2008). *Feminism and war: Confronting U.S. imperialism.* London: Zed Books.

Roberts, D. (1997). *Killing the black body.* NY: Pantheon.

Roth, B. (2004). *Separate roads to feminism.* New York: Cambridge University Press.

Russell, D. (1990). *Rape in marriage.* New York: Collier.

Saltzman, L. E., Fanslow, J. L., McMahon, P. M., Shelley, G. A. (2002). Intimate partner violence surveillance: Uniform definitions and recommended data elements, Version 1.0, Atlanta, GA: National Center for Injury Prevention and Control, Centers for Disease Prevention.

Sampselle, C. M. (1991). The role of nursing in preventing violence against women. *Journal of Obstetric and Gynecological Nursing, 20,* 481–487.

Schram, D. (1978). Rape. In J. R. Chapman & M. Gates (Eds.). *The victimization of women* (pp. 53–79). Beverly Hills: Sage.

Schrock, D., & Schwalbe, M. (2009). Men, masculinity, and manhood acts. *Annual Review of Sociology, 35*(1), 277–295.

Shapiro, T. M. (1985) *Population control politics: Women, sterilization and reproduction choice.* Philadelphia: Temple University Press.

Sharps, P. W., Campbell, J. C., Campbell, D. W., Gary, F. A., & Webster, D. (2001). The role of alcohol use in intimate partner femicide. *The American Journal on Addictions 10,* 122–135.

Shepard, M. (2005). Twenty years of progress in addressing domestic violence: An agenda for the next 10. *Journal of Interpersonal Violence, 20*(4), 436–441.

Sherriff, N. (2007). Peer group cultures and social identity: An integrated approach to understanding masculinities. *British Educational Research Journal, 33*(2), 349–370.

Shiu-Thornton, S., Senturia, K., & Sullivan, M. (2005). "Like a bird in a cage": Vietnamese women survivors talk about domestic violence. *Journal of Interpersonal Violence, 20*(8), 959–976.

Silliman, J. M., & King, Y. (Eds.). (1999). *Dangerous intersections: Feminist perspectives on population, environment, and development*. Boston: South End Press.

Smith, M. D. (1987). The incidence and prevalence of woman abuse in Toronto. *Violence & Victims, 2*(3), 173–188.

Sokoloff, N. J., & Dupont, I. (2005). Domestic violence: Examining the intersections of race, class and gender—An introduction. In N. J. Sokoloff & C. Pratt (Eds.), *Domestic violence at the margins: Readings on race, class, gender and culture* (pp. 1–13). New Brunswick, NJ: Rutgers University Press.

Stanley, J., Bartholomew, K., Taylor, T., Oram, D., & Landolt, M. (2006). Intimate violence in male same-sex relationships. *Journal of Family Violence, 21*(1), 31–41.

Stark, E. (2007). *Coercive control: How men entrap women in personal life*. Oxford, UK: Oxford University Press.

Straus, M. (1980). Wife-beating: How common and why? In M. A. Straus & G. T. Hotaling (Eds.), *The social causes of husband-wife violence* (pp. 23–38). Minneapolis: University of Minnesota Press.

Straus, M., & Gelles, R. J. (1990). *Physical violence in American families*. New Brunswick, NJ: Transaction.

Swain, J. (2003). How young schoolboys become somebody: The role of the body in the construction of masculinity. *British Journal of Sociology of Education, 24*(3), 299–315.

Swan, S. C., & Snow, D. L. (2003). Behavioral and psychological differences among abused women who use violence in intimate relationships. *Violence against Women, 9*(1), 75–109.

Talle, A. (2007). Female circumcision in Africa and beyond: The anthropology of a difficult issue. In Y. Hernlund & B. Shell-Duncan (Eds.), *Transcultural bodies: Female genital cutting in global context.* (pp. 91–106). New Brunswick: Rutgers University Press.

Taylor, J. Y. (2004). Moving from surviving to thriving: African American women recovering from intimate partner abuse. *Research and Theory for Nursing Practice: An International Journal, 18*(1), 35–50.

Testa, M., & Leonard, K. E. (2001). The impact of husband physical aggression and alcohol use on marital functioning: Does alcohol "excuse" the violence. *Violence and Victims, 16* (5), 507–516.

Thompson, R. S., Bonomi, A. E., Anderson, M., Reid, R. J., Dimer, J. A., Carrell, D., et al. (2006). Intimate partner violence: Prevalence, types, and chronicity in adult women. *American Journal of Preventive Medicine, 30*(6), 447–457.

Tiger, L. (1969). *Men in groups*. NY: Random House.

Tjaden, P., Thoennes, N., & Allison, C. J. (1999). Comparing violence over the life span in samples of same-sex and opposite-sex cohabitants. *Violence & Victims, 14*(4), 413–426.

Tjaden, P., & Thoennes, N. (2000). *Full report of the prevalence, incidence, and consequences of violence against women*. Washington, D.C.: National Institute of Justice. NCJ-183781.

Toby, J. (1966). Violence and the masculine ideal: Some qualitative data. *Annals of the American Academy of Political and Social Science, 364*, 19–27.

Turell, S. C. (2000). A descriptive analysis of same-sex relationship violence for a diverse sample. *Journal of Family Violence, 15*(3), 281–293.

Ulrich, Y. C. (1991). Women's reasons for leaving abusive spouses. *Health Care for Women International, 12*, 465–473.

Ulrich, Y. C., Mckenna, L. S., King, C., Campbell, D. W., Ryan, J., Torres, S., et al. (2006). Postpartum mothers' disclosure of abuse, role, and conflict. *Health Care for Women International, 27*(4), 324–343.

United Nations. (2009). *World Population Prospects: The 2008 Revision, Highlights*. United Nations, Department of Economic and Social Affairs, Population Division.

Varcoe, C., & Irwin, L. G. (2004). "If I killed you, I'd get the kids": Women's survival and protection work with child custody and access in the context of woman abuse. *Qualitative Sociology, 27*(1), 77–99.

Waldner-Haugrud, L. K., Gratch, L. V., & Magruder, B. (1997). Victimization and perpetration rates of violence in gay and lesbian relationships: Gender issues explored. *Violence & Victims, 12*(2), 173–184.

Walker, L. E. (1984). *The battered woman syndrome*. NY: Springer.

Walker, L. E. (1979). *The battered woman*. NY: Harper and Row.

Warshaw, C., & Ganley, A. (1998). *Improving the health care response to domestic violence: A resource manual for health care providers*. San Francisco: Family Violence Prevention Fund.

Weber, L. (2006). Reconstructing the landscape of health disparities research: promoting dialogue and collaboration between feminist intersectional and biomedical paradigms. In: A. J. Schultz & L. Mullings (Eds.), *Gender, race, class and health: Intersectional approaches* (pp. 21–59). San Francisco, CA: Jossey-Bass.

Weber, L., & Parra-Medina, D. (2003). Intersectionality and women's health: Charting a path to eliminating health disparities. In M. T. Segal, V. Demos & J. J. Kronefeld (Eds.), *Gender perspectives on health and medicine, Volume 7: Advances in gender research* (pp. 181–230). Bingley, UK: Emerald Group Publishing.

West, C. M. (2002). Lesbian intimate partner violence: Prevalence and dynamics. *Journal of Lesbian Studies, 6*(1), 121–127.

West, C. M. (1998). Lifting the "political gag order:" Breaking the silence around partner violence in ethnic minority families. In J. L. Jasinski & L. M. Williams (Eds.), *Partner violence: A comprehensive review of 20 years of research* (pp. 184–209). Thousand Oaks, CA: Sage.

Weston, R., Temple, J. R., & Marshall, L. L. (2005). Gender symmetry and asymmetry in violent relationships: Patterns of mutuality among racially diverse women. *Sex Roles, 53*(7–8), 553–571.

WHO. (2008). Eliminating female genital mutilation: an interagency statement UNAIDS, UNDP, UNECA, UNESCO, UNFPA, UNHCHR, UNHCR, UNICEF, UNIFEM, WHO. Geneva: World Health Organization.

WHO (2009). Retrieved from http://www.who.int/violenceprevention/approach/ecology/en/index.html.

Wood, K., & Jewkes, R. (2001). Dangerous love: Reflections on violence among Xhosa township youth. In R. Morrell (Ed.) *Changing men in Southern Africa* (pp. 317–336). Pietermaritzburg, SA: University of Natal Press.

Wuest, J., Ford-Gilboe, M., Merritt-Gray, M., & Berman, H. (2003). Intrusion: The central problem for family health promotion among children and single mothers after leaving an abusive partner. *Qualitative Health Research, 13*(5), 597–622.

Wuest, J., & Merritt-Gray, M. (1999). Not going back: Sustaining the separation in the process of leaving abusive relationships. *Violence Against Women, 5*(2), 110–133.

Wuest, J., & Merritt-Gray, M. (2001). Beyond survival: reclaiming self after leaving an abusive male partner. *Canadian Journal of Nursing Research, 32*(4), 79–94.

Wuest, J., Merritt-Gray, M., & Ford-Gilboe, M. (2004). Regenerating family: strengthening the emotional health of mothers and children in the context of intimate partner violence. *Advances in Nursing Science, 27*(4), 257–274.

Xu, X., Campbell, J. C., & Zhu, F. (2001). Domestic violence against women in China: Prevalence, risk factors and health outcomes. Paper presented at the Annual American Public Health Association. Atlanta, GA.

Zambrana, R. E. (1987). A research agenda on issues affecting poor and minority women: A model for understanding their health needs. *Women & Health, 12*(3–4), 137–160.

Zink, T., Elder, N., & Jacobsen, J. (2003). How children affect the mother/victim's process in intimate partner violence. *Archives of Pediatrics and Adolescent Medicine, 157*(6), 587–592.

4

Theories and Research on Child Maltreatment

Susan J. Kelley, PhD, RN, FAAN

EPIDEMIOLOGY

Child maltreatment (CM) is a serious social and public health concern that occurs globally, with serious health and legal implications. The term child maltreatment encompasses physical, sexual, and psychological abuse as well as neglect. During 2007, the most recent year that federal data were available, there were 3.2 million referrals to child protective services (CPS) for cases of suspected maltreatment in the United States involving 5.8 million children (Children's Bureau, 2009). Of these referrals, 794,000 cases of child maltreatment were confirmed by CPS, representing a decrease from the previous year's estimate of 905,000 victims of child maltreatment in 2006, representing a 12% decrease (Children's Bureau, 2008). It is important to note that the actual numbers of children who experience child maltreatment is believed to be considerably higher because only a small proportion of cases are actually reported to CPS.

The younger the child, the greater the risk of child maltreatment, with children under the age of 1 year having the highest rate of victimization at 21.9 per 1,000 children (Children's Bureau, 2009). Slightly more than half (51.5%) were females. Approximately one-half of all victims were Caucasian (46.1), 21.7% were African American, and 20.8% were Hispanic. While physical and sexual abuses often receive the most attention in the media and other public venues, neglect is, by far, the most common form of CM involving nearly 60% of all cases. It is followed by physical abuse (10.8%), sexual abuse (7.6%), and psychological abuse (4.2%) in terms of prevalence.

It is estimated that 1,760 children died from either neglect or physical abuse in 2007, with neglect being the more common cause. Of these child fatalities, children younger than 4 years are at greatest risk and involved more than three-quarters (75.7%) of the cases. Of children in this age group, those 1 year of age and younger are of greatest risk, with boys being at the highest risk for fatalities (Children's Bureau, 2009). An analysis of longitudinal data was conducted to determine whether low-income children, who survived a first incident of reported child maltreatment, were at higher risk of later childhood death compared to a matched comparison group of low-income children without reports of maltreatment (Jonson-Reid, Chance, & Drake, 2007). In contrast to the comparison group, children in the maltreatment group had about twice the risk of death before age 18. Among children with maltreatment reports, median time from first report to subsequent death was 9 months. The majority of deaths among children in the maltreatment group were due to accidents or recurrent maltreatment, as opposed to serious illness.

Nearly 80% of perpetrators of CM are parents, and another 6.6% were other relatives of the victim. Women comprised a larger percentage of all perpetrators than men with 56.5% compared to 42.4%. This finding is not surprising given that mothers tend to spend much more time with their children than do fathers. Nearly 17% (16.8%) were maltreated by both parents.

HISTORICAL CONTEXT

It is important to place the phenomenon of child maltreatment in a historical context. The first well-known case of child maltreatment in the United States involved a child in New York City named Mary Ellen Connolly in the late 1800s who had been severely beaten. Because there were no laws protecting children, her legal case was brought before the New York Society for the Prevention of Cruelty to Animals. The public outcry this case received in the public arena led to the establishment of the New York Society for Prevention of Cruelty to Children, the first of its kind in the United States. By the early 1900s there were 161 such organizations in the United States.

It is important to note that it was not until the 1940s that the Supreme Court determined that states have the authority to protect children. By 1967, 44 states had implemented mandatory child abuse-reporting laws. In 1974, the federal government passed the Child Abuse Prevention and Treatment Act (CAPTA) requiring states to adopt mandatory reporting laws in order to qualify for federal funds for the investigation of CM. It also required immunity for mandated reporters.

Caffey's 1946 classic article "Multiple Fractures in the Long Bones of Infants Suffering from Chronic Subdural Hematoma" was the first article in a medical journal to question the occurrence of these injuries together, as well as their cause (Caffey, 1946). Caffey had the insight to suggest that the fractures in the long bones may have been caused by the same traumatic forces that were responsible for the traumatic brain injuries and implied that infliction by parents may have been a possibility. Although not labeled "child abuse" per se, Caffey's paper was the first to suggest the possibility of severe abuse of children by caregivers. In 1962, physician C. Henry Kempe and colleagues published a seminal paper in the *Journal of the American Medical Association* entitled "The Battered-Child Syndrome" (Kempe, Silverman, Steele, Droegemueller, & Silver, 1962). In it, they estimated that as many of 500 children in the United States were abused each year. This paper created the first professional awareness of physical abuse of children.

THEORETICAL FRAMEWORKS

A number of theoretical frameworks have been postulated to explain the complex phenomenon of CM. Psychological or pathologic conceptualizations focus on caregiver characteristics, while sociological perspectives are based on factors such as poverty and violent environments. More recent theoretical modes of CM are multifactorial and take into account parental, child, and environmental variables.

Ecological Model

A multifactorial model of CM is the developmental–ecological perspective proposed by Belsky (1993). It grew out of the ecological model first proposed by Bronfenbrenner (1979) who offered a framework for organizing sets of environmental systems. He proposes four contexts, or layers, which range from the most immediate settings, such as the family or peer group, to the more remote contexts in which the child is not directly involved, such as local government. This model is widely used by researchers and clinicians in the field of family violence (Almgren, 2005; Casey & Lindhorst, 2009; Freisthler, Merritt, & LaScala, 2006; Mohr & Tulman, 2000; Little & Kantor, 2002).

The developmental–ecological perspective conceptualizes CM as a social and psychological phenomenon determined by multiple forces acting within the individual, family, community, and culture. Thus, it is multiply determined by a variety of factors operating

---

EXHIBIT 4.1 | *Overview of Theoretical Frameworks and Models of Child Maltreatment*

Ecological Model of Child Maltreatment (CM)
Determined by multiple forces within the:
- Individual
- Family
- Community
- Culture

Transactional processes of analysis in context of parent–child interaction
- Balance of potentiating and compensatory factors determines whether CM occurs
- No single cause and no single solution to problem

Stress and Coping Model
Caregiver's cognitive appraisal and coping strategies play important role in occurrence of CM
- Four major components:
  - Potential stressors, including child, parental, and ecological
  - Cognitive appraisals
  - Coping resources
  - Caregiver behaviors
- Components linked by multiple pathways

Developmental Victimology
Examines victimization and other negative experiences across childhood
- While children can experience the same victimizations as adults, they differ primarily by their status as dependents.
- Children are the most criminally victimized people in society due to:
  - Immaturity in controlling own behavior
  - Weak sanctions concerning offenses against children
  - Children's inability to control with whom they interact

Attachment Theory
Used extensively to explain development and potential disruptions in relational processes
- Attachment emerges in a consistent series of steps in first 6 months of life
- During second 6 months of life, infant forms specific attachments to caregivers
- Infants and toddlers who are maltreated form insecure attachments
- Many aspects of social, emotional, and cognitive development are related to early attachment profiles, with insecure attachments predicting negative outcomes

through transactional processes at various levels of analysis in the broad ecology of parent–child interactions.

The first level of analysis involves individual characteristics of the parent and child. At the parent level, risk factors include parental distress, including depression, substance abuse, parental history of CM and corporal punishment, and poor impulse control. Unrealistic and distorted expectations of children can lead to abuse through a caregiver's lack of knowledge of normal, age-appropriate child behaviors. For example, some abusive parents believe that young infants cry for attention because they are "spoiled." Crowded or inadequate housing, and unemployment can also enhance a parent's potential for abuse. Child risk factors include age of child, with younger children at greatest risk; developmental delays; and chronic illness. At the family level, CM is more likely to occur in families experiencing poverty, interpersonal violence, social isolation, and stress (Mohr & Tulman, 2000). At the community level, risk factors include high levels of neighborhood crime and violence, as well as high levels of drug and alcohol abuse. At the societal level, influences include government resources for families living in poverty, laws and policies aimed at protecting children, professional attitudes, and the current economy.

According to this model, the balance of stressors and supports—that is, the balance of potentiating (risk) and compensatory (preventive) factors, determines whether maltreatment occurs. When stressors outweigh supports, or when potentiating factors are not balanced by compensatory ones, the probability of CM increases. Thus, there is no single cause of CM and no single solution to the problem.

Stress and Coping Model

Another comprehensive conceptualization of CM is the stress and coping model proposed by Hillison and Kuiper (1994). This model documents the various ways in which stress levels may become increased in caregivers and thus contribute to the likelihood of CM. According to this model, caregiver's cognitive appraisals and coping strategies are believed to play an important role in the occurrence of CM as shown in Figure 4.1.

The four major components of the stress and coping model are (1) potential stressors, including parental, child, and ecological; (2) cognitive appraisals, including primary and secondary; (3) coping resources; and (4) caregiver behaviors that include facilitative behaviors, as well as neglectful and abusive behaviors. These components are linked by multiple pathways, reflecting the interactive and dynamic nature of the various elements of the stress and coping process. The model acknowledges the multideterminate nature of maltreatment, beginning with the need for continuous monitoring of parental, child, and ecological factors as potential stressors. Whether these factors are stressful is determined by primary cognitive appraisals. If these primary appraisals indicated the presence of a stressor, secondary appraisals are used to determine what internal and external resources are available to the caregiver to cope with it.

The type of coping behavior that is sought from the caregiver depends on the outcome of the primary and secondary appraisals, with the coping response determined, in part, by the caregivers' coping dispositions or tendencies. Caregiver's coping strategies may be facilitative and not result in maltreatment, or may be less facilitative and result in child neglect. Coping responses such as those that focus on emotions and venting of emotions may be quite maladaptive and result in child abuse.

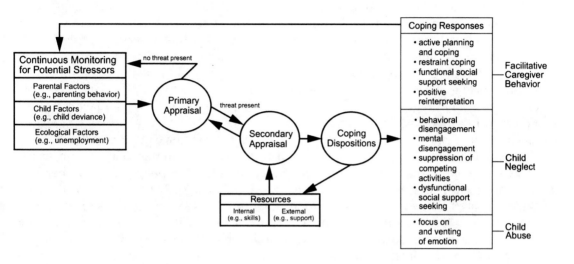

FIGURE 4.1 Stress and coping model. *Source:* Hillison, J. K. C. & Kuiper, N. A. (1994). A stress and coping model of child maltreatment. *Clinical Psychological Review, 14,* 261–285. Reprinted with permission from Elsevier.

Developmental Victimology

More recently, Finkelhor (2008) has proposed the concept of developmental victimology. Developmental victimology looks at child victimization across childhood and is concerned with negative life experiences that stand apart from other life events. While children can experience the same victimizations as adults do, such as homicides, robberies, sexual assault, children differ from adults in their victimization experiences, primarily because of their status as dependents. The types of victimization that children suffer can be arrayed on a continuum of dependency, according to the degree to which they violate a child's dependency status. This comprehensive approach encompasses the prevention, treatment, and study of child victims, unifying conventional subdivisions such as child sexual and physical abuse, bullying, and exposure to community violence.

Finkelhor (2008) effectively argues that children are the most criminally victimized people in society. Their increased vulnerability is attributed to several factors: (1) children's developmental immaturity in controlling their own behavior, (2) society's tolerance for or weak sanctions concerning offenses against children, and (3) children's lesser ability to regulate and choose who they associate and interact with.

Attachment Theory

Attachment theory has been used extensively to explain the development and potential disruption in relational processes, especially as it pertains to child maltreatment (Cicchetti, Rogosch, & Toth, 2006; Morton & Browne, 1998). It is based on the early work of Bowlby (1982) who posited that attachment is the result of a set of instinctual responses that are important for the protection and survival of the species. Infant behaviors, such as crying, smiling, clinging, and following, elicit necessary parental care and protection for the infant and promote physical and emotional contact between the mother and infant. As a result of these biologically based systems, mothers and infants develop mutual attachments to each other. Almost all infants become attached to their primary caregivers, even when the caregivers are abusive or neglectful. However, not all attachment relationships foster positive development.

Attachment emerges in a consistent series of steps in the first 6 months of life. Initially, the infant is attracted to all social objects and comes to prefer human to inanimate objects. Next, the infant learns to discriminate familiar and unfamiliar people. Finally, the infant develops the capacity to form a special relationship with specific individuals with whom the infant actively seeks to maintain contact. During the second 6 months of life, the infant begins to form specific attachments. Infants learn to differentiate the mother from others and must become aware that people and objects still exist even when not visible. When mothers are sensitive and responsive to their infants' cues and respond promptly and consistently, they form secure attachments with their infants. When mothers are either insensitive or unresponsive, their infants will learn to avoid them by looking away or refusing their attempts to interact.

Studies have shown that despite their experiences with abuse and neglect, infants and toddlers develop an attachment, although insecure in most cases, with their parents, with the majority of research focusing on mothers (Cicchetti et al., 2006; Morton & Browne, 1998; Zeanah & Smyke, 2005). These children typically develop a disorganized, insecure attachment pattern with their primary caregiver (Cicchetti et al., 2006). Based on an analysis of the research literature on attachment and maltreatment, Morton and Browne (1998) concluded that (1) quality of infant attachment is most dependent upon the sensitiveness of the mother, (2) maltreated children are less securely attached to their mothers than nonmaltreated children, and (3) this early mother–infant relationship is internalized by the child and consequently forms a prototype by which all future relationships are assimilated leading to problems forming relationships with peers, partners, and their own children. The authors postulate that this is the primary process by which child maltreatment continues from one generation to the next.

In a study involving 137 maltreated 1-year olds, mothers in the maltreatment group, relative to the nonmaltreatment group of mothers, reported greater abuse and neglect in their own childhoods, more insecure relationships with their own mothers, more maladaptive parenting attitudes, more parenting stress, and lower family support, and they were observed to show lower maternal sensitivity (Cicchetti et al., 2006). Infants in the maltreatment groups had significantly higher rates of disorganized attachment than children in the comparison group.

Longitudinal studies that have addressed the relation between early attachment and later social functioning in preschool, school, and other social settings have demonstrated that many aspects of social, emotional, and cognitive development are related to early attachment profiles (Carson, Sroufe, & Egeland, 2004; Schneider, Atkinson, & Tardif, 2001). Research findings have demonstrated the negative long-term impact of insecure and disorganized attachments into adulthood (Cicchetti et al., 2006; Schneider et al., 2001).

RISK FACTORS FOR CHILD MALTREATMENT

Research findings indicate that certain societal, community, family, parental, and child characteristics are associated with an increased risk for CM (Exhibit 4.2).

A combination of individual, familial, community, and societal factors contributes to the likelihood that a caregiver will abuse a child. Parental factors that contribute to the potential for abuse include parenting stress and belief in the value of corporal punishment (Crouch & Behl, 2001). Other parental risk factors include unrealistic expectations of children, role reversal, lack of preparation for the parenting role, lack of empathy, and poor parental role models. Psychological factors may include poor impulse control, cognitive disorders, substance abuse disorder, and depression or other mental health

---

EXHIBIT 4.2 | *Risk Factors For Child Maltreatment*

Societal factors:
- Laws and policies intended to protect children
- State of the economy
- Lack of adequate resources for economically challenged families
- Weak norms and sanctions against violence

Community risk factors:
- High levels of drug use and alcohol availability in neighborhood
- High levels of violence in community

Family risk factors:
- Substance abuse
- Social isolation; lack of family support
- Intimate partner violence/domestic violence
- Poverty (major single risk factor for neglect)
- Economic pressures and other stressors
- Crowded or inadequate housing

Parental risk factors associated with child maltreatment:
- Low self-esteem
- Mental health issues
- Social isolation
- Belief in physical punishment
- Unrealistic expectations of children
- Parental role reversal
- Lack of empathy to child's needs
- Childhood history of abuse
- Depression or other mental health disorder
- Substance abuse
- History criminal activity or incarceration
- Young mothers ($\leq$18 years)

Child risk factors associated with child maltreatment:
- Premature birth
- Prenatal drug exposure
- Developmental disability
- Physical disability
- Chronic illness
- Product of a multiple birth

disorders. Neglectful parents are often economically disadvantaged, socially isolated, lack adequate social support, and have low self-esteem.

Children whose mothers are physically abused by their husbands or other intimate partners are themselves clearly at increased risk of physical abuse. Researchers found that 92% of couples who reported physical aggression between the partners also reported severe aggression toward a child (Smith Slep & O'Leary, 2005). Other studies have demonstrated that children in families in which IPV has occurred are between two and four times more likely to be abused subsequently than children in families without IVP (Casanueva, Martin, & Runyan, 2009; Cox, Kotch, & Everson, 2003; Lee, Kotch, & Cox, 2004). Furthermore, children reported to CPS whose mothers experience intimate partner violence (IPV) are twice likely to be rereported for subsequent abuse (Casanueva et al., 2009). (Please refer to chapter 11 for an in-depth discussion on children of mothers who experience IPV). Other child risk factors for maltreatment include prematurity, chronic illness, developmental delays, and behavior problems. Child maltreatment needs to be considered within its cultural context as child-rearing practices can vary greatly across various cultural and ethnic groups.

Physical abuse may consist of excessive corporal punishment. Parents who over-discipline their children cross the fine line between what some would consider acceptable forms of physical discipline and what the law would consider a reportable case of abuse. The abuse may take place while parents are attempting to "teach the child a lesson" in order to change what they perceive as unacceptable or bad behavior. Unrealistic and distorted expectations of children can lead to abuse through a caregiver's lack of knowledge of normal, age-appropriate child behaviors. For example, some abusive parents believe that young infants cry for attention because they are "spoiled."

Intergenerational Transmission of Child Maltreatment

While the early experience of abuse or harsh punishment is regarded as a potential vehicle for the transmission of abusive behavior, it is important to note that a history of maltreatment in childhood does not necessarily lead to parents who are abusive or neglectful of their own children (Kolko, 2002). In what is now considered a classic paper, Widom (1989) reviewed three decades of research on the so-called "intergenerational transmission of child maltreatment" and concludes that most children who are abused do not subsequently abuse their own children. It is estimated that only 30% of abused children become abusive parents (Kaufman & Zigler, 1987). Subsequent involvement in emotionally supportive relationships decreases the likelihood that an abused child will become a maltreating parent.

TYPES OF MALTREATMENT

Child maltreatment is generally divided into four major categories: (1) physical abuse, (2) sexual abuse, (3) psychological abuse, and (4) neglect. Each state's child protective reporting law provides definitions of physical abuse, sexual abuse, and neglect, with these definitions varying slightly from one state to another. The following are generally accepted definitions.

EXHIBIT 4.3 | *Types of Maltreatment*

Physical abuse
- Physical injury intentionally inflicted on child younger than 18 years by parent or other caregiver
- Includes being hit with hand or object or being kicked, shaken, thrown, burned, stabbed or choked

Sexual abuse
- Any sexual activity between a child and adult (or considerably older child)
- Can involve force, persuasion, or coercion

Psychological maltreatment
- Parental behaviors that include spurning, degrading, terrorizing, isolating, exploiting, corrupting, or rejecting
- Can occur through acts of commission or omission

Neglect
- Caregiver's failure to meet a child's basic needs, including needs for:
  - Food
  - Protection
  - Shelter
  - Clothing
  - Health care
  - Education
  - Safety

Physical Abuse

Physical abuse refers to physical injury intentionally inflicted on a child younger than 18 years by a parent or caregiver through the use of excessive and inappropriate physical force. This may include being hit with a hand or other object, or having been kicked, shaken, thrown, burned, stabbed, or choked.

Sexual Abuse

Sexual abuse refers to any sexual activity between a child and an adult (or considerably older child), where consent is not or cannot be given. Sexual abuse can involve force, persuasion, or coercion. It can include acts such as penetration, sexual touching, or non-contact sexual acts such as exhibitionism, using sexually explicit language, showing children sexually explicit materials, involving children in the production of sexually explicit materials, and voyeurism.

Psychological Maltreatment

Psychological maltreatment involves parental behaviors that include spurning, degrading, terrorizing, isolating, exploiting/corruptive, or rejecting. It can include perpetrator acts of commission or omission.

Neglect

Neglect refers to the caregiver's failure to meet a child's basic needs, including its needs for food, protection, shelter, clothing, health care, education, and safety. Unlike physical abuse, neglect typically involves acts of omission rather than commission and may, or may not, be intentional.

Although the behaviors that characterize these forms of maltreatment are distinct from each other, it is important to note that multiple types of child maltreatment often occur simultaneously or over the course of childhood.

CHILD MALTREATMENT IN THE CONTEXT OF SUBSTANCE ABUSE

Children in the United States are at risk of being impacted by drug or alcohol abuse within the family. For instance, 23.8% of children live in a household where a parent or other adult is a binge or heavy drinker, and 12.7% live in a household where a parent or other adult uses illicit drugs (National Center on Addiction and Substance Abuse, 2005). Recognition of the serious role that substance abuse plays in child maltreatment is growing, as evidenced by the emerging body of research linking substance abuse and CM.

While the association between prenatal substance abuse and negative birth outcomes has received considerable attention in the research literature over the past two decades, the caregiving environment after birth has received far less attention. The caregiving environment of children exposed prenatally to substances of abuse is often far more detrimental to child outcomes than the actual prenatal exposure to drugs. Numerous studies have found a strong association between child maltreatment and substance abuse (Besinger, Garland, Litrownick, & Landsverk, 1999; Hanson, Self-Brown, Fricker-Elhai, Kilpatrick, Saunders, & Resnick, 2006; Kelleher, Chaffin, Hollenberg, & Fisher, 1994; Nair, Schuler, Black, Kettinger, & Harrington, 2003; Sprang, Clark, & Bass, 2005).

One study, in which researchers analyzed data from the National Institute of Mental Health (NIMH) Epidemiological Catchment Area Study, found that even after controlling for household factors and Diagnostic and Statistical Manual-Axis II disorders, any alcohol or drug use disorder was associated with increased maltreatment and, in fact, tripled the risk of maltreatment (Kelleher et al., 1994). In a study of 639 children removed from their homes because of CM, evidence of caregiver substance abuse was found in 79% of the cases (Besinger et al., 1999). Hanson et al. (2006) examined data from a nationally representative sample of 4,023 adolescents who participated in the National Survey of Adolescents. The researchers found physical abuse to be 2.0 and 2.4 times more likely among families in which alcohol and drug use were present.

Substance abuse appears to contribute to parental characteristics such as low frustration tolerance, disinhibited aggression, interference with good judgment, and preoccupation with alcohol and drug-seeking behaviors (Kelley, 2002). The co-occurrence of mental health disorders in parents who are substance abusers may also place them at risk for maltreating behaviors. Furthermore, substance-abusing families are less likely than nonsubstance-abusing families to comply with interventions aimed at protecting their children.

Numerous studies have found a co-occurrence of mental health disorders in substance-abusing mothers who abuse or neglect their children (Chaffin, Kelleher, Hollenberg, 1996; Espinosa, Beckwith, Tyler, & Swanson, 2001; Nair et al., 2003). For instance in the study by Nair et al., 70% of participants reported depressive symptomatology. These findings related to the co-occurrence of substance abuse and mental health disorders in parents who maltreat children, underscore the need for widespread screening for depression and other psychological disorders, as well as for substance abuse in high-risk populations. Screening for depression and substance abuse is relatively inexpensive in terms of cost and time and can be easily conducted by health and social service professionals using standardized measures.

As noted above, there has been considerable attention given to prenatal use of illicit drugs. Alcohol, however, appears to have the direst consequences of all forms of prenatal substance abuse. It is the only prenatal substance of abuse that has proven to have irreversible negative effects, including intellectual impairment, neurological deficits, facial anomalies, and growth retardation. An estimated 12,000 infants are born each year with fetal alcohol syndrome. A much greater number of infants suffer from more subtle effects of prenatal alcohol exposure. It is important to note that many infants exposed to alcohol in utero are also exposed to illicit drugs.

An often overlooked consequence of parental substance abuse is the direct exposure of children to substances *after* birth. The literature contains numerous reports of children being exposed to illicit drugs beyond the neonatal period. Reports indicate that children living with substance-abusing parents are at risk for passive exposure to marijuana, methamphetamines, phencyclidine (PCP), and crack cocaine when these substances are smoked (Kelley, 2002). Signs and symptoms of passive inhalation of cocaine and PCP can include ataxia, epistaxis, hypotonia, dehydration, lethargy, nystagmus, vomiting, diarrhea, seizures, apnea, coma, and death (Henretig, Paschall, & Donaruma-Kwoh, 2009). Clinical manifestations of passive inhalation to marijuana/THC include ataxia, sluggish pupils, lethargy, hyperactivity, and irritability (Henretig et al., 2009). Children have also been known to die from intentional and unintentional ingestion of illicit drugs.

Exposure to methamphetamine in the home has become a significant health hazard for children. So-called "mom and pop" labs for manufacturing the drug have spread from west to east and can now be found in almost every state (National Center on Addiction and Substance Abuse, 2005). The materials and chemicals used to make the drug are highly explosive and toxic, and the fumes that emanate from the lab can cause significant physical damage or death. In 2003, 8,000 methamphetamine labs were raided, with 3,300 children found. Forty-eight children were burned, or injured, and one killed during lab explosions (National Center on Addiction and Substance Abuse, 2005). Unfortunately, it is all too common for adults who make this drug in their homes to store the materials or drug itself in places such as the kitchen or garage, where there is ample opportunity for children to access the drug and accidentally ingest it.

In 2005, federal and state governments spent at least $3.3 trillion to operate government and provide public services such as education, health care, income assistance, child welfare, mental health, law enforcement and justice services, transportation, and highway safety. Embedded in this spending was $373.9 billion, or 11.2%, that was spent on problems associated with tobacco, alcohol, and other drug abuse. It is noteworthy that only 1.9% of funds spent on substance abuse and addiction are spent on prevention or treatment of addiction (National Center on Addiction and Substance Abuse, 2009).

EFFECTS OF CHILD MALTREATMENT

Research has clearly established that CM has serious immediate and long-term consequences. It negatively affects the cognitive, emotional, social, and in some instances physical development of children, and often with negative impact across the life span.

Consequences in Childhood

Numerous studies have documented the relationship between various types of CM and psychological harm in childhood (Cicchetti et al., 2006; Holbrook, Hoyt, Coimbra, Potenza, Sise, & Anderson, 2005; Pears, Kim, & Fisher, 2008; Ward & Haskett, 2008). CM is also associated with lower performance on tests of intelligence, developmental delays, behavioral and emotional problems, and poor academic performance (Daignault & Herbert, 2009; Holbrook et al., 2005; Kendall-Tackett & Eckenrode, 1996; Shonk & Cicchetti, 2001). Maltreatment also is associated with disruptions in several stage-salient areas of development, including emotion regulation, the formation of secure attachment relationships, development of an autonomous and integrated self-system, effective peer relationships, and successful adaptation to school (Flores, Cicchetti, & Rogosch, 2005).

Neurobiological research has shown that early abuse results in altered physiological response to stressful stimuli, a response that negatively affects the child's subsequent socialization (Stirling & Amaya-Jackson, 2008). Children who have suffered early abuse or neglect may later present with significant behavior problems including emotional difficulties, depression, and aggressive or violent behaviors. Problematic behavior may continue long after the abuse or neglect has ended, even when they are living in supportive environments such as in foster care or an adoptive home.

In cases of child abuse or neglect in which the stress is typically prolonged, long-term stress reactions are common and can be particularly damaging. In children suffering from the sequelae of early stress, the offending stimulus, even when seemingly minor, can produce a dramatic emotional reaction that is disproportionate to the provocation. Stimuli that produce such reactions are referred to as traumatic reminders and may take on many forms. Symptoms can be grouped into three main clusters: (a) re-experiencing

---

EXHIBIT 4.4 | *Effects of Childhood Maltreatment*

Consequences in childhood:
- Altered physiological response to stressful stimuli
- Behavior problems
- Attachment disorders
- Depression
- Posttraumatic stress disorder

Consequences in adulthood:
- Substance abuse disorders
- Depression
- Anxiety
- Posttraumatic stress disorder
- Suicidality

through intrusive thoughts, dreams, and flashbacks; (b) avoidance of reminders and numbing of responsiveness, including social withdrawal; and (c) physiological hyper-arousal in the form of hypervigilance and exaggerated startle response, attention problems, and sleep disturbance (Stirling & Amaya-Jackson, 2008). These systems in abused and neglected children are consistent with posttraumatic stress disorder (PTSD), which can lead to anatomical differences including smaller brain volumes and size differences in limbic system, the area of the brain that supports a variety of functions such as emotion, behavior, and long-term memory. Trauma in childhood is also associated with prolonged exposure to cortisol, which is critical to the body's stress response. The exaggerated behavioral responses to complex PTSD have durable anatomical and physiological underpinnings resulting in behavioral and developmental consequences and can be very difficult to change (Stirling & Amaya-Jackson, 2008).

While most physical injuries resulting from child abuse will heal with relatively little long-term physical disability, some inflicted injuries can lead to permanent and severe neurological problems, including motor deficits, blindness, seizure, cerebral palsy, or permanent cognitive impairment (Rubin, Feinstein, & Berkowitz, 2009). Death from inflicted head injuries is reported to occur in approximately 13% to 36% of cases, exceeding the 6% to 12% mortality rate for noninflicted head injuries (Rubin et al., 2009).

Intervention with Maltreated Children

Although research has documented that children suffer short- and long-term consequences of maltreatment, most abused children do not receive therapy. Children who have experienced any form of maltreatment should be referred for a psychological evaluation to determine whether there is a need for therapy. Those who have been severely abused may need in-patient treatment. Because child maltreatment most often occurs in the family setting, therapy must address not only the child's individual needs, but family dysfunction as well.

Treatment modalities frequently used with abused children include individual therapy, group therapy, family therapy, play therapy, and art therapy. A core tenet of contemporary approaches to therapy for maltreated children, adolescents, and adults is that it should be trauma-focused and incorporate a cognitive behavioral approach. Evidence-based, trauma-focused therapy borrows from a wide variety of behavioral, cognitive, systemic, and dynamic therapeutic techniques. It is based on the concept that abuse is a form of victimization by the powerful of the relatively powerless and that the sequelae of abuse are readily understandable if not expected "normal" adaptations to abnormal experiences. Trauma-focused therapy emphasizes describing, exploring, and comprehending the individual's experience of the abuse.

Long-Term Consequences

Over the past three decades, researchers have identified the long-term adverse impact of child maltreatment and adult psychological and physical health (Anda et al., 2002; Banyard, Williams, Saunders, & Fitzgerald, 2008; Chapman, Whitfield, Feletti, Dube, Edwards, & Anda, 2004; Edwards, Holden, Feletti, & Anda, 2003; Roberts, O'Connor, Dunn, & Golding, 2004). The mental health consequences include PTSD, depression, anxiety, dissociative disorder, suicidality, nonsuicidal self-injurious behaviors, and substance abuse disorders (Afifi, Boman, Fleisher, & Sareen, 2009; Anda, Whitfield, Feletti, et al, 2002; Edwards et al., 2003; Yates, Carlson, & Egeland, 2008; Schumm, Briggs-Philip, & Hobfoll, 2006).

In a large study of low-income, urban-dwelling women, those with histories of child maltreatment or adult rape were six times more likely to develop PTSD symptoms than those without such a history (Schumm et al., 2006). Participants who experienced both child abuse and adult rape had PTSD rates 17 times the comparison group. In another significant study, researchers using a prospective cohort of maltreated children, ages 0–11, were matched with nonmaltreated children and followed into adulthood (Wilson & Widom, 2008). Early sexual contact, promiscuity, and prostitution were assessed through in-person interviews and official records for prostitution. Results indicated that child maltreatment was associated with prostitution and early sexual contact. Furthermore, participants in the maltreated group were twice as likely as the controls to test positive for HIV in middle adulthood.

Researchers tested the hypothesis that children who are maltreated earlier in life are at greater risk for poor psychological function in adulthood, compared to those maltreated later in life (Kaplow & Widom, 2007). They prospectively examined onset of maltreatment at three time classifications: (1) continuous from ages 0–11; (2) dichotomous (early, 0–5 years, vs later, 6–11 years); and (3) developmental (infancy, 0–2 years; preschool 3–5 years; early school age, ages 6–8 years, and school age, 9–11 years). Individuals with documental cases of maltreatment ($N = 496$) were followed-up and assessed in adulthood. Results indicated that earlier onset of maltreatment, measured dichotomously and developmentally, was predictive of more symptoms of anxiety and depression in adulthood.

Recent research confirms the fundamental hypothesis that childhood victimization leads to increased vulnerability for subsequent revictimization in adolescence and adulthood. Using a prospective cohort design, researchers studied participants with documented past histories of childhood physical and sexual abuse and neglect comparing them to participants with no known history of child maltreatment (Widom, Czaja, & Dutton, 2008). Both groups were interviewed in person using an instrument to assess lifetime trauma and victimization history. Abused and neglected individuals reported a higher number of traumas and victimization experiences than comparisons. All types of childhood maltreatment were associated with increased risk for lifetime revictimization. Childhood victimization increased the risk for physical and sexual assault/abuse, kidnapping/stalking, and having a family friend murdered or commit suicide, but not for general traumas, witnessing trauma, or crime victimization. The authors conclude that the finding provides strong support for the need for early intervention with abused and neglected children and their families to prevent subsequent exposure to traumas and victimization experiences.

Over the past decade, a body of research has emerged that demonstrates an association between childhood maltreatment and chronic physical health conditions (Corso, Edwards, Fang, & Mercy, 2008; Prosser & Corso, 2007; Rodgers, Lang, Laffaye, Satz, Dresselhaus, & Stein, 2004). There is evidence that child maltreatment can cause an increase in risky behavior later in life such as smoking, alcoholism, drug use, eating disorders, obesity, and sexual promiscuity that can certainly contribute to chronic physical health problems (Prosser & Corso, 2007). In a study involving 221 female participants attending a primary care clinic, researchers found that sexual, physical, and emotional abuse and emotional neglect were related to different health behaviors (Rodgers et al., 2004).

Sexual abuse was associated with current use of tobacco and alcohol, having driven while intoxicated, and being younger at first pregnancy and first consensual intercourse. Physical abuse was related to engaging in less frequent exercise, alcohol use, smoking during pregnancy, and younger age at both first pregnancy and consensual intercourse. The more types of childhood maltreatment participants were exposed to the more likely they were to have problems with substance abuse and risky sexual behaviors in adulthood.

Researchers, comparing health-related quality of life of 2,812 adults maltreated in childhood to 3,356 adults with no history of child maltreatment, found that persons who experienced childhood maltreatment had significant and sustained losses in health-related quality of life relative to persons who did not experience maltreatment (Corso et al., 2008). Other researchers examined the association between self-reported health and physical and/or sexual abuse experience before age 18 years in a sample of 3,568 of women, aged 18–64 years, and enrolled in a prepaid health care plan (Bonomi, Cannon, Anderson, Rivara, & Thomson, 2008). Poorest health status was found in women with a history of both physical and sexual abuse. Women with both abuse types had increased prevalence of moderate and severe depression, physical symptoms from joint pain to nausea, and poorer overall health. Women with physical abuse only or sexual abuse only also had higher prevalence of symptoms and lower overall health scores, but the associations were not as strong.

Resilience to Maltreatment

There are various definitions and uses of the terms resiliency and resilience. Because resiliency infers an enduring characteristic or personality trait, most researchers prefer to use the term resilient. In the context of child maltreatment, it refers to the minority of child victims who display little or no symptomatology compared to other maltreated children. While the majority of research on child maltreatment over the past three decades has focused on its negative sequelae, a smaller number of studies have reported that a minority of individuals exposed to child maltreatment manifest little or no negative outcomes. Extant studies on resilience to child maltreatment are often challenged by lack of standard definitions for resilience, risk, competence, and child maltreatment (Heller, Larrieu, D'Imperio, & Boris, 1999). As noted by McGloin and Widom (2001), research on resilience needs to be broadly encompassing and has the ability to capture the dynamic nature of development. Absence of a single negative outcome such as depression or a "snapshot" of the person at one point in time does not provide an adequate determination of outcomes related to child maltreatment. Therefore, research on the long-term consequences of early child maltreatment needs to examine resilience across a variety of domains of functioning including psychiatric, emotional, and behavioral.

In one well-designed study, researchers used a number of domains and time periods to determine the extent to which maltreated children demonstrate resilience later in life (McGloin & Widom, 2001). They matched substantiated cases of physical abuse and neglect on gender, age, race, and social class with nonabused and nonneglected children and followed them prospectively into young adulthood. Between 1989 and 1995, 676 abused and neglected and 520 control participants were administered a 2-hour in-person interview that included a psychiatric assessment. In order to meet the criteria of resilience, participants needed to meet the criteria for success across six of eight domains of functioning, which included employment, homelessness, education, social activity, psychiatric disorder, substance abuse, and two domains assessing criminal behavior. Results indicate that 22% of abused and neglected individuals met the criteria for resilience. Females were more successful across the individual domains of function, had a higher mean number of domains in which success was met, and were more likely to meet the criteria for overall resilience than males in the sample. The authors speculate that, beyond the risk of child maltreatment, males may be inherently more vulnerable to maladaptive outcomes related to stress than females.

In a study of resilience in socioeconomically challenged Latino children, researchers examined multiple aspects of functioning, personal resources, and relationship features in school-age maltreated and nonmaltreated children (Flores et al., 2005). Maltreated Latino children were found to have fewer areas of resilient functioning than nonmaltreated children. Ego-resilience and ego-control, as personal resources, and the ability to form a positive relationship with an adult figure outside of the immediate family predicted resilience. However, certain aspects of interpersonal functioning were differentially related to resilience for maltreated and nonmaltreated Latino children. Twice as many Latino maltreated children as nonmaltreated Latino children were found to be functioning maladaptively. In terms of gender differences, findings were similar to the McGloin and Widom (2001) study described above. Being female was associated with higher levels of resilient functioning in Latino children.

Economic Consequences of Child Maltreatment

A body of research is currently emerging that identifies the enormous economic consequences of child maltreatment. Corso and Lutzker (2006) provide a strong rationale for the need for economic analysis in research on child maltreatment prevention programs. They contend that economic analysis fits well in the public health model for preventing child maltreatment, complementing work in etiology, efficacy, effectiveness, implementation, and dissemination. Economic analysis includes a variety of methods to assess systematically the impact that intervention policies and programs have on outcomes and costs. The most widely used methods include cost of illness/injury (COI) analysis, program cost analyses, and economic evaluation methods, including cost-benefit analysis (CBA), cost-effectiveness analysis (CEA), and cost-utility analysis (CUA). See Corso and Lutzker (2006) for descriptions of each.

Despite our knowledge regarding economic analysis methods as used routinely in public health, a paucity of data regarding the application of these methods to child maltreatment prevention continues despite the fact that there has been widespread implementation of home visitation prevention programs. Corso and Lutzker (2006) argue that robust effectiveness data represent only one piece of the puzzle and that economic analysis is a key component of child maltreatment prevention research and should be included in policy making, funding decisions, or national recommendations.

In a study designed to examine long-term health care utilization and costs associated with childhood physical and sexual abuse of females, researchers found that significantly higher annual health care use and costs were observed for women with a child abuse history compared to women without comparable abuse histories (Bonomi et al., 2008). The most pronounced use and costs were observed for women with a history of both physical and sexual abuse. Total adjusted annual health care costs were 36% higher for women with both types of abuse, 22% higher for women with physical abuse only, and 16% higher with sexual abuse only. The authors emphasize that screening for past abuse should be routinely explored by health care professionals, especially for women with high health care utilization.

Prevent Child Abuse America estimates that the annual direct cost of child maltreatment is $103.8 billion in 2007 value (Holton & Wang, 2007). The greatest costs are for child protective service systems to investigate cases and intervene in cases of child maltreatment services, followed by costs for hospitalization of abused children, mental health treatments, and law enforcement. It is important to note that these costs do not necessarily take into consideration the impact of the pain, suffering, and reduced quality of life that child victims experience.

Mental Health of Children in Foster Care

Because a significant minority of maltreated children enter foster care through the CPS system or by informal family arrangements, it is important to be knowledgeable with regard to the issues confronted by children in foster care. An extensive body of research indicates that children in foster care are at risk for significant mental heath concerns (Leslie, Gordon, Meneken, Premji, Michelmore, & Ganger, 2005; McMillen, Zima, Scott, Auslander, Munson, Ollie, & Spitznagel, 2005). Most studies demonstrate comparable rates of mental health issues in children placed in both relative and nonrelative foster care (Leslie et al., 2005; McMillen et al., 2005). In a study of more than 1,500 young children removed from their homes for allegations of maltreatment, researchers found no differences in prevalence of mental health issues at time of placement between children subsequently placed with relative and nonrelative foster parents (Leslie et al., 2005). McMillen et al. (2005) reported similar findings in a study involving 373 adolescents in foster care. No differences were found in prevalence of psychiatric disorders between those in relative care and those in nonrelative foster care. Overall, 61% of the youths qualified as having at least one psychiatric disorder during their lifetime, with 37% meeting the criteria for a psychiatric disorder during the past year. In contrast, European researchers examining behavior problems in 214 foster care children found that those in kinship care had fewer emotional and behavioral problems than those in nonkinship care (Holtan, Ronning, Handegard, & Sourander, 2004). Both groups, however, had relatively high proportions of children scoring in the clinical range on the Child Behavior Checklist (CBC) (Achenbach, 1991) with 36% of those in kinship care and 52% in nonkinship care scoring in the clinical range on total behavior problems.

Several studies have examined the prevalence of mental health disorders in children raised in kinship care (Dubowitz, Feigelman, Harrington, Starr, Zuvarin, & Sawyer, 1994; Dubowitz, Zuvarin, Starr, Feigelman, & Harrington, 1993; Holtan et al., 2004). Researchers examining the emotional status of 288 children aged 4 to 18 years and residing in kinship care found that 26% scored in the clinical range on total and externalizing behavior problems, with 14% scoring in the clinical range on internalizing behaviors (Dubowitz et al., 1994). The authors note that these proportions are considerably higher than the 10% found in the normative population for each of these domains. While almost half (47%) of participants resided with grandparents, no comparisons were made between those residing with grandparents and those residing with other relatives. In a related study involving 346 children in kinship care, 35%, 24%, and 18% had scores in the clinical range for total, externalizing, and internalizing behaviors, respectively (Dubowitz et al., 1993).

Children Raised by Grandparents

An ever-growing number of children are being raised by grandparents in parent-absent homes. Since 1990, the number of children living in households maintained by their grandparents has increased 30% (U.S. Bureau of Census, 2003). According to the 2000 U.S. Census, more than 6 million children in the United States are currently living in grandparent-headed households (U.S. Bureau of Census, 2003). Of these, 2.4 million children are being raised solely by grandparents.

The emotional well-being of these children is of particular concern given that most have been abused, neglected, or abandoned by birth parents (Kelley, Whitley, Sipe, & Yorker, 2000). Although a considerable body of literature exists that describes the emotional and behavioral problems of children in foster care, empirical studies of the well-being of grandchildren in kinship care are limited. Placement of children with grandparents can occur abruptly or after a long and difficult period with the biological parents. The reasons why children are raised by grandparents are multiple and often times interrelated. The most commonly reported reasons are parental substance abuse, child maltreatment, abandonment, mental illness, incarceration, and homicide (Kelley et al., 2000). Thus, many children raised by grandparents have experienced multiple adverse events that place them at increased risk for emotional and behavioral problems. Furthermore, when birth parents are no longer present in their lives, children experience significant disruptions in key attachment relationships which are critical to their later social and emotional development (Poehlmann, 2003).

Despite the fact that the number of children raised by grandparents is increasing, we know little about their emotional well-being. The few studies that are available involve relatively small samples and are retrospective (Ghuman, Weist, & Shafer, 1999; Edwards, 2006; Campbell, Hu, & Oberle, 2006). In a chart review of child and adolescent clients treated at a community mental health center in Baltimore, researchers found that 22% of the 233 youths in the sample were being raised by grandparents (Ghuman, Weist, & Shafer, 1999). A disproportionate number of the youth raised by grandparents were African American, male, and younger when compared to other clients. The most frequent psychiatric diagnoses included oppositional defiant, depressive, and anxiety disorders.

In a study comparing 54 African American school-aged children being raised by grandparents with a matched group of children raised by birth parents, investigators asked teachers to rate behavior problems using the Child Behavior Checklist (Edwards, 2006). Results showed that children raised by grandparents were reported to have significantly more internalizing and externalizing behavior problems than those in the comparison group. On total behavior problem scores, 44% of children living with grandparents scored in the clinical range compared with only 13% of the participants raised by birth parents.

Researchers conducting a retrospective study of 66 adolescents in the juvenile justice system found that those raised by grandparents were more likely to have risk factors associated with reoffending when compared to youth in parent-headed families (Campbell, Hu, & Oberle, 2006). More specifically, youth in grandparent-headed households had higher rates of mental health issues, school problems, deviant peer relationships, and poor supervision. They were also more likely to have had a serious prior adjudication and to have committed their first delinquent offence before the age of 12. While these studies suggest that children raised by grandparents are at increased risk for behavioral health issues, the investigations are limited both in number and by either small samples or use of retrospective data collection.

Grandparents raising grandchildren often face considerable challenges in their parenting roles, raising concerns regarding the caregiving environment of the children. In one study, researchers found a greater proportion (19%) of families in which grandparents are raising grandchildren live in poverty compared with other types of family structures that include children (14%) (Hayslip & Kaminski, 2005). Other researchers estimate that as many as 30% of custodial grandparents live in poverty, with at least 40% having cared for their grandchildren 5 or more years (Simmons & Dye, 2003). In a population-based study, researchers found that African American custodial grandparents were more likely than noncaregiving grandparents to be living in poverty and receiving public assistance (Minkler & Fuller-Thomson, 2005).

Another challenge faced by grandparents is their health, both physical and mental. A substantial body of literature indicates that grandparents experience significant psychological distress, including depression (Fuller-Thomson & Minkler, 2000; Kelley et al., 2000; Scarcella, Ehrle, & Geen, 2003). For instance, researchers, using data from the National Survey of Families and Households, determined that in comparison to noncustodial grandmothers, custodial grandmothers are more likely to have significantly higher levels of depressive symptomatology (Fuller-Thomson & Minkler, 2000). In another national study, researchers found that nearly one-third of grandchildren were raised by grandparents experiencing poor mental health (Scarcella et al., 2003). Factors that have been found to be predictive of increased psychological distress in grandparent caregivers include lack of economic resources, physical health challenges, and, to a lesser extent, lack of social support (Kelley et al., 2000).

Additionally, many grandparents raising grandchildren experience significant physical health problems (Fuller-Thomson & Minkler, 2000; Minkler & Fuller-Thomson, 2005; Okagbue-Reaves, 2005; Whitley, Kelley, & Sipe, 2001). Using both objective and subjective data, researchers studying 100 African American grandparents found that almost one-quarter had diabetes and high cholesterol, over one-half had hypertension, and over three-quarters had cardiovascular compromise related to obesity (Whitley et al., 2001). When compared with a normative population on a standardized measure of self-reported health, participants scored significantly worse on the following health attributes: general health, physical functioning, bodily pain, role functioning, and social functioning. Only 7% described their health as excellent, with the remaining describing it as good (48%), fair (41%), or poor (4%).

An intervention designed by a team of nurses and social workers appears to be effective in improving the outcomes of grandparents raising grandchildren (Kelley et al., 2007). The intervention, based on an empowerment model, consists of home visitation by nurses to provide developmental and health screenings, monitoring of chronic health conditions, as well as health education and referrals. Case management by social workers, which includes addressing housing issues, adequate household resources, including food, parenting strategies, and referrals to community resources, is also conducted in the home. In addition, the intervention model involves grandparent support groups, parenting classes, early intervention services, as well as referrals for pro bono legal assistance related to a variety of issues, including custody and adoption.

SUMMARY

Child maltreatment is a significant public health and societal issue that does not receive the attention and resources it warrants given its vast societal costs. Over the past three decades, the scientific knowledge base related to child maltreatment has grown exponentially, especially our knowledge regarding its consequences, both immediate and long term. There is now evidence that maltreatment in childhood, in the majority of cases, negatively impacts its victims across the life span with enormous economic consequences. Efforts to reduce the burden of child maltreatment require a health care workforce that is knowledgeable regarding the manifestation and treatment of all forms of child maltreatment. The existing body of scientific knowledge on child maltreatment underscores the need for early identification and intervention with abused and neglected children and their families to ameliorate the negative sequelae and prevent subsequent exposure to trauma. Nurses and other health care professionals are in key positions to identify child maltreatment and assure that its victims receive early intervention and protection. In addition, nurses can work directly with parents to formulate effective coping strategies and to mobilize community resources.

REFERENCES

Achenbach, T. M. (1991). *Manual for the Child Behavior Checklist-4-18 and the 1991 Profile*. Burlington, VT: University of Vermont, Department of Psychiatry.

Afifi, T. A., Boman, J., Fleisher, W., & Sareen, J. (2009). The relationship between child abuse, parental divorce, and lifetime mental disorders and suicidality in a nationally representative adult sample. *Child Abuse & Neglect, 33,* 139–147.

Almgren, G. (2005). The ecological context of interpersonal violence: From culture to collective efficacy. *Journal of Interpersonal Violence, 20,* 218–224.

Anda, R. F., Whitfield, C. L., Feletti, V. L., Chapman, D., Edwards, V. J., Dube S. R., et al. (2002). Adverse childhood experiences, alcoholic parents, and later risk of alcoholism and depression. *Psychiatric Services, 53,* 1001–1009.

Banyard, V. L., Williams, L. M., Saunders, B. E., & Fitzgerald, M. M. (2008). The complexity of trauma in the lives of women in families referred for family violence: Multiple mediators of mental health. *American Journal of Orthopsychiatry, 78,* 394–404.

Belsky, J. (1993). Etiology of child maltreatment: A developmental–ecological analysis. *Psychological Bulletin, 114,* 413–434.

Besinger, B., Garland, A. F., Litrownick, A. J., & Landsverk, J. (1999). Caregiver substance abuse among maltreated children placed in out-of-home care. *Child Welfare, 78,* 221–239.

Bonomi, A. E., Cannon, E. A., Anderson, M. L., Rivara, F. P., & Thomson, R. S. (2008). Association between self-reported health and physical and/or sexual abuse experienced before age 18. *Child Abuse & Neglect, 32,* 693–701.

Bowlby, J. (1982). Attachment and loss. *American Journal of Orthopsychiatry, 52,* 664–678.

Bronfenbrenner, U. (1979). *The ecology of human development: Experiments by nature and design.* Cambridge, MA: Harvard University Press.

Caffey, J. I. (1946). Multiple fractures in the long bones of infants suffering from chronic subdural hematoma. *American Journal of Roentgenology, 56,* 163–173.

Caffey, J. (1972). On the theory and practice of shaking infants: Its potential residual effects of permanent brain damage and mental retardation. *American Journal of Diseases of Children, 124,* 161–169.

Campbell, L. R., Hu, J., & Oberle, S. (2006). Factors associated with future offending: Comparing youth in grandparent-headed homes with those in parent-headed home. *Archives of Psychiatric Nursing, 20,* 258–267.

Carson, E. A., Sroufe, L. A., & Egeland, B. (2004). The construction of experience: A longitudinal study of representation and behavior. *Child Development, 75,* 66–83.

Casey, E. A., & Lindhorst, T. P. (2009). Toward a multi-level, ecological approach to the primary prevention of sexual assault. *Trauma, Violence, & Abuse, 10,* 91–114.

Casanueva, C., Martin, S., & Runyan, R. K. (2009). Repeated reports for child maltreatment among intimate partner violence victims: Findings from the National Survey of Child and Adolescent Well-Being. *Child Abuse & Neglect, 33,* 84–93.

Chaffin, M., Kelleher, K., & Hollenberg, J. (1996). Onset of physical abuse and neglect: Psychiatric substance abuse and social risk factors from prospective community data. *Child Abuse & Neglect, 20,* 191–203.

Children's Bureau (2008). *Child maltreatment 2006.* Washington, DC: Administration for Children and Families, DHHS.

Children's Bureau (2009). *Child maltreatment 2007.* Washington, DC: Administration for Children and Families, DHHS.

Cicchetti, D., Rogosch, R. A., & Toth, S. L. (2006). Fostering secure attachment in infants in maltreating families through preventive interventions. *Development and Psychopathology, 18,* 623–649.

Chapman, D. P., Whitfield, C. L., Feletti, V. J., Dube, S. R., Edwards, V. J., & Anda, R. F. (2004). Adverse childhood experiences and the risk of depressive disorders in adulthood. *Journal of Affective Disorders, 82,* 217–225.

Corso, P. S, Edwards, V. J., Fang, X., & Mercy, J. A. (2008). Health-related quality of life among adults who experienced maltreatment during childhood. *American Journal of Public Health, 98,* 1094–1100.

Corso, P. S., & Lutzker, J. R. (2006). The need for economic analysis in research on child maltreatment. *Child Abuse & Neglect, 30,* 727–738.

Cox, C. E., Kotch, J. B., & Everson, M. D. (2003). A longitudinal study of modifying influences in the relationship between domestic violence and child maltreatment. *Family Violence, 18,* 5–17.

Crouch, J. L., & Behl, L. E. (2001). Relationships among parental beliefs in corporal punishment, reported stress, and physical abuse potential. *Child Abuse & Neglect, 25,* 413–419.

Daignault, I. V. & Herbert, M. (2009). Profiles of school adaptation: Social, behavioral and academic functioning in sexually abused girls. *Child Abused & Neglect, 33,* 102–115.

Dubowitz, H., Feigelman, S., Harrington, D., Starr, R., Zuvarin, S., & Sawyer, R. (1994). Children in kinship care: How do they fare? *Children and Youth Services Review, 16,* 85–106.

Dubowitz, H., Zuravin, S., Starr, R. H., Feigelman, S., & Harrington, D. (1993). Behavior problems of children in kinship care. *Journal of Developmental and Behavioral Pediatrics, 14,* 386–393.

Edwards, O. W. (2006). Teacher's perceptions of the emotional and behavioral functioning of children raised by grandparents. *Psychology in the Schools, 43,* 565–572.

Edwards, V. J, Holden, G. W., Feletti, V. J. & Anda, R. F. (2003). Relationship between multiple forms of childhood maltreatment and adult mental health in community respondents: Results from the adverse childhood experiences study. *American Journal of Psychiatry, 160,* 1454–1460.

Espinosa, M., Beckwith, J. H., Tyler, R., & Swanson, K. (2001). Maternal psychopathology and attachments in toddlers of heavy cocaine-using mothers. *Infant Mental Health Journal, 22,* 316–333.

Finkelhor, D. (2008). *Childhood victimization: Violence, crime and abuse in the lives of young people.* New York, NY: Oxford University Press.

Flores, E., Cicchetti, D., & Rogosch, F. A. (2005). Predictors of resilience in maltreated and nonmaltreated Latino children. *Developmental Psychology, 41,* 238–351.

Freisthler, B., Merritt, D. H., & LaScala, E. A. (2006). Understanding the ecology of child maltreatment: A review of the literature and directions for future research. *Child Maltreatment, 11,* 263–280.

Fuller-Thomson, E., & Minkler, M. (2000). The mental and physical health of grandmothers who are raising their grandchildren. *Journal of Mental Health and Aging, 6,* 311–323.

Ghuman, H. S., Weist, M. D., & Shafer, M. E. (1999). Demographic and clinical characteristics of emotionally disturbed children being raised by grandparents. *Psychiatric Services, 50,* 1496–1498.

Hanson, R. F., Self-Brown, S., Fricker-Elhai, A. E., Kilpatrick, D. G., Saunders, B. E., & Resnick, H. S. (2006). The relations between family environment and violence exposure among youth: Findings from the national survey of adolescents. *Child Maltreatment, 11,* 3–5.

Hayslip, B., & Kaminski, P. L. (2005). Grandparents raising their grandchildren: A review of the literature and suggestions for practice. *The Gerontologist, 45,* 262–269.

Hillison, J. K. C., & Kuiper, N. A. (1994). A stress and coping model of child maltreatment. *Clinical Psychological Review, 14,* 261–285.

Heller, S. S., Larrieu, J. A. D'Imperio, R., & Boris, N. W. (1999). Research on resilience to child maltreatment: Empirical considerations. *Child Abuse & Neglect, 23,* 321–338.

Henretig, F. M., Paschall, R. T., & Donaruma-Kwoh, M. M. (2009). Child abuse by poisoning. In R. M., Reece & C. W. Christian (Eds.), *Child abuse: Medical diagnosis and treatment* (3rd ed., pp. 549–599). Chicago: American Academy of Pediatrics.

Holbrook, T. L., Hoyt, D. B., Coimbra, R., Potenza, B., Sise, M., & Anderson, J. P. (2005). Long term trauma persists after major trauma in adolescents: New data on risk factors and functional outcome. *Journal of Trauma, 58,* 764–771.

Holtan, A., Ronning, J. A., Handegard, B. H., & Sourander, A. (2004). A comparison of mental health problems in kinship and nonkinship foster care. *European Child and Adolescent Psychiatry, 14,* 200–207.

Holtan, J., & Wang, C. T. (2007). *Total estimated cost of child abuse and neglect in the United States.* Chicago: Prevent Child Abuse America.

Jonson-Reid, M., Chance, T., & Drake, B. (2007). Risk of death among children reported for nonfatal maltreatment. *Child Maltreatment, 12,* 86–95.

Kaufman, J., & Zigler, E. (1987). Do abused children become abusive parents? *American Journal of Orthopsychiatry, 57,* 186–192.

Kaplow, J. B., & Widom, C. S. (2007). Age of onset of child maltreatment predicts long-term mental health outcomes. *Journal of Abnormal Psychology, 116,* 176–187.

Kelleher, K., Chaffin, M., Hollenberg, J., & Fisher, E. (1994). Alcohol and drug disorders among physically abusive and neglectful parents in a community-based sample. *American Journal of Public Health, 84,* 1586–1590.

Kelley, S. J. (2002). Child maltreatment in the context of substance abuse. In J. E. B. Meyers, L. Berliner, J. Briere, C. T. Hendrix, C. Jenny, & Reid, T. A. (Eds.), *The APSAC Handbook on Child Maltreatment* (2nd ed., pp. 105–118). Thousand Oaks, CA: Sage Publications.

Kelley, S. J., Whitley, D. M., & Sipe, T. A, (2007). Results of an interdisciplinary intervention to improve the psychosocial well-being and physical functioning of African American grandmothers raising children. *Journal of Intergenerational Relations, 5,* 45–64.

Kelley, S. J., Whitley, D. M., Sipe, T. A., & Yorker, B. C. (2000). Psychological distress in grandmother kinship care providers: The role of resources, social support and physical health. *Child Abuse & Neglect, 24,* 311–321.

Kempe, C. H., Silverman, F. N., Steele, B. F., Droegemueller, W., & Silver, H. K. (1962). The battered-child syndrome. *Journal of the American Medical Association, 182,* 17–24.

Kendall-Tackett, K., & Eckenrode, J. (1996). The effects of neglect on academic achievement and disciplinary problems: A developmental perspective. *Child Abuse & Neglect, 20,* 161–169.

Kolko, D. J. (2002). Child physical abuse. In J. E. B. Meyers, L. Berliner, J. Briere, C. T. Hendrix, C. Jenny, & Reid, T. A. (Eds.), *The APSAC Handbook on Child Maltreatment* (2nd ed., pp. 21–54). Thousand Oaks, CA: Sage Publications.

Lee, L. C., Kotch, J. B., & Cox, C. E. (2004). Child maltreatment in families experiencing domestic violence. *Violence and Victims, 19,* 573–591.

Leslie, L. K., Gordon, J. N., Meneken, L., Premji, K., Michelmore, K., & Ganger, W. (2005). The physical, developmental, and mental health needs of young children in child welfare by initial placement type. *Journal of Developmental and Behavioral Pediatrics, 26,* 177–185.

Little, L. & Kantor, G. K. (2002). Using ecological theory to understand intimate partner violence and child maltreatment. *Journal of Community Health Nursing, 19,* 133–145.

McGloin, J. M., & Widom, C. S. (2001). Resilience among abused and neglected children grown up. *Developmental and Psychopathology, 13,* 1021–1038.

McMillen, J. C., Zima, B. T., Scott, L. D., Auslander, W. F., Munson, M. R., Ollie, M. T., & Spitznagel, E. L. (2005). Prevalence of psychiatric disorders among older youths in the foster care system. *Journal of the American Academy of Child and Adolescent Psychiatry, 1,* 88–95.

Minkler, M., & Fuller-Thomson, E. (2001). Physical and mental health status of American grandparents providing extensive child care to their grandchildren. *Journal of the American Medical Women's Association, 56,* 199–205.

Minkler, M., & Fuller-Thomson, E. (2005). African American grandparents raising grandchildren: A national study using the census 2000 American community survey. *Gerontological Society of America, 60B,* S82–S92.

Mohr, W. K., & Tulman, L. J. (2000). Children exposed to violence: Measurement considerations with an ecological framework. *Advances in Nursing Science, 23,* 59–68.

Morton, N., & Browne, K. D. (1998). Theory and observation of attachment and its relation to child maltreatment: A review. *Child Abuse & Neglect, 22,* 1093–1104.

Nair, P., Schuler, M. E., Black, M. M., Kettinger, L., & Harrington, D. (2003). Cumulative environmental risk in substance abusing women: Early intervention, parenting stress, child abuse potential, and child development. *Child Abuse & Neglect, 27,* 997–1017.

National Center on Addiction and Substance Abuse (March, 2005). *Family matters: Substance abuse and the American family.* New York: Columbia University. Online at: www.casacolumbia.org.

National Center on Addiction and Substance Abuse (May, 2009). *Shoving up II: The impact of substance abuse on federal, state, and local budgets.* New York: Columbia University. Online at: www.casacolumbia. org/su2report.

Okagbue-Reaves, J. (2005). Kinship care: Analysis of the health and well-being of grandfathers raising grandchildren using the grandparent assessment tool and the Medical Outcomes Trust SF-36 Health Survey. *Journal of Family Social Work, 9,* 47–66.

Pears, K. C, Kim, H. K., & Fisher, P. A. (2008). Psychosocial and cognitive functioning of children with specific profiles of maltreatment. *Child Abuse & Neglect, 32,* 958–971.

Poehlmann, J. (2003). An attachment perspective on grandparents raising their young grandchildren: Implications for intervention and research. *Infant Mental Health Journal, 24,* 149–173.

Prosser, L. A., & Corso, P. S. (2007). Measuring health-related quality of life for child maltreatment: A systemic literature review. *Health Quality Life Outcomes, 5,* 42.

Rodgers, C. R., Lang, A. J., Laffaye, C., Satz, L. E., Dresselhaus, T. R., & Stein, M. B. (2004). The impact of individual forms of childhood maltreatment on health behaviors. *Child Abuse & Neglect, 28,* 575–586.

Roberts, R., O'Connor, T., Dunn, J., & Golding, J. The effects of child sexual abuse in later life; mental health, parenting and adjustment of offspring. *Child Abuse & Neglect, 28,* 525–545.

Rubin, D., Feinstein, J. A., & Berkowtiz, C. D. (2009). Medical and psychological sequelae of child abuse and neglect. In R. M., Reece & C. W. Christian (Eds.), *Child abuse: Medical diagnosis and treatment* (3rd ed., pp. 853–875). Chicago: American Academy of Pediatrics.

Scarcella, C. A., Ehrle, J., & Geen, R. (2003). Identifying and addressing the needs of children in grandparent care. *Urban Institute: New Federalism: National Survey of America's Families,* Series B., No. B-55, August, 1–7.

Schneider, B. H., Atkinson, L., & Tardif, F. (2001). Child–parent attachment and children's peer relations: A quantitative review. *Developmental Psychology, 37,* 86–100.

Schumm, J. A., Briggs-Philip, M., & Hobfoll, S. E. (2006). Cumulative interpersonal traumas and social support as risk and resiliency factors in predicting PTSD and depression among inner city women. *Journal of Traumatic Stress, 19,* 825–836.

Shonk, S. M., & Cicchetti, D. (2001). Maltreatment, competency deficits, and risk of academic and behavioral maladjustment. *Developmental Psychology, 37,* 3–17.

Simmons, T., & Dye, J. L. (2003). *Grandparents living with grandchildren: 2000.* Census 2000 Brief.

Smith Slep, A. M., & O'Leary, S. G. (2005). Parent and partner violence in families with young children: Rates, patterns, and connections. *Journal of Consulting and Clinical Psychology, 73,* 435–444.

Sprang, G., Clark, J. J., & Bass, S. (2005). Factors that contribute to child maltreatment severity: A multimethod and multidimensional investigation. *Child Abuse & Neglect, 29,* 335–350.

Stirling, J., & Amaya-Jackson, L. (2008). Understanding the behavioral and emotional consequences of child abuse. *Pediatrics, 122,* 667–673.

U.S. Bureau of Census. (October, 2003). *Grandparents Living with Grandchildren: 2000; Census 2000 Brief.* Washington, DC: U.S. Bureau of the Census.

Ward, C. S., & Haskett, M. E. (2008). Exploration and validation of clusters of physically abused children. *Child Abuse & Neglect, 32,* 577–588.

Widom, C. S. (1989). Does violence beget violence? A critical examination of the literature. *Psychological Bulletin, 106,* 3–28.

Widom, C. S., Czaja, S. J., & Dutton, M. A. (2008). Childhood victimization and lifetime revictimization. *Child Abuse & Neglect, 32,* 785–796.

Wilson, H. W., & Widom, C. S. (2008). An examination of risky sexual behavior and HIV in victims of child abuse and neglect: A 30 year follow-up. *Health Psychology, 27,* 149–159.

Whitley, D. M., Kelley, S. J., & Sipe, T. A. (2001). Grandmothers raising grandchildren: Are they at increased risk of health problems? *Health & Social Work, 26,* 105–114.

Yates, T. M., Carlson, E. A, & Egeland, B. (2008). A prospective study of child maltreatment and self-injurious behavior in a community sample. *Development and Psychopathology, 20,* 651–671.

Zeanah, C. H., & Smyke, A. T. (2005). Building attachment relationship following maltreatment and severe deprivation. In L. J. Berlin, Y. Ziv, L. Amaya-Jackson, & M.T, Greenberg (Eds.), *Enhancing early attachments: Theory, research intervention, and policy* (pp. 195–216). New York: Guilford Press.

5

Intimate Partner Violence and Nursing Practice

Marilyn Ford-Gilboe, RN, PhD
Colleen Varcoe, RN, PhD
Judith Wuest, RN, PhD
Marilyn Merritt-Gray, MN, RN

INTRODUCTION

Intimate partner violence (IPV) is a global health and social problem, which occurs in all countries and in all economic, social, religious, and cultural groups, and results in tremendous personal and social costs (World Health Organization, 2002, 2005). Reducing these costs, including long-term health consequences, is a complex problem which requires collaboration among policy makers and service providers in health, domestic violence, social service, and legal sectors, community stakeholders, and women themselves. The response should focus both on preventing IPV by working to address its root causes and addressing the consequences of IPV by supporting women who have experienced IPV to reduce the violence, gain access to needed resources, and strengthen their personal capacities.

Health professionals in every area of practice have an important role to play in making the health care system an "empowerment zone" for women who have experienced IPV (Campbell, 1998). However, comprehensive approaches for addressing IPV and its consequences have yet to be widely integrated into health care. There is a substantial body of theory, research, and practice knowledge on which to base trauma-informed clinical approaches for identifying and responding to women who have experienced IPV. By trauma-informed, we mean practice informed by an understanding of the dynamics and consequences of violence, including the notion that IPV can be thought of as chronic traumatization (Kaysen, Resick, & Wise, 2003).

In this chapter, we explore the nurse's role in relation to IPV. First, we provide an understanding of IPV as it exists within broader gendered social, political, and economic contexts and summarize what is known about women's experiences of living with, leaving, and recovering from violence, as well as the health, social, and economic impacts of violence. Drawing on this understanding, we suggest a set of "best practices" to guide nurses in working with women who have experienced IPV, in preventing IPV, and in strengthening health care and other systems and policies so that women's needs are more effectively addressed.

THE COMPLEXITY OF WOMEN'S EXPERIENCES OF INTIMATE PARTNER VIOLENCE IN CONTEXT

Women in every society endure high levels of violence. Nursing practice should be based on understanding both the prevalence of violence and the dynamics that shape experiences of violence. According to the World Health Organization (2002), IPV is any behavior within an intimate relationship that causes physical, psychological, or sexual harm to those in the relationship. These behaviors include physical assault, sexual abuse or forced sex, psychological abuse and/or controlling behaviors. IPV occurs in all types of intimate partner relationships and varies in intensity and severity. Johnson (2006) argued that there are different types of violent relationships and that distinguishing between the types is important. According to Johnson, "Situational couple violence" is characterized by lower-level *conflict* within a relationship that may be bilateral and which escalates to violence, but does not include the use of control. In contrast, "intimate terrorism" is more severe physical and/or sexual violence, almost always directed toward a woman by a male partner in order to maintain *power* and *control*. This gender-specific pattern of deliberate, repeated physical and/or sexual assault within the context of coercive control has also been called "battering" (Campbell & Humpheys, 1993 ; WHO, 2005). Control tactics used by abusive men, including threats, verbal abuse, forced isolation or imprisonment, humiliation, stalking, monitoring of activities, control of money, and denial of access to services or assistance (Tjaden & Thoennes, 2000), create a traumatic context for women who live in fear of their abusive partners (Kaysen, Reswick, & Wise, 2003). In this chapter, we focus on trauma-informed nursing practice with women who have experienced IPV characterized by coercive control.

The causes of IPV and the responses of women, those in their social networks, health care providers, and other helpers are shaped by broader social forces and structures, including gender role norms and expectations, tolerance for violence in society, economic and social resources, community services, and the policies which govern them. The ecological model developed by the World Health Organization (2002) positions violence against women as a complex, multidimensional problem rooted in the interactions among biological, social, cultural, economic, and political factors. In this model, the woman is positioned at the center of a nested series of family, community, and societal factors, which interact with each other to affect her experiences of violence (Figure 5.1). This lens underscores how the causes of violence against women are interconnected, suggesting that IPV is more than an individual woman's problem.

A woman's "choices" for addressing IPV and its consequences are shaped by the intersection of her history of other forms of violence, her social location (i.e., by ability, class, ethnicity, and place), and environmental factors, such as the availability of needed services. IPV occurs in the context of multiple forms of violence common in western societies: child abuse, bullying, sexual assault, workplace violence, racism, and various forms of harassment. Women's lifetime experiences of physical, sexual, and emotional abuse-related trauma influence the outcomes of IPV (Humphreys, Sharps, & Campbell, 2005). Individual women's social locations are shaped by broad social determinants. So, although economic resources are powerful determinants of whether women enter, remain

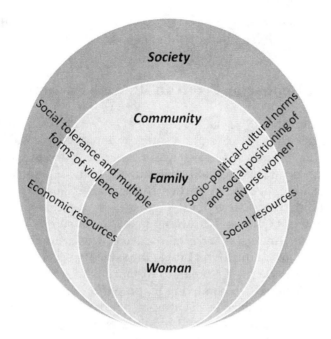

FIGURE 5.1   An ecological view of violence against women.

in, or leave abusive partners (Anderson & Saunders, 2003; Goeckermann, Hamberger, & Barber, 1994; Lambert & Firestone, 2000), different challenges will be faced, for example, by a middle class suburban woman, a rural woman living in poverty, or a woman living on the street in an inner city core.

The broader social and policy context shapes how IPV is publically understood, including ideologies regarding the causes and who is held responsible for violence (Paterson, 2009), arrest policies and how they are applied (e.g., Buzawa & Buzawa, 1993), women's access to social assistance and housing policies (Barron, 2005), and child custody policies and practices (Hardesty, 2002; Varcoe & Irwin, 2004; Wuest, Ford-Gilboe, Merritt-Gray, & Lemire, 2006). Strategies for improving women's safety and supporting their ability deal with the impacts of IPV must take this broader context into account.

WOMEN'S EXPERIENCES OF VIOLENCE

Women's experiences of violence vary in severity and form, and often change over the course of a relationship. Within an intimate partner relationship, violence is not the only feature. Commitment to the relationship, community, and religious norms, including those about gender roles, family ties, and children are all factors that shape how women deal with violence, including if and when they chose to disclose violence to others and/or attempt to leave their abusive partners. Leaving an abusive partner is the dominant, socially sanctioned solution to IPV (Brown, 1997), and most women do eventually separate from their abusers or manage to make the violence end (Campbell & Soeken, 1999). However, leaving is a complex process that often occurs over a long period of time. IPV tends to continue and intensify with significant health consequences after women leave, although, eventually, both the violence and the health problems improve (Anderson &

Saunders, 2003; Campbell, Rose, Kub, & Nedd, 1998; Logan, Walker, Jordan, & Campbell, 2004; Tjaden & Thoennes, 2000; Wuest, Ford-Gilboe, Merritt-Gray, & Berman, 2003).

The Process of Disengaging From an Abusive Partner

Much has been written about the challenges of leaving an abusive partner. In quantitative studies, women's access to external resources, particularly employment and/or a reasonable income (including social assistance or "welfare"), and to a lesser extent, child-care, transportation, social support, and commitment to the relationship have been the best predictors of leaving the abusive partner (Anderson & Saunders, 2003).

In qualitative studies, the process of leaving has been depicted as complex and tenuous, with some women leaving and returning many times before separating from their partners (see review by Anderson & Saunders, 2003). These studies highlight women's agency in making changes in their lives but, at the same time, show how personally and practically difficult it can be for a woman to distance herself from an abusive partner. Landenburger (1989) studied women living in, preparing to leave, and exiting abusive relationships and identified a process of entrapment and recovery (Figure 5.2).

The four stages of that process, named binding, enduring, disengaging, and recovering, guided the development of a clinical tool, the Domestic Violence Survivor Assessment (DVSA), which can be used by nurses, domestic violence advocates, and other health care providers to help the woman identify her stage of change in the process of leaving (Dienemann, Campbell, Landenburger, & Curry, 2002). Merritt-Gray and Wuest (1995) and Wuest and Merritt-Gray (1999, 2001) studied women leaving abusive partners, considering how economic, personal, and social circumstances affect that process. Their theory of reclaiming self addresses not only the process of leaving but also how women sustain the separation and establish a life distinct from the abuser through processes of counteracting abuse, breaking free, not going back, and moving on. The findings of

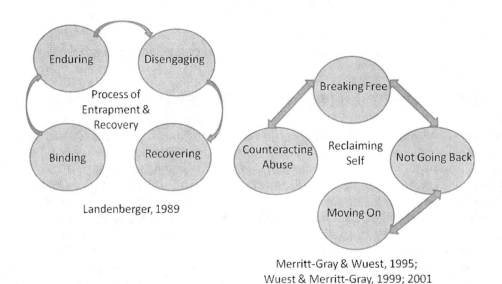

FIGURE 5.2 Two theories about leaving abusive partners.

these studies help nurses to consider when and how they might be helpful to women in abusive relationships, during the crisis of leaving, and when struggling to sustain the separation and moving on.

Landenburger (1989) described the initial development of the relationship as binding, where the woman's desire for a loving relationship overrides any warning signs of abuse. Over time, women endure by consciously blocking out the abuse by concentrating on the good, placating, and publicly covering up abuse with a consequence of experiencing a shrinking self. Similarly, Merritt-Gray and Wuest (1995) noted that women relinquished parts of self in the process of counteracting abuse. However, they also found that women as survivors actively resisted abuse by protecting, reasoning, and sometimes fighting back, strategies supported in independent research by Campbell and colleagues (1998). Women were fortified when they survived crises, distanced themselves, enhanced their personal capabilities, and experienced caring relationships. Opportunities for personal development through education, recreation, new employment challenges, or volunteering were pivotal for fortifying women's confidence and capabilities. Importantly, helpers at this stage could undermine or enhance this fortifying process. As women recognized that the abuse was continuing or getting worse no matter what they did, their increased confidence helped them to break free of their abusive partner. Landenburger noted that disengaging included identifying oneself as abused, seeking help, and making attempts to leave. Through disengagement, women learned that leaving was very difficult and potentially more dangerous than staying especially when abuse escalated in response to their efforts (Merritt-Gray & Wuest 1995).

After leaving, women struggled in a process that Wuest and Merritt-Gray (1999) called "not going back." The social expectation to maintain marriages forced women who left to constantly justify their actions to family members and social agencies from whom they sought help. Women worked hard to establish themselves separately from the abuser through relocating themselves socially and physically. This required gaining control of their finances and safety, a process frequently challenged by escalating abuse, unsympathetic financial institutions, and a bewildering justice system. This process is captured in Landenburger's (1989) description of recovering or readjustment after leaving, which included struggling for survival as well as grieving and searching for meaning. According to Wuest and Merritt-Gray (2001), these last two processes occur over many years as women move on. Moving on involved shedding the identities of "victim" and "survivor" by settling on why the abuse happened, putting the abuse "in its rightful place," taking on a new image, and sometimes launching new relationships.

Nurses need to recognize the process of separating from an abusive partner, and recovering from trauma takes place over many years with women frequently taking "one step forward and two steps back." Their progress depends not only on their own actions but also on how family, friends, justice, social and health systems reinforce or undermine their efforts to disengage, take control, and move on.

Staying and Working to Eliminate the Violence

There is growing evidence that some abusive relationships change and become nonviolent (Bell, Goodman, & Dutton, 2007; Campbell et al., 1998). Wuest and Merritt-Gray (2008) found that, similar to women who leave, women whose relationships eventually became nonviolent moved through the stages of counteracting abuse and breaking free.

Leaving or shifting the pattern of abusive control in relationships was tied to women's fortifying activities, leading to life skills that helped them develop personal autonomy and economic security. In relationships that became nonviolent, abusive men took notice of women's efforts to counteract abuse by backing off, ceasing physical abuse, and in some cases getting help or otherwise investing in this nonviolent relationship. In contrast, in relationships where women eventually left, men responded to women's efforts to counteract abuse by escalating the abuse. Thus, how an abusive partner reacts to a woman's efforts to increase autonomy and set limits may be a good indicator of whether there is potential for the abuser to become nonabusive.

Importantly, few domestic violence services adequately support women who stay and work to eliminate the violence (Yoshioka & Choi, 2005; Dunn & Powell-Williams, 2007). For some women, this is a viable, but difficult, alternative to separation. Offender intervention programs are available in most communities, and evaluations show they are useful for some abusers (Gondolf, 2002). A challenge for nurses is to understand the complexity of women's lives and to foreground support for women's decisions. The overly simplistic notion that women "should just leave" is not useful for nursing practice.

Beyond the Crisis of Leaving

Women leave to escape the violence and to create a better life for themselves and for their children, but there has been limited attention in practice or policy to what actually happens to women and their children beyond the initial crisis of leaving. Understanding how mothers and their children navigate this journey can help nurses anticipate needs and be prepared to offer targeted support. The grounded theory, *Strengthening Capacity to Limit Intrusion* (Ford-Gilboe, Wuest, & Merritt-Gray, 2005; Wuest et al., 2003), was developed based on interviews with 40 mothers who had left an abusive partner up to 18 years previously. In this theory, *Intrusion* makes it difficult for women to create a better life after leaving (see Figure 5.3). Intrusion is unwanted interference from ongoing harassment or abuse, cumulative physical and mental health consequences of abuse, reduced economic and social circumstances after leaving, and the "costs" of getting help (i.e., stress and conflict related to bureaucratic process and expectations of "helpers").

Leaving is a proactive, risk-taking act of positioning for the future, but soon after leaving, intrusion increases and forces women to focus on immediate priorities through surviving. Depending on the level of intrusion, women cycle back and forth from surviving to positioning for the future as they attempt to address four priorities:

1. *Providing* involves meeting basic needs of symptom relief, sleep, medication, food, safe housing, household necessities, and child care. Stability in providing for basic needs allows women to purposefully take risks to improve their future prospects for providing (for example, quitting jobs and going back to school, or incurring debt to acquire permanent housing). Safe and affordable housing is often crucial in women's ability to break free (Pavao, Alvarez, Baumrind, Induni, & Kimerling, 2007).
2. *Regenerating family* entails developing a storyline that helps the woman, her children, and others make sense of her current situation and gives purpose to developing daily routines, rules for avoiding conflicts, and new roles for daily functioning so that they can survive despite intrusion. As they gain confidence in working together, women and children identify and try to live by new standards for relationships that replace

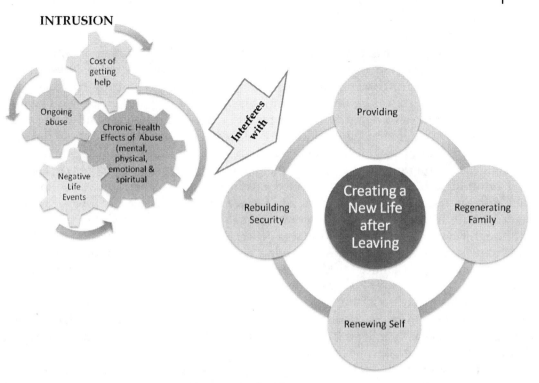

INTRUSION

Cost of getting help

Ongoing abuse

Chronic Health Effects of Abuse (mental, physical, emotional & spiritual)

Negative Life Events

Interferes with

Providing

Rebuilding Security

Creating a New Life after Leaving

Regenerating Family

Renewing Self

FIGURE 5.3 Theory of strengthening capacity to limit intrusion.

the destructive interactions of the abusive past. Women's ability to parent effectively during this period makes a great deal of difference to how well their children thrive after leaving (Berman, 1999; Humphreys, 1995) (see also chapter 11).

3. *Rebuilding security* involves safeguarding from threats to physical and emotional safety through vigilance, self-imposed isolation, and pulling back from others. As women gain confidence in their ability to keep themselves and their children safe, they position for the future by cautiously connecting with the larger community. This involves weighing the benefits and costs of relationships in terms of what they provide for the woman/family versus the demands or conditions that might come with these contacts.

4. *Renewing self* is a process of individual restoration and realization of potential. Feeling unworthy, lacking confidence, and struggling with pervasive health problems, women and their children initially are almost disoriented by the freedom to do and be as they wish. Over time, they recognize that simply having freedom is not enough and begin to purposefully focus on their needs for health, healing, and realizing their potential in the future.

Strengthening capacity to limit intrusion does not follow a predetermined trajectory but is an incremental process of change over time that is characterized by ongoing shifts between surviving and positioning in response to intrusion and the most significant priorities at a particular point in time. This theory has provided the basis for a nursing intervention, which is in the early stages of testing (see section on *Comprehensive Nursing Approaches*).

Summary

Collectively, these theories help us to understand that deciding whether or not to leave, staying, and leaving and creating a new life after separation are normal and proactive responses to very complex and challenging situations. They provide a basis for nurses to critically reflect on their assumptions about leaving and creating a new life after leaving, and to question how their own practices might be helpful rather than "intrusive" to women and their children. Furthermore, nurses can use these theories about the process of leaving or staying to help women "frame" their experiences of ambivalence, continuing love or commitment to their partners, and a pattern of leaving and returning multiple times as expected acts of change. Furthermore, these theories can help the nurse avoid the tendency to focus on leaving as the goal for all women and, instead, focus on supporting women's goals and decisions on their own terms. Although women's lives and experiences differ, nurses may draw on these theories to anticipate some of the challenges of leaving or sustaining a life without their partner and offering support tailored to the issues which women typically face at a particular stage.

Much of this literature positions women as "survivors" rather than "victims." This is a conscious effort to bring attention to women's strengths and their potential to move beyond the abuse in their lives. It is important to note that not all women see themselves in this way. The language of "survivor" emphasizes women's agency and choices, that, while intended to absolve women of responsibility for the violence perpetrated against them and emphasize strengths, paradoxically, attributes more responsibility to them (Dunn & Powell-Williams, 2007).

This label may also imply that the violence has ended, when in fact, many women experience ongoing abuse and harassment after leaving (Davies, Ford-Gilbe, & Hammerton, 2009). Health care providers should be cautious in the use of any language that can label and strive to recognize that, while women have agency, their choices are often severely constrained. In practice, the nurse may want to introduce the "survivor" language to abused women, sharing that some women find it helpful in thinking about themselves differently, but ask the woman to chose whether this concept fits for her or not.

HEALTH, SOCIAL, AND ECONOMIC CONSEQUENCES OF INTIMATE PARTNER VIOLENCE

Substantial health, social, and economic consequences of IPV arise from the complex intersections of social, political, cultural, and economic influences. These consequences affect women, their families, and society.

Health Consequences of Intimate Partner Violence

There is substantial evidence that IPV has significant, negative implications for women's physical and mental health (e.g., Campbell, 2002; Campbell & Kendall-Tackett, 2005; Coker, Hopenhayn, DeSimone, Bush, & Crofford, 2009; Ellsberg, Jansen, Heise, Watts, & Garcia-Moreno, 2008; Dutton, et al., 2006; Plichta, 2004).

Health Problems Are Both Acute and Chronic

IPV-related health problems may be immediate or chronic, and are due both to injuries, often untreated and/or unhealed, and to women's physical and psychological responses to trauma (Plichta, 2004; Sutherland, Bybee, & Sullivan, 2002; Wuest et al., 2009). Furthermore, IPV trauma may lead to increased health risk behaviors such as smoking, or substance abuse, or risk factors for HIV and/or sexually transmitted infections (STIs) that contribute to further health problems (U.S. Centers for Disease Control and Prevention [CDC], 2008; Weaver & Resnick, 2004).

Injuries are a direct cause of both acute and chronic health problems. Abused women are more likely than nonabused women to sustain injuries to the head, neck, and face most commonly from a punch or slap (Corrigan et al., 2003; Muelleman, Lenaghan, & Pakiesier, 1996; Plichta, 2004; Sheridan & Nash, 2007). Traumatic brain injury (TBI), a consequence of head injury, is often undiagnosed in abused women and confused with symptoms of posttraumatic stress disorder (Banks, 2007). Among women attending family practice clinics, those with a history of abuse had higher odds than nonabused women for migraines, epilepsy, and seizure disorders (Coker, Smith, & Fadden, 2005), symptoms consistent with long-term effects of TBI and/or attempted strangulation or "choking" (Smith, Mills, & Taliaferro, 2001). Neurological problems subsequent to head injury or attempted strangulation can be mistaken for mental health symptoms, reminding nurses of the importance of a thorough trauma history in sorting out the causes and management of symptoms.

Importantly, physical health problems may be associated not only with assaultive IPV but also with psychological IPV (Follingstad, 2009; Wuest et al., 2008). IPV also leads to myriad health effects that are not directly attributable to specific injuries, but rather arise from living under conditions of chronic stress. Women with a history of IPV are more likely than nonabused women to experience heart disease or heart attack, arthritis, fibromyalgia, asthma, stroke (CDC, 2008), chronic pain (Campbell et al., 2002; Coker, Smith, Bethea, King, & McKeown, 2000), disability related to chronic pain (Coker, Smith, & Fadden, 2005; Weinbaum et al., 2001), and cervical cancer (Coker et al., 2009). In clinical populations of women, lifetime physical and/or sexual abuse has been associated with gastrointestinal disorders and symptoms (Leserman & Drossman, 2007) and with pelvic pain (Leserman, Zolnoun, Meltzer-Brody, Lamvu, & Steege, 2006).

Women who have been sexually assaulted by their intimate partners have more gynecological problems than those who have not experienced forced sex (Campbell, 2002; Eby, Campbell, Sullivan, & Davidson, 1995; Campbell & Soeken, 1999) and may experience vaginal and anal tearing, bladder and urinary tract infections, pelvic pain, and sexual dysfunction (Campbell & Alford, 1989; Campbell et al., 2002) (see chapter 2 for more detailed physiological explanations of some of the stress-related symptoms).

Compared to nonabused women, those with a history of IPV also have higher rates of many mental health problems including clinical depression, acute and chronic symptoms of anxiety, protracted disabling sleep disturbances, symptoms consistent with PTSD, substance use and dependence, and thoughts of suicide (Carbone-López, Kruttschnitt, & MacMillan, 2006; Golding, 1999; Humphreys & Lee, 2005; Mechanic, Weaver, & Resick, 2008; Woods, 2000; Zlotnick, Johnson, & Kohn, 2006). PTSD is an often debilitating mental health consequence of IPV that is poorly understood by health professionals, including nurses (see Exhibit 5.1 and chapter 2).

EXHIBIT 5.1 | *Posttraumatic Stress Disorder (PTSD)*

PTSD** is an often misdiagnosed anxiety disorder that develops after being exposed to a severely traumatic event/s. About one in four people exposed to a traumatic event will develop PTSD, but all trauma survivors are at high risk. Women are twice as likely as men to experience PTSD over their life time and are four times more likely to develop PTSD when exposed to the same trauma. This gender difference is thought to be due to women's higher lifetime exposure to interpersonal trauma, including IPV. In a meta-analysis, Golding (1999) estimated the weighted mean prevalence of PTSD among female survivors of IPV to be 63.8% (range 31% to 84.4%). Cumulative traumas, particularly across the life span, are believed to increase the risk for and severity of PTSD symptoms. Symptoms of PTSD can vary from mild to severe. About 50% of those diagnosed with PTSD recover within a few months, while others experience years of incapacity.

Diagnostic Symptom Profile
 I. Clients identify that they have had a traumatic experience (i.e., one which is horrific, unpredictable, life altering/threatening, and/or beyond the person's control).
 II. Symptoms from each of the following clusters, lasting more than 1 month, are present:
   A. *Intrusion:* Client continues to relive aspects of the trauma experience, through intrusive thoughts, dreams, or images but not necessarily flashbacks; has marked distress in reaction to internal or external triggers or cues.
   B. *Numbing:* Client repeatedly, consciously or unconsciously, avoids trauma-related stimuli and has a general numbing of responsiveness, not just to traumatic triggers but to situations in general (e.g. systematically avoids, has poor recall, has marked loss of interest, feels isolated and detached, emotions blunted)
   C. *Hyperarousal:* Client reports at least two hyperarousal symptoms not experienced as problematic prior to the trauma (e.g., insomnia, poor concentration, extreme vigilance, exaggerated startle response).

Treatment: Psychological therapies for PTSD are rapidly evolving with current best evidence recommending a three-phase approach to treatment (stabilization, trauma reprocessing, maintenance).

Nursing Role: The therapeutic focus is one of secondary prevention. Within generalist practice, the nurse uses Phase 1 treatment strategies: early identification of symptoms; helping clients to name what they are experiencing and understand that PTSD is a common response to past trauma; supporting clients to link their symptoms to current triggers and manage intrusive hyperarousal symptoms (e.g., insomnia, anxiety), and assisting them to reconnect to social supports and re-engage in daily routines and physical activities. A detailed discussion and reprocessing of the traumatic events would not be initiated. Clients needing these Phase 2 treatment approaches, or who have comorbid psychiatric symptoms, should be referred for specialist intervention.

**NOTE: In recent years, the diagnosis of *Complex PTSD* has been presented as being more representative of women's experiences of trauma, particularly when both child and adult abuse are present. Currently, *Complex PTSD* is not a diagnosis used in generalist practice (Hegadoren, Lasik, & Coupland, 2006).

Sources: Morrison, J. (1995). *DSM-IV Made Easy.* New York: The Guilford Press.
Foa, E.B., Keane, T. & Friedman (2000). Guidelines for treatment of PTSD. *Journal of raumatic Stress*, 13(4), 539–588.

Importantly, regardless of whether women's health problems have been diagnosed or not, those with IPV histories report more physical symptoms/health problems than other women (Campbell et al., 2002; Plichta, 2004; Sutherland, Sullivan, & Bybee, 2001). These symptoms or health problems include low energy, fatigue, sleep problems, pain, swollen joints, sore muscles, faintness, dizziness, memory loss, difficulty concentrating, ringing in ears, indigestion, and appetite loss. These symptoms often are nonspecific and cross diagnostic boundaries (Woods, Hall, Campbell, & Angott, 2008), yet interfere with women's daily lives. Among women who had recently separated from their abusive partners, Wuest et al. (2007) found that women reported an average of 12 health current problems and 3 diagnoses by health professionals, and had taken 3 prescription medications in the past month.

Physical and Mental Health Consequences of Intimate Partner Violence Are Interrelated

Physical health problems are often linked to injuries but are also thought to result from a complex biopsychosocial response to trauma (Chapman, Tuckett, & Song, 2008) which, in turn, results in longer-term physical and mental health problems (see Figure 5.4). Chronic exposure to repeated violence, within an environment of humiliation, coercion, and control, provokes an acute stress response (Carlson & Dahlenberg, 2000). Chemical mediators are secreted by the sympathetic nervous system, hypothalamic–pituitary–adrenal (HPA) axis, or immune system to protect vital body functions in a process of allostasis (MacEwen, 2007). When these protective mediators are chronically elevated, such as in IPV, pathophysiological changes (i.e., allostatic overload) can result. Posttraumatic stress disorder (PTSD) symptoms are an indicator of allostatic overload (Friedman & McEwan, 2004).

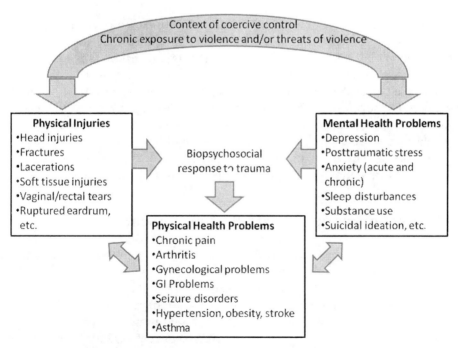

FIGURE 5.4   Interrelated health problems following IPV.

PTSD has been proposed as a major pathway by which physical health is affected by trauma (Green & Kimmerling, 2004) and, specifically, by IPV (Dutton, 2009). Symptoms of PTSD have been found to mediate the relationships between partner abuse and (a) altered immune function (increased levels of proinflammatory cytokines) (Woods et al., 2005), (b) physical health symptoms (Taft, Vogt, Mechanic, & Resick, 2007), and (c) chronic pain (Wuest et al., 2009). Symptoms of PTSD have been found to predict symptoms of stress and neuromuscular, gynecologic, and sleep problems (Woods et al., 2008) (see chapter 2 for a more in-depth discussion of PTSD and physiological effects).

Health Problems Often Persist After "Leaving"

Many of the physical and mental health problems experienced by abused women may persist after leaving. In one qualitative study (Wuest et al., 2003), women's health problems persisted for as long as 20 years after leaving their abusive partners. In one of the few longitudinal studies (Campbell & Soeken, 1999), women's mental health improved over a 3.5-year period only for women who reported that they were no longer experiencing abuse. In our current study of women who had been separated from their abusive partners an average of 20 months, women reported poorer physical and mental health than the general population, experienced high levels of chronic disabling pain (33%), symptoms of depression (58%) and PTSD (48%), cardiovascular risk factors, including smoking and high BMI, and a pattern of health service use considerably higher than that of Canadian women of comparable age (Ford-Gilboe et al., 2009; Scott-Storey, Wuest, & Ford-Gilboe, 2009; Wuest et al., 2007, 2008; Wuest et al., 2009). Current and past year IPV has been associated with more severe and more costly physical and mental health problems than lifetime IPV (Snow-Jones et al., 2006; Woods, 2000). There is evidence that health care utilization decreases over time after IPV ends, although in an HMO sample, it was still significantly higher for abused versus nonabused women 5 years after the abuse had ended (Rivara et al., 2007).

In summary, we need to better understand the conditions which lead to improvements as well as continued problems in abused women's health so that appropriate supports and interventions may be developed. A challenge for practitioners is to recognize that, in addition to supporting and providing safety planning and health interventions for women who are currently experiencing abuse, many women with past histories of IPV also need ongoing support and interventions to address enduring health consequences. A further challenge is to understand that past experiences of child abuse, sexual assault, and workplace violence along with current harassment may compound the health effects of IPV. The research summary presented in Exhibit 5.2 illustrates the complex relationships between trauma and health outcomes, using chronic pain as an exemplar.

Social Consequences of Intimate Partner Violence

IPV erodes women's natural support networks making them less available to support their health (Ford-Gilboe et al., 2009). Abusers may isolate women or limit their contact with family members and friends; these potential supports may also avoid contact with the woman out of fear for their own safety. Separation from an abusive partner may further reduce social networks due to relocation or alignment of friends with the abusive partner (Walker, Logan, Jordan, & Campbell, 2004; Wuest et al., 2003), while forging new networks or continuing supportive connections from family and friends can enhance the

EXHIBIT 5.2 | *Research Highlight: Chronic Pain and IPV*

Despite extensive literature that child and adult abuse experiences, abuse-related injury, depressive symptoms and posttraumatic stress disorder (PTSD) each influence the severity of chronic pain *individually* (Campbell, Greeson, Bybee, & Raja, 2008; Coker, Smith, & Fadden, 2005; Walsh, Jamieson, MacMillan, & Boyle, 2007; Woods et al., 2005; Wuest et al., 2008), how these factors *together* influence chronic pain severity in abused women has seldom been studied.

Using data collected from a community sample of 309 women who had been living separately from their abusive partners for an average of 20 months, we examined how PTSD symptom severity, depressive symptom severity, and lifetime abuse-related injury affected the relationships of child abuse severity, assaultive IPV (physical and sexual) severity, and psychological abuse severity with chronic pain severity (Wuest et al., unpublished manuscript). We found that 40% of the variance in chronic pain severity was accounted for by a model containing the following pathways:

• Child abuse severity affected chronic pain severity indirectly through lifetime abuse-related injury, PTSD symptom severity, and depressive symptom severity
• Assaultive IPV severity affected chronic pain severity indirectly through lifetime abuse-related injury
• Psychological IPV severity affected chronic pain severity directly

Why are these findings important to clinicians?
The findings suggest that:

1. Chronic pain severity in abused women must be understood in the context of the severity of assaultive and psychological IPV, and past child abuse, as well as women's lifetime abuse-related injuries and the severity of their PTSD and depressive symptoms. While depression is commonly identified in abused women, often PTSD is not. In this sample, although almost 50% of the women had symptoms consistent with a diagnosis of PTSD, only 7% reported a PTSD diagnosis (Wuest et al., 2007). Assessment of child abuse history may provide opportunities to affirm women's experiences and help them consider its role in her current health and social context (Wuest et al., 2008).
2. Early assessment, treatment, and follow-up of child abuse are vital to prevent long-term effects on physical health in adulthood through biophysical changes associated with mental health and injury.
3. Timely treatment and follow-up of IPV injuries is critical to prevent chronic pain in abused women. Currently, fewer than 50% of women seek help for abuse-related injuries (Campbell & Kendall-Tackett, 2005).
4. Contrary to common assumptions, psychological IPV directly affects chronic pain severity. Chronic traumatization through coercion, threats, and control has potential to directly affect physical health symptoms and should be taken seriously.

health of women who have experienced IPV (Coker, Watkins, Smith, & Brandt, 2003). Both support from other women who share a history of IPV (Wang & McKinney, 1997) and from family members and friends (Campbell et al., 1995; Humphreys, Lee, Neylan, & Marmer, 2001) have been associated with a reduction in physical and/or psychological distress among women who have experienced IPV. Furthermore, there is evidence that social support mediates the relationship between changes in abuse and depression over time (Beeble, Bybee et al., 2009) and that practical help mediates the impact of sexual or physical assault on PTSD symptoms (Glass, Perrin, Campbell, & Soeken, 2007).

At the same time, however, there often are *costs* associated with social relationships. Given that many women who experience IPV also have histories of child abuse, relationships with extended family members, who may have been perpetrators or witnesses of the abuse, may be strained. Family members, friends, and neighbors are often helpful in providing refuge, linkages to resources, practical help, and emotional support, but they may also undermine women's decision making by minimizing, blaming, and maintaining secrecy (Rose, Campbell, & Kub, 2000; Merritt-Gray & Wuest, 1995). Offers of help may also come with conditions which rob women of control over decisions or force them to take actions with which they do not agree (Lempert, 1997; Wuest et al., 2003). For example, a woman's mother might provide child care on the condition that she end the relationship with her abusive partner (when she may not be ready to do so); offers of public housing may come with the condition that women go to a shelter; seeking support for parenting from community agencies may lead others to question the woman's competence and open the woman up to surveillance and scrutiny by child protection services; in the United States, a history of IPV may lead to increased insurance costs (Grim, 2009).

In general, the costs and conflict inherent in relationships are better predictors of health outcomes than perceived social support (Stewart & Tilden, 1995). Among women who had left an abusive partner, the positive impact of social support on mental and physical health was diminished when social conflict was high (Guruge et al., 2009). In practice, nurses must be mindful of the benefit and costs of relationships, help women to evaluate their relationships, and to maintain or re-establish contact with supportive networks. Furthermore, nurses must work to ensure that their interactions with women do not contribute to the social costs of IPV.

Economic Consequences of Intimate Partner Violence

Being in an abusive relationship typically restricts women's economic independence, making employment difficult (Davis, 1999; Swanberg, Logan, & Macke, 2005; Tolman & Rosen, 2001), limiting access to income, and impeding women's self-sufficiency (Moe & Bell, 2004). After leaving, willingness to give up financial support or marital assets in exchange for greater custody and less visitation (Davis, 1999) and the costs of multiple moves, legal bills, security measures, counseling, medications, and debts incurred by ex-partners (Varcoe & Irwin, 2004; Wuest et al., 2003) erode women's financial resources further. The stress associated with financial problems may lead to or exacerbate health problems (Sutherland et al., 2001; Carlson, McNutt, Choi, & Rose, 2002).

These costs for individual women translate into significant costs for society. In the United States (National Center for Injury Prevention and Control, 2003), Australia (VicHealth, 2004), the United Kingdom (Walby, 2004), and Canada (Greaves, Hankivsky, & Kingston-Riechers, 1995; Varcoe et al., 2009), research has shown that IPV accounts for significant state expenditures in criminal justice, social welfare, child welfare, and health care. Health care costs in the United States and Canada are higher for abused versus nonabused women (Rivara et al., 2007; Snow-Jones et al., 2006; Varcoe et al., 2009).

HEALTH CARE AND INTIMATE PARTNER VIOLENCE

Nurses are in an ideal position to support women in relation to IPV, whether women are seeking routine care (for example, related to childbirth or cancer screening), care for injuries directly related to IPV, or care for health problems that may be a consequence of, or exacerbated by, living with violence (for example, gastrointestinal problems, migraines). There is good evidence that women who have experienced violence make more visits to health care providers than those who do not have this history (Plitcha, 2007; Ulrich et al., 2003) and that a history of more severe abuse is associated with greater use of services (Duterte et al., 2008; Ford-Gilboe et al., 2009). Although women's contact with the health care system provides an opportunity for support and intervention, health care systems provide limited support for such care.

Capacity of the Health Care System to Address Intimate Partner Violence

To date, the health care response to IPV has been less than adequate. Women exposed to IPV have unmet care needs and face barriers in accessing health and other services (Ford-Gilboe et al., 2009; Plichta, 2007). Research consistently has shown that health professionals often fail to identify IPV, and when abuse is recognized, their responses can be negative, inappropriate, or even harmful (Bacchus, Mezey, & Bewley, 2003; Gerbert, Abercrombie, Caspers, Love, & Bronstone, 1999; Kramer, Lorenzon, Mueller, 2004; Humphreys & Thiara, 2003; McCloskey & Grigsby, 2005; Plichta, 2007). For example, health professionals sometimes inaccurately assume that IPV is primarily a problem for poor and racialized women (Varcoe, 2001) and respond to women in ways which are unsympathetic, disempowering and victim-blaming, and focused on treating physical injuries as quickly and efficiently as possible, rather than addressing the wider context of women's lives (Gerbert et al., 1996; McMurray & Moore, 1994; Varcoe, 2001). This makes it difficult for women to trust health care providers (Kramer et al, 2004). Although Tower (2007) concluded that nurses and other health care providers often lack knowledge about IPV, have attitudes and values that inhibit an effective response, and think they have no time to respond, there is evidence that health professionals can suitably identify women who have experienced IPV if they use appropriate strategies (Rhodes et al, 2006). In large-scale surveys (e.g., Gielen et al., 2006; Sachs, Koziol-McLain, Glass, Webster, & Campbell 2002), the majority of women who disclosed IPV to a health care provider reported that they found the response helpful, while only 17% found it unhelpful. A challenge for practitioners is to develop the knowledge, attitudes, and skills needed to provide sensitive and effective care to women who have experienced IPV.

Successful practice changes also require support from health care systems and organizations. However, a focus on medically defined problems, along with organization of services by body systems (for example, Respiratory Care), age, or life event (for example, Palliative Care), has meant that IPV is not seen as a priority for most practitioners and does not have a specific place in health care. Attention to IPV in particular areas (such as emergency or maternity care) has developed primarily because IPV is often more visible in these settings. Within the context of competing priorities, administrative support for addressing IPV has been lacking. In Emergency Department (ED) settings, nurses who reported that their employers expected them to assess for IPV were more likely to incorporate routine assessment of IPV and follow-up into their practice (Hollingsworth & Ford-Gilboe, 2006). Similarly, Campbell, Coben and colleagues (2001) found that training of ED physicians and nurses in the United States, along with environmental prompts, history form changes, and administrative support, increased routine assessment of IPV and improved women's satisfaction with their experiences. Clearly, developing an effective health care response to IPV requires a commitment from both practitioners and from the systems in which they deliver care.

Beyond the "Screening Debate"

A major recommendation for health care professionals has been to universally *screen* for violence, but this is an area of controversy, some or which arises from the term "screening." Screening has its origins in a disease model and, not surprisingly, this has led some to define screening as including the *identification* of IPV but not follow-up or intervention. For nurses, this can set up an expectation that all a nurse has to do is "Ask the Question," while minimizing the responsibility to provide an appropriate response and to be well prepared to do so. Furthermore, a narrow definition of screening has meant that some health care organizations put minimal resources into dealing with IPV, focusing only on training related to the use of screening tools. The term "screening" suggests that IPV is akin to an illness which can be "treated"; medicalizing IPV has the potential to overlook women's self-determination and rob women of control over their own decisions.

An emerging shift from *screening for IPV* to *Routine Assessment and Response* terminology expands the role of health care providers in a meaningful way by reinforcing the notion that identification and follow-up are essential components of an appropriate health care response to IPV. The Family Violence Prevention Fund (FVPF) now uses this terminology in their guidelines for Health Professionals (FVPF, 2004). This change acknowledges the inadequacy of asking about IPV with no systematic plan for follow up and holds health professionals accountable for ensuring that they have the requisite knowledge and skills to ethically carry out these activities.

It also reflects that, in the United States, "screening" terminology has come to refer to medical tests for various conditions (e.g., mammograms, PSAs), which necessitate cost-benefit analyses to be sure the benefits of such tests (i.e., finding the disease and having a demonstrated effective treatment for it) are worth the monetary and human costs (e.g., pain) associated with it. Assessment (or inquiry in the United Kingdom) language is now applied to questions that accurately identify psychosocial issues, such as depression or substance abuse. Importantly, *Routine Assessment and Response* moves us toward integrating care for women who have experienced IPV into everyday practice, rather than seeing this as a separate activity.

In order to recommend routine assessment for a condition, the review of evidence (clinical trials) needs to show that the condition is sufficiently widespread and is associated with sufficiently detrimental health outcomes to warrant routine inquiry. The U.S. Preventive Task Force (USPTF) stated that IPV meets both of these conditions (Nelson, Nygren, McInerny, Klein, & U.S. Preventive Services Task Force, 2004). However, the USPTF and a separate review by the Canadian Task Force for Preventive Medicine (Wathen, MacMillan, & Canadian Task Force on Preventive Health Care, 2003) both reached the conclusion that there is insufficient evidence on which to base a recommendation to implement *universal* screening for IPV in health care settings. In both reviews, this recommendation was based on the lack of clinical trial evidence for interventions to which women could be referred and the lack of evidence about harms associated with routine inquiry for IPV. In another systematic review, Ramsay et al. (2002) found that screening resulted in better detection of abused women and increased referral to outside agencies, but there was no evidence of changes in key health outcomes, such as mental health or quality of life.

In general, screening intervention studies have used weak study designs and have not included some of the most salient outcomes for women or measured potential harms associated with screening. In a recent Canadian randomized controlled trial examining the effectiveness of screening for IPV in health care settings, MacMillan et al. (2009) found that screening was not associated with harms but that the benefits were modest when carried out in the context of current practice, rather than under ideal conditions. In this study, each woman completed a screening tool, with a positive result placed on the chart for follow-up by the health care provider using usual practice.

However, less than half (44%) of women who screened positive reported having their abuse experiences discussed by their health care provider. All women were given information about domestic violence services by the research team. Eighteen months after screening, women in the screen and no screen groups both experienced a reduction in exposure to IPV and improvement in quality of life, but there were no significant differences between the groups. Similarly, a clinical trial of screening plus a telephone support intervention (McFarlane, Groff, O'Brien, & Watson, 2006) showed that both groups improved on violence and mental health outcomes, and again, both groups were asked about abuse and given referrals, leading some to suggest that assessment of IPV with referral *may* be helpful. While the merits of implementing large-scale screening programs without further evidence of effectiveness has been questioned, some (e.g., Alpert, 2007) have argued that these programs should continue while clinical trials are being mounted to demonstrate intervention efficacy (Moracco & Cole, 2009). Clearly, there are many challenges to implementing screening in practice (see Exhibit 5.3).

There is a critical need to develop effective health care responses to identify and support women who have experienced IPV. More comprehensive interventions are being

---

EXHIBIT 5.3 | *Some Challenges to Screening for Abuse Include:*

- Women experiencing violence may not identify their experiences as abuse
- Women experiencing violence may be ashamed or anticipate judgment by care providers
- Privacy for disclosure may not be available in health care settings
- Women may fear health care provider responses, including acts that will increase their risks, such as increasing danger for themselves or family members, or risk that their children might be apprehended
- Health care providers may ask screening questions more often of women of color or poor women, further perpetuating stereotypes of abuse and overlooking abuse experiences of other women
- Providers may lack the knowledge and skills to respond to women in an appropriate way following disclosure
- Organization support for the time and resources needed for screening and follow-up may be lacking

developed and tested by nurses and others in a variety of settings. In the absence of evidence that routine assessment and response is effective or the availability of well-tested interventions, nurses still have an ethical responsibility to provide safe and supportive care to women who have experienced IPV and to work toward making wider improvements in health care responses to women. Practice in relation to IPV must be grounded in adequate knowledge, skills, and experience (FVPF, 2004).

NURSING PRACTICE IN THREE CONTEXTS

Based on previous review of theory and research, and our collective experiences of working with women who have experienced IPV, we outline a set of implications for nursing practice in three contexts:

- when the woman's history of IPV is not known;
- in the immediate period when IPV is identified;
- longer-term or more extensive follow-up of women who have experienced IPV as they seek to improve their safety and/or make changes in their lives.

In each of these contexts, we make some key assumptions about IPV and about nursing practice in relation to women who have experienced IPV (Ford-Gilbe, Wuest, Varcoe, & Merritt-Gray, 2006). Specifically, we assume that the experiences of particular women must be at the center of health care related to IPV. Although women have many commonalities, they are diverse, and each woman and her experiences of IPV and health are unique. Furthermore, we understand women's health to be socially determined by income and social status, education, social support, employment and working conditions, social environment, physical environment, personal health practices and coping skills, health services, childhood development, gender, and culture (Health Canada, 2003; Moss, 2002). Experiences of IPV often erode the determinants of health which are modifiable, reinforcing the need for intersectoral collaboration in creating services and programs, which are helpful to women. Access to high-quality, relevant, affordable health care is an important part of a larger system of services, and nurses have a key role to play in developing, providing, and evaluating these services.

In this process, nursing approaches that emphasize collaboration with women and other providers focus on capacities and strengths, and view women in the context of family and community (e.g., Allen & Warner, 2002; Doane & Varcoe, 2005; Ford-Gilboe, 2002) are particularly important in conveying respect for women's wisdom and enhancing her control. Principles to Guide Collaborative Nursing Practice With Women Who Have Experienced IPV are shown in Exhibit 5.4.

Creating a Context for Safe and Responsive Health Care: Providing Care When Intimate Partner Violence Is Not Known

Given what we know about the prevalence of IPV and other types of traumas among women, the reality that women choose when and to whom they disclose a history of IPV, and that women with histories of IPV are high users of health services, nurses should understand that many of the women they encounter will have experienced or are experiencing

EXHIBIT 5.4 | *Principles to Guide the Collaborative Nursing Practice*

With Women Who Have Experienced IPV

- The woman's emotional and physical safety will be promoted in all interactions
- The woman's physical, mental, emotional, and spiritual health will be prioritized
- The experiences of the woman and other women who have experienced IPV will be used as a key source of knowledge to help the woman reflect on, talk about, and name her experiences, concerns, and priorities
- The woman's context of family and close relationships as she defines them will be taken into account
- The woman will be supported to assess, judge, and take calculated risks
- The costs of getting help, including from the nurses and the intervention, will be assessed and limited as much as possible
- The woman's strengths and capacities will be recognized, drawn upon, and further developed
- The woman will direct the pace, what is given priority within the intervention, and who is involved
- The woman will be helped to seek and obtain support from her community and services, and to deal with the barriers she encounters
- The nurse will work to advocate for improved system responses to women receiving the intervention as they are variously situated within broad social systems of inequity

IPV. Women are experts in working to keep themselves safe and may have a vested interest in keeping their experiences of IPV private. Even when asked directly, some women will deny experiences of IPV. The reasons for this are complex and include: (a) the woman may not yet have "named" her experiences as abuse, (b) fear that her abuser may discover the disclosure, (c) previous experiences with health care or other providers that lead her to anticipate judgmental or unhelpful responses, and (d) fear that she will be reported to child protective services and may lose custody of her children. In reality, a nurse may never know the extent of IPV or trauma any particular woman has experienced.

A major challenge for health care providers is to provide care in a way that is *trauma-informed* without necessarily knowing that violence is a current or past issue for a particular woman. The nurse can begin to create a practice climate, which is empowering for women by treating every woman as though she may have a history of trauma. This is akin to taking "universal precautions" in dealing with blood products or infection. To do this, the nurse must work to ensure that *all* health care encounters are conducted in such as way as to avoid triggering a trauma response and/or re-victimizing women by making women's physical and emotional safety, and her sense of control, a priority. What would this look like in practice?

First, it is helpful to understand responses to trauma and how these can be triggered by a health care encounter. Responses to trauma are best understood in terms of anxiety, which varies in intensity from signs of mild to moderate distress (such as increased heart rate and respirations, sudden displays of fear or anger, restlessness, sweating, startle response) to dissociation. Although dissociation is very rare and may be difficult to recognize, the nurse may observe that a woman is not fully aware of her surroundings, is unable to follow instructions, respond to communication and/or concentrate (Schachter,

Stalker, Teram, Lasiuk, & Danilkewich, 2008). When providing care to a woman in this state, it is important to think of trauma first, rather than dismissing the behavior as related to drugs and alcohol. Even when drug or alcohol use is part of a woman presentation, trauma is likely an underlying issue.

Trauma responses can be "triggered" by sensations (i.e., sights, sounds, touch, smells, tastes), which are linked to the abuse and which evoke emotional responses, and memories or flashbacks of the abuser, the abuse experience, or the context. Many experiences in health care settings can serve as triggers. The general health care environment with its lack of personal space, privacy and control, intrusive questioning, and constant monitoring can set the survivor on edge. Additionally, the smell of cigarette smoke or cologne, hearing someone cry or call out, noise from equipment, dark examining rooms or locked doors, gel or other solutions, and unexpected or sudden touch can serve as triggers. These vary from woman to woman, and many are difficult to anticipate and avoid.

Most abused women do not have problematic anxiety reactions during health care encounters even when discussing the violence. They may cry when talking about their experiences but generally do not become overly anxious, even when they have PTSD. Even so, taking steps to minimize the intrusiveness of each health care encounter is important. Concern for a woman's comfort sends a message that the nurse is "in tune" with and respectful of her experiences. In this sense, nurses should seek to enhance *all* women's safety and comfort by:

- Ensuring privacy in all interactions;
- Explaining what you would like to do in detail, before and during a procedure, and ensuring free consent to treatment;
- Asking each woman about her level of comfort/discomfort and what might increase her comfort;
- Providing options and choices to enhance comfort (e.g., keeping lights dimmed; having a support person accompany her; etc);
- Avoiding common triggers over which the nurse has control, such as those which involve body space or physical touch (e.g., asking permission to touch any woman but not avoiding touch entirely as it can be therapeutic);
- Being mindful of each woman's responses, particularly to signs of distress and/or potential dissociation;
- Supporting each woman to deal with trauma responses if they occur, in a way that helps her regain her composure and sense of control and minimizes any embarrassment she may feel (see Exhibit 5.5).

A trauma-informed approach to practice is important because it puts the issue of IPV on the nurse's "radar" and reinforces the need to be mindful of potential signs, which could indicate IPV in everyday practice. Developing a heightened index of suspicion about women's exposure to IPV is an important part of identifying women who have experienced abuse. It also helps the nurse to frame many of the problems for which women seek care as potential consequences of abuse (for example, problems ranging from substance use to head injury, to migraines), raises awareness about how care may trigger trauma responses and provides a basis for minimizing harms to women. Furthermore, a trauma-informed approach is the basis for developing relationships with women that are fortifying and which encourage women to return for care, regardless of disclosure. Finally, it sets the conditions for safe disclosure if and when the woman is ready. Women

---

EXHIBIT 5.5 | *Tips for Supporting Women After an Extreme Trauma Response*

- Orient the woman to the present (time, place, context).
- Encourage slow, rhythmic breathing, and/or offer a glass of water.
- Offer verbal reassurance in a calm voice. Avoid touching her.
- Ask simple questions to help the woman connect (e.g. "Are you with me"?).
- Allow time and space to regain her composure.
- Frame her experience as a common response to abuse (if abuse was disclosed) or the anxiety that some people feel in health care settings (if no disclosure).
- Ask if she would like to contact someone to be with her and/or accompany her home.
- Explore her desire for ongoing support. Offer to connect her to an appropriate support (i.e., community agency, counselor, or other professional support).

Source: Schachter, C.L., Stalker, C.A., Teram, E., Lasiuk, G.C., Danilkewich, A. (2008). Handbook on sensitive practice for health care providers: Lessons from adult survivors of child sexual abuse. Ottawa: Public Health Agency of Canada.

---

will be more likely to disclose abuse if they feel they will not be judged or pressured to take actions they do not want to take (Catallo, 2009).

Assessing for Intimate Partner Violence and Providing Follow-Up Care

Knowing about IPV can strengthen the nurse's ability to provide more comprehensive and appropriate care to women. Assessing whether women have experienced IPV and providing follow up care after a disclosure must be a core part of health care for all women.

Routine Assessment Versus Case Finding

There are two main schools of thought about when and how often to ask women about their experiences of IPV: routine assessment and case finding. Routine assessment entails asking all women who present to health care settings about their experiences of IPV, *regardless of the reason for seeking care*, as part of the normal health history. The main rationale for routine assessment is that the prevalence of IPV among women and its impact are substantial enough to warrant a broad approach in order to identify those who are living with violence. Published recommendations for how often routine assessment should be conducted often vary by clinical site and the reason for the health care visit (e.g., at every visit to the ED versus each initial visit and comprehensive health assessment in primary care) (FVPF, 2004).

In contrast to routine assessment, *case finding* involves assessing for IPV only when certain "warning signs" or "cues" are present. These cues are potential indicators of abuse and should lead the clinician to have *high index of suspicion* about IPV, and subsequently, to inquire about the woman's history of abuse. The success of case finding depends on health professionals having a relatively sophisticated understanding of IPV and its consequences, the critical awareness that abused women come from all walks of life, and the ability to not make unconscious assumptions based on women's backgrounds about the possibility of IPV, the ability to listen carefully and observe for cues, and to link these cues to possible IPV. In practice, this means that whenever a woman presents with injuries consistent with IPV, chronic mental and/or physical health problems, which have been associated with IPV (e.g., insomnia, chronic pain, depression, substance use, generalized aches, and pains), or factors known to increase the woman's vulnerability to IPV (e.g., disabilities, social isolation, marital conflict, economic dependence), the nurse should inquire about her history of abuse. It could be argued that gender alone is a strong enough risk factor for IPV to justify routine assessment of all women for IPV.

Is there an optimal strategy? In reality, routine assessment and case finding are concerned with the same goal (i.e., the effective identification and support of women who have experienced IPV), use similar approaches in asking about IPV and providing initial support, and value the role of clinical judgment in guiding this process. The main point of disagreement is how often and under what conditions to assess for IPV. As noted, identification of IPV and providing either follow-up referrals or brief supportive interventions, have both been associated with a reduction in violence and other desired outcomes, such as safety behaviors (McFarlane et al., 2006; McFarlane, Parker, Soeken, Silva, & Reed, 1998), although we do not have strong research evidence to support the effectiveness of either routine assessment or case finding for IPV in comparison to doing nothing (i.e., control). Therefore, a reasonable approach should emphasize:

➤ *Continuing education of nurses and other health care providers.* If effective practices related to IPV are to be developed and integrated into health care, each nurse has a responsibility to ensure that he or she has the knowledge and skills needed for safe inquiry and follow-up before engaging in these practices.
➤ *Encouraging nurses who have developed such expertise to integrate assessment of IPV and follow-up into their everyday practice* in a way that is thoughtful, reflects their practice style, draws on their clinical judgment, and is appropriate to their practice setting. Nurses also need to know about and be able to carry out local protocols for assessing and responding to women who have experienced IPV. Where no protocols exist, the nurse should work with members of the health care team to develop local, evidence-based guidelines for practice.
➤ A commitment to continually update and improve local protocols based on reflective practice and new evidence is critical.

This approach moves beyond "Asking the Question" and may incorporate elements of both routine assessment and case finding. As noted later in this chapter, there is reasonably good evidence to support of use of routine assessment and follow-up during pregnancy (Tiwari et al., 2005). In other areas of practice, indicator-based approaches may be more appropriate. Integrating assessment of IPV into everyday practice reinforces its importance to other practitioners, to the public, and to women, who may identify health professionals as a source of help for themselves or for other women in the future.

Strategies for Assessing Intimate Partner Violence

There is no one *right* way to inquire about IPV. It is important that the nurse develop an approach that works for him or her, while respecting the safety, privacy, confidentiality, and autonomy of the woman. Family members or friends who accompany the woman to the visit should be respectfully asked to leave the room for a short period of time in order to complete her health assessment. An abusive partner may be reluctant to honor this request. While it may be possible to fabricate an excuse which provides a valid reason for the separation (e.g., woman needs to go for a special test or partner needs to complete paperwork), the nurse should be aware that insisting on separation might anger an abusive partner and increase the woman's risk of harm when she leaves the health care setting. A high level of controlling behavior in a partner is an important indicator of possible abuse. In this situation, the nurse should adopt strategies to ensure that the woman is assessed elsewhere or at a later, but not too distant time.

The issue of IPV can be introduced in subtle or more direct ways. For example, a nurse may wish to frame questions by talking about how relationships can affect health, noting that most relationships have positives and negatives associated with them (e.g., "How are things at home?", "How supportive is your partner in relation to [your health problem]", "How are decisions made in your home?", "How do you and your partner deal with conflict?", "Does a conflict ever get physical?"). Another option is to be more direct and comment on the link between IPV and health as the reason for including it in a health care visit (e.g., "Because abuse from a partner is so common and we know that it has major impact on a woman's mental and physical health, I would like to ask you a few questions about your relationship with your partner."). Finally, when women present with health problems or injuries that are consistent with IPV, questions about abuse can be linked to the reason for seeking care (e.g., "Some of the health problems you are experiencing, such as chronic pain, are more common in women who have had injuries or are living with stress because of abuse from a partner or someone close to them. This is very common. Is this something you have experienced?"). This approach can help raise women's awareness about the impact of abuse on their health.

Examples of direct questions can be found in published screening Guidelines (FVPF, 2004; Registered Nurses Association of Ontario, 2005) or clinical tools, such as the Abuse Assessment Screen. This screening tool, developed by Helton and McFarlane, has been widely used in health care settings (Rabin, Jennings, Campbell, & Blair-Merritt, 2009) and is available in English and Spanish at http://www.nnvawi.org). See Exhibit 5.6 below.

When assessing for IPV, paying attention to language is important. Since a woman may not identify their experiences as abusive, it is best to ask whether she has experienced particular abusive acts, rather than whether she has been *abused*. As noted earlier, the definition of IPV is broader than physical or sexual assault and IPV ranges in intensity. Sexual coercion needs to be asked about in the language of "forced sex" rather than sexual assault or rape as women associate such terms with stranger rape. There is also some evidence that psychological abuse (i.e., repeated actions to maintain power, control, and fear, systematic patterns of degrading verbal attacks) may be at least as harmful as physical and sexual violence. For these reasons, a thorough assessment of IPV must address varied types of abuse (physical or sexual violence, or the threat of such violence, and psychological or emotional abuse, including threats, stalking, and coercive control, including restricting access to material assets and employment).

Providing Follow-Up Care

It is critical that the nurse be respectful of women's responses to questions about IPV, including whether she discloses IPV and, if so, the extent to which she wants to share these experiences with the nurse. An effective response to a disclosure of IPV should incorporate the following:

EXHIBIT 5.6 | *Abuse Assessment Screen (AAS)*

1. Have you ever been emotionally or physically abused by your
   partner or someone important to you?   Yes   No
2. Within the last year, have you been hit, slapped, kicked, or
   otherwise physically hurt by someone?   Yes   No
   If yes, by whom? _____
   Total number of times:____
3. Since you have been pregnant, have you been hit, slapped,
   kicked, or otherwise physically hurt by someone?   Yes   No
   If yes, by whom? _____
   Total number of times: ____

Mark area of injury on the body map.
Score each incident according to the following scale: **SCORE**

   1 = Threats of abuse, including use of a weapon   _____
   2 = Slapping, pushing; no injuries and/or
       lasting pain   _____
   3 = Punching, kicking, bruises, cuts, and/
       or continuing pain
   4 = Beaten up, severe contusions, burns,
       broken bones   _____
   5 = Head, internal, and/or permanent injury   _____
   6 = Use of weapon, wound from weapon   _____

If any of the descriptions for the higher number apply,
use the higher number.

4. Within the past year, has anyone forced you to
   have sexual activities?   Yes   No

   If yes, by whom? _____
   Total number of times:____
5. Are you afraid of your partner or anyone you listed above?   Yes   No

Developed by the Nursing Research Consortium on Violence and Abuse.
Readers are encouraged to reproduce and use this assessment tool www.nnvawi.org

---

1. *Listen to her story in a nonjudgmental way without interrupting.* Being present to witness and believe the woman's account is one of the most powerful and helpful things a nurse can do for women who have previously encountered disbelief, blame, or judgment from others (Lempert, 1997). The use of open-ended questions may help the woman feel in more control. Sharing complete details or the full abuse story is not essential for recovery or healing. What is critical is that the woman feels heard and validated.
2. *Affirm that she is not to blame and help her place her experience in context.* Women who have experienced IPV repeatedly have been told that the abuse is their fault and often come to internalize this belief. Let her know that abuse is never right, and no woman deserves to be abused. Unconditional acceptance and positive regard are the foundation

for developing trust. It may be helpful to share information about IPV with woman at this point in order to help validate her feelings and experiences (e.g., many women feel confused or afraid about what to do about the violence; they may feel trapped, angry, hopeless, and have mixed feelings about the abuser, including commitment. Most just want the abuse to end, not the relationship, at least at first).

3. *Document the woman's story in her health record.* The nurse should record as much of the woman's story as possible, using her own words whenever possible. Documenting should not interfere with her ability to actively listen and attend to the woman. Taking short notes and constructing a note immediately after the interaction is recommended. An accurate record may be useful to the woman in court as documentation of abuse, but nurses should find out how medical records are used in courts (particularly those dealing with child custody disputes) in their jurisdictions. Based on knowing about the particular jurisdiction, the nurse should talk to the woman about how the documentation may be helpful to her, and explain the limits to confidentiality of medical records, and how she can access this information in future.

4. *Assess her level of risk and discuss safety strategies.* At a minimum, the nurse should inquire about her current safety risks and discuss possible safety strategies with her. Because women often underestimate their risk, using a tool such as the *Danger Assessment* (Campbell, Webster, & Glass, 2009) can be useful in helping women think about risk in a new way (for more information, see http://nnvawi.org/assessment.htm, www.dangerassessment.org and Appendix B).

Identify how she has managed to keep herself and/or her children safe and who she can go to for emotional support and practical help. Discuss any services she has used in the past and her experiences using these services. Share strategies other women have used to enhance their safety by completing a safety plan (Exhibit 5.7).

5. *Conduct a thorough health assessment.* Use this time as an opportunity to explain that abuse has a wide range of health consequences. Identify and document any health concerns and explore with the woman how her health problems may be linked to abuse and particular health issues she may want to proactively pay attention to in the future.

6. *Ask the woman what she needs now, what would be helpful to her.* Work with the woman to identify options that fit with her needs and preferences. Offer information about services, which can provide more in-depth support or assistance as appropriate (e.g., shelter, domestic violence program, the nurse, or other health professional in the agency). Respect her choices—do not try to convince her to take another route. Help her problem solve how to get the support she needs for the decision she has made.

7. *Discuss referral if the woman is interested.* Offer to directly facilitate her access to services. This type of active referral might involve staying with her while she calls the provider from the health care agency, or if the program is on-site, accompanying her to meet the person who will follow-up. Based on the premise that witnessing IPV is harmful to child safety and well-being, in many jurisdictions, a disclosure of IPV also requires that the health care provider make a report to child protective services. The requirements and conditions for reporting vary by jurisdiction from a duty to report all instances of IPV to only those where there is obvious evidence of negative impact on the child/ren (e.g., acting out or aggression, school difficulties, anxiety or

---

EXHIBIT 5.7 | *Basic Safety Planning Strategies*

Safety at Home
- Identify an escape route(s) for each room and practice getting out quickly.
- Keep your purse/wallet and keys handy and in the same place so that you can locate them easily if you need to leave in a hurry.
- Hide a second set of keys in case your partner takes the first set.
- Keep copies of important documents such as birth certificates and Medicare cards for you and your children and extra clothing/personal items in a safe place (e.g., with a friend).
- Keep change for telephone calls with you at all times.
- If you need to keep your plans from your partner, use a pay phone or borrow one from a friend (contacts can be traced).
- Internet use and email can also be traced—use a computer that he cannot access (e.g., library) and/or erase or clear the history from computers you use.
- If possible, remove weapons (including guns) from the home.
- Put a little money aside each week (e.g., open a bank account in your name only).
- Teach your children how to call 911, when to leave the house, and where to go.
- Get legal advice from a lawyer who understands woman abuse.
- Call the police (they can be helpful and must lay charges against the partner if there is evidence of assault).
- Tell someone you trust about the violence and ask them to call the police if they think you are in (e.g., hear strange noises or some other signal, like an outside light which is turned on).
- Have a code word to use with friends, children, or family members if you need them to call for help.
- Know that fighting back with violence could result in being charged with a criminal offence.

Leaving Home
- Identify safe places to go for a few hours or a few days (e.g., family member, shelter, etc.).
- Do not tell the partner that you are leaving face to face.
- If you leave when he is not home, you could leave note or call him later.
- Have a plan for getting to a safe place in an emergency (e.g., taxis often take women to a shelter free of change)
- If you have time, take important items with you (i.e., identification/passports; copy of protection orders; school and health records; medications; driver's license; money and/or bank/credit cards and passwords for accounts; legal documents, such as marriage/separation, deed to property, lease agreement); address book; pictures/photos (other items of sentimental value); children's favorite toy/blankets; recent photo of partner that would help identify him to neighbors, teachers, police, etc.

---

depression, change in usual behavior or affect, etc.). The nurse must be aware of local requirements and the processes used to make reports. In cases where reporting is required, the nurse should share information about the requirement and the reason for it (i.e., concern for the welfare of children). Whenever possible, offering women the option of making the call themselves, with support from the nurse, may help her maintain some control of the situation.

8. *Leave the door open to further contact.* Inviting the woman back for health concerns is good practice, whether a disclosure of violence has occurred or whether or not violence is a suspected issue. The FVPF (2004) suggests scheduling at least one follow-up appointment after initial support for a disclosure. However, such follow up must fit with the woman's goals and needs for safety.

Nurses' responses to disclosures need to be "fortifying." This can be a particular challenge when a woman does not make the choices the nurse would make for her or thinks she should make. The woman should leave the interaction feeling listened to and validated, knowing that you were genuinely concerned, particularly about her emotional and physical safety. She should have at least a rudimentary safety plan, information about services, and some options in place. In most cases, it is impossible to address all of the considerations listed above in one contact. When possible, a more thorough assessment of safety and discussion of options can occur at subsequent visits.

Comprehensive Nursing Approaches to Supporting Women Who Have Experienced Intimate Partner Violence

The development of interventions to support women who have experienced violence has been identified as a priority for research, yet few such interventions exist (Wathen & MacMillan, 2000). As previously noted, within health care systems, attention to IPV has largely focused on the issue of universal screening and referral to support services associated with the crisis of leaving abusive partners. Less attention has been granted to developing interventions that address women's safety and the complex health and social issues which they face while with the abusive partner or, for some women, after leaving. The "empowerment intervention" or "10-minute intervention" as it is sometimes called, was developed by McFarlane and Parker and is available through the March of Dimes. It is a brief, brochure-driven nursing intervention, which includes an assessment of danger, choices of strategies to address the violence, and brief safety planning. The research supporting the intervention is quasiexperimental in the United States, but it has been tested in a clinical trial in Hong Kong (Tiwari et al., 2005) and showed significant improvements in psychological and physical abuse as well as depression and functioning among women attending prenatal clinics.

In a systematic review of advocacy interventions for women who had experienced IPV, Ramsay et al. (2009) concluded that there is evidence to support an improvement in quality of life, safety actions, social support and access to services and a reduction in violence for women who had sought help, particularly through shelters, when an advocacy intervention was delivered. While a brief empowerment and safety planning intervention (Tiwari et al., 2005) delivered by nurses also resulted in a reduction in depressive symptoms, a postshelter system navigation intervention delivered by paraprofessionals (Sullivan & Bybee, 1999; Sullivan, Bybee, & Allen, 2002) did not. These findings suggest that services focusing on support, safety, and system navigation are important for women who have left abusive partners but may not be sufficient to address the mental health consequences of violence.

There is considerable potential to develop more comprehensive health care responses aimed at supporting women who have experienced IPV. Nurses have an important role to play in these interventions since client trust is often high, and as the largest group of health professionals, they come in regular contact with women in all types of health care settings. Furthermore, nurses' knowledge and skills related to therapeutic relationships, symptom management, health promotion and disease prevention, supportive counseling, and system navigation fit well with many women's needs.

In particular, a focus on symptom management and referrals for health care is an area not well addressed by domestic violence services and requires expertise that nurses can provide, both to support women in developing strategies for managing distressing symptoms and to tap into formal and informal networks in the health care sector in order to expedite referrals and service delivery (Ford-Gilboe, Wuest, Merritt-Gray, & Varcoe, 2006). Assisting women to reduce distressing symptoms can lead to general improvements in health and strengthen personal resources (i.e., energy, ability to concentrate) needed to deal with violence on an ongoing basis.

Thus, successful symptom management may indirectly affect a woman's level of safety. Given the complexity of IPV and the fact that changes in a woman's life typically occur as a process over time, the greatest opportunities to develop more comprehensive interventions may be in clinical contexts where nurses have ongoing relationships with women, such as in community health, primary care, or mental health practice.

A number of health interventions for women who have experienced IPV are in the early stages of development and testing. Most of these emerging interventions are community based and, since IPV is a complex issue with broad consequences for women's lives, incorporate collaboration with and/or referral to services in other sectors. Emerging interventions vary in their theoretical grounding, intervention approach, and in the women they seek to serve. Two examples of developing interventions are described below briefly as a way of stimulating thinking about how we might develop nursing practice in relation to IPV.

Extending Community Nursing Practice With Pregnant and Parenting Women: The DOVE Intervention

Although 3% to 19% of pregnant women experience IPV, few evidence-based strategies exist for preventing or reducing adverse outcomes of IPV for pregnant women and infants. The Domestic Violence Enhanced Home Visitation (DOVE) intervention was developed by a team led by nursing researchers (Phyllis Sharps, Linda Bullock, Jacquelyn Campbell) with the goal of reducing victimization among women and infants in homes in which IPV has been identified. The DOVE intervention incorporates identification of IPV and safety planning using a more intensive and sustained approach than found in previous screening and referral interventions.

Delivered during six home visits (three prenatal, three postpartum), DOVE was designed to enhance the usual nurse home visiting practice. Nurses use a specific empowerment and educational protocol to increase pregnant women's awareness of IPV and enhance their ability to make and implement a safety plan for themselves and their infants. The effectiveness of the DOVE intervention is being tested in a randomized controlled trial in health departments in two states and as an enhancement to an established nurse home visitation program for women with young children (the Nurse Family Partnership). If shown to be effective, DOVE could be integrated into existing perinatal home visiting programs, providing a direct and immediate model for enhancing nursing practice in relation to IPV.

Supporting Women After Leaving: The i-HEAL Intervention

In contrast to the DOVE intervention, the Intervention for Health Enhancement after Leaving (i-HEAL) is a complex, primary health care intervention designed to enhance women's health and quality of life in the early years after leaving an abusive partner by (a) reducing abuse-related *intrusion*, and (b) increasing the capacities and external resources women need to limit and manage the *intrusion* in their lives. Since 2006, we have been engaged in designing this intervention based on the theory of *strengthening capacity to limit intrusion*, the early findings of our study of the health and economic effects of intimate partner violence after leaving, and health promotion interventions more generally (Ford-Gilboe et al., 2006).

The i-HEAL is delivered by a nurse in collaboration with a domestic violence advocate over a period of 6 months through approximately 12 to 14 face-to-face meetings in women's homes or other safe locations. Eight principles (see Exhibit 5.4) guide the interventionist in working through six intervention components: *safeguarding, managing basics, managing symptoms, renewing self,* and *regenerating family, cautious connecting* (Exhibit 5.8). Each component is addressed during the intervention, but the timing and emphasis are tailored to women's priorities. The nurse and advocate are guided by a standardized process and draw on a toolkit, which contains information, assessment, and strategy tools. For example, for the component of managing symptoms, the toolkit includes information tools regarding what is known about common symptoms experienced by women, including chronic pain, sleep problems, symptoms of depression, and symptoms of PTSD; assessment tools, including a symptom diary, to identify the characteristics and patterns of the women's symptoms; and strategy guidelines for managing specific health problems.

EXHIBIT 5.8 | *Six Components of the i-Heal Intervention*

1. *Safeguarding* involves limiting the exposure of the woman and her family to people or circumstances that threaten their physical and emotional safety. It focuses on assessing her sense of physical and emotional safety and feeling safe and developing strategies to manage risks and build her sense of security.
2. *Managing basics* involves getting material and economic resources, energy, and skills needed to have a quality life as the woman defines it.
3. *Managing symptoms* entails the identification and testing of various approaches to reducing the distress associated with symptoms, both those that the woman can direct herself and those that require support from other professionals.
4. *Renewing self* involves identifying personal needs, desires, feelings and abilities, and enhancing her capacity to make time and space for herself.
5. *Regenerating family* focuses on taking stock of family patterns of interaction and developing strategies to enhance family routines, rules and roles, and reinforce standards for relating to one another that are important to the family.
6. *Cautious connecting* entails supporting women to evaluate the costs and optimize the benefits of current and potential relationships with peers, extended family, social networks, or formal service agencies in order to gain a sense of belonging, emotional support, social interaction, and/or practical aid.

Pilot testing of i-HEAL is being conducted with a community sample of women who have left abusive partners to examine the feasibility, relevance and efficacy of this new intervention. Follow-up studies are planned to examine efficacy in larger, more diverse groups of women (e.g., aboriginal women in urban settings) and effectiveness (i.e., impact when integrated into an existing system of care) in varied contexts (e.g., as an enhancement to outreach services in the domestic violence sector).

What Can We Learn From These Emerging Intervention Studies?

Research in the area of intervention related to IPV is in its infancy. However, important direction can already be derived from this ongoing work. Nurses should:

- Be creative in thinking about how to support women;
- Acknowledge and assess for abuse across the life span, not only current or recent IPV;
- Focus on partnerships between women, health care providers, and others, including DV services. For example, nurses from community health settings, labor and delivery units and emergency units have partnered with service providers in women's shelters to provide services to women who are living in shelter and to develop outreach programs;
- Consider a range of roles, such as case management, to help women navigate complex systems of care and to advocate for access to services. Moreover, a case management model would build in continuity and connections for women to help reduce fragmentation of services and provide a contact to help women access supports and services in the future;
- Engage in wider system change.

NURSES' ROLE IN POLITICAL ADVOCACY AND SYSTEM CHANGE

Nurses must act at levels beyond their individual patients if intimate partner violence is to be responded to more effectively, prevented, and its prevalence lowered. First, the social and health care response to IPV must be strengthened. Nurses can have a profound impact by lobbying for (a) better education of health care providers regarding IPV, (b) resources in health care settings to support more effective responses to IPV, (c) better collaboration across sectors (for example, between health care agencies and antiviolence agencies and services, and (d) the development of policies based on understanding of the dynamics of violence in areas such as social assistance and child welfare.

Second, the root causes and factors influencing the prevalence of violence must be addressed. Using the idea of pulling drowning victims from the water, without going upstream to see who is pushing people in the water, Butterfield (1990) argues that nurses must look "upstream" at health problems. This is particularly crucial in relation to intimate partner violence. Nurses can have a powerful role in lobbying against factors that promote violence (such as war or media depictions of women that promote tolerance of violence) and for factors which mitigate violence (such as any factors that promote gender or racial equity). Nurses can lobby in their everyday lives, on a daily basis in their work lives or through professional nursing associations, or take on a wider role by joining with others in their communities who work against violence.

CULTURAL CONSIDERATIONS IN ASSESSMENT AND INTERVENTION

Culture is a process that happens between people in specific social, historical, and political contexts. Rather than just being the values, beliefs, and practices of particular groups of people, culture is a continuously evolving process, with as much diversity occurring within groups as between them. Lay understandings often confuse "culture" with "ethnicity" and emphasize the idea that culture is a static "thing" that people have, rather than as a dynamic process. In this confusion, people are thought to "have" culture associated primarily with their country of birth or that of their ancestors (for example, Vietnamese culture, Chinese culture), or associated with their physical features (for example, black culture), without considering how cultures are multifaceted and produced within a complex network of power dynamics unfolding historically in an ongoing process. For example, in the United States, African American culture is not related to particular physical characteristics, but rather arises from a history of power, oppression, and resistance.

With respect to IPV and culture, violence is often understood in racialized ways—that is to say, the prevalence of IPV among certain groups is erroneously assumed to be inherent to the biology of those groups, rather than recognizing that experiences of violence are shaped by multiple factors. Despite widespread understanding that (a) IPV crosses all cultures, classes, nations, and ethnicities and (b) race has no biological basis (Henry & Tator, 2006; United Nations Educational Scientific and Cultural Organization, 1952), there is a tendency in public media, research, and social institutions such as health care, to understand violence in relation to "race" without considering power dynamics and oppression. For example, news media report violence in ways that promote racial stereotypes (e.g., Meyers, 2004; Wilcox, 2005). In providing nursing care related to IPV, nurses can contribute to or work against stereotyping and discrimination.

Cultural considerations in relation to providing nursing care related to IPV include three key elements. First, nurses should *understand how the dominant culture shapes violence* in their particular contexts. For example, IPV is shaped by militarization and war in a range of ways, including increasing tolerance for violence generally and through the exposure of military personnel to violence (Adelman, 2003; Okazawa-Rey, 2002; Tambiah, 2005).

Second, nurses should *critically reflect on their understanding and assumptions* regarding (a) intimate partner violence, (b) how social factors (such as poverty, where people live, age) shape exposure to and experiences of violence, (c) dominant sociocultural responses to violence (such as a primary emphasis on women "leaving," and (d) how stereotyping (such as stereotypes about violence related to race, ethnicity, gender, class, sexual orientation) can further victimize people who experience violence. For example, if nurses see violence as something that is more common to certain ethnocultural communities, they may tend to have a higher index of suspicion with some groups of people and overlook cues with other groups.

Third, understanding how violence is shaped by broader social features, nurses can engage with individuals with *greater awareness of how those individuals' experiences are shaped by their social circumstances.* So, for example, with a greater understanding of how economic resources shape options for leaving abusive partners, nurses can better attend to the needs of individuals, rather than providing care based on assumptions that any given person has the required resources to "leave." Nurses operating with a better sense of how racism limits employment options or housing options can similarly work to develop more realistic and effective safety plans.

Finally, as we have argued, nurses have an obligation to engage in political advocacy and system change. Better understanding on how dominant culture fosters violence, including violence against women and racism, and how these forms of violence intersect, will allow nurses to more effectively engage politically. Whether nurses take action at an individual level (for example, countering a colleague's erroneous assumption that members of a certain group are inherently "more violent") or at an organizational level (for example, by lobbying against depictions of women in media that promote tolerance

---

EXHIBIT 5.9 | *Resources: Materials on Partner and Family Violence*

Best Practice Guidelines: Registered Nurses Association of Ontario. http://www.rnao.
   org/Storage/12/655_BPG_Women_Abuse.pdf
Center for Disease Control: Intimate Partner Violence Prevention resources http://
   www.cdc.gov/ViolencePrevention/intimatepartnerviolence/index.html
End Violence Against Women: Tools and guidelines for gender-based violence
   programs. http://www.infoforhealth.org/endvaw/resources/tools.shtml#tools_
   intersection
Hot Peach Pages, International Directory of Domestic Violence Services: Canada http://
   www.hotpeachpages.net/canada/canada1.html United States http://www.
   hotpeachpages.net/usa/index.html Mexico http://www.hotpeachpages.net/
   camerica/camerica1.html#Mexico
Violence Against Women Online Resources: Materials on domestic violence, sexual assault,
   and stalking for criminal justice professionals, sexual assault, and domestic violence
   victim advocates, and other multidisciplinary professionals and community partners
   who respond to these crimes. http://www.vaw.umn.edu/
MINCAVA Electronic Clearing House, Minnesota Center Against Violence and Abuse:
   Materials on family violence. http://www.mincava.umn.edu/
National Health Resource Center on Domestic Violence, Family Violence Prevention Fund:
   Downloadable health materials (brochures, videos, training materials, guidelines)
   index http://endabuse.org/section/programs/health_care/_health_material
National Online Resource Center on Violence Against Women: Online resources for
   advocates working to end domestic violence, sexual assault, and other violence in
   the lives of women and their children. http://www.vawnet.org/
Nursing Network on Violence Against Women International: Assessment tools. *http://www.
   nnvawi.org/assessment.htm*
Public Health Agency of Canada: Downloadable materials on violence against women.
   http://www.phac-aspc.gc.ca/ncfv-cnivf/publications-eng.php
US Federal Government Source for Women's Health Information related to Violence: Includes
   state listings, brochures, and links to other sites http://www.womenshealth.gov/
   Violence/
US National Domestic Violence Hotline: 800-799-SAFE (7233), 800-787-3224 TYY.

of violence), a deeper understanding of culture as a dynamic process in which we all participate will inform such actions.

CONCLUSION

Nursing can make a significant contribution to the health of women who have experienced IPV and can work toward decreasing violence in society. Basing practice on evidence regarding the complexity and effects of violence and a stronger understanding of how those dynamics play out in individual lives will allow nurses to more effectively promote women's health and contribute to a wider community response to intimate partner violence.

See Exhibit 5.9 for a list of resources for materials on partner and family violence.

REFERENCES

Adelman, M. (2003). The military, militarism, and the militarization of Domestic Violence. *Violence Against Women, 9*(9), 1118–1152.

Allen, M., & Warner, M. (2002). A developmental model of health and nursing. *Journal of Family Nursing, 8*(2), 96–135.

Alpert, E. (2007). Addressing domestic violence: The long road ahead. *Annals of Internal Medicine Med., 147,* 666–667.

Anderson, D., & Saunders, D. (2003). Leaving an abusive partner: An empirical review of predictors, the process of leaving, and psychological well-being. *Trauma, Violence, & Abuse, 4*(2), 163–91.

Campbell, J. C., & Humpreys, J. (1993). *Nursing care of survivors of family violence.* St. Louis: Mosby.

Bacchus, L., Mezey, G., & Bewley, S. (2003). Experiences of seeking help from health professionals in a sample of women who experienced domestic violence. *Health & Social Care in the Community, 1*(1): 10–8.

Banks, M. E. (2007). Overlooked but critical: Traumatic brain injury as a consequence of interpersonal violence. *Trauma, Violence & Abuse, 8*(3), 290–298.

Barron, J. (2005). Multiple challenges in services for women experiencing domestic violence. *Housing, Care and Support, 8.1,* 11–15.

Beeble, M., Bybee, D., Sullivan, C., & Adams, A. (2009). Main, mediating, and moderating effects of social support on the well-being of survivors of intimate partner violence across 2 years. *Journal of Consulting and Clinical Psychology, 77,* 718–729.

Bell, M., Goodman, L., & Dutton, M. A. (2007). The dynamics of staying and leaving: Implications for battered women's emotional well-being and the experiences of violence at the end of a year. *Journal of Family Violence, 22,* 413–428.

Berman, H. (1999). Health in the aftermath of violence: A critical narrative study of children of war and children of battered women. *Canadian Journal of Nursing Research, 31*(3), 89–109.

Brown, J. (1997). Working toward freedom from violence: The process of change in battered women. *Violence Against Women, 3*(1), 5–26.

Butterfield, P. G. (1990). Thinking upstream: Nurturing a conceptual understanding of the social context of health behavior. *Advances in Nursing Science, 12*(2), 1–8.

Buzawa, E. S., & Buzawa, C. G. (1993). The impact of arrest on domestic violence. *American Behavioral Scientist, 36*(5), 558–574.

Campbell, J. C. (Ed.) (1998). *Empowering survivors of abuse: Health care for battered women and their children.* Newbury Park, CA: Sage.

Campbell, J. C. (2002). Health consequences of intimate partner violence. *The Lancet, 359,* 1331–1336.

Campbell, J. C., & Alford, P. (1989) The dark consequences of marital rape. *American Journal of Nursing, 89,* 946–949.

Campbell, J. C., Coben, J., Dearwater, S., McLoughlin, E., Glass, N., & Nah, G. (2001). Evaluation of a system change training model to improve ED response to battered women. *Academic Emergency Medicine, 8,* 131–138.

Campbell, J. C., & Kendall-Tackett, K. (2005). Intimate partner violence: Implications for women's physical and mental health. In K. Kendall-Tackett (Ed.), *Handbook of women, stress, and trauma* (pp. 123–158). New York: Brunner-Routledge.

Campbell, J. C., Rose, L., Kub, J., & Nedd, D. (1998). Voices of strength and resistance: A contextual and longitudinal analysis of women's responses to battering. *Journal of Interpersonal Violence, 13*(6), 743–762.

Campbell, J. C., Snow-Jones, A., Dienemann, J., Kub, J., Schollenberger, J., O'Campo, P., Carlson-Gielen, A. (2002). Intimate partner violence and physical health consequences. *Archives of Internal Medicine, 162,* 1157–1163.

Campbell, J. C., & Soeken, K. L. (1999). Forced sex and intimate partner violence: Effects on women's risk and women's health. *Violence Against Women, 5,* 1017–1035.

Campbell, J. C., & Soeken, K. (1999). Women's responses to battering: A test of the model. *Research in Nursing and Health, 22,* 49–58.

Campbell, J. C., Webster, D. W., & Glass, N. E. (2009). The Danger Assessment: Validation of a lethality risk assessment instrument for intimate partner femicide. *Journal of Interpersonal Violence, 24,* 653–674.

Campbell, R., Greeson, M., Bybee, D., & Raja, S. (2008). The co-occurrence of childhood sexual assault, adult sexual assault, intimate partner violence, and sexual harassment: A mediation model of post-traumatic stress disorder and physical health outcomes. *Journal of Consulting and Clinical Psychology, 76,* 194–207.

Campbell, R., Sullivan, C., & Davidson, W. (1995). Women who use domestic violence shelters: Changes in depression over time. *Psychology of Women Quarterly, 19,* 237–255.

Carbone-López, K., Kruttschnitt, C., & MacMillan, R. (2006). Patterns of intimate partner violence and their associations with physical health, psychological distress, and substance use. *Public Health Reports, 121*(4), 382–392.

Carlson, E., & Dalenberg, C. (2000). A conceptual framework for the impact of traumatic experiences. *Trauma Violence & Abuse, 1,* 4–28.

Carlson, B., McNutt, L., Choi, D., & Rose, I. (2002). Intimate partner violence and mental health. *Violence Against Women, 8,* 720–745.

Catallo, C. (2009). *Disclosure of intimate partner violence: A mixed methods study.* Unpublished doctoral dissertation, McMaster University, Hamilton, ON.

Chapman, C. R., Tuckett, R., & Song, C. W. (2008). Pain and stress in a systems perspective: Reciprocal neural, endocrine and immune interactions. *Journal of Pain, 9,* 122–145.

Coker, A. L., Hopenhayn, C., DeSimone, C. P., Bush, H. M., & Crofford, L. (2009). Violence against women raises risk of cervical cancer. *Journal of Women's Health, 18*(8), 1179–1185.

Coker, A., Smith, P., Bethea, L., King, M., & McKeown, R. (2000). Physical health consequences of physical and psychological intimate partner violence. *Archives of Family Medicine, 9,* 451–457.

Coker, A., Smith, P., & Fadden, M. P. (2005). Intimate partner violence and disabilities. *Journal of Women's Health, 14,* 829–838.

Coker, A., Watkins, K., Smith, P., & Brandt, H. (2003). Social support reduces the impact of partner violence on health: Application of structural equation models. *Preventive Medicine, 37,* 259–67.

Corrigan, J. D., Wolfe, M., Mysiw, W. J., Jackson, R. D., & Bogner, J. A. (2003). Early identification of mild traumatic brain injury in female victims of domestic violence. *American Journal of Obstetrics and Gynecology, 188*(5), S71–S76.

Davies, L., Ford-Gilboe, M., & Hammerton, J. (2009). Gender inequality and patterns of abuse post leaving. *Journal of Family Violence, 24,* 27–39.

Davis, M. (1999). The economics of abuse: How violence perpetuates women's poverty. In R. A. Brandwein (Ed.), *Battered women, children and welfare reform: The ties that bind* (pp. 17–30). Thousand Oaks, CA: Sage.

Dienemann, J., Campbell, J., Landenburger, K., & Curry M. A. (2002). The domestic violence survivor assessment: A tool for counseling women in intimate partner violence relationships. *Patient Education & Counseling, 46*(3), 221–228.

Doane, G., & Varcoe, C. (2005). *Family nursing as relational inquiry: Developing health promoting practice.* Philadelphia: Lippincott, Williams and Wilkins.

Dunn, J. L., & Powell-Williams, M. (2007). "Everybody makes choices." *Violence Against Women, 13,* 977–1001.

Duterte, E. Bonomi, A., Kernic, M. A., Schiff, M. A., Thompson, R. S., & Rivara, F. P. (2008). Correlates of medical and legal help seeking among women reporting intimate partner violence. *Journal of Women's Health, 17*(1), 85–95.

Dutton, M. (2009). Pathways linking intimate partner violence and posttraumatic stress disorder. *Trauma, Violence, & Abuse, 10*, 211–224.

Dutton, M., Green, B., Kaltman, S. Roesch, D., Zeffiro, T., & Krause, E. (2006). Intimate partner violence, PTSD, and adverse health outcomes. *Journal of Interpersonal Violence, 21*(7), 955–968.

Eby, K., Campbell, J., Sullivan, C. & Davidson, W. (1995). Health effects of experiences of sexual violence for women with abusive partners. *Health Care for Women International, 16*, 563–576.

Ellsberg, M., Jansen, H., Heise, L., Watts, C., & Garcia-Moreno (2008). Intimate partner violence and women's physical and mental health in the WHO multi-country study on women's health and domestic violence: An observational study. *Lancet, 371*, 1165–1172.

Family Violence Prevention Fund. (2004) National consensus guidelines for identifying and responding to domestic violence victimization in health care settings. San Francisco, CA: Family Violence Prevention Fund.

Follingstad, D. (2009). The impact of psychological aggression on women's mental health and behavior: The status of the field. *Trauma, Violence & Abuse, 10*, 271–289.

Ford-Gilboe, M. (2002). Developing knowledge about family health promotion by testing the developmental health model. *Journal of Family Nursing, 8*(2), 140–156.

Ford-Gilboe, M., Hammerton, J., Burnett, C., Wuest, J., & Varcoe, C. (2009). *Patterns of service use among women who have left an abusive partner.* Manuscript submitted for publication.

Ford-Gilboe, M., Wuest, J., & Merritt-Gray, M. (2005). Strengthening capacity to limit intrusion: Theorizing family health promotion in the aftermath of woman abuse. *Qualitative Health Research, 15*(4), 477–501.

Ford-Gilboe, M., Wuest, J., Varcoe, C., & Merritt-Gray, M. (2006). Knowledge Translation: Developing an evidence-based health advocacy intervention for women who have left abusive partners. *Canadian Journal of Nursing Research, 38*(1), 147–167.

Ford-Gilboe, M., Wuest, J., Varcoe, C., Davies, L., Merritt-Gray, M. Campbell, J., & Wilk, P. (2009). Modelling the effects of intimate partner violence and access to resources on women's health in the early years after leaving an abusive partner. *Social Science & Medicine, 68*, 1021–1029.

Friedman, M., & McEwan, B. (2004). Posttraumatic stress disorder, allostatic load, and medical illness. In P. Schnurr & B.Green (Eds.). *Trauma and health: Physical consequences of exposure to extreme stress.* (pp. 157–188). Washington, DC: APA.

Gielen, A., Campbell, J., Garza, M., O'Campo, P., Dienemann, J., Kub, J., Snow Jones, A., & Lloyd, D. (2006). Domestic Violence in the military: Women's policy preferences and beliefs concerning routine screening and mandatory reporting. *Military Medicine, 171*(8), 29–735.

Gerbert, B., Johnston, K., Caspers, N., Bleecker, T., Woods, A., & Rosenbaum, A. (1996). Experiences of battered women in health care settings: A qualitative study. *Women & Health, 24*(3), 1–17.

Gerbert, B., Abercrombie, P., Caspers, N., Love, C., & Bronstone, A. (1999). How health care providers help battered women: The survivor's perspective. *Women & Health, 29*(3), 115–135.

Glass, N., Perrin, N., Campbell, J., & Soeken, K. (2007). The protective role of tangible support on posttraumatic stress disorder symptoms in urban women survivors of violence. *Research in Nursing & Health, 30*, 558–568.

Goeckermann, C. R., Hamberger, L. K., & Barber, K. (1994). Issues of domestic violence unique to rural areas. *Wisconsin Medical Journal, 93*(9), 473–479.

Golding, J. (1999). Intimate partner violence as a risk factor for mental disorders: A meta-analysis. *Journal of Family Violence, 14*, 99–132.

Gondolf, E. W. (2002). *Batterer intervention systems. Issues, outcomes, and recommendations.* Beverly Hills, CA: Sage Publication.

Greaves, L., Hankivsky, O., & Kingston-Riechers, J. (1995). *Selected estimates of costs of violence against women.* London, ON: Centre for Research on Violence Against Women and Children.

Green, B., & Kimerling, R. (2004). Trauma, posttraumatic stress disorder and health status. In P. Schnurr & B.Green B. (Eds.). *Trauma and health: Physical consequences of exposure to extreme stress.* (pp. 13–37). Washington, DC: APA.

Grim, R. (2009). When getting beaten by your husband is a pre-existing condition. *Huffington Post.* Retrieved September 18, 2009, from http://www.huffingtonpost.com/2009/09/14/when-getting-beaten-by-yo_n_286029.html.

Guruge, S., Ford-Gilboe, M., Wuest, J., Varcoe, C., Samuels-Dennis, J., & Wilk, P. (2009). *The impact of social support and social conflict on women's health after leaving an abusive partner*. Manuscript submitted for publication.

Hardesty, J. L. (2002). Separation assault in the context of post divorce parenting: An integrative review of the literature. *Violence Against Women, 8*(5), 597–626.

Health Canada (2003). "The Social Determinants of Health: An Overview of the Implications for Policy and the Role of the Health Sector."

Henry, F., & Tator, C. (2006). *The colour of democracy: Racism in Canadian society* (3rd ed.). Toronto, ON, Canada: Nelson Thomson.

Hollingsworth E., & Ford-Gilboe M. (2006). Registered nurses' self-efficacy for assessing and responding to woman abuse in emergency department settings. *Canadian Journal of Nursing Research, 38*(4), 54–77.

Humphreys, C., & Thiara, R. (2003). Mental health and domestic violence: 'I call it symptoms of abuse'. *The British Journal of Social Work, 33*(2), 209–226.

Humphreys, J. (1995). The work of worrying: Battered women and their children. *Scholarly Inquiry for Nursing Practice, 9*(2), 127–145.

Humphreys, J., & Campbell, J. C. (2004). *Family violence and nursing practice*. Philadelphia: Lippincott.

Humphreys, J., & Lee, K. (2005). Sleep disturbances in battered women living in transitional housing. *Issues Ment Health Nurs, 26*, 771–780.

Humphreys, J., Lee, K., Neylan, T., & Marmer, C. (2001). Psychological and physical distress of sheltered battered women. *Health Care for Women International, 22*, 401–414.

Humphreys, J., Sharps, P., & Campbell, J. (2005). What we know and what we still need to learn. *Journal of Interpersonal Violence, 20*(2), 182–187.

Johnson, M. (2006). Conflict and control: Gender symmetry and asymmetry in domestic violence. *Violence Against Women, 12*(11), 1203–1218.

Kaysen, D. Resick, P., & Wise, D. (2003). Living in danger: The impact of chronic traumatisation and the traumatic context on posttraumatic stress disorder. *Trauma, Violence & Abuse, 4*(3), 247–264.

Kramer, A., Lorenzon, D., & Mueller, G. (2004). Prevalence of intimate partner violence and health implication for women using emergency departments and primary health clinics. *Women's Health Issues,* (14), 19–29.

Lempert, L. B. (1997). The other side of help: Negative effects in the help-seeking processes of abused women. *Qualitative Sociology, 20*(2), 289–309.

Landenburger, K. (1989). A process of entrapment in and recovery from an abusive relationship. *Issues in Mental Health Nursing, 10*, 209–227.

Leserman, J., & Drossman, D. (2007). Relationship of abuse history to functional gastrointestinal disorders and symptoms: Some possible mediating factors. *Trauma Violence & Abuse, 8*, 331–343.

Leserman, J., Zolnoun, D., Meltzer-Brody, S., Lamvu, G., & Steege, J. (2006). Identification of diagnostic subtypes of chronic pelvic pain and how subtypes differ in health status and trauma history. *American Journal of Obstetrics & Gynecology, 196*, 554–561.

Logan, T., Walker, R., Jordan, C., & Campbell, J. (2004). An integrative review of separation in the context of victimizaton: Consequences and implications for women. *Trauma, Violence, & Abuse, 5*(2), 143–193.

MacEwen B. (2007). Physiology and neurobiology of stress and adaptation: Central role of the brain. *Physiology Review, 87*, 873–904.

McFarlane, J., Groff, J., O'Brien, J., & Watson, K. (2006). Secondary prevention of intimate partner violence. *Nursing Research, 55*(1), 52–61.

McFarlane, J., Parker, B., Soeken, K., Silva, C. & Reel, S. (1998). Safety behaviours of abused women after an intervention during pregnancy. *Journal of Obstetrics, Gyencological and Neonatal Nursing, 27*, 64–69.

MacMillan, H., Wathen, C., Jamieson, E., Boyle, M., Shannon H., Ford-Gilboe, M., Worster, A., Lent, B., Coben, J., Campbell, J. C., McNutt, L. A., and the McMaster Violence Against Women Research Group (2009). Screening for intimate partner violence in health care settings: A randomized trial. *JAMA, 302*(5), 493–501.

McCloskey, K., & Grigsby, N. (2005). The ubiquitous clinical problem of adult intimate partner violence: The need for routine assessment. *Professional Psychology: Research and Practice, 36*(3), 264–275.

McMurray, A. & Moore, K. (1994). Domestic violence: Are we listening? Do we see? *The Australian Journal of Advanced Nursing, 12*(1), 23–28.

Mechanic, M., Weaver, T., & Resick P. (2008). Mental health consequences of intimate partner abuse: A multidimensional assessment of four different forms of abuse. *Violence Against Women, 14,* 634–654.

Merritt-Gray, M., & Wuest, J. (1995). Counteracting abuse and breaking free: The process of leaving revealed through women's voices. *Health Care for Women International, 16,* 399–412.

Meyers, M. (2004). African American women and violence: gender, race, and class in the news. *Critical Studies in Media Communication, 21*(2), 95–118.

Moe, A. & Bell, M. (2004). Abject Economics: The Effects of Battering and Violence on Women's Work and Employability. *Violence Against Women, 10,* 29–55.

Moracco, B., & Cole, T. (2009). Preventing intimate partner violence: Screening is not enough. *JAMA, 302*(5) 588–569.

Moss, N. E. (2002). Gender equity and socioeconomic inequality: A framework for the patterning of women's health. *Social Science and Medicine, 54*(5), 649–661.

Muelleman, R., Lenaghan, P., & Pakieser, R. (1996). Battered women: Injury locations and types. *Annals of Emergency Medicine, 28,* 486–492.

Murray, C., & Lopez, A. (1996). *The global burden of disease.* Cambridge, MA: Harvard University Press.

National Center for Injury Prevention and Control (2003). *Costs of intimate partner violence against women in the United States.* Atlanta, GA: Centers for Disease Control and Prevention.

Nelson, H., Nygren, P., McInerney, Y., and Klein, Y., & U.S. Preventive Services Task Force (2004). Screening women and elderly adults for family and intimate partner violence: A review of the evidence for the U.S. Preventive Services Task Force. *Annals of Internal Medicine, 140*(5), 387–396.

Okazawa-Rey, M. (2002). Warring on women: Understanding complex inequalities of gender, race, class, and nation. *Affilia, 17*(3), 371–383.

Paterson, S. (2009). (Re) Constructing women's resistance to woman abuse: Resources, strategy choice and implications of and for public policy in Canada. *Critical Social Policy, 29,* 121–145.

Pavao, J., Alvarez, J., Baumrind, N., Induni, M., & Kimerling, R. (2007). Intimate partner violence and housing instability. *American Journal of Preventative Medicine, 32*(2), 143–146.

Plichta, S. (2004). Intimate partner violence and physical health consequences: Policy and practice implications *Journal of Interpersonal Violence, 19*(11), 1296–1323.

Plichta, S. B. (2007). Interactions between victims of intimate partner violence against women and the health care system: policy and practice implications. *Trauma Violence & Abuse, 8*(2), 226–39.

Rabin, R., Jennings, J., Campbell, J. C., & Bair-Merritt, M. (2009). How should health care providers ask about intimate partner violence? A systematic review of intimate partner violence screening questionnaires tested in health care settings. *American Journal of Preventive Medicine, 36*(5), 439–445.

Ramsay, J., Carter, Y., Davidson, D., Eldridge, S., Feder, G., Hegarty, K., Rivas, C., Tuft, A., & Warburtan, A. (2009). Advocacy interventions to reduce or eliminate violence and protect the physical and psychosocial well-being of women who experienced intimate partner violence. *Cochrane Database of Systematic Reviews, 3,* Art No. CD005043. DOI: 10.1002/14651858.CD005043.pub2.

Ramsay, J. Richardson, J., Carter, Y., Davidson, L., & Feder, G. (2002). Should health professionals screen women for domestic violence? Systematic review. *BMJ, 325*(7359), 314.

Registered Nurses Association of Ontario (RNAO) (2005). Woman abuse: Screening, identification, and initial response. Toronto, ON: RNAO. Retrieved September 19, 2009, from http://www.rnao.org/Storage/12/655_BPG_Women_Abuse.pdf .

Rhodes, K. V., Drum, M., Anliker, E., Frankel, R., Howes, D., & Levinson, W. (2006). "Lowering the threshold for discussions of domestic violence: a randomized controlled trial of computer screening." *Archives of Internal Medicine, 166*(10), 1107–1114.

Rivara, F. P., Anderson, M. L., Fishman, P., Bonomi, A. E., Reid, R. J., Carrell, D., et al. (2007). Healthcare utilization and costs for women with a history of intimate partner violence. *American Journal of Preventive Medicine, 32*(2), 89–96.

Rose, L, Campbell, J., & Kub, J. (2000). The role of social support and family relationships in women's responses to battering. *Health Care for Women International, 21,* 27–39.

Sachs, C. J., Koziol-McLain, J., Glass, N. E., Webster, D., & Campbell, J. C. (2002). A population-based survey assessing support for mandatory domestic violence reporting by healthcare personnel. *Women and Health, 35,* 121–134.

Schachter, C. L., Stalker, C. A., Teram, E., Lasiuk, G. C., & Danilkewich, A. (2008). *Handbook on sensitive practice for health care providers: Lessons from adult survivors of child sexual abuse.* Ottawa: Public Health Agency of Canada.

Scott-Storey, K., Wuest, J., & Ford-Gilboe, M. (2009). Intimate partner violence and cardiovascular risk: Is there a link? *Journal of Advanced Nursing, 65*(10), 2186–2197.

Sheridan, D., & Nash, K. (2007). Acute injury patterns of intimate partner violence victims. *Trauma, Violence, & Abuse, 8*(3), 282–289.

Smith, D., Mills, T., & Taliaferro, E. (2001). Frequency and relationship of reported symptomology in victims of intimate partner violence: The effect of multiple strangulation attacks. *The Journal of Emergency Medicine, 21*(3), 323–329.

Snow-Jones, A., Dienemann, J., Schollenberger, J., Kub, J., O'Campo, P., Gielen, A. C., et al. (2006). Long-term costs of intimate partner violence in a sample of female HMO enrollees. *Women's Health Issues: Official Publication of The Jacobs Institute of Women's Health, 16*(5), 252–261.

Stewart, M., & Tilden, V. (1995). The contributions of nursing science to social support. *International Journal of Nursing Studies, 32*, 535–544.

Sullivan, C. M., & Bybee, D. I. (1999). Reducing violence using community-based advocacy for women with abusive partners. *Journal of Consulting & Clinical Psychology, 67*(1), 43–53.

Sullivan, C. M., Bybee, D. I., & Allen, N. E. (2002). Findings from a community-based program for battered women and their children. *Journal of Interpersonal Violence, 17*, 915.

Sutherland, C., Bybee, D., & Sullivan, C. (2002). Beyond bruises and broken bones: The joint effects of stress and injuries on battered women's health. *American Journal of Community Psychology, 30*(5), 609–636.

Sutherland, C., Sullivan, C., & Bybee, D. (2001). Effects of intimate partner violence versus poverty on women's health. *Violence Against Women, 7*(10), 1122–1143.

Swanberg, J. E., Logan, T., & Macke, C. (2005). Intimate partner violence, employment, and the workplace: Consequences and future directions. *Trauma, Violence & Abuse, 6*(4), 286-312.

Tambiah, Y. (2005). Turncoat bodies: Sexuality and sex work under militarization in Sri Lanka. *Gender and Society, 19*(2), 243–261.

Taft, C., Vogt, D., Mechanic, M., & Resick, P. (2007). Posttraumatic stress disorder and physical health symptoms among women seeking help for relationship aggression. *Journal of Family Psychology, 21*, 354–362.

Tiwari, A., Leung, W. C., Leung, T. W., Humphreys, J., Parker, B., & Ho, P. C. (2005). A randomized controlled trial of empowerment training for Chinese abused pregnant women in Hong Kong. *British Journal of Obstetrics and Gynecology, 112*, 1–8.

Tolman, R. M., & Rosen, D. (2001). Domestic violence in the lives of women receiving welfare: Mental health, substance dependence and economic wellbeing. *Violence Against Women, 7*(2), 141-158.

Tower, M. (2007). Intimate partner violence and the health care response: a postmodern critique. *Health Care for Women International, 28*(5), 438–452.

Tjaden, P., & Thoennes, N. (2000). *Full report of the prevalence, incidence, and consequences of violence against women*. Washington: National Institute of Justice.

Ulrich, Y., Cain, K., Sugg, N., Rivara, F., Rubanowice, D., & Thompson, R. (2003). Medical care utilization patterns in women with diagnosed domestic violence. *Am J Prev Med. 24*(1), 9–15.

United Nations Educational Scientific and Cultural Organization (1952). *The race question in modern science: the results of an inquiry—The concept of race.* Paris: United Nations Educational, Scientific and Cultural Organization.

U.S. Centers for Disease Control and Prevention (2008). Adverse health conditions and health risk behaviors associated with intimate partner violence—United States, 2005. *Morbidity and Mortality Weekly Report Feb 8, 57*(5), 113–117.

Varcoe, C. (2001). Abuse obscured: an ethnographic account of emergency nursing in relation to violence against women. *Can J Nurs Res, 32*(4), 95–115.

Varcoe, C., Hankivsky, O., Ford-Gilboe, M., Wuest, J., Wilk, P., & Hammerton, J. (2009). *The health-related economic costs of violence against women after leaving: Building evidence for better prevention and supportive policies and practices*. Manuscript submitted for publication.

Varcoe, C., & Irwin, L. (2004). "If I killed you, I'd get the kids": Women's survival and protection work with child custody and access in the context of woman abuse. *Qualitative Sociology, 27*(1), 77–99.

VicHealth (2004). The health costs of violence: Measuring the burden of disease caused by intimate partner violence, from www.vichealth.vic.gov.au.

Walby, S. (2004). The cost of domestic violence: Women and equality unit.

Walker, R., Logan, T. K., Jordan, C., & Campbell, J. (2004). An integrative review of separation in the context of victimization. *Trauma, Violence, & Abuse, 5*(2), 143–193.

Walsh, C., Jamieson, E., MacMillan, H., & Boyle, M. (2007). Child abuse and chronic pain in a community survey of women. *Journal of Interpersonal Violence, 22*, 1536–1554.

Wathen, N. C. & MacMillan, H. L. (2000). Interventions for violence against women: Scientific review. *JAMA, 289(5)*, 589–600.

Wathen, N. C., MacMillan, H. L., & Canadian Task Force on Preventive Health Care (2003). Prevention of violence against women: Recommendation statement from the Canadian Task Force on Preventive Health Care. *CMAJ, 169(6)*, 582–584.

Weaver, T., & Resnick, H. (2004). Toward developing complex multivariate models for examining intimate partner violence–physical health relationship. *Journal of Interpersonal Violence, 19(11)*, 1342–1349.

Weinbaum., Z., Stratton, T. L., Chavez, G., Motylewski-Link, C., Barrera, N., Courtney, J., & California Department of Health Services Women's Health Survey Group. (2001). Female victims of intimate partner physical domestic violence (IPP-DV), California 1998. *American Journal of Preventive Medicine, 21(4)*, 313–319.

Wilcox, P. (2005). Beauty and the beast: Gendered and raced discourse in the news. *Social & Legal Studies, 14(4)*, 515–532.

Woods, A., Page, G., O'Campo, P., Pugh, L, Ford, D., & Campbell, J. (2005). The mediation effect of post-traumatic stress disorder symptoms on the relationship of intimate partner violence and IFN-γ levels. *American Journal of Community Psychology, 36(1/2)*, 159–175.

Woods, S. (2000). Prevalence and patterns of posttraumatic stress disorder in abused and post-abused women. *Issues in Mental Health Nursing, 21*, 309–324.

Woods, S., Hall, R., Campbell, J., & Angott, D. (2008). Physical health and post-traumatic stress disorder symptoms in women experiencing intimate partner violence. *Journal of Midwifery and Women's Health, 53(6)*, 538–546.

World Health Organization (2002). *World report on violence and health.* Geneva, WHO.

World Health Organization (2005). *WHO multi-country study on women's health and domestic violence: Report of initial results on prevalence, health outcomes and women's responses.* Geneva: WHO.

Wuest, J., Ford-Gilboe, M., Merritt-Gray, M., & Berman, H. (2003). Intrusion: The central problem for family health promotion among children and single mothers after leaving an abusive partner. *Qualitative Health Research, 13(5)*, 597–622.

Wuest, J., Ford-Gilboe, M., Merritt-Gray, M., & Lemire, S. (2006). Using grounded theory to generate a theoretical understanding of the effects of child custody policy on women's health promotion in the context of intimate partner violence. *Health Care for Women International, 27*, 490–512.

Wuest, J., Ford-Gilboe, M., Merritt-Gray, M, Varcoe, C., Lent, B., Wilk, P., & Campbell, J. C. (2009). Abuse-related injury and symptoms of posttraumatic stress disorder as mechanisms of chronic pain in survivors of intimate partner violence, *Pain Medicine, 10(4)*, 739–747.

Wuest, J., Ford-Gilboe, M., Merritt-Gray, M., Wilk, P., Campbell, J., Lent, B., Varcoe, C., & Smye. V. (2009). *Pathways of chronic pain in survivors of intimate partner violence: Considering abuse-related injury, symptoms of posttraumatic stress disorder, depressive symptoms, and child abuse.* Manuscript submitted for publication.

Wuest, J., & Merritt-Gray, M. (1999). Not going back: Sustaining the separation in the process of leaving abusive relationships. *Violence Against Women, 5*, 110–133.

Wuest, J., & Merritt-Gray, M. (2001). Beyond survival: Reclaiming self after leaving an abusive male partner. *Canadian Journal of Nursing Research, 32(4)*, 79–94.

Wuest, J., & Merritt Gray, M. (2008). A theoretical understanding of abusive intimate partner relationships that become non-violent: Shifting the pattern of abusive control. *Journal of Family Violence, 23*, 281–293.

Wuest, J., Merritt-Gray, M., Ford-Gilboe, M., Lent, B., Varcoe, C., & Campbell, J. C. (2008). Chronic pain in women survivors of intimate partner violence. *J Pain, 9*, 1049–1057.

Wuest, J., Merritt-Gray, M., Lent, B., Varcoe, C., Connors, A., & Ford-Gilboe, M. (2007). Patterns of medication use among women survivors of intimate partner violence. *Can J Public Health, 98*, 460–464.

Yoshioka, M., & Choi, D. (2005). Culture and interpersonal violence research: Paradigm shift to create a full continuum of domestic violence services. *Journal of Interpersonal Violence, 20*, 513–519.

Zlotnick, C., Johnson, D., & Kohn, R. (2006). Intimate partner violence and long-term psychosocial functioning in a national sample of American women. *Journal of Interpersonal Violence, 21*, 262–275.

6

Intimate Partner Violence During Pregnancy

Tina Bloom, PhD, MPH, RN
Linda F. C. Bullock, PhD, RN, FAAN
Phyllis Sharps, PhD, RN, CNE, FAAN
Kathryn Laughon, PhD, RN
Barbara J. Parker, RN, PhD, FAAN

INTRODUCTION

Pregnancy is a time when friends, family, and health professionals expect a woman's partner to be particularly concerned about and attentive to her health and well-being. It is difficult to imagine that anyone, let alone the father of the baby, would intentionally injure a pregnant woman, thereby jeopardizing her health and the health of the fetus. However, intimate partner violence (IPV, commonly called domestic violence) is more common in pregnancy than placenta previa, gestational diabetes, or pregnancy-induced hypertension (Gazmararian et al., 2000). The purpose of this chapter is to summarize current research on IPV during pregnancy and to provide guidance to nurses who work with pregnant women who may experience such violence.

Nurses, nurse-midwives, and nurse practitioners can play a crucial role in breaking the cycle of violence in the lives of pregnant women. Pregnancy may be the only time an abused woman has frequent, ongoing contact with someone capable of assisting her. The nursing process, as applied to survivors of IPV, includes identification, assessment, planning, intervention, and follow-up. The primary role of the nurse specific to IPV is that of advocate. Advocacy with the abused woman includes providing accurate information regarding abusive relationships, domestic abuse laws, resources, and options, and providing ongoing emotional support regardless of the choices she makes.

Abuse during pregnancy has been a topic of a significant amount of nursing research and clinical interventions. Early research on this topic focused on establishing the rate of IPV in pregnancy and comparing disclosure rates using different instruments, and different modalities (interview versus written questionnaire). Subsequent research established the effects of IPV during pregnancy on maternal and infant health, and predictors of IPV in pregnancy. Later research validated previous findings, included new variables, and tested nursing interventions. This growing body of research provides a strong basis for nursing practice with abused pregnant women.

DEFINITION OF INTIMATE PARTNER VIOLENCE

Intimate partner violence occurs between intimate partners (current or former spouses or unmarried partners). It is defined by the Centers for Disease Control and Prevention as follows: physical or sexual violence or threat of such violence; or psychological/emotional abuse and/or coercive tactics when there has previously been physical and/or sexual violence between partners (Saltzman, Fanslow, McMahon, & Shelley, 1999). IPV is characterized by a pattern of assault and coercive behaviors enacted by one intimate partner with the purpose of gaining control over the other. These behaviors may include inflicted physical injuries, emotional and sexual abuse, progressive isolation, deprivation, stalking, intimidation, and threats (Family Violence Prevention Fund, 2004).

RATES OF INTIMATE PARTNER VIOLENCE DURING PREGNANCY

Early researchers noted that abuse often began or escalated during pregnancy. However, for the largest proportion of women abused during pregnancy, the abuse began prior to conception (McFarlane, Parker, Soeken, Silva, & Reed, 1999; Martin, Mackie, Kupper, Buescher, & Moracco, 2001; Saltzman, Johnson, Gilbert, & Goodwin, 2003), but the woman might have been motivated by pregnancy to disclose abuse and seek care to protect her unborn child. Congruent with such findings, in many studies, abuse before pregnancy seems to be the best predictor of abuse during pregnancy (Martin et al., 2001; Saltzman et al., 2003).

In a large review of studies in the United States, Gazmararian and colleagues (2000) found an incidence range of abuse during pregnancy between 0.9% and 20.1%, with most estimates between 4% and 8%, which translates into approximately 156,000 to 332,000 pregnant women who experience violence each year. Differences may exist by ethnicity; for example, McFarlane et al. (1999) and Campbell et al. (1999) found rates of abuse to be lower in first-generation Hispanic women compared to African American or Caucasian women; however, in Campbell's sample (1999), Puerto Rican women had a significantly higher prevalence of abuse during pregnancy than any of the other groups.

Abuse during pregnancy is a red flag for a particularly dangerous abuser. McFarlane et al. (1999) reported greater severity on each of five severity measures for women who were abused both before and during the pregnancy than women abused only before or only during the pregnancy. Similarly, Macy et al. (2007) found that women who experienced physical violence from a partner in the first 6 months of pregnancy also had higher mean rates of physical, sexual, and emotional IPV before and after pregnancy, suggesting greater severity of violence.

IPV in pregnancy may also indicate increased risk for lethal violence. Women in the United States are nine times more likely to be murdered by an intimate partner or ex-partner than a stranger (Fox & Jawitz, 2004), and the majority of these murders (65% to 70%) occur in relationships in which the woman has been abused (Campbell et al., 2003). In the Campbell and colleagues intimate partner femicide study, women who were murdered by an abusive partner (n=437) were compared with randomly identified abused women living in the same metropolitan area (n=384) (McFarlane, Campbell, Sharps, &

Watson, 2002). As in other research, women abused during pregnancy endured significantly higher levels of violence. Additionally, after adjusting for significant demographic factors, such as age, ethnicity, education, and relationship status, abuse during pregnancy increased the risk of being murdered by an intimate partner threefold (AOR 3.08, 95% adjusted CI 1.86, 5.10). African American women abused during pregnancy had even higher risk (AOR 3.6, 95% adjusted CI 2.4, 5.5) compared with white women.

Comprehensive reviews of medical records and death certificates have revealed that up to one fifth of pregnancy-associated deaths are the result of murder (Horon & Cheng, 2001; Krulewitch, Pierre-Louis, de Leon-Gomez, Guy, & Green, 2001). Violence may be responsible for many cases of maternal mortality, including those for which no clear cause is identified (Horon & Cheng, 2001; Krulewitch et al., 2001). Such findings underscore the significance of IPV in pregnancy, the importance of nurses as advocates for abused pregnant women, and the importance of including IP homicide cases in maternal mortality reviews.

THEORETICAL ASPECTS

Reasons for Intimate Partner Violence in Pregnancy

Theories of why some men abuse women during pregnancy vary widely. The most commonly cited reason for abuse during pregnancy is jealousy. The abuser may view the fetus as a competitor for the woman's attention or as an intruder in their relationship (Campbell, Oliver, & Bullock, 1998). He may resent the woman's increased contact with friends, family, and health care providers during pregnancy. Many women report the abuser's response to the pregnancy is to deny paternity and to accuse her of infidelity (McFarlane, Parker, & Moran, 2007). In such cases, the abuse may reflect sexual jealousy, a hallmark of abusive men.

In a retrospective cohort study of 1,468 pregnant or postpartum women who received inpatient or emergency department care following intimate partner assault, Nannini et al. (2008) documented that the leading injury women sustained was to the head and neck. However, abdominal injuries occurred twice as often during pregnancy, compared to the postpartum period (22% versus 9%). In the third trimester, 25% of injuries documented were to the abdomen. Blows directed at the abdomen of a pregnant woman may represent a form of prenatal child abuse. The abuse may be a conscious or unconscious attempt to terminate the pregnancy or kill the fetus. A number of women in one study reported abdominal beatings they believe were deliberate attempts to induce abortion because the abuser did not want the child to be born (Brendtro & Bowker, 1989; Campbell, Oliver, & Bullock, 1998).

Although each of the foregoing explanations of abuse during pregnancy may apply in any single abuse situation, none alone explains all cases of abuse during pregnancy. Campbell, Oliver, and Bullock (1998) questioned women about their perceptions of why the abuse occurred. Their replies varied. Twenty percent reported the abuse was directed toward the baby, as an instance of the abuser not wanting the baby to be born, and another 20% believed that the abuse was pregnancy-related, resulting from her feeling ill or the stress of another child. This latter group thought the violence was directed at them, rather than at the baby. Another group of women cited jealousy as a factor. In the majority of cases, however, abuse during pregnancy was simply the continuation of ongoing violence ("business as usual") and was unrelated to the pregnancy itself.

A final explanation for why some women experience increased abuse during pregnancy has been noted in families with concurrent substance abuse. This is particularly true for women who choose to abstain from drugs and alcohol during pregnancy, while their partner continues to abuse drugs and alcohol. These men often get high with their friends and are subsequently unhappy when they return home to a sober partner, particularly if she is perceived as critical of his intoxication (McFarlane et al., 2007).

Ultimately, it is the abuser's desire for power and control, and his belief that violence and coercion are legitimate means to achieve these ends that prompt him to abuse his partner. This is true both during and outside of pregnancy.

Pregnant Women's Responses to Intimate Partner Violence

A number of theories have been advanced to explain how women's responses to IPV may differ in pregnancy. More research is needed in this area, particularly in terms of how culture, race/ethnicity, or other factors may additionally influence pregnant women's decision making. However, overall, the research, so far, indicates that an abused woman's resistance and response to IPV is influenced by both social contexts and the need to balance care for her and for others. Landenburger's (1989, 1998) process theory of intimate partner violence describes how abused women struggle to make sense of the abuse and interpret the mixed messages they receive from their partner, their families, and the community. Landenburger suggests that abused women experience an initial binding phase in the relationship, in which they work toward constructing a loving relationship, overlook warning signals, and shoulder the blame for the abuse. This phase may or may not be followed by subsequent phases, described as enduring, disengaging, and recovering. The binding phase is accompanied by an altered self-identity in which women experienced feelings of powerless, loss of control, isolation, and a sense of living in two worlds—one in which the positive aspects of her relationship were acknowledged and another reality in which abuse occurred. The theory has been supported as applying to pregnant women (see chapter 2 for further discussion of Landenburger's theory.)

Indeed, in research studies, pregnant abuse survivors describe a sense of "dual self" in which they feel torn between the public image of expectant motherhood and a happy family, and the positive aspects of their relationship—and a private reality of violence. Feelings of shame and fear are common, and pregnant women may continuously weigh the benefits and costs of disclosing the abuse, versus keeping silent (Libbus et al., 2006; Lutz, 2004; Lutz, Curry, Robrecht, Libbus, & Bullock, 2006; Ulrich et al., 2006). They may fear abuse disclosure will bring judgment (Lutz, 2005) and unwanted pressure to stay in the relationship (Rose, Campbell, & Kub, 2000) or to leave it (Curry, Durham, Bullock, Bloom, & Davis, 2006; Lutz et al., 2006). Abused pregnant women may conclude that no one can really help them (Lutz, 2005). This may be a particularly salient factor for women who rely on the abusive partner for tangible resources, such as financial support, housing, transportation, health insurance, or other vital resources (Cloutier et al., 2002; Libbus et al., 2006).

However, the decision-making process may ultimately be different for women who are pregnant (Libbus et al., 2006). Lutz et al. (2006) analyzed qualitative data from two studies of racially and geographically diverse abused pregnant women. Exemplars consistent with the tasks of motherhood and becoming a mother within the context of abuse were identified. The themes illustrated the difficult choices that abused pregnant women made and how those choices were embedded within an ecological context of limited resources and the need for both emotional and tangible support in order to seek safe passage. Pregnancy itself constricted the economic choices available to these women, many of whom already faced limited resources.

Lutz et al. (2006) proposed a conceptual framework called "double-binding" to explain the particular impact of violence upon pregnant women. The conceptual framework of double-binding combines aspects of Landenburger's work and maternal role theory (Rubin, 1984), in which the mother is bound to the partner as she bonds to her child. An overarching theme was the abused pregnant woman doing what she perceived as best for the baby, even at cost to herself, including concealing the abuse and/or staying with the abusive partner if she felt the benefits to the child outweighed the risks. This sometimes took the form of protecting the fetus from abuse (for example, by directly shielding her abdomen from physical abuse or by placating her partner to keep things "smooth" and prevent violent incidents).

Allowing women to talk about their difficulties without having to identify themselves as abused may be particularly important for pregnant women who are in a "double-bind" situation. Ulrich et al., (2006) conducted interviews in an urban postpartum unit with 30 newly delivered white, African American, and Latina women who screened positive for violence. Although women reported abusive behaviors, the majority (57%) did not define their relationship as abusive. Women felt that their relationships were not abusive because the abuse was infrequent, was normal or expected behavior from men, because they were satisfied with the relationship, or because she stood up for herself and hit back. However, women did want to talk about their intimate relationships and conflicts, even in an inpatient, immediate postpartum setting.

THE ECOLOGICAL CONTEXT OF INTIMATE PARTNER VIOLENCE IN PREGNANCY

As previously noted, abuse before pregnancy seems to be the best predictor of abuse during pregnancy (Martin et al., 2001; McFarlane et al., 1999). Nurses are cautioned to recall the abused pregnant woman's sense of "dual self" and desire to preserve external appearances of the "happy family," and to avoid clinical decision making based on erroneous stereotypes or assumptions about who among their patients may, or may not be, experiencing violence. It is more reasonable to assume that we cannot always know who among our patients may be experiencing violence—particularly if we fail to routinely ask.

With that caution in mind, nurses should be aware that some populations of women have increased vulnerability to violence and its effects. Violence against women occurs not in a vacuum, but in an ecological context, in which every individual woman and her family are also situated within the community and society. Multiple factors contribute to her experience of violence and her access to interpersonal and tangible resources such as the level of social support, employment, degree of economic autonomy (Dutton, Goodman, Lennig, Murphy, & Kaltman, 2005). Abused pregnant women who are otherwise vulnerable (i.e., those of low socioeconomic status, minority status, rural residence, young age) may be disparately impacted by the effects of IPV. Further, these categories of vulnerability are not mutually exclusive, but may substantially overlap.

Women of Low Socioeconomic Status

For poor women, violence can limit their ability to escape from poverty, and poverty, in turn, makes it more difficult to escape the violence and recover from the damage done by it. Consistent associations have been found between IPV in pregnancy and socioeconomic factors that increase risk and/or limit women's resources and options for escaping violence. These include low income, low educational attainment, young age, unemployment, and living in substandard or overcrowded housing (Bohn, Tebben, & Campbell, 2004; Bowen, Heron, Waylen, & Wolke, 2005; Bullock, Bloom, Curry, Davis, & Kilburn, 2006; Datner, Wiebe, Brensinger, & Nelson, 2007; Gazmararian et al., 1995).

For example, in a prospective, longitudinal cohort study of 7,591 women (Bowen et al., 2005), the numbers of "social adversities" or social risk factors faced by a pregnant woman were assessed: single, having her first child at a young age, low education, financial difficulties, inadequate housing, mental illness, substance abuse, trouble with the law, or lack of social support. These social risk factors predicted not only current abuse, but also future victimization up to 3 years later. A better understanding is needed of how abused pregnant women navigate these multiple and intersecting issues in their decision-making process. Research has suggested that for pregnant women experiencing IPV and contending with multiple other issues (e.g., poverty, discrimination, housing problems, depression, addiction), the violence may not be her most pressing priority (Curry et al., 2006; Lutz et al., 2006).

Racial and Ethnic Minority Women

For women who are not pregnant, some evidence suggests that patterns of violence may differ across racial and ethnic groups. Violence against women of color, in general, and during pregnancy, in particular, is a complex and understudied issue. Patterns of IPV characteristic of racial/ethnic groups are inconsistent between studies, and may depend on the setting, the sample, and the type of analysis used. In addition, racial and ethnic categories used to collect and analyze data often are broad. For example, in federal guidelines used to collect national data, "Latina" can refer to women of many diverse subgroups, (e.g., of Mexican, Puerto Rican, Dominican, Spanish, Cuban, Central American, Brazilian, Chilean, or Argentinean origin) who may have very different backgrounds, socioeconomic levels, experiences, and prenatal outcomes.

Studies have found higher rates of IPV among pregnant women of color, particularly African-American women (Bullock et al., 2006; Campbell, Sharps, Gary, Campbell, & Lopez, 2002; Certain, Mueller, Jagodzinski, & Fleming, 2008; Goodwin, Gazmararian, Johnson, Gilbert, & Saltzman, 2000). In contrast, McFarlane, Parker, and Soeken. (1996a), who assessed for IPV three times during pregnancy among a stratified sample of 1,203 women attending prenatal clinics in the southwestern United States, found that African American and White women were abused at a similar rate (18% and 17%, respectively). However, the white women reported the most episodes of abuse and the greatest percentage of severe episodes.

Patterns of abuse may vary among Latina subgroups based upon cultural factors. Torres et al. (2000) found Puerto Rican women reported abuse during pregnancy in a significantly greater proportion than other Latina groups. Higher levels of acculturation to U.S. society was associated with more physical abuse during pregnancy, as were several of the indicators of cultural norms, such as belief in wife/mother role supremacy for women and cultural group belief in the acceptability of men hitting women. Other studies have also found Puerto Rican women to have a significantly higher prevalence of abuse during pregnancy than other Hispanic (Mexican-American, Central American, Cuban American groups) with African American and white women between (Campbell, 1998; Mattson & Rodriquez, 1999).

Few if any studies have had sufficient proportions of Native American women to determine if the abuse during pregnancy prevalence is higher than other groups as it is in nonpregnant women (Tjaden & Thoennes, 2000). However, Bohn (2002) studied 30 urban pregnant Native American women in the Midwest and found high levels of recent violence exposure. In this study, 60% of women were currently in a relationship where they had been abused, and 33% reported abuse during the index pregnancy.

Other studies have found no relationship between IPV and race or ethnicity (Bacchus, Mezey, & Bewley, 2004; Martin et al., 2001). Therefore, how minority racial and/or ethnic status affects IPV in pregnancy is unclear, and more research into risk, prevalence, and protective factors for IPV in pregnancy for women of color is needed. What is quite clear from the literature, however, is that abuse and minority status may intersect in the health system. They may have more reasons not to ask health care providers for help, including reduced trust, cultural, institutional, or language barriers, and fear of racism and racial stereotyping (Campbell et al., 2002; Hampton, Oliver, & Magarian, 2003; McFarlane, Soeken, Reel, Parker, & Silva, 1997; West, 1996).

Adolescent Mothers

IPV is highly prevalent among young women. In data from the 2001 National Youth Behavior Risk Survey, approximately one in five sexually active teenagers (17.7%) reported past-year physical violence from a dating partner (Silverman, Raj, & Clements, 2004). Adolescent pregnancy may result from coercion or manipulation from an abusive partner. For example, in a recent study, Miller et al. (2007) describe qualitative interviews with 53 girls aged 15–20 years, in which some participants describe how their abusive partners had made explicit statements about wanting them to become pregnant and had manipulated and sabotaged use of condoms and birth control use. The finding of a significant association of IPV and unintended pregnancy is well established (Palitto, Campbell, & O'Campo, 2005).

Teen dating violence is also associated with rapid repeat pregnancy. In a prospective study, Jacoby, Gorenflo, Black, Wunderlich, and Eyler (1999) found within 12 months of giving birth, 43.6% of the participants who were abused became pregnant again. Within 18 months, 63.2% of the abused participants had experienced at least one additional pregnancy. The investigators also found an association between current abuse and the presence of at least one spontaneous abortion in the obstetrical history ($p = 0.007$).

Some adolescents may be partnered with adult men, increasing the risk of power imbalances within the relationship, which increase the potential for violent victimization. For example, Harner (2004) interviewed 86 pregnant adolescents in the postpartum unit and found an overall 13% rate of violence perpetrated by the father of the baby. Those teens whose partner was an adult male (4 or more years older) reported over twice the rate of abuse as those who were partnered with peer-age partners (21% versus 9%), although the difference was not statistically significant in this study.

For some teens, intimate partner violence may be part of a lifelong cycle of violence exposures. Abused pregnant teens in Renker's research (2002, 2003) commonly described unstable and chaotic family lives, and often experienced substantial past-year violence exposures within their families of origin (from parents, stepparents, or siblings) and/or sexual violence from acquaintances in addition to IPV. Data from a 14-year longitudinal study of 229 adolescent mothers suggest that, for these young women, having been in a violent relationship as an adolescent was associated with an increased likelihood of adult IPV (Lindhorst & Oxford, 2008). Such findings suggest a critical role for nurses who can connect with these vulnerable teens and provide empathy, advocacy, and support to help end the cycle of violence in their lives.

Rural Women

Rural women are another vulnerable group at high risk for IPV (Bailey & Daugherty, 2007; Kershner, Long, & Anderson, 1998). These women may face additional, unique layers of difficulty that increase their vulnerability to IPV, such as increased isolation, lack of transportation, employment and health care, and low socioeconomic status. Bhandari et al. (2008) conducted a qualitative analysis of interviews with a group of rural pregnant smokers, which illustrate the high stress levels and vulnerability of these women. In addition to the stress of the abuse, women who were experiencing IPV also described more financial strain, lack of social support, legal issues, and transportation issues, than rural nonabused women.

HEALTH CONSEQUENCES OF ABUSE DURING PREGNANCY

For nurses who care for pregnant women and their infants, overlooking IPV in their patients' lives means missing a critical piece of the clinical puzzle. IPV is associated with substantial health consequences for pregnant women and their infants (Boy & Salihu, 2004; Campbell, 2002); see also Table 6.1. These health effects may be due to the acute and long-term effects of traumatic injury, as well as indirect effects related to neuroendocrine dysregulation associated with maternal stress, depression, and posttraumatic stress disorder, and attendant behavioral sequelae (e.g., increased maternal smoking).

Physical Health Consequences for the Mother

Women who experience IPV, in general, are often subjected to sexual abuse and diminished ability to negotiate safer sex practices and contraception, and as mentioned previously, IPV has been strongly associated with unplanned pregnancy (Gazmararian et al., 1995; Goodwin et al., 2000; Palitto, Campbell, & O'Campo, 2005). Bourassa and Bérubé (2007) found significantly higher rates of past-year IPV among women seeking elective termination of pregnancy compared to women continuing pregnancy (25.7% versus 9.3%, $p<0.0001$). In a study of 304 HIV-positive women (Lang, Salazar, Wingood, DiClemente, & Isis, 2007), 10% of the women screened positive for physical or sexual abuse from a partner in the previous 3 months. Of these women, 31% reported they were threatened, and 27% reported they had been hit when asking their partner to use a condom. Pregnancy may also result when abusers coerce their partner into becoming pregnant, or from forced sex. In a 2005 study, two thirds (67%) of physically abused women reported sexual assault by their intimate partner, and most reported repeated sexual assault; 26% experienced a rape-related pregnancy (McFarlane et al., 2005).

IPV has also been linked with increased risk for miscarriage. The degree of risk is likely underestimated in current research, due to no standardized reporting of fetal deaths with a maternal death, and because few research studies, to date, account for fetal losses under 20 weeks gestation (El Kady, 2008). Using data from the Chicago Women's Health Risk Study, Morleand et al. (2008) compared women who had a past-year live birth ($n=88$) with those that had a miscarriage ($n=30$). Women who had a miscarriage were significantly more likely to report IPV, and furthermore, the likelihood of miscarriage versus live birth increased significantly as the severity of violence increased ($\chi^2=12.40(2), p=0.002$).

Evidence is less consistent for some other maternal child outcomes, and more research is needed. Nonetheless, direct assaults on pregnant women are estimated to increase the risk of maternal mortality 19-fold, and the risk of uterine rupture (which have a nearly 100% fetal mortality rate) up to 46-fold (El Kady, 2008). Violence in pregnancy has been linked in studies with poor maternal weight gain and anemia, bleeding, placental abruption, uterine rupture, chorioamnionitis, vaginal infections, and kidney infection (Berenson, Wiemann, Wilkinson, Jones, & Anderson, 1994; Cokkinides, Coker, Sanderson, Addy, & Bethea, 1999; Curry, Perrin, & Wall, 1998; El-Kady, Gilbert, Xing, & Smith, 2005; El Kady, 2008; Greenberg, McFarlane, & Watson, 1997; McFarlane et al., 1996a).

Early and consistent prenatal care may help prevent some of these outcomes, as it allows ongoing assessment of maternal and fetal well-being, detection of actual or potential problems, and interventions to prevent, modify, or correct pregnancy complications. However, abuse survivors often do not receive adequate care, and the care they receive may not address IPV directly. Abused women may delay entry into care and miss scheduled appointments (Curry, et al., 1998; Long & Curry, 1998; McFarlane et al., 1996a; Taggart & Mattson, 1996). Women may miss appointments because their abuser will not let them leave the house, denies her access to transportation, or purposely detains her. Ambivalence, denial, or the "dual self" (Lutz et al., 2006) may also lead women to avoid prenatal care to conceal abuse. The abused woman or her partner may decide she should miss an appointment if trauma injuries are evident. Abused women who use or abuse substances during pregnancy may avoid prenatal care because of shame, guilt, or fear of repercussions. Finally, the woman may fear she could lose her children if the abuse becomes known. In contrast, Attala's (1994) survey of 400 women participating in the Women, Infants, and Children (WIC) supplemental food program showed no relationship between a history of physical abuse and delay in seeking prenatal care.

In nonpregnant women, IPV has been associated with high utilization of medical services (Campbell, 2002). Similarly, while some abused pregnant women may have delayed entry into prenatal care or not obtained care at all, some data suggests others may present to health care services (including prenatal care, emergency departments, and labor and delivery) more frequently than pregnant women who are not abused (Bloom, Curry, & Durham, 2007; Webster, Chandler, & Battistutta, 1996). This high utilization of medical services may continue in the postpartum; Ellis et al. (2008) found that among a sample of rural mothers, abused women ($n=211$) utilized health care for their infants significantly more often than the nonabused women ($n=405$; Pearson $\chi^2=4.89; p=0.027$).

This provides multiple opportunities for nurses to connect with abused women, assess for violence exposures, and intervene.

Mental Health Outcomes

Over their lifetime, women are more likely than men to be diagnosed with depression, anxiety, and posttraumatic stress disorder (PTSD), perhaps related to their higher risk for exposure to lifetime trauma and abuse. Chronic stress, depression, and PTSD are deleterious to maternal–child health through a number of pathways, including both direct effects via neuroendocrine dysregulation, and indirect effects via behavioral effects, including disordered eating and self-medication via tobacco, alcohol, and drugs. IPV in pregnancy has been strongly associated with high rates of stress and emotional distress, antepartum and postpartum depression, anxiety, and PTSD. For pregnant women, depression, anxiety disorders, and posttraumatic stress disorder are often correlated and co-occurring (Campbell, Poland, Waller, & Ager, 1992).

Depression in pregnant women has been linked to dysregulated neuroendocrine profiles in pregnant women, including elevated cortisol and lower levels of dopamine and serotonin. These neuroendocrine disruptions may at least partially explain research findings that demonstrate an association between prenatal depression and obstetric complications including low birth weight and preterm delivery (Bacchus et al., 2004; Field, Diego, & Hernandez-Reif, 2006; Kelly et al., 2002). The definitive association between IPV and postpartum depression was recently noted in a population-based study (MMWR, 2008), but the neurophysiological linkages have yet to be demonstrated.

Posttraumatic stress disorder, or PTSD, is not a normal reaction to an extreme stressor. Rather, it is a distinct, chronic, and debilitating reaction that occurs among a subset of trauma survivors. PTSD is estimated to affect 3% to 8% of pregnant women, and may be

TABLE 6.1 *Intimate Partner Abuse and Maternal Health Consequences*

Types of Abuse	Health Consequences
Physical Abuse Beating, biting, burning, choking, hitting, kicking, pushing, shaking, stalking, and assault with a weapon	• Maternal injuries • Placental injuries or bleeding • Preterm labor • Preterm delivery • Premature rupture of membranes
Sexual Abuse Forced sex, unsafe sex, inability to use contraception, sexually degrading activities	• HIV/AIDS • Reproductive organ injuries • Sexually transmitted diseases
Emotional/Psychological Abuse Verbal threats, intimidation, social isolation, exploitation	• Poor maternal–fetal attachment • Poor maternal–infant attachment • Poor maternal–infant interaction
Intimate Partner Abuse Any combination of physical, emotional/psychological or sexual abuse	• Late entry into prenatal care • Inconsistent prenatal care pattern of use • Poor weight gain • Eating disorders—including not taking prenatal vitamins and/or iron supplements • Poor mental health, including depression, PTSD, substance misuse/abuse

comorbid with anxiety or depression (Loveland-Cook et al., 2004; O'Campo et al., 2006). PTSD is characterized by intrusive re-experiencing symptoms (e.g., flashbacks, nightmares, unwanted memories, emotional, or physical reactions to reminders of trauma), avoidance and numbing (avoiding reminders, detachment, amnesia about traumatic events), and hyperarousal symptoms (irritability, exaggerated startle, insomnia). Pregnant women with PTSD may also experience somatization, dissociation, and interpersonal sensitivity (e.g., difficulty with boundaries, relationships, or trust), and associated behavioral features such as self-harm or suicidal behaviors, substance abuse, and disordered eating (Seng, Low, Sparbel, & Killion, 2004).

The neuroendocrine and behavioral sequelae of PTSD are substantial and may increase the risk of ectopic pregnancy, miscarriage, hyperemesis, preterm contractions, and fetal growth disturbances as well as isolation, depression, anxiety, and suicidality. In a study that compared 455 women with PTSD to 638 without PTSD, Seng et al. (2001) found that women with PTSD had significantly elevated risk for ectopic pregnancy, spontaneous abortion, hyperemesis, preterm contractions, and excessive fetal growth.

A dose–response relationship has been demonstrated between women's mental health outcomes and their number of lifetime exposures to violence (Golding, 1999; McCauley et al., 1998; Nicolaidis, Curry, McFarland, & Gerrity, 2004; Romito, Turan, & De Marchi, 2005). For example, Lindhorst and Oxford (2008) conducted a 14-year longitudinal study of 229 adolescent mothers and found that the highest mean levels of depressive symptoms were among women who reported both adolescent and adult IPV. An analysis of PRAMS data from 17 states found abuse increasing the risk of postpartum depression in every state, even adjusting for other risk factors (MMWR, 2008). In a meta-analysis of research with abused women, Golding (1999) found that there was a temporal relationship between women's depressive symptoms and IPV. In other words, the longer the time elapsed since the health effects, the fewer depression symptoms women had. Clearly, nursing interventions that connect women to mental health treatment and services to decrease their ongoing exposure to IPV will decrease the health consequences for women and children.

Smoking and Other Substance Abuse

Increased rates of tobacco, alcohol, and drug use in pregnancy have been linked to IPV exposure (Campbell et al., 1992; Curry et al., 1998; Flynn, Walton, Chermack, Cunningham, & Marcus, 2007; Koenig et al., 2006). Substance abuse may be an antecedent risk factor which increases women's vulnerability to violence, as well as sequelae of violence. For many women, the use of tobacco, alcohol, and/or drugs may be a way of self-medicating the pain and/or associated mental health sequelae of an abusive relationship. Some adolescent women experiencing violence may also be wrestling with substantial drug and alcohol issues (both their own, and their partner's) (Renker, 2002).

Smoking during pregnancy is associated with a number of adverse effects on the fetus and developing child. These outcomes include LBW, intrauterine growth retardation, ear and lower respiratory tract infections, negative behaviors and behavioral problems, miscarriage or fetal death, stillbirth, and SIDS (Fried, Watkinson, & Gray, 1998; Griesler, Kandel, & Davies, 1998; Lipscomb et al., 2000; Thomas, 2001; Varisco, 2001). In the most recent national data, the infant mortality rate among mothers who were smokers was 70% higher than for nonsmokers (11.4 per 1,000 versus 6.54) (Mathews & MacDorman, 2007).

Alcohol consumption during pregnancy, especially if chronic or heavy, is associated with numerous fetal/infant problems. These problems may include growth and neuro-development disorders and deficits, LBW, microcephaly, behavioral, facial, limb, cardiac, genital, and neurological abnormalities and other anomalies and problems frequently associated with fetal alcohol syndrome or fetal alcohol effect (Lipscomb et al., 2000; Shu, Hatch, Mills, Clemens, & Susser, 1995).

Maternal problems related to drug use during pregnancy may include miscarriage, abruptio placentae, delayed prenatal care, and parenting problems (Brady, Posner, Lang, & Rosati, 1994). Polysubstance use may be particularly harmful (Chasnoff, Neuman, Thornton, Callaghan, & Angela, 2001). While there is some debate about the relative effects of drug, alcohol, and tobacco exposure during pregnancy (Frank, Augustyn, Knight, Pell, & Zuckerman, 2001), negative fetal/infant effects of maternal drug use may include LBW, preterm birth (PTB), congenital malformation, intrauterine growth retardation, intrauterine fetal demise (IUFD), asphyxia, sudden infant death syndrome (SIDS), seizures, hyaline membrane disorders, abnormal behavior and state control, mental retardation, cerebral infarcts and withdrawal symptoms (Delaney-Black et al., 2001; Wilbourne, Dorato, Yeo, & Curet, 2000).

In summary, abused pregnant women with co-occurring alcohol or substance abuse and mental health issues represent a particularly vulnerable group of women. The combined stigma of these issues in pregnancy likely represents a tremendous barrier to seeking help.

Health Consequences for the Child

The interrelated issues of preterm delivery and low birth weight (LBW) represent leading factors for infant morbidity and mortality in the United States. In the most recently available (2004) data, preterm delivery and/or low birth weight caused 15.7% of infant

---

EXHIBIT 6.1 | *Intimate Partner Abuse and Infant Health Consequences*

Growth Consequences
- Intrauterine growth retardation (IUGR)
- Low birth weight (LBW)
- Very low birth weight (VLBW)
- Poor breastfeeding patterns (may be related to interference or maternal mental health)

Birth Consequences
- Preterm labor
- Preterm birth

Mortality Consequences
- Intrauterine fetal demise
- Stillbirth
- Sudden Infant Death (SIDS)

Behavioral Consequences
- Poor attachment
- Poor interaction
- Sleep disturbances
- Clinginess
- Irritability/fretfulness

mortalities overall, second only to congenital/genetic defects as a cause of infant deaths (20.5%) (Mathews & MacDorman, 2007). The most common cause of LBW/VLBW is a short gestation (i.e., preterm birth), but it can also result from intrauterine growth restriction or IUGR. IUGR infants may be born at full term, or they may be born preterm (Inst Med 2006).

IPV has been associated with preterm labor (Berenson et al., 1994; Cokkinides et al., 1999; El-Kady et al., 2005; Neggers, Goldenberg, Cliver, & Hauth, 2004). Some of the most consistent evidence regarding fetal effects of IPV are related to its impact upon birth weight. Bullock and McFarlane (1989) were the first to describe the relationship between violence and low birth weight (LBW). This association has been validated repeatedly across multiple studies (Curry et al., 1998; El-Kady et al., 2005; Lipsky, Holt, Easterling, & Critchlow, 2003; McFarlane et al., 1996a; Renker, 1999; Yost, Bloom, McIntire, & Leveno, 2005). Some studies have not replicated these findings, but a in recent systematic review and a meta-analysis of eight studies (Boy & Salihu, 2004), Murphy et al. (2001) concluded that women reporting physical, emotional, or sexual violence had 1.4 times greater odds of giving birth to a LBW infant than nonabused women (95% CI 1.1–1.8).

Mediating or moderating factors may account for studies in which this association has not been replicated. Maternal low weight gain, smoking, or both may mediate the relationship between IPV and low birth weight (McFarlane et al., 1996b). Abusers might pressure their wives or girlfriends not to gain weight, or the stress from abuse could lead to smoking and low weight gain (Campbell, 2002; Curry et al., 1998).

In three major nursing studies, both physical and nonphysical abuse were significant risk factors for LBW for the term but not the preterm infants, but the risk estimates became nonsignificant in the adjusted statistical models (Campbell et al., 1999; Curry et al., 1998; Parker, McFarlane, Soeken, 1994). This again suggests a confounding or mediating effect of other abuse-related maternal health problems (notably low weight gain and poor obstetrical history) and further describes the path by which abuse affects birth weight.

An extensive review of the affects of IPV on children is beyond the scope of this chapter (see chapter 11); however, nurses should be aware that IPV has implications for children's health after delivery as well. The majority of abused women care deeply about their children's well-being (Campbell, 1998; Schechter & Edleson, 1999). Pregnant women who are living with violence often base their decisions on the safety needs or best interests of their children, not themselves (Libbus et al., 2006; Lutz, 2005; Lutz et al., 2006; Tilley & Brackley, 2004).

One negative effect of IPV during the postpartum period is interference with breastfeeding. In addition to the well-known benefits of breastfeeding for mothers and babies, some evidence suggests that breastfeeding is neuroprotective for infants of depressed mothers. Jones et al. (2004) found that while infants of depressed mothers may have abnormal EEG patterns that mimic those of chronically depressed adults, those that were breastfed had normal EEG patterns. This has implications for children in violent homes, given the substantially increased risk of depression among mothers experiencing IPV. However, abused women are overrepresented among those who wean their infants early or never breastfeed in population-based data from Pregnancy Risk Assessment Monitoring System (PRAMS). Women who reported experiencing IPV in the year prior to or during pregnancy were approximately 35–52% less likely to breastfeed their infants and 41–71% more likely to wean by 4 weeks postpartum (Silverman, Decker, Reed, & Raj, 2006). Preterm delivery and LBW, as well as a partner who considers her breasts "his," may add to abused mothers' barriers to breastfeeding (Kendall-Tackett, 2007).

IPV potentially affects children of mothers experiencing domestic violence in other ways. Witnessing violence can have an adverse psychological impact on children, with attendant behavioral issues. Lemmey et al. (2001) found that 72% of abused mothers reported "distress-indicating" behaviors by their children, most commonly sleep disturbances, clinging, and fretful behaviors. Levendosky et al. (2003) found that IPV exposure negatively affected young children's behaviors and was *positively* associated with maternal–child attachment and parenting effectiveness scores, suggesting that mothers appeared to be compensating for the violence by being more effective and responsive to their children. These findings clearly underscore the importance of nurses as advocates, to connect with abused mothers and link them to the help and support they need to overcome the effects of violence in their lives and the lives of their children.

IMPLICATIONS FOR NURSING PRACTICE

The review of evidence thus far demonstrates clearly that IPV has substantial health implications for pregnant women and their children, born and unborn. Nurses play a critical role in offering empathy, advocacy, and support to abused women, and providing her links to needed services. Because IPV impacts the lives and health of so many pregnant women, identification and assessment of and intervention with women experiencing abuse must become a routine part of prenatal care.

Nurses' Interactions With Survivors of Intimate Partner Violence

For nurses to become effective agents in ending the cycle of violence in women's lives, they must accept two basic premises. The first premise is that IPV is a serious public health problem, rather than a private problem, that therefore falls within the purview of nursing. The second premise is that no woman, under any circumstances, deserves to be physically, sexually, or emotionally abused.

Nurses must take care to maintain empathy and support for their patients, refrain from judgment, and remember that escaping from violence is a process, not an event. Gentle, sincere statements to the abuse survivor that she is a worthwhile person and does not deserve to be hurt can be extremely empowering to a woman in a vulnerable position. She has undoubtedly been told by her abuser that no one will believe her and that she deserves the abuse, and she may have come to believe this herself.

The Nursing Role and Intimate Partner Violence

The nurse's tasks when dealing with abused women are to (1) identify the presence of abuse, (2) assess the nature, severity, and potential lethality of the abuse, and the impact it has had on the woman's health, (3) plan intervention strategies, (4) intervene through referrals, information sharing, safety planning, and support, and (5) follow-up or assess the effectiveness of interventions. Throughout the nursing process, the primary role of the nurse is that of advocate. Advocacy includes assisting the battered woman to make informed decisions by information sharing and providing continued support, regardless of the decisions and choices that are made.

Identification/Screening

There are three methods that are useful in identifying IPV in a medical setting: observing, chart reviews, and direct questioning.

Early signs of abuse take many forms. These include warning signs like the partner being overly possessive and jealous, being threatened by the woman's success or pregnancy, being highly controlling, or being cruel and violent in other relationships. Observations of the woman and her partner during clinic visits, in childbirth classes, and during hospital stays for pregnancy complications or labor and delivery may also provide clues to the presence of abuse. These methods must not be used to replace, but rather, should be used in conjunction with direct questioning.

Chart reviews may only provide clues to past abuse (see the display that follows). There are a number of "red flag" items that may be encountered in a woman's medical record. These are listed in Exhibit 6.2, "Identifying Battered Women."

EXHIBIT 6.2 | *Identifying Battered Women*

Chart Review
- Assault, regardless of the assailant's stated identify
- Injuries inflicted by weapons
- Injuries consistent with assault that are inadequately explained
- Multiple medical visits for injuries or anxiety symptoms
- Injury or assault during pregnancy
- History of depression, drug use, or suicide attempts
- Sex-specific or disfiguring injuries, such as to the face, breasts, or genitals
- Eating disorders
- Unexplained somatic symptoms, such as back, chest, or pelvic pain, or choking sensations
- Tranquilizer or sedative use

Obstetrical/Gynecological History
- Elective abortions
- Sexually transmitted infections
- Sexual assault
- Late or inadequate prenatal care
- Substance use during pregnancy
- Preterm labor or preterm bleeding
- Low birth weight
- Unexplained fetal injuries, present at birth
- Unexplained intrauterine fetal demise
- Abruptio placentae
- Suicide attempts during pregnancy
- Poor weight gain during pregnancy
- Trauma injuries during pregnancy

Observations During Clinic Visits
- Partner is conspicuously unwilling to leave the woman's side
- Partner speaks for the woman or belittles what she says
- Partner makes derogatory comments about the woman's appearance or behavior
- Partner is over solicitous with care providers
- Partner is emotionally absent or out of tune with the woman
- Woman is obviously afraid of her partner

Certainly, not all survivors of domestic abuse have medical histories or have partners who behave so that nurses have reason to suspect abuse. For this reason, all women must be assessed for abuse.

Direct questioning for abuse should be conducted separately and not be limited to one question in a list of previous medical conditions. Multiple abuse-focused questions should be asked because women, who often deny abuse with the first question, often answer positively to subsequent questions. The Abuse Assessment Screen (see Appendix A) is a useful, evidence-based set of questions which can be used to screen for IPV in approximately the same amount of time it takes to obtain a blood pressure. Several recent studies suggest that using a computerized assessment may be preferable to women to out loud screening (MacMillan et al., 2006; Trautman, McCarthy, Miller, Campbell, & Kelen, 2007).

It is important to remember that some battered women may deny abuse during an initial assessment because of guilt, denial, shame, the belief that the abuse is somehow her fault, and the desire to preserve the "public face" of the happy pregnancy. She may also fear losing her children if she reveals the abuse. Later in the woman's pregnancy, after rapport has been established, she may be more willing to reveal past or current abuse.

Assessment

When IPV is identified, further assessment is needed. Nurses should assess the history and course of the abuse, including how long it has been occurring, the severity and frequency of the abuse, injuries and other health problems the woman believes have resulted from the abuse, and whether the abuse is escalating. Nonphysical and sexual abuse must also be explored. Women should be asked what resources (police, shelters, clergy, family, etc.) they have used and how helpful these individuals or organizations have been. Nurses should also enquire about the use of the court system and protective orders.

All assessments must be thoroughly documented. This can be time-consuming, but can be invaluable for the woman in future legal proceedings (e.g., custody hearings). Details should be documented in the woman's own words as much as possible and with photographs and body maps where appropriate. Chapter 13 in this volume provides in-depth information about how to document IPV.

Planning

Safety planning with women experiencing IPV consists of determining available options and the benefits and risks of each option. Two factors are important in this phase of the nursing process: (1) What does the woman want to do or have happen; and (2) What is her level of current danger? Determining the woman's current level of danger in her relationship is a crucial part of assessment. Most abuse survivors are "tuned in" to their immediate risk of harm. In addition, the Danger Assessment should be administered (see Appendix B). This research and clinical instrument is a widely used, evidence-based set of questions that assesses the risk that the abused woman will face severe or lethal violence from an abusive partner (Campbell, Soeken, McFarlane, & Parker, 1998; Campbell et al., 2003). Training in the use and interpretation of the Danger Assessment is available online at http://www.dangerassessment.org.

Abused women essentially have three options: (1) stay with the abuser, (2) leave for a safe place, or (3) have the abuser removed from the place of residence. In some cases, only the first two options are available. The role of the nurse in the planning phase of the nursing process is to provide the woman with the information necessary to make informed decisions. Ultimately, the most effective responses to IPV are those that are multidisciplinary and coordinated across all levels of the community (i.e., health care, victim services, child welfare and protective service agencies, and the civil and criminal justice systems) (Family Violence Prevention Fund, 2004). Help is also available via the National Domestic Violence Hotline, 1-800-799-SAFE.

Staying With the Abuser

An abused woman, particularly one who is pregnant, may choose to stay with or return to an abusive partner for many complex reasons. She stays or returns for many of the same reasons women stay in nonabusive but difficult relationships: financial constraints, societal and familial pressures, and because of the children. For many women, staying in the relationship may be preferable to single parenthood, inadequate housing, and financial deprivation.

If a woman chooses to stay with her partner, she can develop a safety or exit plan to be used if she feels in danger. She should have knowledge of where to go, phone numbers, and transportation plans. If possible, a bag with clothing, rent and utility receipts, birth certificates, toys, money, and extra car keys should be kept in a safe place. Encourage her to tell friends, family, and neighbors about the abuse so that they may be able to assist her in the future if necessary.

Leaving

If the pregnant woman chooses to leave her abuser, she must decide where she will go and have a clear idea of how safe she will be there. The evidence is clear that leaving the abuser is typically a particularly dangerous time for abused women, when they may be at elevated risk for serious harm or death (Campbell et al., 2003). If the woman has scored high on the Danger Assessment, her risk may be especially great. She should be counseled that she must never tell the abuser of her intention to leave. Instead, she must leave in secret and only go back to get her belongings accompanied by police or family or friends so that she is not alone with the abuser. Nurses should advise women to take their children with them when they leave. If they do not, they may have great difficulty obtaining legal custody in the future. This is even more crucial if the partner is also abusing the children. Abused children are more likely to remain in their mother's custody if she removes them from the violent situation. Shelter workers can often arrange to have children brought to the shelter from school or elsewhere.

If the abuse survivor stays somewhere other than a shelter, she should have a plan of action should her partner locate her. She should consult a domestic violence advocate regarding issues such as protecting her children from being abducted by the abuser and protecting herself at work and in the home.

Removing the Abuser From the Home

The woman's partner may move out willingly or may be forced to leave by a vacate or protective order. This is generally a temporary order, and it is most likely to be granted if the woman's name is on the lease or title for the residence or if the woman is unable to enter a shelter because they are full. If the partner leaves, safety issues should be discussed. The woman should have all locks changed and obtain an order for protection if she has not already done so.

For nurses to provide accurate information to battered women, they must become familiar with state laws concerning domestic violence, sexual assault, and protective orders, as well as what domestic violence resources are available in their community. Advocates from women's shelters are willing to provide such education personally and often also have written material available. Although laws vary from state to state, domestic violence is illegal nationwide and can be (although it is not always) prosecuted in the same way as assault by a stranger. Many battered women are not aware of this. Marital rape is illegal in most states, and rape outside of marriage is illegal in all.

The abuse survivor is often the best judge of her own safety. Nurses and advocates can help her plan what she would do if her partner comes to her door. She or her children should call 911 and report "some man" is at the door or trying to break in. If she reports that the man is her husband or boyfriend, police response time may be longer.

Follow-Up and Evaluation

In some cases, there will be no further contact between the nurse and the abuse survivor. This may occur if the intervention takes place postpartum in the hospital or if the woman changes location, or if she does not return to the clinic. In such cases, nurses receive no feedback on their interventions. A phone call to the woman inquiring about her welfare is often welcomed.

When there is continuing contact, nurses should provide continued support and encouragement. The nurse should let the abused woman know she is still willing to discuss this issue by asking the woman how things are going. Praise her accomplishments, no matter how small. Continue to encourage her to obtain counseling or join a support group if she has not done so already.

For women who leave their abusers, there is much grieving that must be done. The woman may have lost a husband, a father for her children, perhaps her home, friends, and family. It may take time for her to work through the grief process and to begin making concrete future plans. For many women, it takes years before they fully realize the impact of the abuse on their lives.

Tested Nursing Interventions

In a prospective cohort study, Parker et al. (1999) tested an intervention that they delivered three times during pregnancy to prevent further abuse to pregnant women and found that the intervention significantly increased safety behaviors. The intervention was "brochure based" and is titled *"Cycle of Abuse Pamphlet."* The brochure is available in English and Spanish at the Nursing Network on Violence Against Women, International Web site (http://www.nnvawi.org/assessment.htm). The specific topics included in the brochure is information on the cycle of violence; information on applying for legal protection orders and filing criminal charges; and community resource phone numbers such as shelters, hot lines, and law enforcement.

The Domestic Violence Enhanced Home Visitation (DOVE, NINR/NIH, R01 NR009093-01A2) is another nursing intervention designed to test the effectiveness and efficacy of a structured IPV intervention delivered by prenatal home visitors for abused pregnant women and their infants/toddlers. The DOVE intervention is brochure based (adapted from the Parker et al., 1999 study tested brochure), delivered in an interactive manner. Each woman is encouraged to describe her experiences and choose her own options as they proceed. The brochure includes the four major intervention components: (a) Cycle of Abuse and IPV information, (b) Danger Assessment, (c) Safety Planning, and (d) Resources. Participants receive three prenatal and three postpartum sessions. It is expected that the DOVE intervention will have less frequent and less severe IPV, improved parenting knowledge, attitudes and practices, less parenting stress, increased use of safety behaviors and better mental health outcomes.

Sample recruitment and DOVE intervention is ongoing; however, baseline sample data suggest differences in demographics (i.e., ethnic/racial background, marital status, educational levels), self-reported IPV, physical and mental health that varied by rural and urban settings. This ongoing study is an example of how nursing science has been developed from description to intervention testing, followed by intervention testing in other settings, leading to the improved health and increased safety of women and children.

SUMMARY

Nurses, nurse-midwives, and nurse practitioners can play a crucial role in breaking the cycle of violence in the lives of pregnant women. Pregnant women who are living with IPV are with us wherever we practice as nurses—in clinics, hospitals, and public health practices. Nurses must acquire a working knowledge concerning abusive relationships, the health effects of violence against pregnant women and their children, and the resources and options available to survivors of domestic violence, if they are to be able to intervene effectively.

Violence against women is a serious public health problem that requires a coordinated community response, which includes the advocacy, support, and services of health care professionals. Because nurses are trained in a holistic approach to health, they are uniquely well suited to the task of providing an effective health care response to domestic violence. By working closely with abused women's services outside of the medical community, nurses can be an effective force in ending the violence in the lives of the women they serve.

REFERENCES

Attala, J. M. (1994). Risk identification of abused women participating in a women, infants, and children program. *Health care for women International, 15,* 587–597.

Bacchus, L., Mezey, G., & Bewley, S. (2004). Domestic violence: Prevalence in pregnant women and associations with physical and psychological health. *European Journal of Obstetrics & Gynecology and Reproductive Biology, 113*(1), 6–11.

Bailey, B. A., & Daugherty, R. A. (2007). Intimate partner violence during pregnancy: incidence and associated health behaviors in a rural population. *Maternal and Child Health Journal, 11*(5), 495–503.

Berenson, A. B., Wiemann, C. M., Wilkinson, G. S., Jones, W. A., & Anderson, G. D. (1994). Perinatal morbidity associated with violence experienced by pregnant women. *American Journal of Obstetrics and Gynecology, 170*(6), 1760–1766; discussion 1766–1769.

Bhandari, S., Levitch, A. H., Ellis, K. K., Ball, K., Everett, K., Geden, E., et al. (2008). Comparative analyses of stressors experienced by rural low-income pregnant women experiencing intimate partner violence and those who are not. *Journal of Obstetric, Gynecologic, & Neonatal Nursing, 37*(4), 492–501.

Bloom, T., Curry, M. A., & Durham, L. (2007). Abuse and psychosocial stress as factors in high utilization of medical services during pregnancy. *Issues in Mental Health Nursing, 28*(8), 849–866.

Bohn, D. K. (2002). Lifetime and current abuse, pregnancy risks, and outcomes among Native American women. *Journal of Health Care for the Poor and Underserved, 13*(2), 184–198.

Bohn, D. K., Tebben, J. G., & Campbell, J. C. (2004). Influences of income, education, age, and ethnicity on physical abuse before and during pregnancy. *Journal of Obstetrical, Gynecological, and Neonatal Nursing, 33*(5), 561–571.

Bourassa, D., & Bérubé, J. (2007). The prevalence of intimate partner violence among women and teenagers seeking abortion compared with those continuing pregnancy. *Journal of Obstetrics and Gynaecology of Canada, 29*(5), 415–423.

Bowen, E., Heron, J., Waylen, A., & Wolke, D. (2005). Domestic violence risk during and after pregnancy: findings from a British longitudinal study. *BJOG: An International Journal of Obstetrics and Gynaecology, 112*(8), 1083–1089.

Boy, A., & Salihu, H. M. (2004). Intimate partner violence and birth outcomes: a systematic review. *International Journal of Fertility and Women's Medicine, 49*(4), 159–164.

Brady, J. P., Posner, M., Lang, C., & Rosati, M. J. (1994). *Risk and reality: The implications of prenatal exposure to alcohol and other drugs.* Retrieved May 21, 2009, from www.aspe.hhs.gov/hsp/cyp/drugkids.htm

Brendtro, M., & Bowker, L. H. (1989). Battered women: how can nurses help? *Issues in Mental Health Nursing, 10*(2), 169–180.

Bullock, L., Bloom, T., Curry, M. A., Davis, J., & Kilburn, E. (2006). Abuse disclosure in private and Medicaid funded pregnant women. *Journal of Midwifery and Women's Health, 51*(5), 361–369.

Bullock, L. F., & McFarlane, J. (1989). The birth-weight/battering connection. *American Journal of Nursing, 89*(9), 1153–1155.

Bureau of Justice Statistics. (2007). *Intimate partner violence in the United States.* Washington, DC: US Department of Justice, Office of Justice Programs. http://www.ojp.usdoj.gov/bjs/intimate/ipv.htm. Accessed August 20, 2008.

Campbell, D. W., Sharps, P. W., Gary, F. A., Campbell, J. C., & Lopez, L. M. (2002). Intimate partner violence in African American women. *Online Journal of Issues in Nursing, 7*(1), 5.

Campbell, J., Poland, M., Waller, J., & Ager, J. (1992). Correlates of battering during pregnancy. *Research in Nursing and Health, 15*(219–226).

Campbell, J. C. (1998). Abuse during pregnancy: progress, policy, and potential. *American Journal of Public Health, 88*(2), 185–187.

Campbell, J. C. (2002). Health consequences of intimate partner violence. *Lancet, 359*(9314), 1331–1336.

Campbell, J. C., ,Oliver, C., & Bullock, L. (1998). The dynamics of battering during pregnancy: Women's explanations of why. In J. C. Campbell (Ed.) *Empowering survivors of abuse: Health care for battered women and their children* (pp. 81–89). Thousand Oaks, CA: Sage.

Campbell, J. C., Ryan, J., Campbell, D. W., Torres, S., King, C., Stallings, R., et al. (1999). Physical and nonphysical abuse and other risk factors for low birthweight among term and preterm babies. *American Journal of Epidemiology, 150*, 714–726.

Campbell, J. C., Soeken, K., McFarlane, J., & Parker, B. (1998). Risk factors for femicide among pregnant and nonpregnant battered women. In J. C. Campbell (Ed.), *Empowering survivors of abuse: Health care for battered women and their children* (pp. 90–97). Thousand Oaks, CA: Sage.

Campbell, J. C., Webster, D., Koziol-McLain, J., Block, C., Campbell, D., Curry, M. A., et al. (2003). Risk factors for femicide in abusive relationships: Results from a multisite case control study. *American Journal of Public Health, 93*(7), 1089–1097.

Certain, H. E., Mueller, M., Jagodzinski, T., & Fleming, M. (2008). Domestic abuse during the previous year in a sample of postpartum women. *Journal of Obstetric, Gynecologic, and Neonatal Nursing, 37*(1), 35–41.

Chasnoff, I. J., Neuman, K., Thornton, C., Callaghan, M. A., & Angela, A. (2001). Screening for substance use in pregnancy: A practical approach for the primary care physician. *American Journal of Obstetrics & Gynecology, 184*(4), 752–758.

Cloutier, S., Martin, S. L., Moracco, K. E., Garro, J., Clark, K. A., & Brody, S. (2002). Physically abused pregnant women's perceptions about the quality of their relationships with their male partners. *Women & Health, 35*(2–3), 149–163.

Cokkinides, V. E., Coker, A. L., Sanderson, M., Addy, C., & Bethea, L. (1999). Physical violence during pregnancy: maternal complications and birth outcomes. *Obstetrics & Gynecology, 93*(5 Pt 1), 661–666.

Curry, M. A., Durham, L., Bullock, L., Bloom, T., & Davis, J. (2006). Nurse case management for pregnant women experiencing or at risk for abuse. *Journal of Obstetric, Gynecologic, and Neonatal Nursing, 35*(2), 181–192.

Curry, M. A., Perrin, N., & Wall, E. (1998). Effects of abuse on maternal complications and birth weight in adult and adolescent women. *Obstetrics & Gynecology, 92*(4 Pt 1), 530–534.

Datner, E. M., Wiebe, D. J., Brensinger, C. M., & Nelson, D. B. (2007). Identifying pregnant women experiencing domestic violence in an urban emergency department. *Journal of Interpersonal Violence, 22*(1), 124–135.

Delaney-Black, V., Nordstrom-Klee, B., Covington, C., Templin, T., Ager, J., & Sokol, R. (2001). Prenatal drug exposure and growth to age 7. *American Journal of Obstetrics and Gynecology, 184*(1), S169.

Dutton, M. A., Goodman, L., Lennig, D., Murphy, J., & Kaltman, S. (2005). *Ecological Model of Battered Women's Experience over Time* (No. 213713): National Institute of Justice Office of Justice Programs.

El-Kady, D., Gilbert, W. M., Xing, G., & Smith, L. H. (2005). Maternal and neonatal outcomes of assaults during pregnancy. *Obstetrics & Gynecology, 19*(4), 357–363.

El Kady, D. (2008). Perinatal outcomes of traumatic injuries during pregnancy. *Clinical Obstetrics and Gynecology, 50*(3), 582–591.

Ellis, K. K., Chang, C., Bhandari, S., Ball, K., Geden, E., Everett, K. D., et al. (2008). Rural mothers experiencing the stress of intimate partner violence or not: Their health concerns. *Journal of Midwifery and Women's Health, 53*(6), 556–562.

Family Violence Prevention Fund, N. C. G. o. i. a. r. t. i. p. v. i. h. c. s. (2004). *National Consensus Guidelines on identifying and responding to intimate partner violence in health care settings*. San Francisco, CA: Family Violence Prevention Fund.

Field, T., Diego, M., & Hernandez-Reif, M. (2006). Prenatal depression effects on the fetus and newborn: A review. *Infant Behavior & Development, 29*, 445–455.

Flynn, H. A., Walton, M. A., Chermack, S. T., Cunningham, R. M., & Marcus, S. M. (2007). Brief detection and co-occurrence of violence, depression, and alcohol risk in prenatal care settings. *Archives of Women's Mental Health, 10*, 155–161.

Fox, G. L., & Jawitz, M. W. (2004). *Homicide trends in the United States*. Washington, DC: US Department of Justice: Bureau of Justice Statistics.

Frank, D. A., Augustyn, M., Knight, W. G., Pell, T., & Zuckerman, B. (2001). Growth, development, and behavior in early childhood following prenatal cocaine exposure: A systematic review. *Journal of the American Medical Association, 285*(12), 1613–1625.

Fried, P. A., Watkinson, B., & Gray, R. (1998). Differential effects on cognitive functioning in 9-12 year olds prenatally exposed to cigarettes and marijuana. . *Neurotoxicology & Teratology, 20*(3), 293–306.

Gazmararian, J. A., Adams, M. M., Saltzman, L. E., Johnson, C. H., Bruce, F. C., Marks, J. S., et al. (1995). The relationship between pregnancy intendedness and physical violence in mothers of newborns. The PRAMS Working Group. *Obstetrics & Gynecology, 85*(6), 1031–1038.

Gazmararian, J. A., Petersen, R., Spitz, A. M., Goodwin, M. M., Saltzman, L. E., & Marks, J. S. (2000). Violence and reproductive health: Current knowledge and future research directions. *Maternal and Child Health Journal, 4*(2), 79–84.

Golding, J. M. (1999). Intimate partner violence as a risk factor for mental disorders: A meta-analysis. *Journal of Family Violence, 14*(2), 99–132.

Goodwin, M. M., Gazmararian, J. A., Johnson, C. H., Gilbert, B. C., & Saltzman, L. E. (2000). Pregnancy intendedness and physical abuse around the time of pregnancy: findings from the pregnancy risk assessment monitoring system, 1996–1997. PRAMS Working Group. Pregnancy Risk Assessment Monitoring System. *Maternal and Child Health Journal, 4*(2), 85-92.

Greenberg, E. M., McFarlane, J., & Watson, M. G. (1997). Vaginal bleeding and abuse: assessing pregnant women in the emergency department. *MCN: American Journal of Maternal Child Nursing, 22*(4), 182–186.

Griesler, P. C., Kandel, D. B., & Davies, M. (1998). Maternal smoking in pregnancy, child behavior problems, and adolescent smoking. *Journal of Research on Adolescence, 8*(1), 159–185.

Hampton, R., Oliver, W., & Magarian, L. (2003). Domestic violence in the African American community. *Violence Against Women, 9*, 553–557.

Harner, H. M. (2004). Domestic violence and trauma care in teenage pregnancy: Does paternal age make a difference? *Journal of Obstetric, Gynecologic, and Neonatal Nursing, 33*, 312–319.

Horon, I. L., & Cheng, D. (2001). Enhanced surveillance for pregnancy-associated mortality—Maryland, 1993–1998. *Journal of the American Medical Association, 285*(11), 1455–1459.

Jacoby, M., Gorenflo, D., Black, E., Wunderlich, C., & Eyler, A. E. (1999). Rapid repeat pregnancy and experiences of interpersonal violence among low-income adolescents. *American Journal of Preventative Medicine, 16*(4), 318–321.

Jones, N. A., McFall, B. A., & Diego, M. A. (2004). Patterns of brain electrical activity in infants of depressed mothers who breastfeed and bottle feed: The mediating role of infant temperament. *Biological Psychology, 67*, 103–124.

Kelly, R. H., Russo, J., Holt, V. L., Danielsen, B. H., Zatzick, D. F., Walker, E., et al. (2002). Psychiatric and substance use disorders as risk factors for low birth weight and preterm delivery. *Obstetrics & Gynecology, 100*(2), 297–304.

Kendall-Tackett, K. A. (2007). Violence against women and the perinatal period: The impact of lifetime violence and abuse on pregnancy, postpartum, and breastfeeding. *Trauma, Violence, & Abuse, 8*(3), 344–353.

Kershner, M., Long, D., & Anderson, J. E. (1998). Abuse against women in rural Minnesota. *Public health Nursing, 15*(6), 422–431.

Koenig LJ, Whitaker DJ, Royce R. A., Wilson T. E., Callahan M. R., Fernandez M. I. (2006). Physical and sexual violence during pregnancy and after delivery: A prospective multistate study of women with or at risk for HIV infection. *American Journal of Public Health, 96*, 1052–1059.

Krulewitch, C. J., Pierre-Louis, M. L., de Leon-Gomez, R., Guy, R., & Green, R. (2001). Hidden from view: Violent deaths among pregnant women in the District of Columbia, 1988–1996. *Journal of Midwifery and Women's Health, 46*(1), 4–10.

Landenburger, K. A. (1989). Process of entrapment in and recovery from an abusive relationship. *Issues in Mental Health Nursing, 10*, 209–227.

Landenburger, K. A. (1998). Exploration of women's identity: Clinical approaches with abused women. In J. C. Campbell (Ed.), *Empowering survivors of abuse* (pp. 61–69). Thousand Oaks, CA: Sage.

Lang, D. L., Salazar, L. F., Wingood, G. M., DiClemente, R. J., & Isis, M. (2007). Associations between recent gender-based violence and pregnancy, sexually transmitted infections, condom use practices, and negotiation of sexual practices among HIV-positive women. . *Journal of Acquired Immune Deficiency Syndromes, 46*(2), 216–221.

Lemmey, D., McFarlane, J., Wilson, P., & Malecha, A. (2001). Intimate partner violence: Mother's perspectives of effects on their children. *American Journal of Maternal Child Nursing, 26*(2), 98–103.

Levendosky, A. A., Huth-Bocks, A. C., Shapiro, D. L., & Semel, M. A. (2003). The impact of domestic violence on the maternal–child relationship and reschool-age children's functioning. *Journal of Family Psychology, 17*(3), 275–287.

Libbus, M. K., Bullock, L. F., Nelson, T., Robrecht, L., Curry, M. A., & Bloom, T. (2006). Abuse during pregnancy: Current theory and new contextual understandings. *Issues in Mental Health Nursing, 27*(9), 927–938.

Lindhorst, T., & Oxford, M. (2008). The long-term effects of intimate partner violence on adolescent mothers' depressive symptoms. *Social Science and Medicine, 66*, 1322–1333.

Lipscomb, L. E., Johnson, C. H., Morrow, B., Gilbert, B. C., Ahluwalia, I. B., Beck, L. F., et al. (2000). *PRAMS 1998 surveillance report.* Atlanta, GA: Division of Reproductive Health, National Center for Chronic Disease Prevention and Health Promotion, Centers for Disease Control and Prevention.

Lipsky, S., Holt, V. L., Easterling, T. R., & Critchlow, C. W. (2003). Impact of police-reported intimate partner violence during pregnancy on birth outcomes. *Obstetrics & Gynecology, 102*(3), 557–564.

Long, C. R., & Curry, M. A. (1998). Living in two worlds: Native American women and prenatal care. *Health Care for Women International, 19*(3), 205–215.

Loveland-Cook, C. A., Flick, L. H., Homan, S. M., Campbell, C., McSweeney, M., & Gallagher, M. E. (2004). Posttraumatic stress disorder in pregnancy: prevalence, risk factors, and treatment. *Obstetrics & Gynecology, 103*(4), 710–717.

Lutz, K. F. (2004). Living two lives: A grounded theory of abuse during pregnancy. *Communicating Nursing Res, 37,* 101, 103–109.

Lutz, K. F. (2005). Abuse experiences, perceptions, and associated decisions during the childbearing cycle. *Western Journal of Nursing Res, 27*(7), 802–824; discussion 825–830.

Lutz, K. F., Curry, M. A., Robrecht, L. C., Libbus, M. K., & Bullock, L. (2006). Double binding, abusive intimate partner relationships, and pregnancy. *Canadian Journal of Nursing Research, 38*(4), 118–134.

Macmillan, H. L., Wathen, C. N., Jamieson, E., Boyle, M., McNutt, L. A., Worster, A., Lent, B., & Webb, M. (2006). Approaches to screening for intimate partner violence in health care settings. *JAMA, 296*(5), 530–536.

Macy, R. J., Martin, S. L., Kupper, L. L., Casanueva, C., & Guo, S. (2007). Partner violence among women before, during, and after pregnancy: Multiple opportunities for intervention. *Women's Health Issues, 17*(5), 290–299.

Martin, S. L., Mackie, L., Kupper, L. L., Buescher, P. A., & Moracco, K. E. (2001). Physical abuse of women before, during, and after pregnancy. *JAMA, 285*(12), 1581–1584.

Mathews, T. J., & MacDorman, M. F. (2007). Infant mortality statistics from the 2004 period linked birth/infant death data set. *National Vital Statistics Reports* (Vol. 55). Hyattsville, MD: National Center for Health Statistics.

Mattson, S., & Rodriguez, E. (1999). Battering in pregnant Latinas. *Issues in Mental Health Nursing, 20,* 405–422.

McCauley, J., Kern, D. E., Kolodner, K., Dill, L., Schroeder, A. F., DeChant, H., Ryden, J., Bass, E. B., & Derogatis, L. R., Kern, D. E., Kolodner, K., Derogatis, L. R., & Bass, E. B. (1998). Relation of low-severity violence to women's health. *Journal of General Internal Medicine, 13*(687–691).

McFarlane, J., Campbell, J. C., Sharps, P., & Watson, K. (2002). Abuse during pregnancy and femicide: urgent implications for women's health. *Obstetrics & Gynecology, 100*(1), 27–36.

McFarlane, J., Malecha, A., Gist, J., Watson, K., Batten, E., Hall, I., et al. (2005). Intimate partner sexual assault against women and associated victim substance use, suicidality, and risk factors for femicide. *Issues in Mental Health Nursing, 26*(9), 953–967.

McFarlane, J., Parker, B., & Moran, B. (2007). *Abuse during pregnancy: A Protocol for Prevention and Intervention* (3rd edition). White Plains: March of Dimes.

McFarlane, J., Parker, B., & Soeken, K. (1996a). Abuse during pregnancy: associations with maternal health and infant birth weight. *Nursing Research, 45*(1), 37–42.

McFarlane, J., Parker, B., & Soeken, K. (1996b). Physical abuse, smoking, and substance use during pregnancy: Prevalence, interrelationships, and effects on birth weight. *Journal of Obstetric, Gynecologic, and Neonatal Nursing, 25*(4), 313–320.

McFarlane, J., Parker, B., Soeken, K., Silva, C., & Reed, S. (1999). Severity of abuse before and during pregnancy for African American, Hispanic, and Anglo women. *Journal of Nurse-Midwifery, 44*(2), 139–144.

McFarlane, J., Soeken, K., Reel, S., Parker, B., & Silva, C. (1997). Resource use by abused women following an intervention program: associated severity of abuse and reports of abuse ending. *Public Health Nursing, 14*(4), 244–250.

Miller, E., Decker, M. R., Reed, E., Raj, A., Hathaway, J. E., & Silverman, J. G. (2007). Male partner pregnancy-promoting behaviors and adolescent partner violence: Findings from a qualitative study with adolescent females. *Academic Pediatrics, 7*(5), 360–366.

MMWR. (2008). Prevalence of self-reported postpartum depressive symptoms in 17 states, 2004–2005. *MMWR,57*(14), 361–366.

Morleand, L. A., Leskin, G. A., Block, C. R., Campbell, J. C., & Friedman, M. J. (2008). Intimate partner violence and miscarriage: Examination of the roles of physical and psychological abuse and post-traumatic stress disorder. *Journal of Interpersonal Violence, 23*(5), 652–669.

Murphy, C. C., Schei, B., Myhr, T. L., & Du Mont, J. (2001). Abuse: A risk factor for low birth weight? A systematic review and meta-analysis. *Canadian Medical Association Journal, 164*(11), 1567–1572.

Nannini, A., Lazar, J., Berg, C., Barger, M., Tomashek, K., Cabral, H., et al. (2008). Physical injuries reported on hospital visits for assault during the pregnancy-associated period. *Nursing Research, 57*(3), 144–149.

Neggers, Y., Goldenberg, R., Cliver, S., & Hauth, J. (2004). Effects of domestic violence on preterm birth and low birth weight. *Acta Obstetricia et Gynecologica Scandinavica, 83*(5), 455–460.

Nicolaidis, C., Curry, M., McFarland, B., & Gerrity, M. (2004). Violence, mental health, and physical symptoms in an academic internal medicine practice. *Journal of General Internal Medicine, 19*(8), 819–827.

O'Campo, P., Kub, J., Woods, A., Garza, Snow-Jones, Gielen, A. C., et al. (2006). Depression, PTSD, & co-morbidity related to IPV in civilian and military women. *Brief Treatment and Crisis Intervention, 6,* 99–110.

Palitto, C. C., Campbell, J. C., & O' Campo, P. (2005). Is intimate partner violence associated with unintended pregnancy? A review of the literature. *Trauma, Violence, & Abuse, 6,* 217–235.

Parker, B., McFarlane, J., & Soeken, K. (1994). Abuse during pregnancy: Effects on maternal complications and birth weight in adult and teenage women. *Obstetrics & Gynecology, 84*(3), 323–328.

Parker, B., McFarlane, J., Soeken, K., Silva, C., & Reel, S. (1999). Testing an intervention to prevent further abuse to pregnant women. *Research in Nursing and in Health, 22*(1), 59–66.

Renker, P. R. (1999). Physical abuse, social support, self-care, and pregnancy outcomes of older adolescents. *Journal of Obstetric, Gynecologic, and Neonatal Nursing, 28*(4), 377–388.

Renker, P. R. (2002). "Keep a blank face. I need to tell you what has been happening to me": Teens' stories of abuse and violence before and during pregnancy. *American Journal of Maternal Child Nursing, 27*(2), 109–116.

Renker, P. R. (2003). Keeping safe: teenagers' strategies for dealing with perinatal violence. *Journal of Obstetric, Gynecologic, and Neonatal Nursing, 32*(1), 58–67.

Romito, P., Turan, J. M., & De Marchi, M. (2005). The impact of current and past interpersonal violence on women's mental health. *Social Science & Medicine, 60,* 1717–1727.

Rose, L. E., Campbell, J., & Kub, J. (2000). The role of social support and family relationships in women's responses to battering. *Health Care for Women International, 21*(1), 27–39.

Rubin, R. (1984). *Maternal identity and the maternal experience.* New York: Springer.

Saltzman, L. E., Fanslow, J. L., McMahon, P. M., & Shelley, G. A. (1999). *Intimate partner violence surveillance: Uniform definitions and recommended data elements, Version 1.0.* Atlanta, GA: National Center for Injury Prevention and Control, Centers for Disease Control and Prevention.

Saltzman, L. E., Johnson, C. H., Gilbert, B. C., & Goodwin, M. A. (2003). Physical abuse around the time of pregnancy: An examination of prevalence and risk factors in 16 states. *Maternal and Child Health Journal, 7,* 31–42.

Schechter, S., & Edleson, J. L. (1999). Effective intervention in woman battering and child maltreatment cases: Guidelines for policy & practice (The Greenbook).

Seng, J. S., Low, L. K., Sparbel, K. J., & Killion, C. (2004). Abuse-related post-traumatic stress during the childbearing year. *J Adv Nurs, 46*(6), 604–613.

Seng, J. S., Oakley, D. J., Sampselle, C. M., Killion, C., Graham-Bermann, S., & Liberzon, I. (2001). Posttraumatic stress disorder and pregnancy complications. *Obstetrics & Gynecology, 97*(1), 17–22.

Shu, X. O., Hatch, M. C., Mills, J., Clemens, J., & Susser, M. (1995). Maternal smoking, alcohol drinking, caffeine consumption, and fetal growth: Results from a prospective study. *Epidemiology and Community Health, 6*(2), 115–120.

Silverman, J. G., Decker, M. R., Reed, E., & Raj, A. (2006). Intimate partner violence around the time of pregnancy: Association with breastfeeding behavior. *Journal of Women's Health, 15*(8), 934–940.

Silverman, J. G., Raj, A., & Clements, K. (2004). Dating violence and associated sexual risk and pregnancy among adolescent girls in the United States. *Pediatrics, 114,* e220–e225.

Soeken, K., McFarlane, J., Parker, B., & Lominak, M. (1998). The Abuse Assessment Screen: A clinical instrument to measure frequency, severity and perpetrator of abuse against women. In J. Campbell (Ed.), *Empowering survivors of abuse: health care for battered women and their children* (pp. 195–203). Thousand Oaks: Sage.

Taggart, L., & Mattson, S. (1996). Delay in prenatal care as a result of battering in pregnancy: Cross-cultural implications. *Health Care for Women International, 17,* 25–34.

Thomas, J. C. (2001). Maternal smoking during pregnancy associated with negative toddler behavior and early smoking experimentation [Electronic Version]. *IDA Notes, 16* from http://165.112.78.61/NIDA_Notes/NNVol16N1/Maternal.html.

Tilley, D. S., & Brackley, M. (2004). Violent lives of women: Critical points for intervention—Phase I focus groups. *Perspectives in Psychiatric Care, 40*(4), 157–166, 170.

Tjaden, P. & Thoennes, P. (2000). *Extent, nature, and consequences of physical violence: Findings from the National Violence Against Women Survey*. Washington, D.C.: National Institute of Justice and Centers for Disease Control and Prevention.

Torres, S., Campbell, J. C., Campbell, D. W., Ryan, J., King, C., Price, P., et al. (2000). Abuse during pregnancy: Prevalence and cultural correlates. *Violence and Victims, 15*(3), 303–322.

Trautman, D., McCarthy, M. L., Miller, N., Campbell, J. C., & Kelen, G. (2007). Intimate partner violence and Emergency Department screening: Computerized screening versus usual care. *Annals of Emergency Medicine, 49*, 526–534.

Ulrich, Y. C., McKenna, L. S., King, C., Campbell, D. W., Ryan, J., Torres, S., et al. (2006). Postpartum mothers' disclosure of abuse, role, and conflict. *Health Care for Women International, 27*(4), 324–343.

Varisco, R. (2001). Drug abuse and conduct disorder linked to maternal smoking during pregnancy [Electronic Version]. *NIDA Notes, 15* from http://165.112.78.61/NIDA_Notes/NNVol15N5/Drug.html.

Webster, J., Chandler, J., & Battistutta, D. (1996). Pregnancy outcomes and health care use: Effects of abuse. *American Journal Obstetric and Gynecology, 174*(2), 760–767.

West, C. M. (1996). Lifting the "political gag order": Breaking the silence around partner violence in ethnic minority families. In J. L. Jasinski & L. M. Williams (Eds.), *Partner violence: A comprehensive review of 20 years of research*. Thousand Oaks, CA: Sage.

Wilbourne, P. I., Dorato, V., Yeo, R., & Curet, L. B. (2000). Relationship of social, medical and substance use characteristics to gestational age in poly-substance using women. *American Journal of Obstetrics and Gynecology, 182*(1, part 2), S156.

Yost, N. P., Bloom, S. L., McIntire, D. D., & Leveno, K. J. (2005). A prospective observational study of domestic violence during pregnancy. *Obstetrics Gynecology, 106*, 61–65.

7

Nursing Care of Women With Disabilities Who Experience Abuse

Dena Hassouneh, PhD, RN
Mary Ann Curry, DNSc, RN

INTRODUCTION

Interpersonal violence (IPV) of women with disabilities is defined as a pattern of co-ercive and oppressive behavior that is harmful to their emotional, social, or physical well-being (Hassouneh-Phillips & McNeff, 2004). This definition is broad enough to en-compass the many forms of IPV women with disabilities experience, including psycho-logical, physical, sexual, and financial abuse, as well as disability-related types of IPV, such as destruction of assistive devices (Curry, Powers, & Oschwald, 2003; Curry et al., 2009; McFarlane et al., 2001; Nosek, 1996). The perpetrators may be intimate partners, family members, friends, caregivers, health care providers, transportation providers, and other service providers (Copel, 2006; Hassouneh-Phillips & McNeff, 2004; Milberger et al., 2003; Nosek, Howland, Rintala, Young, & Chanpong, 1997).

Whereas many of the forms of IPV women with disabilities experience are identical to those experienced by nondisabled women, the nature of their disabilities may place them at additional risk. Women with disabilities are more likely than nondisabled women to be abused by multiple perpetrators and to stay in abusive situations for longer periods of time (Nosek et al., 1997). Additionally, women with disabilities who depend on others for essential personal care may experience disability-related forms of IPV, such as others threatening to or actually denying essential personal care, intentionally placing belong-ings out of reach, or refusing to provide food and water (Powers et al., 2002; Saxton et al., 2001). Unfortunately, because health care providers are often uninformed about the patterns and types of IPV women with disabilities experience, appropriate assessment and intervention with this population in clinical settings is often lacking.

Prevalence

Women with disabilities comprise a major proportion of the noninstitutionalized civil-ian U.S. population. Almost 18% of women between the ages of 16 and 64 and 43% of women 65 and older experience a disability (Waldrop & Stern, 2003). Population-based studies (Barrett, O'Day, Roche, Carlson, 2009; Brownridge, 2006; Casteel, Martin, Smith, Gurka, & Kupper, 2008; Cohen, Forte, DuMont, Hyman, & Romans, 2005; Martin et al., 2006; Smith, 2008) provide growing evidence that women with disabilities experience significantly more IPV than women without disabilities. These studies, while an extremely important breakthrough in understanding the prevalence of IPV among women with disabilities in the general population, do have limitations that need to be acknowledged. The measurement of disability and IPV varied across studies, and the types of IPV were limited to emotional, financial, physical, and sexual abuse. The time reference for the IPV ranged from "ever" to the past year, and the perpetrator ranged from intimate partner to "anyone." Consequently, the reported differences in IPV between women with and without disabilities were very different. For example, when the time frame was "ever" abused, Barrett and colleagues (2009) found 33.2% of women with disabilities reported some type of IPV compared to 21.2% among nondisabled women. However, when the time frame was the past 5 years, the rates of physical abuse among women with disabilities varied from 9.1% to 11.9% compared to 7.8% among nondisabled women (Brownridge, 2006; Cohen et al., 2005). When the time frame was the past year, the overall rates for all types of IPV were much lower for both groups. and the primary difference between the groups was that women with disabilities reported more sexual abuse (Casteel et al., 2008; Martin et al., 2006). An unavoidable limitation in all of these studies was the use of telephone interviews, which excludes many women with disabilities who do not have land-based telephones, cannot participate in telephone interviews because of their disability, or were afraid to disclose IPV because their perpetrator was present during the call.

These population-based studies support the findings from clinical studies of women with disabilities that also reported high incidences of IPV (Curry et al., 2003; Curry et al., 2009; Hassouneh, Hanson, McNeff, & Perrin, 2008; McFarlane et al., 2001; Millberger et al., 2003; Powers et al., 2002; Oktay & Tompkins, 2004). As with the larger studies, the clinical studies also have limitations, including differences in the definition of IPV, time frame for exposure, type of perpetrator, and the data collection method. When the time frame for exposure was lifetime experience of IPV by anyone, the rates range from 53% for sexual abuse and 67% for physical abuse when data were collected by nonconfidential telephone interviews (Powers et al., 2002) to 60% when physical, sexual, emotional, and disability types of abuse were measured by anonymous telephone interviews (Oktay & Tompkins, 2004). Millberger and colleagues (2003) reported 89% of their sample of 177 women with physical disabilities reported IPV since the age of 18 when participants were offered a choice of phone, mail, fax, or online data completion. Hassouneh and colleagues (2008) reported 53% of their sample of 166 women with physical disabilities reported IPV since the age of 18 and after the onset of disability using confidential face-to-face interviews. When the time reference was the past year, McFarlane and colleagues reported a 9.8% rate when physical, sexual, and two types of disability-related IPV were measured among 511 women with physical disabilities who were personally interviewed. However, Curry et al. (2009) found a 68% rate of past year IPV among 305 women with diverse disabilities when 17 types of IPV were measured using an anonymous computer-assisted interview.

Information regarding the prevalence and experience of IPV among men with disabilities is just beginning to emerge. A qualitative study of 76 men with diverse disabilities found participants experienced various forms of IPV from caregivers, including not showing up for work, physical abuse, neglect, and financial and emotional abuse (Saxton et al., 2001). A telephone survey administered to 342 men with diverse disabilities found

65% experienced lifetime physical abuse by anyone, with 55% experiencing the abuse since acquiring their disability (Powers et al., 2008). Overall, 24% reported some type of sexual abuse during their lifetime, but 52% reported sexual abuse since acquiring their disability. Past year physical abuse was reported by 18.4% of the men, and 31.3% reported past year sexual abuse, both of which are higher than past year intimate partner violence reported by men without disabilities (Tjaden, 2005). A second study using confidential face-to-face interviews with 125 men with physical disabilities found similarly high rates with 55% reporting any abuse within the past year and 63% prior to the past year (Hassouneh et al., 2008). Only abuse experienced age 18 and older after the onset of disability was included in the analysis. With regard to specific types of abuse, 37% reported psychological, 11% sexual, 16% physical, 34% financial, and 43% disability-related abuse within the past year. Prevalence rates reported prior to the last year for these same categories were 46%, 14%, 27%, 41%, and 45%, respectively.

Theoretical Frameworks

Three theoretical approaches have been developed for use with women with disabilities who experience abuse. These include: ecological, social justice, and experiential models. A brief description of each approach is provided below.

Ecological Model

Curry, Hassouneh-Phillips, and Johnston-Silverberg (2001) were among the first to apply an ecological model to abuse of women with disabilities. Their model examines *environmental and cultural factors*, and *victim* and *perpetrator* characteristics that increase vulnerability to abuse. *Environmental and cultural factors* include pervasive discrimination, stigma, and marginalization of women with disabilities in institutions and in society at large. *Characteristics that increase women's vulnerability to abuse* include dependence on others for essential personal care, lack of education about appropriate sexual behaviors, a learned dissociation from any physical sensation as a result of perceiving their bodies marked as "public" by health providers, and a belief that experiencing any feelings, even if painful, is better than not feeling anything at all. Women with cognitive disabilities who use concrete thinking have limited experience or ability to use problem-solving skills and lack assertiveness, language, and/or communication skills may also be at risk. Finally, *characteristics of potential offenders* included in the model are the need for control, low self-esteem, exposure to abusive models, poor impulse control, anxiety, and antisocial behavior.

Several studies provide support for components of Curry and colleague's (2001) model. Devaluation of women with disabilities has been identified as a factor affecting women's relationship decision making, access to domestic violence services, and ability to access quality health care (Hassouneh-Phillips & McNeff, 2005; Hassouneh-Phillips, McNeff, Powers, & Curry, 2005). Dependence on others for essential personal care has also been identified in several qualitative and quantitative studies as a major factor that places women with disabilities at risk for abuse (Gilson, Cramer, & Depoy, 2001; Hassouneh-Phillips & McNeff, 2004; Nosek, Foley, Hughes, & Howland, 2001; Saxton et al., 2001). Mobility disability in particular has been identified as a marker for risk (Nosek, Hughes, Taylor, & Taylor, 2006). With regard to offender characteristics,

---

EXHIBIT 7.1 | *Overview of Theoretical Frameworks and Models of Abuse of Women With Disabilities*

Ecological Model
Environmental and cultural factors:
- Discrimination
- Stigma
- Marginalization

Characteristics that increase women's vulnerability to abuse:
- Dependence on others for essential personal care
- Lack of education about appropriate sexual behaviors
- Dissociation from any physical sensation
- Belief that experiencing any feelings, even if painful, is better than not feeling anything at all
- Concrete thinking
- Limited experience or ability to use problem-solving skills
- Lack assertiveness, language and/or communication skills

Characteristics of potential offenders:
- Need for control
- Low self-esteem
- Exposure to abusive models
- Poor impulse control
- Anxiety and antisocial behavior

Social Justice Models
Intersecting Systems of Oppression:
- Social Model of Disability defines disability as a system of oppression (i.e., Disability is Disablism)
- Disablism is often experienced in conjunction with other forms of oppression
- Intersecting systems of oppression reinforce and perpetuate violence against women with disabilities

Experiential/Abuse Pathways Model
- Getting in
- Experiencing abuse
- Lack of intervention
- Staying in
- Breaking point
- Building support and gaining strength
- Getting out

Brownridge (2006) reported that male partners of women with disabilities are significantly more likely to behave in a patriarchal dominating manner and engage in sexually proprietary behaviors than partners of nondisabled women, increasing the risk of this population.

Social Justice Models

Social Justice Models theorize the influence that systems of oppression have on abused women's live. Theorists who focus on social justice specific to women with disabilities often rely on the social model of disability as a central construct. The social model of disability distinguishes between impairment and disability, with impairment being conceptualized as biological and disability as sociocultural in nature. The memorable disability rights slogan "disabled by society not by our bodies" sums up this distinction (Shakespeare, 2006). Although the social model offers distinct advantage as a political strategy and has opened up new lines of academic inquiry, the model's rigid distinction between impairment and disability is being increasingly cited as limiting (Dewsbury, Clarke, Randall, Rouncefield, & Summerville, 2004; Shakespeare, 2006). Despite this growing critique, however, the social model has proven useful to authors seeking to theorize abuse of women with disabilities within a social justice framework. These approaches generally combine disability and feminist theory to theorize the gendered experiences of disability and abuse.

In an analysis of evolving theoretical models, Nixon (2009) noted that experiences of disability are gendered and that women with disabilities experience oppression in multiple ways:

> Disabled people often experience disablism in conjunction with other forms of oppression which may be linked to issues of class, race, gender, sexuality or other facets of identity. This dynamic has implications for the complexity of disabled survivors' experiences of violence as well as for the recognition of the abuse of disabled women as a pressing social issue. (p. 85)

The paper goes on to argue that women with disabilities who are vulnerable to experiencing abuse may be silenced by the intersection of disablism, sexism, ageism, and other aspects of oppression within organizations, social movements, and the broader social world. Similarly, Mays (2006) advocated combining material feminism and the social model of disability to inform understandings of abuse of women with disabilities stating that "domestic violence against women with a disability needs to be understood in terms of the relationship to gendered power relations and historical, social, and material conditions that perpetuate and reinforce violence" (p. 152). Using this feminist-disability framework, Mays argued against analyses that include examination of individual factors suggesting that this reinforces the tendency to pathologize abused women and portray women with disabilities as a special needs group.

Experiential Model

Experiential models of abuse of women with disabilities have emerged from qualitative studies of the phenomenon. The most comprehensive experiential model currently available, the *Abuse Pathways Model*, describes the processes women go through as they enter, stay, and leave abusive relationships (Hassouneh-Phillips, 2005). The social context of disability, vulnerability factors for abuse, and concomitant negative health outcomes are linked with the abuse trajectory described in the model. Stages included in this trajectory are *getting in, experiencing abuse, lack of intervention, staying in, breaking point, building support and gaining strength, and getting out.* Components of the *Abuse Pathways* Model are supported by findings from several other published qualitative studies of abuse of women with disabilities (Copel, 2006; Gilson et al., 2001; Hassouneh-Phillips, 2005; Hassouneh-Phillips & McNeff, 2005; Saxton et al., 2001). The vulnerability factors and health outcomes identified in the model were also supported by findings from a quantitative study of individuals with physical disabilities (Hassouneh et al., 2008). A brief overview of the *Abuse Pathways* Model is provided below.

Getting in describes women with physical disabilities' processes of and risk factors for, entering into abusive relationships. Women, particularly women with mobility limitations, often have limited options for intimacy. When abusers offer the opportunity for intimate partner relationships, many women may be willing to ignore warning signs in order to experience intimacy. Women's risk factors for entering into an abusive relationship cited in the model include a history of childhood abuse, history of intimate partner abuse prior to the onset of disability, substance abuse, fear of being alone, poor parental relationships, comorbid mental heath disorders, institutionalization, and dependency on others for essential personal care. Experiencing abuse denotes the types of abuse women with disabilities experience. These include emotional, physical, sexual, financial, and disability-related forms of abuse. Specific examples of various types of abuse include name-calling, theft of medication, forced sex, and abandonment or threat of abandonment to maintain power and control.

Once a woman with a disability experiences abuse, she often has nowhere to turn. In most areas, systems that address abused women with disabilities' specific needs are not in place. Lack of Intervention, describes the inadequacy of care systems to identify and intervene with women with physical disabilities. Common barriers to help-seeking identified by the model include lack of emergency back up caregivers, lack of availability of caregivers in general, inaccessible shelters, inaccessible mental health services, and lack of awareness on the part of law enforcement, health care, and social service providers.

The problem of inadequate care systems is reflected in the factors that place women with disabilities at risk for remaining in abusive relationships for extended periods of time. *Staying in* describes these factors which include low self-esteem, lack of social support, lack of resources, and receipt of essential personal care from an intimate partner.

The violence literature indicates that at some point most women eventually leave their abusers. *Breaking point* refers to the point in time when women begin to contemplate terminating their abusive relationships. This occurs when the harm associated with remaining in an abusive relationship outweighs any potential benefits. Sadly, many women may be willing to accept a certain level of abuse in exchange for intimacy, companionship, and personal care. When the abuse ceases to end and/or escalates to an unacceptable level, this trade-off becomes untenable.

Once a woman has reached the *breaking point*, she likely will begin the process of *building support and gaining strength*. *Building support and gaining strength* refers to a process wherein women begin to build their social networks, gain strength, actively seek safety, and deepen their resolve to leave. Examples of this process include obtaining alternate personal care services, attending support groups or classes to bolster their self-esteem and inner strength, and establishing or strengthening ties with potential allies.

Finally, *getting out* describes the process of leaving. This may mean anything from refusing to utilize the services of a particular transportation worker, to obtaining a divorce. Once out of their abusive relationships, women may then remain abuse-free, re-enter the abusive relationship, or enter into a new relationship with a different abuser.

Health Consequences of Abuse

Scant research on the health consequences of abuse for women with disabilities has been reported. To our knowledge, only four published quantitative studies provide information about the health effects of abuse of women with disabilities. Cohen and colleagues

(2005) examined the physical and psychological sequelae of intimate partner violence in women with activity limitations using data from the Canadian General Social Survey. Analyses were conducted using data from 897 women with and without activity limitations who reported physical and/or sexual violence in the previous 5 years. The authors found that women with activity limitations reported more negative psychological consequences and physical injury from intimate partner violence than women without activity limitations. Women with activity limitations also took more time off from everyday activities and were more likely to report use of medications for sleep, anxiety, and depression. After controlling for the severity of violence, women with activity limitations still reported more psychotropic medication use for sleep, anxiety, and depression compared to women without activity limitations.

Barrett and colleagues (2009) examined the relationship between intimate partner violence, health status, and health care access in women with disabilities in seven states using data from the Behavior Risk Factor Surveillance Survey. Women with disabilities who reported lifetime physical and/or sexual abuse were significantly more likely to rate their general health as poor and to report unmet health care needs compared to nonabused women with disabilities.

Sequeira and colleagues (2003) examined behavioral and psychiatric problems in adults with intellectual disabilities living in residential care. The study used a matched case-control design comparing 54 adults who had experienced sexual abuse with 54 adults with no reported history of abuse. Interviews were conducted with keyworkers and clients identified by managers of charitable and private sector organizations for people with intellectual disabilities in England, Scotland, and Wales. Findings indicated that sexual abuse is associated with increased rates of mental illness and behavioral problems in this population. Psychological responses to abuse were similar to those observed in the general population but with the addition of stereotypical behavior (e.g., repetitive rocking and odd or bizarre behaviors). More serious abuse was associated with more severe symptoms.

Using vulnerability factors and health outcomes identified in the *Abuse Pathways Model*, Hassouneh and colleagues (2008) studied predictors of abuse and health outcomes in abused versus nonabused individuals with physical disabilities in a nonprobability community-based sample (*n*=166 women and 125 men). Health outcomes measured included depression, posttraumatic stress disorder (PTSD), and health promoting behaviors. Although all types of abuse were measured, only adult abuse that occurred while disabled was included in the analysis. The results indicated that participants who had experienced abuse in the past year were significantly more likely to report symptoms of depression and PTSD and were much less likely to report engaging in health-promoting behaviors compared to never abused. Women who reported no abuse in the past year but reported abuse prior to that time were also significantly more likely to report symptoms of depression and PTSD compared to never abused women, indicating that the health effects of abuse continue even after the abuse has ended.

SCREENING AND ASSESSMENT

The routine screening and assessment of women with disabilities for past and current IPV has not been a priority for disability and domestic-violence advocates, or health care professionals. Advocates and professionals in the disability community have historically focused on obtaining access to basic health and social services and only recently have begun to address problems related to IPV. Similarly, the domestic-violence community has primarily focused on outreach to and services for nondisabled women. Health care professionals have not typically paid attention to screening for IPV among women with disabilities, as they are more likely to focus on the health issues they assume are directly related to the disability. However, in some instances, these health issues are caused or worsened by violence and are not necessarily the result of disability.

Methods of Screening

Women with disabilities generally have frequent contact with a wide variety of health professionals and disability and social-service providers. Thus, there are many opportunities for case finding and screening for abuse. Nurses are uniquely positioned to provide leadership in this area because of their diversity of roles and presence in multiple workplaces, such as hospitals, rehabilitation centers, skilled nursing facilities, outpatient clinics, and home health.

Case finding may be achieved by obtaining a good history via chart review and clinical interview, careful clinical observation, and/or physical examination (see Table 7.1), and use of a screening tool. We encourage the simultaneous use of all methods whenever possible. For example, a nurse in an outpatient clinic may note some "red flags" in the clinical record, such as repeated requests for wheelchair repair, actually observe the partner of the woman handle her roughly during a transfer, and then use a screening tool to ask specific questions. Because of the frequency of abuse against women with disabilities and its health consequences, all women with disabilities should be screened using one or more of the questions described in a following section. It is imperative to recognize that women with disabilities are exposed to many potential perpetrators, not just intimate partners. Thus, it is necessary to screen for abuse by paid and unpaid caregivers, family members, friends, health care providers, and disability service providers, such as transportation drivers.

Barriers to Abuse Disclosure

It is important for nurses to recognize that women with disabilities experience significant barriers to disclosing abuse in the health care setting, even though screening by health providers, particularly nurses, has been reported as important by women with disabilities (Powers et al., 2002). Some barriers are directly related to previous negative experiences in the health care setting, such as being ignored or "talked over," having pain minimized, being pushed beyond physical limits, handled roughly, and being touched inappropriately (Hassouneh-Phillips, McNeff, Powers, & Curry, 2005; Powers et al., 2002), resulting in a distrust of the health system and health providers. This distrust is compounded by lack of attention to abuse of women with disabilities and failure to screen on the part of health care providers. In a study of 305 women with diverse disabilities, Curry et al. (2009) found that only 15% reported that a health provider had ever discussed abuse and personal safety. The women who were most likely to have been screened by a health provider were younger, reported their disabilities as mild, and either reported never experiencing abuse or abuse that occurred prior to the past year (*n*=96) (Curry et al., 2009).

Other barriers are similar to those experienced by nondisabled women. In Curry et al. (2009) study, the most highly endorsed barrier to disclosing abuse to a professional

---

EXHIBIT 7.2 | *Clinical Indicators of Abuse*

Data Obtained From Patient History and Chart Review
- Prior history of abuse or neglect
- History of unexplained bruises, fractures, and other injuries
- Involvement with Adult Protective Services
- Frequently missed or cancelled appointments
- Delay in seeking treatment
- Unexplained deterioration of health condition (e.g., uncontrolled diabetes, pressure sores, seizure disorder)
- History of depression, drug use, suicide attempts
- Unexplained weight loss or malnutrition
- Frequent requests for medication refills due to loss or theft
- Unusual number of requests for equipment repair or replacement
- Reports of caregivers who are drunk or high on the job

Data Obtained From Clinical Observation and/or Physical Examination
- Partner or caregiver speaks for woman, contradicts, or minimizes what she says
- Partner or caregiver oversolicitous with care providers
- Partner or caregiver unwilling to leave woman alone
- Partner or caregiver pushes woman beyond her physical limits (e.g., makes her stand long periods beyond her comfort level)
- Woman obviously afraid of her partner or caregiver
- Woman's appearance is unkempt
- Injuries or bruises
- Malnutrition

---

was women preferring to wait until they were sure it was abuse. This uncertainty can be exacerbated by isolation and repeated exposure to abuse, leaving some women unable to recognize they have been abused. Consequently, it is imperative that multiple examples of abusive behaviors, including disability-related types of abuse, such as destruction of equipment, are described during screening. Other barriers endorsed in the study included fear abuse would get worse if reported, fear of what would happen if police were notified, shame and embarrassment, loss of something important like personal care, and fear of being injured or killed. Nearly 20% of women in the study said there was no point in reporting the abuse because nothing could be done to change it. Although women who reported the most past-year IPV and the most dangerous perpetrators endorsed more barriers and fewer facilitators, these women were also more likely to have disclosed abuse to a professional. Overall, the main facilitators to disclosing abuse related to the extent to which women believed they would be seen as credible and would receive tangible and emotional support, which illustrates the importance of creating a safe and supportive environment when asking about IPV.

Screening Instruments

Recent collaborations by nursing and disability researchers have resulted in two screening tools designed specifically for women with disabilities. Both tools, the Abuse Assessment Screen-Disability (*AAS-D*) (McFarlane et al., 2001) and the Safer and Stronger

Abuse Measure (*SSAM*), (Curry et al., 2009) were developed using qualitative interviews with women with disabilities.

The *AAS-D* was developed and tested with 511 ethnically diverse women with physical disabilities (McFarlane et al., 2001). Interviewers orally administered the four-item tool, which included two questions from the Abuse Assessment Screen that ask about physical and sexual abuse and two disability-related questions. The disability-related questions asked if anyone prevented participants from using assistive devices (e.g., cane or wheelchair) or had refused to provide an important personal need such as helping to take medication or get out of bed. Overall, 9.8% ($n = 50$) reported abuse; 7.8% ($n = 40$) reported physical or sexual abuse, and an additional 2% ($n = 10$) reported disability-related abuse. The primary perpetrator of physical or sexual abuse was an intimate partner, although health providers and family members were also identified. However, health professionals, intimate partners, and caregivers were equally named as perpetrators of disability-related abuse.

The *SSAM* has 17 dichotomous (yes/no) questions that were administered during the *Safer and Stronger Program*, an audio Computer-Assisted Self-Interview created specifically for women with diverse disabilities, including physical, cognitive, and sensory disabilities (Oschwald et al., 2009). An iterative process was used to develop the questions, which included review and refinement by women with disabilities (see Appendix A). The questions included items related to emotional abuse, threats of and actual physical and sexual abuse, financial abuse, and disability-related abuse such as refusing or forgetting to help with an important personal need and breaking or withholding assistive devices, such as a walker or cane (Curry et al., 2009). A total of 305 women completed the interview. Most women ($n = 208$; 68%) endorsed one or more items in the past year, which is similar to the results found by Curry and colleagues (2003) using an eight-item disability-specific tool. The most commonly endorsed items were emotional abuse (51%) and feeling unsafe (38%). Nearly a quarter of the women reported past-year disability-related abuse ($n = 73$; 24.9%), actual sexual abuse ($n = 70$; 22.9%), and/or physical abuse ($n = 68$; 22.2%). Preliminary evidence for the validity and reliability of the questions were found, which can also be administered in person or as a paper–pencil assessment (Curry et al., 2009).

In-Depth Assessment

Once a woman with a disability has been identified as having experienced abuse, additional assessment is required. The type(s), frequency, and severity of abuse; impact on her disability and health; and the identity of the perpetrator(s) need to be assessed. Asking a woman to chronologically describe the abuse helps to identify patterns and possible escalation. It is important to validate her reports of threats of physical harm and threats of abandonment as abuse. For example, threats to refuse to let a woman out of her wheelchair all day or threats to leave a respirator-dependent woman alone at night are persuasive types of controlling and abusive behavior. Another powerful form of intimidation is to threaten to not provide or actually not provide essential personal care needed by a woman's children. If she is dependent on someone else to care for her children, the fear of losing her children makes it extremely difficult for a woman with a disability to seek help.

Risk Assessment

VICTIM CHARACTERISTICS. Assessment of the woman's potential for further harm is a critical component of in-depth assessment. Questions regarding her current living situation need to be asked to determine her potential vulnerability for additional harm. The following five questions administered in the *Safer and Stronger Program* (Oschwald et al., 2009) were found to predict women's increased risk for emotional, disability-related, and financial abuse:

1. Do you need help with important daily activities?
2. Do you depend on one person to assist you and have no one else who can help?
3. Do you use a lot of medical or disability services such as special transportation?
4. Would it be impossible for you to leave or call for help without your assistive devices?
5. Do you have a health problem that can become worse if neglected?

Other predictors of abuse were identified by Hassouneh and colleagues' (2008) study of abuse and health in men and women with physical disabilities. The authors identified three significant risk factors including physical dependency, a history of childhood abuse, and a history of abuse as an adult with a disability prior to the past year. Of note, participants who reported abuse as an adult with a disability prior to the past year were over 58 times more likely to report current abuse than participants who reported no adult abuse history.

PERPETRATOR CHARACTERISTICS. It is also important to assess risk associated with perpetrator characteristics. The 12 perpetrator risk questions in the *SSAM* are based on the Danger Assessment (Campbell, 1995), focus-group data, clinical expertise of disability and domestic-violence advocates, and information from women with disabilities. Factor and latent class analysis of these questions (Curry et al., 2009) found three types of perpetrators: *controlling*, *noncontrolling*, and *low-risk*. Perpetrators in the *controlling* and *noncontrolling* groups were more likely than the *low-risk* group to abuse alcohol/drugs, get jealous and angry, have hurt others, and choked or threatened the participant. However, perpetrators in the *controlling group* were more likely to be the participant's caregiver; control their access to services, including health care; control their access to family and friends; control their daily activities; and escalate the abuse.

Communicating During the Interview

Attending to issues of communication during the clinical interview is critical to appropriate assessment and intervention. All assessments should be conducted privately, without relying on a partner, caregiver, friend, or family member for essential data. Even in cases where dementia or very low IQ makes it difficult to communicate with the woman, some time for private interview should be included in the visit. If women require a professional interpreter, such as a sign-language interpreter, it must be done with the assurance of confidentiality. When talking with women who use wheelchairs, assume a position that allows level eye-contact, minimizing the need for women to look up. It is also important never to assume that because a woman has a physical disability, she also has a cognitive disability.

When working with women with cognitive disabilities, allow them to speak for themselves. Identify yourself, and speak clearly and directly to the woman using short sentences and simple language. Ask "who," "what," or "where" questions, and avoid confusing questions about time, sequences, or reasons for behavior. Be sensitive to guilt, self-blame, and fear of persons in authority. Most important, treat women with cognitive disabilities as adults and be fully present. Unfortunately, there is a misunderstanding that people with cognitive disabilities do not comprehend their experiences and are therefore unreliable reporters of mistreatment. Consequently, after being discounted over time, many women assume they will not be believed and stop trying to disclose abuse. This was illustrated by the data that women with cognitive disabilities reported significantly fewer facilitators and more barriers to disclosing abuse to a professional (Curry et al., 2009). Therefore, it is essential that screening for IPV takes place in an unhurried, trusting, confidential environment and that hurtful experiences, when disclosed, are validated as forms of abuse that the women did not cause or deserve.

Documentation

Documentation of abuse of women with disabilities should include a description of the abuse that has occurred including the name of the perpetrator (if named), the specifics of what occurred (the nature and effects of the assault), where the abuse occurred, and the presence of any witnesses. If the abuse involves theft of medication, the type and amount of medication stolen should be described. When documenting abuse, it is important to avoid using language such as "patient alleges," as this casts doubt on women's reports in the event that the medical record is used as evidence in legal proceedings. If injuries are present, it is important to take photographs and include them in the medical record along with the signed consent authorizing you to do so. Because women with disabilities may experience caregiver abuse and/or may be subject to mandatory reporting requirements, it is important for the nurse to include this information and report appropriately. A record of formal reporting needs to include the agency to which it was reported, the position of the person to whom it was reported, and the person's name.

NURSING INTERVENTION

Evidence Base for Intervention

Safer and Stronger Program

There is beginning evidence that describes the type of safety-promoting behaviors used by women with disabilities. In the *Safer and Stronger* computer-assisted interview, 305 women with diverse disabilities responded to 43 questions regarding a wide range of safety behaviors (Powers et al., 2009). The questions were designed to provide information about the use of safety behaviors as well as collect information about their use. For example, video clips of women introduced each section with examples of how the women had used the behaviors in their own lives (Oschwald et al., 2009). Thus, the questions were intentionally designed to be both an intervention and outcome measure.

Like women without disabilities, participants were more likely to reach out to informal support, such as talking to a friend, than using formal resources such as a domestic violence agency or the police. Participants who had experienced past year abuse and had the most dangerous perpetrators, were more likely to use safety-promoting behaviors, and among those, the women who reported the most severe past-year abuse were the most likely to have talked about or actually obtained a stalking or restraining order. However, compared to women with less severe abuse and less dangerous perpetrators, women with the most severe abuse and dangerous perpetrators were *not* more likely to report using emergency safety planning. This was due in part to the high overall endorsement for many of the items, such as having copies of important papers in a safe place, having a safe place to go, having a list of important names and phone numbers in a safe place, and setting up a way to call for help; behaviors that may have also been related to experiencing a disability. It is also possible that women who reported less abuse did so because they had used safety planning behaviors to prevent and/or reduce the abuse. Nurses can use the emergency safety planning items to reinforce the need to plan for unexpected disability needs as well as safety planning for IPV.

To determine if the *Safer and Stronger Program (SSP)* had an effect on the use of safety-promoting behaviors, women randomized to complete the *SSP* were compared to women who had been randomized to complete a computer-assisted health awareness program. Three months later, the women who completed the *SSP* were significantly more likely to report more abuse awareness behaviors than control women (Hughes & Robinson-Whelen, 2009). These behaviors asked how much in the past few months women had watched the ways they or other people were treated and decided if it were abuse or not; told themselves they had a right to be safe from abuse; thought about ways to be as safe from abuse as possible; thought about ways to be as safe from abuse as possible; and talked to someone about abuse and safety. This provides preliminary evidence that the *SSP* was effective in improving the abuse and safety awareness of participants.

Sexual Abuse Survivor's Group Pilot for Women With Intellectual Disabilities

Peckham, Howlett, and Corbett (2007) conducted a pilot study of a survivors' group (SG) for women with intellectual impairment who had experienced sexual abuse ($n=7$) and a concurrent educational support group (ESG) for their caregivers ($n=7$). The aims of the program were to help participants build trust and rapport, provide them with basic education about sexual abuse designed for their level of ability, and help them re-process the trauma of their sexual abuse. The SG program included 20 sessions delivered weekly over 5 months, and the ESG program occurred concurrently. Results indicated that the program significantly increased both clients' and caregivers' knowledge of sexual abuse. The group was also effective in helping clients reduce traumatic and depressive symptoms, an effect that increased significantly during the 3-month follow-up.

Planning for Safety

Planning and intervention strategies for women with disabilities who experience violence is similar to the process used for nondisabled women, as it consists of determining available options and weighing the benefits and risks of each. However, women with disabilities have fewer options and more challenges to consider, such as severity of the disability, level of dependence on caregivers, and scarce or nonexistent community resources. Critical factors in planning these interventions include:

- Empowering the woman to determine what she wants to do or have happen
- Determining her level of current risk or danger
- Imparting knowledge of available resources and services
- Planning for safety

As with nondisabled women, women with disabilities basically have three options:

- To stay with the abuser
- To have the abuser removed from the place of residence
- To leave the abuser and the place of residence

Staying With the Abuser

If the perpetrator is an intimate partner, the woman may prefer the option of staying in the current relationship, particularly if the intimate partner provides her with essential personal care. It is very likely that the perpetrator has reinforced the belief that s/he is the only option for an intimate relationship, through put-downs about her lack of desirability, the demands of her disability, and her unworthiness (Hassouneh-Phillips & McNeff, 2005).

Other aspects of the intimate partner/caregiver relationship require consideration. If the intimate partner is receiving funding from a state or private agency to provide personal care, there may be overwhelming financial repercussions, as the family income may depend in large part on this funding source. The intimate partner may have legal authority over the joint finances and may be her legal guardian. If the woman and her abuser have children together, the possibility of losing custody to the abuser is very real. All of these factors were identified in a qualitative study of 25 disabled women abused by their intimate partner, who described their helplessness, powerlessness, and inability to leave their abuser because of struggles related to their disability and low sense of self-confidence and energy (Copel, 2006). These women endured the abuse for the sake of survival, rather than clinging to hopes of a happier relationship.

The decision to stay with a perpetrator who provides personal care but is not an intimate partner, is also made with difficulty. Powers and colleagues (2002) identified the primary barriers to leaving an abusive relationship as not having a back up caregiver, shortage of qualified caregivers, and fear of backlash if the abuser were to be reported. Going without essential care, being left all day in a wheelchair because the person from the agency did not show up, having a cell phone taken away as punishment, and being admitted to a nursing home are real considerations in deciding whether to stay. Women may thus prefer to stay with an abusive caregiver. Given these complex potentially life-threatening considerations, it is important for nurses to maintain a nonjudgmental attitude toward women who choose to stay.

When a woman chooses to stay, some form of risk assessment is needed to determine if there is danger of the situation escalating. We recommend using the perpetrator risk characteristic questions from the *SSAM* and the five questions about her current situation described in the assessment section to develop a safety plan for staying with the abuser or, if necessary, to encourage the woman to leave the abuser or have the abuser removed.

Safety planning for the women who choose to stay can begin with determining what they believe they need to do to stay safe, such as having a back up care provider or finding a safe place to hide their medication. Another important step is developing a list of safe people they can talk to about the abuse and providing names and resources of community options such as disability agencies, independent-living centers, and support groups. Obviously, knowledge of these resources is required and may require a fair amount of investigation to uncover, especially if physical accessibility is needed. It is important to remind women that abuse is a crime, and they have the option of calling the police and filing criminal charges. A more extensive guide for personal safety planning for women who are living with their abuser is shown in Exhibit 7.3. It was adapted from materials produced by The Safe Place in Austin, Texas (www.safeplace.org).

Leaving the Abuser

Leaving the abuser is often an emotionally and logistically difficult choice for women generally, and for disabled women, this choice may only become possible after being connected to information and professional help (Copel, 2006). Thus, nurses are uniquely

---

EXHIBIT 7.3 | *Personal Safety Planning for Explosive Events*

Think Ahead and Plan Ahead for Personal Safety
- If cues suggest that the caregiver and/or IP is becoming angry and you feel afraid and/or unsafe, go to a place of safety or call someone you trust to come be with you.
- Plan for caregiver and/or IP to do intimate personal care tasks when it feels safe.
- Try to have your form of mobility available (already be in your wheelchair or have cane close by).
- Stay close to a phone. Keep cell phone safely tucked at side or close by (in wheelchair) with ringer turned off so the abuser does not know you have it.
- If argument seems unavoidable, try to move into a room or area away from dangerous items such as knives or weapons. Try to stay near an exit if possible.
- Get out of an exit if possible. YELL OR MAKE SOME LOUD NOISE IF IT IS SAFE TO DO.
- Practice ahead of time how to get out of the home or get to a phone to call for help.
- Identify a friend or neighbor ahead of time you can call. Memorize their phone number or keep it in a safe place. Ask them to call 911 if they hear a disturbance coming from your house.
- Contact the police when a crisis is not happening. Tell them about your situation. Ask them to send a patrol car by your house as often as possible. Many police will do this if they know you are a person with a disability.
- Figure out a code word or phrases you can use with your children, family, or neighbors to alert them to call 911 if you are in a violent situation.
- Plan ahead for where you will go if you have to leave home (even if you do not think that is possible).
- Use your own judgment and trust your feelings and instincts. If the situation is dangerous, consider giving the abuser what they want, in order to calm them down. You have the right to protect yourself until you are out of danger.

qualified to assist women during this time because of their understanding of the physical and emotional needs of women with disabilities, especially their need for validation and improved self-esteem. Their knowledge of community resources is also crucial. Finding a place to go, though a major consideration is just one of many factors needed to be taken into account. Thus, whenever possible, nurses should encourage women to develop a safety plan in preparation for leaving. These safety planning suggestions in Exhibit 7.3 were adapted from materials produced by The Safe Place in Austin, Texas (www. safeplace.org).

Remain in the Residence

The majority of abused women with disabilities prefer to remain in their own environment with whatever accommodations they require. If the abuser is an intimate partner and is unwilling to voluntarily leave, a Temporary Order to Vacate or an Order of Protection may force the abuser to leave. Getting an order may be required if the abuser is not an IP but has lived in the woman's home as a caregiver. We recommend that, with the woman's consent, nurses work closely with the woman's disability case manager, Adult Protective Services (APS), or both when removing the abuser from the home. This is an extremely complicated issue, which may require legal advice. For example, abusers have used tenant's rights laws to remain in the residence against the victim's wishes.

Once the abuser leaves, safety issues need to be reviewed. All locks should be changed, and the woman should obtain an Order of Protection is she has not already done so, If the abuser is an intimate partner, pressing charges may serve as a deterrent to future violence, and the abuser may be subject to court-mandated treatment programs. If the abuser is a paid caregiver hired through an agency or state provider, the abuse should be reported to the proper authorities. Unfortunately, even when reported, the lack of formal systems for maintaining records often results in these offenders being rehired.

Leave the Residence

If it is not possible to remove the abuser from the residence or if the woman prefers leaving herself, additional considerations are necessary. When developing a safety plan for leaving, the nurse's primary role is that of advocate. The nurse and disabled woman may want to contact her disability case manager at the outset to learn what, if any, resources are available. In some instances, agencies have contracts with Visiting Nurse Associations or other agencies to provide emergency back up caregivers. Unfortunately, this is often not the case, and there may be limited emergency funds available at the local level to assist women in leaving. Reporting the abuse to APS is another option, as in some cases ,this is also an avenue to resources. Nurses need to be aware, however, that many persons with disabilities have a fear of being reported to APS, may have negative past experiences with the agency, and may equate being reported with being put in a nursing home. Thus, unless the nurse is mandated in her jurisdiction to report the abuse to APS, the decision to contact the agency should be jointly made.

The nurse can also offer to call, or assist the woman in calling, local domestic violence shelters and a crisis line to find out about available resources and space. If the shelter is not accessible or does not have immediate space, the people there should be asked if they can issue a hotel or motel voucher for an accessible room. The nurse may also need to assist in finding needed caregivers. If the woman has not made arrangements with family or friends or if it is an emergency, temporary admission to a hospital, nursing home, or skilled-nursing facility may be the only choice.

Other pragmatic issues that may need to be taken into account include accessible transportation, acquisition or transfer of durable medical supplies (such as oxygen or commode), boarding of pets, accommodations in the new facility for a service animal, and access to interpreters. For all these reasons, nurses have to explore every imaginable possibility when assisting a woman when she chooses to leave the abuser. Nurses need to remind themselves and reassure the woman that leaving an abusive relationship may

---

EXHIBIT 7.4 | *Safety Planning When Preparing to Leave*

- Never let the abuser know of plans to leave; don't leave any clues like long-distance phone bills.
- Change your payee (if have one) on SSI/SSDI benefits to a trusted individual. Someone will need to contact Social Security Administration to change the payee name.
- Open a savings account in your name only. Have benefits check directly deposited into that account.
- Plan for personal care needs. Ask several friends, family members, or faith community members to help so one person is not overtaxed.
- Contact your case manager/caseworker to find out about back up care services.
- Obtain a post office box in your own name and hide the key or give to a trusted friend or relative.
- Pack a bag with money, extra keys, medications, prescription numbers, spare adaptive aids or medical supplies, copies of birth certificates for you and your children, and a few spare clothes for you and your children. Leave those items with a trusted friend or relative.
- Figure out who you could stay with (friends, family, etc.) or where you would need to go (accessible hotel or shelter).
- If you drive an adapted vehicle, make sure it is in good repair (make sure the abuser has not tampered with it) and always keep it filled with at least a half a tank of gas.
- Know your transportation options, apply for special transit services if available.
- Call your local domestic violence shelter or the National Domestic Violence Hotline (24/7) at 800-799-7233 and TDD 800-787-3224 to discuss safety planning. Identify yourself as a woman with a disability so they can be the most helpful.
- Memorize your local domestic violence or crisis hotline telephone number. Always carry enough money for a pay phone.
- Call the Adult Protective Services office in your area and report the abuse. Let them know your health and safety are at stake. They must take all self reports. Ask what the investigation process will be like.
- When you leave, write a note to the abuser saying you went to a doctor's appointment or another place that will not make the abuser suspicious in order to buy time.
- If you use a credit card after leaving, make sure the bill will not be sent to the residence where the abuser lives or has access.
- If after you leave you need to telephone anyone who knows the abuser, be careful to block your call.

be one of the most difficult and bravest things the disabled woman has ever done. She needs reassurance that she knows the abuser best and is the authority on the steps that need to be taken.

It is crucial that the nurse advise the woman that the period immediately after leaving may be the most dangerous time for the safety of her and her children. She needs to a have a plan of action if the abuser locates her, threatens her, or stalks her. She may want to obtain an Order of Protection, and the nurse should be prepared to facilitate the process if needed.

Mandatory Reporting

As mandatory reporters, nurses need to be aware of the particular requirements of their own state laws regarding reporting abuse against women with disabilities. In some states, mandated reporters are only obligated to report the abuse of people with developmental disabilities or those receiving state funding for disability services. Nurses need to know how developmental disabilities are defined in each state, as it may vary depending on age of onset of disability, IQ levels, and the current age of the victim. To complicate matters further, there may be several investigative units within one state or jurisdiction depending on the type of disability. Consequently, crimes against people with disabilities remain largely invisible and unappraised. Nurses can play an important role in raising awareness about the magnitude of the problem by diligently fulfilling their professional obligation to report these crimes.

We believe it is crucial to include women with disabilities in the reporting process. If she has not been told that you are a mandated reporter, explain what that means, making it clear that according to the law, the abuse must be reported to the proper authorities. Then, invite her to join in reporting the incident so that she has an opportunity to take control of her situation. Ask her what she needs for you to do, such as talking to a particular case manager or notifying a nonabusing family member.

Barriers to Accessing Services

Services such as those within the justice systems, women's shelters, and health care services frequently present barriers, both physical and attitudinal, that inhibit full access and participation. Barriers to acquiring assistance after abuse identified by the Center for Research on Women with Disabilities (CROWD, 2009) include:

- Women are not believed
- Women are discriminated against
- Transportation is not available
- Referrals are inappropriate
- Services are not accessible

Many programs do not include alternative formats such as Braille for their information. Workers often do not have the necessary skills to adequately serve women with disabilities, and caregiver services are not available. Physical accessibility is often problematic, and some workers may display discriminatory and noninclusive attitudes (Glover-Graf

& Reed, 2006). It is important that nurses be aware of these barriers in order to begin to identify strategies to overcome them.

Follow-Up and Evaluation

Nurses may only have limited contact with the woman, such as during an in-patient hospitalization, or have the opportunity to remain in contact over extended periods of time, such as in a specialty clinic. In the case of limited contact, the evaluation may consist of making sure the woman has a list of community resources and determining if the nurse or another professional such as a community-health nurse, can call the woman to inquire about her well-being. If the woman does agree to subsequent follow-up, it is important to obtain safe phone numbers, good times to call, and a back up plan if the abuser answers the phone or comes into the room during the call.

For cases in which continued follow-up is possible, we recommend that the nurse and the woman jointly decide on realistic goals and the methods of evaluation. For example, a realistic goal for a woman with a cognitive disability may be to develop a plan for staying safe when she commutes from her group home to her sheltered workshop. The goal-setting may include listing safe places to go if harassed and deciding who it is safe to tell if she is in trouble, such as a bus driver or police officer. As another example, a nurse may assist a woman with multiple sclerosis develop a detailed safety plan for leaving an abusive husband who provides essential care. A mutually determined method of evaluation may be that the woman has called area shelters to inquire about physical accessibility, and the nurse has inquired about services available through APS.

Cultural Considerations in Assessment and Intervention

Attending to cultural considerations increases the likelihood that the questions nurses ask women are appropriate and that our understanding of clinical data accurately reflect a woman's situation. For women with disabilities who experience abuse, these considerations require attention to the women's personal identify as well as the meanings of disability and abuse within her ethnic and/or religious cultures. For some women, disability or deaf culture may also play a role in these understandings of self and community. Disability culture has its roots in the disability rights movement in the West and continues to be strongly linked to this social movement. The culture reflects a group identity shared by people with disabilities that is based on common experiences of oppression and resilience as well as art, music, and literature (Brown, 1995). Similarly, Deaf culture is a term applied to the social movement that holds deafness to be a difference in human experience rather than a disability. For this reason, many women who identify with deaf culture do not identify as disabled women.

In addition to promoting accurate and sensitive assessment, attention to cultural considerations also informs patient goal-setting and intervention. For example, women from individualist and collectivist cultures often face different challenges to ending abuse in their lives potentially resulting in the need for different approaches to intervention. In addition, women from specific ethnic backgrounds may benefit from resources in their communities. Women who identify with disability or deaf cultures may also wish to access to resources in their communities. For these women, Independent Living Centers should be considered as a resource for intervention since advocacy and referral services are part of their core mission.

CASE STUDY AND ANALYSIS

The following case study and analysis focuses only on the elements of the history, physical, and treatment plan that apply specifically to instances of violence. Other standard elements of the history, physical, and treatment plan should also be included when working with victims of violence but are not addressed here.

Background/Patient History and Examination

Background

Sandy is a 42-year-old Euro-American female who sustained a C5–6 spinal cord injury at the age of 26. Sandy is a survivor of childhood sexual abuse and IPV prior to the onset of her disability. She has a past and current history of alcoholism and illicit drug use. Sandy presents with complaint of a right shoulder injury following an assault perpetrated by her boyfriend who also serves as her caregiver.

Patient History

The nurse begins the interview by carefully eliciting Sandy's story. The patient reveals that the injury occurred in her van yesterday at noon and that the perpetrators name is George Smith. George was trying to prevent Sandy from driving to the police station and, in doing so, threw her out of her wheelchair and proceeded to beat and choke her. Sandy's shoulder hit the floor of the van when she was thrown out of her wheelchair. She is not sure, but it is possible that she might have hit her head as well. Currently, Sandy's sole abuser is George who is both her caregiver and intimate partner. Sandy relies on George for daily personal care such as toileting and bathing. She reports that George has abused her emotionally, physically, and in ways that are disability-related over the past year. Examples of the abuse she has experienced include name-calling, hitting, confining her to bed, denying her access to her wheelchair, and theft of prescription narcotics. When the nurse asks how the abuse affects Sandy's ability to manage her primary disability, Sandy reports that while partnered to George, she has become increasingly depressed, increased her use of alcohol, experimented with IV drug use (given and administered to her by George), and has unintentionally lost 20 lb. Sandy also reports that she has become increasingly isolated and that she was evicted from two apartments due to her abuser's drug use and violent behavior over the past year. Sandy's lethality assessment reveals that her risk for lethal violence is low.

Physical Examination

After obtaining a careful history, the nurse proceeds to perform a physical examination. In this case, examination of the shoulder, neck, elbow, wrist, back, chest, abdomen, and other proximal extremities looking for hidden injuries is indicated. Because of the possibility of head injury, conducting a thorough neurological examination is also appropriate. During the physical exam, the pattern of injury and the extent to which the injury appears consistent with Sandy's story should also be considered. It will also be important to further assess the extent to which Sandy's injury may affect her ability to use her wheelchair, shift her position in her wheelchair, and perform wheelchair transfers. To ensure that Sandy's injuries are properly documented, the nurse obtains written consent to photograph Sandy's visible injuries. Photographs should include close-up, midrange, and full-body shots using a scale. After completion of the physical exam, the nurse ascertains that Sandy has a right shoulder strain with no other observable injuries and no new neurological deficits. Sandy's ability to use her right arm is reduced, thereby making use of her wheelchair, shifting position in her chair, and wheelchair transfers, painful and difficult.

Patient Goals and Nursing Intervention

Planning with Sandy will include safety and disability-management planning. Providing Sandy with information about the cycle of abuse and its health consequences will be an important component of the teaching plan. Resource information provided should include information about domestic violence and disability community resources, and the accessibility of these resources for women who use wheelchairs and women with sensory loss.

In addition to the standard elements of a safety plan, it is important to discuss other ways to maintain Sandy's safety including reporting the abuser to whatever agency is paying him as her caregiver (with Sandy's agreement), calling 911, changing the locks, and in institutional settings, alerting the staff to the danger the abuser presents. Disability management includes obtaining back up caregiver services, discussing ways that Sandy's care may need to change following her shoulder injury, and arranging primary care follow-up.

To address Sandy's mental health needs, referral to a therapist who specializes in childhood sexual abuse and IPV, and referral to Alcoholics Anonymous or another appropriate substance abuse treatment program should be discussed. Referral to a community-based class on managing personal care assistants, abuse of disabled women, or a support group for women with disabilities would also be appropriate if these resources are available.

Follow-up with Sandy will be critical. Be sure to contact Sandy and assess her safety over the phone at least once a week until her situation has stabilized. Use appropriate judgment when calling Sandy at home. If her abuser answers the phone, refrain from saying or doing anything that will further endanger her safety. Table 7.1 provides details pertaining to nursing assessment, patient goals, and interventions specific to this case.

Evaluation

Criteria that may be useful in evaluating Sandy's case may include ability to verbalize and follow her safety and disability-management plans, staying in contact with the nurse or other designated provider, maintaining social contacts, engaging in self-care activities, following through with mental health and substance abuse referrals, and/or increased

TABLE 7.1   Case Study and Analysis: Patient Goals and Interventions

Patient Goals	Nursing Interventions
Nursing Diagnosis 1. **Adult Violence** Short-term goal: Maintain safety	The nurse will: Provide Sandy with information about the cycle of abuse and its health consequences. Work with Sandy to create an individualized safety plan (see displays 3 and 4). Provide resource information that includes information about domestic violence and disability community resources, and the accessibility of these resources for women who use wheelchairs. Encourage Sandy to call 911 if she fears for her safety. Encourage Sandy to change her locks if she wishes to separate from George.
Long-term goal: Remain free of abuse	Arrange for back up caregiver services to minimize dependence on abusive care providers in the future. Refer Sandy to a domestic violence support group to work through emotional issues related to abusive experiences. Work with Sandy to increase the size of her social network.
Nursing Diagnosis 2. **Impaired Mobility and** **Self-Care Ability** Short-term goal: Promote shoulder healing and self-care activities	The nurse will: Discuss shoulder mobility limitations to avoid aggravation of the injury. Provide shoulder support. Outline potential changes in Sandy's personal care routines based on her new temporary shoulder limitation. Discuss strategies for maximizing Sandy's self-care abilities. Arrange for primary care follow-up for ongoing evaluation and management of Sandy's shoulder injury. Arrange referral to Occupation or Physical therapy if deemed necessary following the initial stages of healing.
Long-term goal: Return shoulder to previous level of function	Reinforce the importance of using her safety plan to reduce the likelihood of future injury.
Nursing Diagnosis 3. **Unmet Personal** **Care Needs** Short-term goal: Obtain immediate personal care assistance services from a safe and competent provider	The nurse will: Assess the level, type, and frequency of personal assistance needed. Explore options for immediate back up caregiving services available in the community. Discuss long-term caregiving resources and options available in the health system and community.
Long-term goal: Obtain personal care assistance from safe and competent providers over the long-term	Refer Sandy to a caregiver management in the community course to promote effective hiring and communication skills for use with future caregivers.
Nursing Diagnosis 4. **Substance Abuse** Short-term goal: Consider treatment options	The nurse will: Discuss the impact of alcohol and drug use on Sandy's health. Encourage Sandy to seek treatment. Discuss treatment options for alcohol and drug treatment available to Sandy. Refer Sandy to an appropriate alcohol and drug treatment center. Provide Sandy with information about Alcoholics Anonymous or 12-step programs in her community. Provide Sandy with information about substance abuse programs specifically designed for people with disabilities available in the community.
Long-term goal: Remain abstinent from alcohol and drugs	Make a commitment to long-term abstinence. Maintain a solid support system. Begin psychotherapy to deal with the traumatic effects of childhood sexual abuse and promote use of healthy coping skills. Avoid spending time with individuals who drink or use drugs excessively.

knowledge and insight about her abuse experiences. It is important not to be discouraged if Sandy allows her abuser to return as her IP and/or caregiver. Consistent support and positive affirmation will be important in helping Sandy to maintain her health and safety over time.

SUMMARY

The seriousness of the problem of abuse of women with disabilities confirms the need for universal screening for abuse with every patient contact in rehabilitation, health care, and other professional settings. In addition to assessment and identification, abuse intervention is also essential. Research investigating abuse of women with disabilities has identified the social context of disability as a factor, which significantly shapes the abuse experiences of this population. Concrete examples of this important context include the problem of inaccessible shelter, home, and community environments and the lack of availability of alternative caregiver services for abused women. Service providers seeking to intervene with abused women must be aware of the resources available in their communities to facilitate appropriate referrals in their local areas while also working to develop and improve services (Nosek, Howland, & Young, 1997; Swedlund & Nosek, 2000). Collaboration with domestic violence shelters to provide caregivers and replace medications and assistive devices left behind when abused women are forced to leave their homes is also necessary. Additionally, collaboration with law enforcement and other professionals should occur to facilitate removal of abusers from women's homes and provide essential personal care services in emergent situations.

In addition to improved services, research is needed to support evidence-based practice with women with disabilities who experience abuse. Future qualitative studies are

---

EXHIBIT 7.5 | *Web Resources*

Abuse Deaf Women's Advocacy Services:
http://www.adwas.org/
Center for Research on Women with Disabilities:
http://www.bcm.edu/crowd/abuse_women/abuse_women.html
Disabled Women's Network Ontario:
http://dawn.thot.net/
Domestic Violence Resource Center:
http://www.dvirc.org.au/Disability/DisabilityIndex.htm
Minnesota Center Against Violence and Abuse Clearinghouse:
http://www.mincava.umn.edu/categories/884
National Center on Abuse and Domestic Violence:
http://www.ncdsv.org/publications_peopledisable.html
Safe Place:
http://www.safeplace.org/site/PageServer?pagename=Homepage
Stop VAW:
http://www.stopvaw.org/Women_with_Disabilities.html
United States Department of Health and Human Services:
http://www.womenshealth.gov/violence/groups/wwd.cfm

needed to investigate the cultural contexts of abuse of women with disabilities both within the dominant culture and within various ethnic cultures. In addition, there is a need for research that focuses specifically on the abuse experiences of women with different types of physical, cognitive, and psychiatric disabilities. Also important, is the need for more information about abuse of women with disabilities within specific settings such as rehabilitation centers, hospitals, clinics, residential care facilities, and private homes. Future quantitative research efforts should include further identification of risk factors for abuse, examination of the direct and indirect effects of abuse on women's health, and development and testing of abuse interventions. Both qualitative and quantitative studies are needed to further develop and test theories of abuse specific to women with disabilities. To ensure that future research findings are accurate and empowering to women with disabilities who experience violence, it is essential that women with disabilities are involved at all levels of this important work.

To conclude, future directions in the care of abused women with disabilities must use a collaborative model, with women with disabilities at the center. Researchers have the obligation to raise the issue of violence against women with disabilities to the same level of public awareness as violence against women in general, and to conduct collaborative research that includes violence and disability researchers, and women with disabilities. Service providers must work to increase the implementation of model programs and improve the quality and accessibility of health care and other services abused women with disabilities need. Educators must work to ensure that content on abuse of women with disabilities, and the social context of disability, is included in nursing school curricula, and further, to provide community education in these important areas. It is incumbent on nursing to be involved in all of these endeavors to ensure that women with disabilities have access to the kind of quality care they deserve, as well as the knowledge and resources needed to end abuse in their lives.

Tools/Resources

Exhibit 7.5 provides a list of Web sites that can serve as useful resources for nurses seeking information about abuse of women with disabilities. The *Safer and Stronger Abuse Measure* questions in Appendix C are also provided as a screening resource.

REFERENCES

Americans with Disabilities Act, 42 U.S.C. 12102 (1990).

Barrett, K., O'Day, B., Roche, A., & Carlson, B. (2009). Intimate partner violence, health status, and health care access among women with disabilities. *Women's Health Issues, 19*, 94–100.

Brown, S. (1995) Disability culture beginnings: A fact sheet. [Online] Available at: http://www.independentliving.org/docs3/brown96a.html

Brownridge, D. (2006). Partner violence against women with disabilities: Prevalence, risk and Explanations. *Violence Against Women, 12*, 805–822.

Campbell, J. C. (1995). Prediction of homicide of and by battered women. In J. C. Campbell (Ed.), *Assessing dangerousness: Violence by sexual offenders, batterers, and child abusers* (pp. 96–113). Thousand Oaks, CA: Sage Publications.

Casteel, C., Martin, S. L., Smith, J. B., Gurka, K. K., & Kupper, L. L. (2008). National study of physical and sexual assault among women with disabilities. *Injury Prevention, 14*, 87–90.

Cohen, M. M., Forte, T., Du Mont, J., Hyman, I., & Romans, S. (2005). Intimate partner violence among Canadian women with activity limitations. *Journal of Epidemiology and Community Health, 59,* 834–839.

Copel, L. (2006). Partner abuse in physically disabled women: A proposed model for understanding intimate partner violence. *Perspectives in Psychiatric Care, 42,* 114–128.

CROWD, (5/25/09). Violence against women with disabilities fact sheet #1 findings from studies 1992–2002. [Online]. Available: http://www.bcm.edu/crowd/?pmid=1409

Curry, M., Hassouneh-Phillips, & Johnston-Silverberg, A. (2001). Abuse of women with disabilities: An ecological model and review. *Violence Against Women, 7*(1), 60–79.

Curry, M. A., Powers, L. E., & Oschwald, M. (2003). Development of an abuse screening tool for women with disabilities. *Journal of Aggression, Maltreatment, and Trauma, 8*(4), 123–141.

Curry, M. A., Renker, P., Hughes, R., Robinson-Whelen, S., Oschwald, M., Swank, P., & Powers, L. (2009). Development of measures of abuse among women with disabilities and the characteristics of their perpetrators. *Violence Against Women, 15* (9), 1001–1025.

Dewsbury, G., Clark, K., Randall, D., Rouncefield, M., & Summerville, I. (2004). The anti-social model of disability. *Disability and Society, 19*(2), 145–158.

Gilson, S., Cramer, E., & DePoy, E. (2001). (Re) Defining abuse of women with disabilities: A paradox of limitation and expansion. *AFFILIA: Journal of Women and Social Work, 16*(2), 220–235.

Glover-Graf, N., & Reed, B. (2006). Abuse against women with disabilities. *Rehabilitation Education, 20*(1), 43–56.

Hassouneh-Phillips, D. (2005). Understanding abuse of women with physical disabilities: An overview of the Abuse Pathways Model. *Advances in Nursing Science, 28*(1), 70–80.

Hassouneh, D., Hanson, G., Perrin, N., & McNeff, E. (2008). Abuse and health in men and women with SCI/D. *Journal of Rehabilitation, 74*(3), 3–9.

Hassouneh-Phillips, D., & McNeff, E. (2004). Understanding care-related abuse and neglect in the lives of women with SCI. *SCI Nursing, 21*(2), 75–81.

Hassouneh-Phillips, D., & McNeff, E. (2005). 'I thought I was less worthy': Low sexual and body esteem and increased vulnerability to intimate partner abuse in women with physical disabilities. *Sexuality and Disability, 23*(4), 227–240.

Hassouneh-Phillips, D., McNeff, E., Powers, L., & Curry, M. (2005). Invalidation: A central process underlying maltreatment of women with disabilities. *Women & Health, 41*(1), 33–50.

Hughes, R. & Robinson-Whelen, S. (May 5, 2009). *Computer Assisted Abuse & Safety Self-assisted abuse and safety interview.* Research presentation for the 2009 National Association of Research and Rehabilitation Training Centers (NARRTC) Annual Conference, Arlington, VA.

Martin, S., Ray, N., Sotres-Alvarez, D., Kupper, L., Moracco, K., Dickens, P., Scandlin, D., et al. (2006). Physical and sexual assault of women with disabilities. *Violence Against Women, 12,* 823–837.

Mays, J. (2006). Feminist disability theory: Domestic violence against women with a disability. *Disability & Society, 21*(2), 147–158.

McFarlane, J., Hughes, R., Nosek, M., Groff, J., Swedland, N., & Mullens, P. (2001). Abuse Assessment Screen-Disability (AAS-D): Measuring frequency, type, and perpetrator of abuse toward women with physical disabilities. *Journal of Women's Health & Gender-Based Medicine, 10,* 861–866.

Milberger, S., Israel, N., LeRoy, B., Martin, A., Potter, L., & Patschak-Schuster, P. (2003). Violence against women with physical disabilities. *Violence and Victims, 18,* 581–591.

Nixon, J., (2009). Domestic violence and women with disabilities: Locating the issue on the periphery of social movements. *Disability & Society, 24*(1), 77–89.

Nosek, M. A. (1996). Sexual abuse of women with physical disabilities. In D. M. Krotoski, M. A. Nosek, & M. A. Turk (Eds.), *Women with physical disabilities: Achieving and maintaining health and well-being.* (pp. 153–173). Baltimore: Paul H. Brooks.

Nosek, M. A., Foley, C. C., Hughes, R. B., & Howland, C. A. (2001). Vulnerabilities for abuse among women with disabilities. Special Issue. *Sexuality and Disability, 19*(3), 177–189.

Nosek, M. A., Howland, C. A., Rintala, D. H., Young, E. M. & Chanpong, G. F. (1997). *National study of women with physical disabilities: Final report.* Houston, TX: Center for Research on Women with Disabilities.

Nosek, M., Howland, C., & Young, M. (1997). Abuse of women with disabilities: Policy implications. *Journal of Disability Policy Studies, 8,* 157–176.

Nosek, M. A., Hughes, R., Taylor, H., & Taylor, P. (2006). Disability, psychosocial, and demographic characteristics of abused women with physical disabilities. *Violence Against Women, 12,* 838–850.

Oktay, J. S., & Tompkins, C. J. (2004). Personal assistance providers' mistreatment of disabled adults. *Health and Social Work, 29,* 177–188.

Oschwald, M., Renker, P., Hughes, R., Arthur, Anne, Powers, L., & Curry, M.A. (2009). Development of an accessible audio computer-assisted self-interview (A-CASI) to screen for abuse and provide safety strategies for women with disabilities. *Journal of Interpersonal Violence. 24,* 795–818.

Peckham, N., Howlett, S., & Corbett, A. (2007). Evaluating a survivor's group pilot for women with significant intellectual disabilities who have been sexually abused. *Journal of Applied Research in Intellectual Disabilities, 29,* 308–322.

Powers, L. E., Curry, M. A., Oschwald, M., Maley, S., Saxton, M., & Eckels, K. (2002). Barriers and strategies in addressing abuse: A survey of disabled women's experiences. *Journal of Rehabilitation, 68*(1), 4–13.

Powers, L., Curry, M.A., McNeff, L., Saxton, M., Powers, J., & Oschwald, M. (2008). End the silence: A survey of abuse against men with disabilities. *Journal of Rehabilitation Medicine, 74,* 41–53.

Powers, L., Renker, P., Robinson-Whelen, S., Oschwald, M., Hughes, R., Swank, P., & Curry, M. A. (2009). Interpersonal violence and women with disabilities: Analysis of safety promoting behaviors. *Violence Against Women, 15* (9), 1040–1069.

Safeplace, (2000). *Stop the violence break the silence* [Online]. Available: http://www.austin-safeplace. org/services/psac/disability/background.htm

Saxton, M., Curry, M., Powers, L. E., Maley, S., Eckels, K., & Gross, J. (2001). "Bring my scooter so I can leave you": A study of disabled women handling abuse by personal assistance providers. *Violence Against Women, 7*(4), 393–417.

Sequeira, H., Howlin, P., & Hollins, S. (2003). Psychological disturbance associated with sexual abuse in people with learning disabilities. *British Journal of Psychiatry, 183,* 451–456.

Shakespeare, T. (2006). *Disability rights and wrongs.* New York: Routledge.

Smith, D. L. (2008). Disability, gender and intimate partner violence: Relationships from the behavioral risk fact or surveillance system. *Sexuality and Disability, 26,* 15–28.

Swedlund, N., & Nosek, M. (2000). An exploratory study on the work of Independent Living Centers to address abuse of women with disabilities. *Journal of Rehabilitation, 66*(4), 57–64.

Tjaden, P. (2005). Defining and measuring violence against women: Background, issues, and recommendations. Paper prepared for the Violence against women: A statistical overview, challenges and gaps in data collection and methodology and approaches for overcoming them, Expert Group meeting organized by U.N. division for the Advancement of Women and Economic commission for Europe and the World Health Organization. Geneva, Switzerland, April 11–14, 2005.

Waldrop, J., & Stern, S. M. (2003). *Disability status 2000.* Washington, DC: US Census Bureau.

8

Nursing Care of Immigrant and Rural Abused Women

Nancy Glass, PhD, MPH, RN, FAAN
Sandra L. Annan, PhD, RN
Shreya Bhandari, PhD, MSW
Tina Bloom, PhD, MPH, RN
Nancy Fishwick, PhD, RN, FNP

INTRODUCTION

As has been noted in previous chapters, intimate partner violence (IPV) is a global health and social problem, which occurs in all countries and in all economic, social, religious, and cultural groups, and results in significant negative health and economic consequences for individuals, families, communities, and society (World Health Organization, 2002, 2005). This chapter on nursing practice with immigrant and rural women will build on previous chapters by integrating theories of IPV (chapter 3), information on long-term health consequences of IPV (chapter 2), and IPV and nursing practice (chapter 5). Specifically, in this chapter, we explore the nurse's role in relation to immigrant and rural abused women. First, we provide an understanding of IPV as it exists within the immigrant population in the United States and summarize what is known about the unique challenges for immigrant women living with and trying to access resources while staying or leaving an abusive relationship. Drawing on this information, we will present a case study to suggest "best practices" to guide the nurse in assessment and response to immigrant women in the health care or home setting as well as guide the nurse in collaboration with the larger immigrant community to raise awareness to prevent and reduce IPV. As immigrants to the United States often live in rural communities, we will also summarize in this chapter the information that exists on IPV within rural communities and the unique challenges for abused women living in rural environments when trying to access resources while staying in, or leaving, an abusive relationship. Again, drawing on this information, we will present a case study to suggest "best practices" to guide the nurse in assessment and response to rural abused women. Lastly, we will discuss the importance of nursing leadership in collaboration between the multiple mainstream systems, including health care, legal, criminal justice, and community-based domestic violence advocacy and culturally competent community leaders and agencies to strengthen the comprehensive community response to vulnerable groups, such as immigrant and rural abused women.

OVERVIEW OF THE U.S. IMMIGRANT POPULATION

United States has seen a stable growth in the immigrant population in the last century with 50% of the immigrants being women (Immigration and Naturalization Services, 1997). At present, 1 in 10 women in this country is an immigrant (U.S. Department of Commerce, Bureau of Census, 2004). Therefore, addressing IPV in immigrant communities is an urgent national health agenda. A higher proportion of immigrants and their U.S.-born children under age 18 live in poverty (16.9% compared with 11.4% for natives and their children), and a much higher proportion of foreign-born individuals lack health insurance (33.8% compared with 13.0% for native-born individuals) (Malone, Baluja, Costanzo, et al., 2003; Family Violence Prevention Fund [FVPF], 2009). These socioeconomic disparities make initiatives to address IPV in immigrant communities compelling and urgent.

CURRENT LITERATURE ON INTIMATE PARTNER VIOLENCE IN THE U.S. IMMIGRANT POPULATION

Very few IPV studies have focused exclusively on U.S. immigrants; most studies focus on specific population groups, such as Latinas and Asian/Pacific Islanders (API) that are known to include a high proportion of foreign-born individuals. Many Latina and Asian ethnic groups have a foreign-born rate of over 60%, compared with the national average of 12.6% (Camarota, 2007, Ramirez, 2004; Reeves & Bennett, 2004). For example, the Asian immigrants in the United States reached 8.2 million in the year 2000, which is 26.4% of the total immigrant population (US Census Bureau, 2000).

Specifically, a recent analysis of the Behavioral Risk Factor Surveillance System (BRFSS) Survey (MMWR, 2008) in 16 states and two territories reported the following estimates of lifetime physical and/or sexual IPV: 20.5% for Hispanic women; 9.7% for Asian women; 29.2% for Black women; and 26.8% for White women. According to a survey of literature conducted by Yoshihama for the Family Violence Prevention Fund Report (March, 2009), although no population-based studies have focused exclusively on immigrant populations, research indicates that lifetime IPV is not more prevalent in immigrant populations as noted above, but rather differences in IPV by race and ethnicity often decrease or disappear when socioeconomic status and partners' substance abuse are included in the analysis (FVPF, 2009).

However, Yoshihama in her contribution to the FVPF report (March, 2009) reported that while nonfatal IPV may be lower for Latinas and Asian immigrants, immigrants of Latino and API descent experience a higher risk of homicide than U.S.-born persons. These higher IPV-related homicide rates may indicate missed opportunities by the health care system and other existing systems, such as criminal justice and domestic violence advocacy to effectively respond to victims and prevent extreme violence.

Another important issue is that the heterogeneity of immigrant groups is often overlooked in research, advocacy, and services. For example, Asian immigrants have diverse immigration history, ethnicity, language, religion, and cultures with the Chinese and

Japanese migrating in the mid-1800s and other groups arriving more recently in the United States (Choi, 2001). The other heterogeneity factor is differences in class, the upper class consisting of wealthy businessmen, middle class comprising of college students and midrange professionals, and the lower class comprising of the low-wage earners, blue-collar workers, and the undocumented workers. Thus, there is an entire segment of immigrant population that may be discounted, such as undocumented workers, as if nonexistent (Abraham, 2000).

THEORETICAL CONSIDERATIONS FOR NURSING CARE OF IMMIGRANT ABUSED WOMEN

Scholarship in the United States that has guided the development of nursing care with abused women has rarely included the experiences of women of racial and ethnic minority (Chow, 1993). An ethnogender perspective or intersectionality approach not only emphasizes the gender inequality but also gives equal importance to racial/ethnicity challenges minority women experience through dual subordination (Abraham, 1995; Kelly, 2009). This perspective advocates the intersection of gender, race, and ethnicity as the cultural differences become an important criteria for the social construction of a national culture in an alien land. Race and ethnicity cuts across socioeconomic class and is usually the most dominant marker of differentiation. Moreover, ethnicity becomes the basis of cohesion for the group in a foreign land (Chow, 1993). Regardless of the class to which the woman belongs in her home country, she faces subordination not only as a woman (gender coming into play) but also as a minority woman in a foreign land. For example, her socialization into rigid gender norms in her home country, on one hand, and the lack of institutional support in a foreign land due to her alien status, on the other hand, expose her to dual marginalization (Kim, 1998). This perspective, thus, raises questions on the construction of gender relations intertwined with the cultural concerns at the individual, organizational, community, and societal level (Abraham, 1995). Any effort to help immigrant women will be futile unless this intersectionality is well understood (also see chapter 3 in the section on intersectionality).

Barriers Experienced by Immigrant Abused Women

Immigrant women in the United States often are economically, socially, psychologically, and legally dependent on their spouses and his family, potentially increasing their risk of experiencing IPV and having limited access to needed resources to increase safety while in the relationship and when leaving the abusive partner. Having migrated to the United States, women leave their social support in their respective country of origin, including their family, coworkers, and friends. Research has demonstrated that abusers isolate their victims from their support systems and families, and this further exacerbates an immigrant woman's situation, hampering her efforts to seek help (Dasgupta & Warrier, 1996; Song, 1996). Moreover, the abuser's coercive control and the woman's limited language skills, coupled with a lack of knowledge of legal rights and services available for IPV survivors, can further isolate immigrant women (Dasgupta, 2000; Mehrotra, 1999). Additional barriers in seeking help, especially among immigrant women, are shame, stigma attached to abuse, fear of the abuser (Bui, 2003), cultural expectations of maintaining familial harmony, and not breaking the marriage (Shiu-Thornton, Senturia, & Sullivan, 2005). For example, the traditional Asian values of privacy, honor, self-control may discourage women from revealing abuse in their lives (Hu & Chen, 1999). Asians are often referred in the U.S. media as a "model minority" due to the rapid economic and social success they have gained in a very a short period of time (Dasgupta, 2000). There also is a misperception that the Asian "community" is free of all social ills including alcoholism, drug addiction to IPV. The Asian community strives to maintain their impeccable image and, in turn, denies any issue that spoils its image, including class and gender inequities.

Another unique barrier for the abused immigrant woman in seeking help is her immigrant status. If the woman is on a dependent immigrant status, she has limited legal rights. The abusers, often times, can use her immigration status as a tool to control her life. The abuser controls her by issuing threats to delay filing for permanent residency, threats to interfere with her access to their children if she seeks help, threats to have family members of uncertain legal status deported, threats to divorce her and keep custody of the children which may be the norm in their country of origin, or to send her "back home" where in some countries she may be "disciplined" by extended family members with impunity. Further, illegal immigrant women are always under the threat of being deported and, hence, fear seeking legal help for abuse (Orloff, 2000). The 1996 Illegal Immigration Reform and Responsibility Act included IPV as grounds for deporting the abuser to his home country. Hence, an immigrant woman may be hesitant in seeking any legal help, as her husband's deportation will hamper her economic well-being and will limit her chances of acquiring American citizenship (Raj & Silverman, 2002). These issues also may be a barrier for immigrant abused women seeking help from the health care system for injuries or health problems related to abuse. Immigrant women are often concerned that health care professionals may report them to immigration authorities, to child protective services, or to the police (Bauer, Rodriguez, Quiroga, Flores-Ortiz, 2000).

The issue of IPV among the immigrant population, thus, is complex with multiple factors such as limited language proficiency, social isolation, disparities in economics and access to social resources, and immigration status that explains women's hesitancy to report IPV to mainstream services, including health care providers (FVPF, 2009).

"BEST PRACTICES" WHEN CARING FOR IMMIGRANT ABUSED WOMEN: A CASE STUDY AND ANALYSIS

The following case study and analysis will focus on "best practices" that acknowledge the unique aspects that the nurses and other health care professionals should be aware of while caring for an immigrant woman.

Background

Niharika, a 27-year-old woman from India, presents to the clinic with concerns of feeling sad, insomnia, lack of appetite, and loss of interest in most areas of her life. Her medical record and stored digital photographs indicate that she sought care in the emergency department with a broken nose 4 months ago that she reported was the result of a fall. Throughout the clinic visit, Niharika's husband was very attentive and resisted leaving her alone during the visit. Niharika had recently moved to the United States and spoke limited English requiring an interpreter. Her husband stated that he must stay with his wife and he was needed to interpret for his wife.

Assessment for Intimate Partner Violence in Private With Professional Interpretation

It is the nurses' responsibility to complete the assessment for IPV in a private setting; this means that no person is in the room with the patient. Even if the patient asks to have a family member or friend in the room, it is important to tell her it is the policy of the clinic to interview all patients in private. The nurse can reassure the patient by being the one to ask the family member or friend to step out of the room and ask them to take the time while the patient is being examined to go make phone calls to others to tell them that she is fine, fill out administrative forms in the waiting room, or get a cup of coffee. Privacy is critical, as the presence of anyone in the exam room may prevent the disclosure of IPV to the nurse or other health care professional. During the private time, the nurse has the opportunity to assess the patient for multiple issues, including using a brief IPV assessment questionnaire that is well-established and has been discussed in detail in chapter 5.

Patient History

The nurse begins the interview by working closely with the professional interpreter to carefully elicit Niharika's story. Niharika appeared to be nervous and frightened. After constant reassurance from the nurse, she agreed to share her story. Niharika was 22 years old when she got married to Suresh, a graduate student, "an intelligent young man with no bad habits," as described by her family. They were married within a few days of their first meeting in India. After arriving in the United States, Suresh seemed to be a completely different man from what little she had seen him in India at the time of their wedding. He was very unsympathetic and prevented her from calling her family back home. It started with verbal abuse where he called her names and accused her of infidelity and purposely not getting pregnant. He hit her with all sorts of objects, repeatedly kicked her, and accused her of not being a good housekeeper. She reported that she has become very isolated and fears talking to anybody in her family or community about Suresh's behavior. She reports feeling hopeless, had lost interest in life, no longer wanted to do the things that she had previously enjoyed, and had difficulty sleeping because of fear that Suresh may attack her while she is asleep. The last time, when he punched her on the nose, he threatened her with dire consequences if she dared to talk to anyone about how the injury happened. Fearing her husband, she lied at the previous health visit and reported to the health care provider that she had taken a fall.

Physical Examination

On examination, the nurse asked Niharika about exposure to physical and sexual violence and nonphysical abuse. The nurse documented multiple bruises on Niharika's abdomen and legs in various stages of healing. Niharika was uncomfortable, reported pain, and was startled easily when touched by the nurse during the exam. The nurse administered a brief assessment for depression and PTSD, as well suicidal ideation. The assessments indicated that Niharika had symptoms consistent with depression and PTSD, but was not suicidal. Niharika reported she has not told anyone about the IPV and does not know about resources in the community to support her safety. The nurse's documentation included the patient's exact words ("Patient states husband has threatened to hurt her if she tells anyone about the physical violence") as well as accurate description of the physical examination.

Nursing Intervention

1. The nurse knows to never use spouses, friends, family members, children, or other patients as interpreters with immigrant women, as it may endanger victim's life. Under Title VI of the Civil Rights Act of 1964, patients with limited English proficiency have the right to receive free professional interpreter services from any health care provider who receives federal financial assistance (Executive Order, 2000). Interpretation services should be provided by trained staff at the health care facility's language bank or by contracted telephone interpreters. The national domestic violence hotline (1-800-799-SAFE) has hotline operators who speak most languages and also know the domestic violence laws related to immigration status and ethnic group-specific domestic violence agencies.

2. Immigrant women may fear dealing with the legal system due to a number of barriers discussed above and that might be a hindrance in disclosing IPV. The nurse knows that it is important to reassure Niharika that nurse–patient confidentiality will be respected and that there are experts on legal issues related to immigration that could help her if needed, and the nurse can assist her in accessing these services. The nurse also knows that the Violence Against Women Act has special provisions for obtaining legal permanent residency for abused women and that the medical documentation of abuse can be crucial in her seeking it (see Exhibit 8.1 for more details).

3. The nurse knows it is important to assess for physical and sexual violence and non-physical types of abuse, including threats of violence, emotional abuse, sexual abuse, stalking, and financial abuse as well as threats of deportation. It is important to define the behaviors of the partner as IPV and begin the process of educating her about IPV and resources/services in the community. It is also important to assess for mental and physical health consequences of IPV.

4. The nurse knows to communicate to that nobody deserves to be abused, the patient is not alone, and IPV is a global phenomenon that affects many women from all cultures. These statements will help to validate the patient's feelings, concerns, and reactions.

5. The nurse knows that evidence-based risk assessment of danger, based on known risk factors for near lethal and lethal IPV, is critical to safety. The nurse will thus follow up with a systematic risk assessment, using the Danger Assessment (www.dangerassessment. org; Campbell, Webster, & Glass, 2009).

6. The nurse knows to briefly explain to the patient the variety of resources and services that may be available to increase her safety. Specifically, the nurse can discuss shelter programs, advocacy programs, and legal options including obtaining a restraining order. The nurse will ask permission from the patient to consult other providers and bring in other clinic and community services to work with her on developing a safety plan regardless if she is returning home with husband or leaving her husband. The additional resources can include a culturally competent community advocate, mental health professional, or social worker to collaboratively work on a plan to increase her health and safety.

7. The nurse knows that providing Niharika with IPV resource information to take with her if she is returning home may increase her risk of violence by her husband. Therefore, the nurse should discuss strategies to safely connect her with local culturally competent resources and/ or organizations that have expertise with immigrant survivors of IPV.

EXHIBIT 8.1 | *Violence Against Women Act Provisions for Immigrant Women*

Under the Violence Against Women Act (WAVA), battered immigrant women can apply for legal permanent residency on the basis of abuse they have endured. It is always safer to consult an immigration expert and/or lawyer on this issue as refraining from doing so might expose the client to undue danger.

What are VAWA Provisions for Immigrant Women?
VAWA was passed by Congress in 1994 and then reauthorized in 2000 and 2005. The Act makes special provisions to protect immigrant survivors of domestic violence and abuse. VAWA allows survivors of domestic violence to self-petition for permanent residency in the United States for themselves and for their children without depending on the abuser.
The options to apply for permanent residency are:

1. To self-petition for legal permanent residency, under the VAWA.
2. Deportation to home country can be cancelled, under VAWA (if the person is already in the deportation process).
3. A crime survivor's visa, called the U Visa could be issued.
4. Asylum could be sought, based on being a victim of domestic violence.

The reauthorizations of VAWA in 2000 and 2005 have further expanded the range of individuals entitled for respite, simplified evidentiary requirements and extended access of abused immigrant women and children to public benefits (Orloff, L & Kaguyutan, J.V., 2002; Lin, J., Orloff, L., & Echavarria, E., 2007).
Some of the respites have been listed below:

"The VAWA 2005 immigration provisions include:

1. Continues to implement VAWA's unique goal by stopping deportation of immigrant victims of domestic violence, sexual assault, or trafficking;
2. Extends immigration relief to larger group of family violence victims;
3. Provides economic stability and security for trafficking victims;
4. Protects safety of victims of domestic abuse, stalking, sexual assault, trafficking;
5. Guaranties economic security for immigrant victims and their children;
6. Improvements in processing VAWA cases and technical amendments; and
7. International marriage broker regulations."

Source: Family Violence Prevention Fund. Background on Laws Affecting Battered Immigrant Women.

---

8. The nurse also knows that a safe way to follow-up with Niharika by phone or other mechanism is needed, as often the abusive partner controls telephone use and contact with services. Developing strategies to maintain contact will allow for ongoing assessment for safety and health needs and provide additional appropriate resources as needed to support the victim's decisions.
9. A visit to the health care clinic may not allow the nurse the time to safely assess and provide information to address the entire complex and multiple needs of the immigrant woman. However, the nurse has the responsibility to begin the assessment and safety planning process by creating a safe, private, and nonjudgmental space for the patient to disclose IPV. By assessing IPV in a respectful and safe manner, Niharika will understand that regardless of her decision on that day, she can seek assistance from

---

EXHIBIT 8.2 | *Web Resources for Immigrant Women*

- **Full list of key resources for working with immigrant women**
  http://www.endabuse.org/section/programs/immigrant_women/_key_resources
- **Legal Momentum's Immigrant Women Program Service Provider Resource Directory**
  http://www.legalmomentum.org/help-center/national-resources-for.html#Legal_Momentums_Immigrant_Women_Program_
- **Compilation of materials, letters, and articles from organizations across the nation working with immigrant women and children**
  http://www.immigrantwomennetwork.org/Resources.htm
- **National Coalition of Domestic Violence**
  http://www.ncadv.org/resources/StateCoalitionList.php
- **List of South Asian women's organizations (in the United States and in home country)**
  http://www.sawnet.org/orgns/#National
- **Partial list of organizations working with the Latino population across the United States**
  http://www.endabuse.org/userfiles/file/ImmigrantWomen/
- **Links to a number of national organizations working at all levels with immigrant women**
  http://www.dvalianza.org/en/dv-links.html

---

the health care clinic in the future (see Exhibit 8.2 for a list of Web-based resources for immigrant women).

Summary of Nursing Care of Immigrant Abused Women

To date, we have limited prevalence information on IPV among immigrant women, and the information we do have primarily focuses on Latino and Asian populations and does not address the heterogeneity within the populations. However, the nurse's understanding of the unique needs of immigrant women, including limited language proficiency, disparities in socioeconomic status, social isolation, and immigration status will assist the nurse, health care, and health organization to develop culturally appropriate strategies that represent best practices for assessment, care, treatment, and referrals for immigrant abused women.

In the following section of the chapter, we will address nursing care of rural abused women.

OVERVIEW OF INTIMATE PARTNER VIOLENCE IN THE CONTEXT OF RURAL ENVIRONMENTS

The term "rural" is defined in a variety of ways for the purpose of population mapping and distribution of federal and state funds. The term implies a low population density in a designated geographic area. The U.S. Census Bureau labels areas as urban when they have more than 2,500 people living in the area, and rural when there are less than 2,500 (U.S. Census Bureau 2005). It is important to realize that quantitative-based definitions do not capture distinctions within and between rural areas. For example, rural Alaska, rural Texas, and rural Vermont are all likely vastly different from one another in populations, political structures, social expectations, and available resources.

The term "rural" also denotes a cultural concept; the notion of "rural people" may raise stereotypical images of people who earn their livelihood from agriculture, forestry, and other natural resources, who reside in clean, peaceful, crime-free environments, and are surrounded by natural beauty. Within the concept of "rural life" lies a diversity of people, geography, livelihoods, and other circumstances—rural populations are comprised of many racial and ethnic groups as well as variety in age, educational achievement, occupation, financial security, and sexual preference.

CURRENT LITERATURE ON INTIMATE PARTNER VIOLENCE AND RURAL WOMEN

Research indicates that lifetime adult IPV prevalence ranges from 7% to 29% within rural populations (Bailey & Daugherty, 2007; Denham, 2003; Denham et al., 2007). As examples, 77% of rural African American women struggling with substance abuse, 15–32% of rural pregnant women, and 19% of Latina migrant farm workers report experiencing IPV (Bhandari et al., 2008; Boyd, Mackey, Phillips, & Tavakoli, 2006; Denham, 2003; Dye, Tolliver, Lee, & Kenney, 1995; Persily & Abdulla, 2000; Van Hightower & Gorton, 1998). This includes not just physical violence, but also psychological/emotional abuse, stalking, forced sex, economic abuse, and forced isolation (Bailey & Daugherty, 2007; Bosch & Bergen, 2006; Krishnan, Hilbert, & VanLeeuwen, 2001; Persily & Abdulla, 2000; Van Hightower & Gorton, 1998).

Although Logan and colleagues (2005) reported similar prevalence of physical and sexual violence and emotional abuse by women in rural and urban communities, they found that rural women were significantly more likely to experience a number of behaviors from their abuser that suggest increased risk for repeat and/or lethal violence. Specifically, Logan et al. (2005) found that rural women were significantly more likely to report stalking, isolation, controlling access to money, abuse of children and/or pets, threatening to hit her, hitting her with an object, breaking her bones or injuring her so severely she required medical care, driving dangerously with her in the car or attempting to run her over with a car, threats with a weapon, and threats to kill. Consistent with such findings, and similar to findings with immigrant women, rates of intimate partner homicide in the United States have been shown to be substantially higher in rural populations compared to metropolitan areas, or areas adjacent to metropolitan areas (Gallup-Black, 2005). Unfortunately, law enforcement personnel are generally more thinly distributed in rural counties, and response times to emergency calls for help may be much longer (Gallup-Black, 2005). These differences may further serve to increase rural women's risk of lethal violence in abusive relationships.

THEORETICAL CONSIDERATIONS WHEN CARING FOR ABUSED RURAL WOMEN

As when providing care to abused immigrant women, nurses and other health care professionals who provide care to rural women must consider the multiple and complex intersection of factors such as gender, race and ethnicity, economics, employment, social support, access to available services, and the culture of rural communities. Some of the factors that rural women may experience as barriers to disclosing IPV and receiving needed resources and services are detailed in the section below.

Barriers Experienced by Rural Abused Woman

Research findings, to date, suggest that rural abused women may face additional, unique layers of difficulty that increase their vulnerability to IPV and their difficulty in finding safety. In addition to geographic isolation, rural women face social or cultural barriers to accessing help, such as adherence to traditional gender stereotypes, lack of anonymity if violence is revealed, and lack of helpful resources (support networks, transportation, access to employment, health care, or formal violence services) (Bosch & Bergen, 2006; Eastman & Bunch, 2007; Evanson, 2006; Gallup-Black, 2005; Johnson, 2000; Logan, Cole, Shannon, & Walker, 2007; Logan, Shannon, & Walker, 2005). For example, Bosch and Schumm (2004) interviewed 56 IPV survivors in 10 rural Kansas counties and found that women resided an average of 78 mi from the nearest domestic violence shelter and had little or no knowledge of formal IPV resources.

Even when rural women are aware of formal IPV resources and attempt to access them, they may find such services are greatly lacking in rural communities. In Kentucky, Logan et al. (2005) compared abused women seeking protective orders in two rural counties ($n = 200$) and one urban county ($n = 250$) over a 2-year period, conducting qualitative interviews with the women and analyzing state data and court dockets. Compared to the urban women in the sample, Logan found rural women faced significant process-related barriers. Rural women were more likely to have to come to court more often and to have to pay to have their protective order served. Nearly half of their cases (46%) ended in nonservice (i.e., authorities did not serve the protective order), compared to 18.2% of urban cases.

Rural residents often have to travel long distances to access social, health care, or legal services. In many rural areas, roads in poor condition and severe weather conditions further complicate travel during certain times of the year. Distance and lack of reliable transportation (public and private) clearly hinder rural women's ability to escape dangerous situations and to access community-based domestic violence-related services. Rural areas rarely have public transportation, taxi service may be sparse, and private transportation may be limited (Bosch & Bergen, 2006; Feyen, 1989; Johnson, 2000; Van Hightower & Gorton, 2002). Rural victims of IPV report limited access to a car or are prevented by the abuser from using their car by tactics such as fuel siphoned from vehicles, car keys hidden, parts removed from car engines, or tires deliberately flattened (Bhandari et al., 2008; Bosch & Bergen, 2006; Logan et al., 2003; Websdale, 1998; Willis, 1998). Further, communication may be limited for rural women, as in many rural areas, women have limited access to mobile phone and internet services to gain information or contact needed services. However, even if health care, domestic violence, and legal services are available and accessible, rural women may avoid their use due to concerns of confidentiality, inability to pay for services, as well as concerns about experiences of stigma from service providers, including nurses (Riddell, Ford-Gilboe, & Leipert, 2009).

Rural communities often have more traditional U.S. values and conservative social beliefs compared to urban communities. Specifically, patriarchy, peer support among males, and traditional gender roles for women found in rural settings may contribute to violence against women (DeKeseredy & Joseph, 2006; Riddell, Ford-Gilboe, & Leipert, 2009; Websdale, 1998). As noted previously, lethal assaults against women, or femicide (murder of women), are more frequent in rural counties compared to urban counties (Gallup-Black, 2005). A gun (both handguns and rifles) in the home is an important predictor of femicide (Campbell, 2001), and guns are often used in rural assaults with rural women more likely to report the use of guns during an assault than urban women

(Logan et al., 2003; Teaster, Roberto, & Dugar, 2006; Websdale & Johnson, 1998). This may be, in part, because rural residents are more likely to engage in hunting than are urban residents, which entails having guns and ammunition in the home.

The smallness of many rural communities often supports a close-knit community. Social ties are such that some form of kinship and/or long-term acquaintanceship with almost everyone is common in rural communities (Ames, Brosi, & Damiano-Teixeira, 2006; Logan et al., 2003). Supportive friends and neighbors have been reported to be most helpful for rural women in abusive relationships (Bosch & Bergen, 2006). In many instances, however, the woman and her abusive partner have made their home within the neighborhood of his family and kin; this serves as a means to keep her isolated from her support network and removed from potential sources of support and assistance. The intimacy of rural communities and the overlap in social and professional roles may make it difficult for abused women and service providers to maintain confidentiality about IPV, and thus may curb women's disclosure even beyond nonrural levels. The likelihood that a rural abused woman would encounter someone she knows, or who knows her abusive partner or family, in the process of disclosing IPV is great. She is aware that her safety may be jeopardized if mutual acquaintances inform the perpetrator of her disclosure of IPV to health care professionals, law enforcement, or other sources of help.

Rural women report that the stress from the barriers identified above, including transportation difficulties, financial concerns, personal legal issues, lack of social support, and abuse from other family members or from strangers (Bhandari et al., 2008) further exacerbates the IPV in their relationship. The way in which these stressors may affect current and long-term health and well-being of women and their children needs further exploration through research.

"BEST PRACTICES" WHEN CARING FOR RURAL ABUSED WOMEN: A CASE STUDY AND ANALYSIS

The following case study and analysis will focus on "best practices" that acknowledge the unique aspects that the nurses and other health care professionals should be aware of while caring for an abused woman from a rural area.

BACKGROUND

Anna Lee, a 31-year-old white woman living in a rural county, is 4 months pregnant with her fourth child. She is being seen in a high-risk clinic because of a history of preterm labor and early delivery with her previous pregnancies. She is accompanied on this visit by her three other children, the oldest of whom is a teenager. She has a boyfriend who is the father of the two youngest children and her current pregnancy. Her partner is not at this visit.

Assessment of Patient in Private

The nurse knows that assessment of IPV in front of the children may prevent Anna Lee from speaking freely, and/or may increase her risk if children inadvertently reveal that she was assessed to an abusive partner. Thus, strategies are needed to talk to Anna Lee alone. After spending a few minutes establishing rapport, the nurse leaves the two younger children in the exam room, supervised by the teenage daughter, and walks Anna Lee to the restroom to collect her urine sample and to assess for IPV in private. Anna Lee responds to the questions casually and somewhat vaguely, by telling the nurse that she and her partner "have a lot of fights," that he is "obnoxious" and her "biggest stressor" but that it is "not a big deal." The nurse asks Anna Lee if she can send the children to the waiting room under the supervision of the teenager, while they take a few minutes to talk privately, and they return to the exam room.

Patient History and Examination

When the children are out of the room, the nurse follows up to elicit a more thorough history. Anna Lee reports that she has been in the relationship for 6 years and that her partner is jealous and "always thinks I am trying to hook up with some other guy." She describes her partner as "mean" and tells the nurse that there has been violence throughout the entire 6-year relationship, including during pregnancy. She adds that he recently tried to suffocate her, "with his hand and mouth over my nose, so I couldn't breathe," then adds, "it's because when I'm pregnant, I get really out of control sometimes." She describes her partner as "the worst boyfriend in the world" and says that she does not love him, but adds that he is a "good dad" and that he stays steadily employed. However, she has recently been in contact with a former boyfriend who recently came into town, and has been fantasizing about leaving her abuser. Her current pregnancy was undesired and was conceived when her partner coerced her into unprotected sex, but she has adjusted to the idea of another child, although she worries about having another preterm delivery. Anna Lee's physical exam is unremarkable, except that the nurse notes that while Anna Lee's children are clean and well-dressed, her own hair is unwashed, she smells like smoke, and she is wearing an oversized man's shirt, which is stained. She also notes that Anna Lee has a somewhat flat affect.

Nursing Intervention

1. The nurse is aware that abused women are often conflicted, embarrassed, fearful, and ashamed about IPV, and that pregnancy may increase the sense of conflict that women feel about disclosing violence. Therefore, as noted in the earlier case study, it is critical to begin the intervention with the patient by showing empathy (but not pity), validating her experience, and acknowledging that IPV is hard to talk about. The nurse also is careful to offer support in keeping Ann Lee and her children safe, to help her understand and deal with the health effects of violence, and to be unconditionally supportive in Anna Lee's immediate and long-term decisions about her relationship.

2. The nurse is aware that IPV during pregnancy is associated with an increased risk for pregnancy complications, including preterm labor and low birth weight. She also knows that most abused women are deeply concerned about the welfare of their children. She therefore knows that helping the patient recognize ways in which abuse may negatively impact her health, and the health of the developing fetus, is important information that will help the patient make informed decisions.

3. The nurse recognizes that Anna Lee's physical appearance is suggestive for significant mental health symptomatology and that antenatal and/or postpartum depression and PTSD are common sequelae of IPV. Thus, assessment and appropriate follow-up of Anna Lee's mental health status are needed. As with the physical sequelae of IPV,

helping her recognize that these symptoms can be a consequence of violence, and can also negatively impact her children, can help the patient make informed decisions.

4. The nurse knows that any abused woman needs evidence-based risk assessment of how dangerous her abuser is, based on known risk factors for near-lethal and lethal IPV. The nurses' level of concern is already elevated because IPV during pregnancy itself already indicates that Anna Lee may be in a particularly dangerous abusive relationship (Campbell et al., 2001; McFarlane et al., 2006). Anna Lee has also mentioned a number of other risk factors that concern the nurse, including extreme jealousy, attempts to strangle or suffocate her, and forced or coerced sex. The nurse will thus follow up with a systematic risk assessment, using the Danger Assessment (www.dangerassessment.org; Campbell, Webster and Glass, 2009)

5. Anna Lee needs referral, and perhaps facilitated referral, to domestic violence resources. This can best be done when the nurse is knowledgeable about services offered by the local/regional domestic violence program and has developed a working relationship with community-based domestic violence advocates. Although domestic violence programs may not be located in the woman's rural community, the regional program may have outreach services for women in remote areas. Advocates may be able to meet with Anna Lee in a safe location, or if a face-to-face meeting is not safe, they can offer support and guidance by telephone. Community-based domestic violence programs that serve remote areas may have established helpful alliances with local law enforcement, attorneys, clergy, and other potential sources of immediate help and safe haven. The nurse can help Anna Lee connect to local resources if these are available, or to the national hotline (1-800-799-SAFE) if they are not available or if the patient's concerns about privacy or confidentiality in a small town make her reluctant to call a local resource. The nurse knows that making these calls can be intimidating and that Anna Lee's partner may control her telephone access or monitor her calls. Therefore, the nurse will encourage her to call from the office and offer to make the call with her if she would like. The nurse reminds Anna Lee that the call is confidential and serves to provide her with information and support, and that no one will pressure her to make any particular decisions or take any particular actions.

6. As a rural health practitioner, the nurse knows that safety planning for rural women may include additional considerations that may not apply to urban abused women. The nurse is aware that the abused rural woman may have minimal financial and social resources, may be very isolated, and may be reluctant to call police due to concerns about privacy and confidentiality. If Anna Lee lives far out in the country and does call the police in an emergency, it may take the police a long time to arrive. The nurse can be instrumental in helping Anna Lee form a safety plan to address this by helping her identify her abuser's "red flags," which indicate that violence may be about to occur, think through the closest safe places that she and the children could go to until police arrive (in the house, or out of it), and plan for additional items that might be important in an emergency bag (e.g., warm clothes, telephone numbers, health-related documents, and financial documents) in the event of leaving by car or foot in the face of danger. Transportation issues are an essential element of safety planning; the nurse and Anna Lee can discuss ideas such as keeping gas in the car if she has access to it, and/or identifying trusted individuals who would respond to her call for a ride if needed (friend, family, neighbor, law enforcement). The nurse explains that, because the time of leaving can be the most dangerous time for abused women and their children, developing strategies for a planned, deliberate departure or for an

---

EXHIBIT 8.3 | *Web Resources for Rural Women and Rural Health Care Professionals*

- **National Coalition Against Domestic Violence**
  http://www.ncadv.org/resources/StateCoalitionList.php
  Links to state organizations, overview of abuse and violence, and safety planning.
- **National Domestic Violence Hotline website**
  http://www.ndvh.org
  Links to the toll-free hotline, information, and resources.
- **Family Violence Prevention Fund**
  http://endabuse.org
  Links to resources for health care professionals in many clinical settings, including those located in rural areas.
- **Rural Health Response to Domestic Violence: Policy and Practice Issues (2000)**
  Federal Office of Rural Health Policy document available online:
  http://ruralhealth.hrsa.gov/pub/domviol.htm
  Compilation of national and state initiatives that address domestic violence in rural areas.

---

emergently dangerous situation, will improve the likelihood of safe outcomes. Linking Anna Lee with the local/regional domestic violence program provides her with a resource for immediate and long-term support and information as her needs evolve over time.

7. Although the nurse values accurate medical record documentation as evidence of care which was rendered to the patient, rural women in abusive relationships may be concerned that the medical record will be seen by others and, if confidentiality is not maintained, may jeopardize her safety if the perpetrator is informed of her disclosure. Similar to urban women, rural women may be concerned that medical record documentation will lead to mandatory reporting to the state's bureau of protective services for domestic violence and/or for child abuse. The benefit of medical record documentation, particularly as evidence for future legal efforts, may not outweigh the perceived risks for rural women. The reader is referred to chapter 14 for suggestions in medical record documentation (see Exhibit 8.3 for a list of Web-based resources for rural women and rural health care professionals).

Summary of Nursing Care for Abused Rural Women

Compared to other populations and settings, relatively little IPV research has focused on rural women (DeKeseredy, 2006; Nolan, 2005). However, research findings, to date, suggest that rural abused women may face additional, unique layers of difficulty that increase their vulnerability to IPV and their difficulty in finding safety. As noted above, rural women are likely to be geographically isolated in areas with few services, and they face social and cultural barriers to accessing help. Lack of anonymity, lack of resources, and lack of reliable transportation are common concerns for rural women who experience IPV. As with immigrant women, understanding the interacting factors that influence rural woman's disclosure of IPV will assist the nurse, health care personnel, and health organizations in the development of culturally appropriate strategies that represent best practices for assessment, care, interventions, and referrals for rural abused women.

NURSE LEADESHIP IN COLLABORATION TO STRENGTHEN THE COMPREHENSIVE COMMUNITY RESPONSE TO IMMIGRANT AND RURAL ABUSED WOMEN

In the previous sections, we have discussed the unique needs of immigrant and rural abused women and best practices for nurses in the provision of care as illustrated through case studies. Nurses and health care systems have multiple opportunities to intervene with abused women in health care and community settings. However, the importance of collaboration between the mainstream systems, including health care, legal, criminal justice, and community-based domestic violence advocacy with culturally competent community leaders and agencies to strengthen the comprehensive community response to vulnerable groups, such as immigrant and rural abused women, must be understood and acted upon by the nurse.

As noted in the FVPF report (2009), abused women must believe that they can be safe if they confront or leave their abusers. Assurance of safety entails provision of culturally competent service providers and programs that can assist in keeping them safe from retaliation; provision of food, shelter, and other basic needs; and assurance that they will not lose their children to the abuser or the child welfare system. To accomplish this, nurse leadership is needed in (1) reforming health care systems to include routine assessment for IPV for every patient and provision of brief interventions, including risk assessment and referrals to appropriate culturally competent resources for those patients who report IPV; (2) advocacy for ongoing and mandatory education and training for health care professionals on assessment, care, treatment, and referral for IPV; (3) advocacy for collaboration with criminal justice, legal, housing, economic empowerment, and advocacy systems to adequately address the multiple and complex, intersecting barriers that prevent abused immigrant and rural women from living free of violence; (4) advocacy for training of mainstream system providers, including police, judges, district attorneys, housing services, welfare and child welfare, as well as domestic violence advocates in providing culturally competent care to immigrant and rural women as well as other vulnerable populations; and (5) developing collaborations with culturally competent programs that can provide expertise on the cultural context of immigrant and rural women and have skilled professionals that can build awareness of IPV in the community and service systems that can be accessed by abused women in their community.

CONCLUSION

Nurses can make a significant contribution to the health and safety of immigrant and rural women who have experienced IPV. Further, nursing leadership is needed in developing collaborations between the multiple mainstream systems and culturally competent services that are needed for immigrant and rural women to feel safe to disclose abuse and decrease the complex and multiple barriers that prevent women from accessing needed resources. This leadership will contribute to the comprehensive and culturally competent community response to intimate partner violence.

REFERENCES

Abraham, M. (1995). Ethnicity, gender and marital violence: South Asian Women's organization in the United States. *Gender and Society, 9*, 450–468.

Abraham, M. (2000). Isolation as a form of marital violence: The South Asian immigrant experience. *Journal of Social Distress and the Homeless, 9*(3), 221–236.

Ames, B. D., Brosi, W. A., & Damiano-Teixeira, K. M. (2006) "I'm just glad my three jobs could be during the day": Women and work in a rural community. *Family Relations, 55*, 119–131.

Bailey, B. A., & Daugherty, R. A. (2007). Intimate partner violence during pregnancy: Incidence and associated health behaviors in a rural population. *Maternal Child Health, 11*, 495–503.

Bauer, H. M., Rodriguez, M. A., Quiroga, S. S., & Flores-Ortiz, Y. G. (2000). Barriers to health care for abused Latina and Asian immigrant women. *Journal of Health Care for the Poor Underserved, 11*, 33–44.

Bhandari, S., Levitch, A., Ellis, K., Ball, K., Everett, K., Geden, E., & Bullock, L. (2008). Comparative analyses of stressors experienced by rural low-income pregnant women experiencing intimate partner violence and those who are not. *JOGNN, 37*, 492–501.

Bosch, K., & Schumm, W. R. (2004). Accessibility to resources: Helping rural women in abusive partner relationships become free from abuse. *Journal of Sex and Marital Therapy, 30*, 357–370.

Bosch, K., & Bergen, M. B. (2006). The influence of supportive and nonsupportive persons in helping rural women in abusive partner relationships become free from abuse. *Journal of Family Violence, 21*, 311–320.

Boyd, M. B., Mackey, M. C., Phillips, K. D., & Tavakoli, A. (2006). Alcohol and other drug disorders, comorbidity and violence in rural African-American women. *Issues in Mental Health Nursing, 27*, 1017–1036.

Bui, H. N. (2003). Help-seeking behavior among abused immigrant women. A case of Vietnamese American women, *Violence Against Women, 2*, 207–239.

Camarota, S. A. (2007) *Immigrants in the United States, 2007: A Profile of America's Foreign-Born Population.* Washington: Center for Immigration Studies.

Campbell, J. C. (2001). *The danger assessment: Research validation from the 12 city femicide study.* Oral Presentation given at Southern Nursing Research Society Annual Conference, February 2001.

Campbell, J. C, Webster, D., & Glass, N. (2009). The Danger Assessment: Validation of a lethality risk assessment instrument for intimate partner femicide. *Journal of Interpersonal Violence, 24*, 653–674.

Choi, N. G. (2001). Diversity within diversity: Research and social work practice issues with Asian American elders. In N. G. Choi (Ed.) *Psychosocial aspects of the Asian-American experience: Diversity within diversity.* New York: Haworth Press, 301–319.

Chow, E. N. L. (1993). The Feminist movement: Where are all the Asian American women? In *Feminist frameworks.* New York: Mc GrawHill.

Dasgupta, S. D., & Warrier, S. (1996). In the footsteps of "Arundhati" Asian Indian Women's experience of domestic violence in the United States. *Violence Against Women, 2*(3), 238–259.

Dasgupta., S. D. (2000). Charting the course: An overview of domestic violence in the South Asian community in the United States. *Journal of Social Distress and the Homeless, 9*(3), 173–185.

Denham, A. C., Frazier, P. Y., Hooten, E. G., Belton, L., Newton, W., Gonzalez, P., et al. (2007). Intimate partner violence among Latinas in Eastern North Carolina. *Violence Against Women, 13*, 123–140.

Denham, S. A. (2003). Describing abuse of pregnant women and their healthcare workers in rural Appalachia. *The American Journal of Maternal Child Nursing, 28*(4), 264–269.

DeKeseredy, W. S., & Joseph, C. (2006). Separation and/or divorce sexual assault in rural Ohio: Preliminary results of an exploratory study. *Violence Against Women, 12*(3), 301–311.

Dye, T., Tolliver, N., Lee, R., & Kenney, C. (1995). Violence, pregnancy and birth outcome in Appalachia. *Paediatric and Perinatal Epidemiology, 9*, 35–47.

Eastman, B. J., & Bunch, S. G. (2007). Providing services to survivors of domestic violence: A comparison of rural and urban service provider perceptions. *Journal of Interpersonal Violence, 22*, 465–473.

Evanson, T. (2006). Intimate partner violence and rural public health nursing practice: Challenges and opportunities. *Online Journal of Rural Nursing and Health Care, 6*(1), 7–20.

Executive Order 13166. (August 11, 2000). "Access to services for persons with limited English proficiency."

Family Violence Prevention Fund (2009). *Background on laws affecting battered immigrant women.* Full list of key resources.

Family Violence Prevention Fund (2009). *Breaking the silence: A training manual for activists, advocates and Latina organizers.* Funded by Office on Violence Against Women, U.S. Department of Justice.

Family Violence Prevention Fund (2009). *Intimate partner violence in the immigrant and refugee community: Challenges, promising practices and recommendations.* A report for the Robert Wood Johnson Foundation.

Feyen, C. (1989). Battered rural women: An exploratory study of domestic violence in a Wisconsin county. *Wisconsin Sociologist, 26*(1), 17–32.

Gallup-Black, A. (2005). Twenty years of rural and urban trends in family and intimate partner homicide: Does place matter? *Homicide Studies, 9*(2), 149–173.

Hu, X., & Chen, G., (1999). Understanding cultural values in counseling Asian families. In J. Carlson (Series Ed.) & K. S. Ng (Vol. Ed.), *The family psychology and counseling series: Vol 2. Counseling Asian families from a systems perspective* (pp. 27–37). Alexandria, VA, American Counseling Association.

Immigration and Naturalization Service. (1997). *1997 statistical yearbook of the Immigration and Naturalization Service.* Washington DC: Author.

Johnson, R. M. (2000). *Rural health response to domestic violence: Policy and practice issues.* Washington, DC: Federal Office of Rural Health Policy, U.S. Department of Health and Human Services.

Kelly, U. (2009). Integrating intersectionality and biomedicine in health disparities research. *Advances in Nursing Science, 32*(2), E42–E56.

Kim, J. H. (1998). *Silence and invisibility: A feminist case study of domestic violence in the lives of five Korean American women* (Doctoral dissertation, University of Illinois at Urbana-Champaign). Ann Arbor, MI: University Microfilms.

Krishnan, S. P., Hilbert, J. C., & Pase, M. (2001). An examination of intimate partner violence in rural communities: Results from a hospital emergency department study from southwest United States. *Family & Community Health, 24*(1), 1–14.

Krishnan, S. P., Hilbert, J. C., & VanLeeuwen, D. (2001). Domestic violence and help-seeking behaviors among rural women: Results from a shelter-based study. *Family and Community Health, 12*(5), 28–38.

Logan, T. K., Walker, R., Cole, J., Ratliff, S., & Leukefeld, C. (2003). Qualitative differences among rural and urban intimate violence experiences and consequences: A pilot study. *Journal of Family Violence, 18*(2), 83–92.

Logan, T. K., Shannon, L., & Walker, R. (2005). Protective orders in rural and urban areas: a multiple perspective study. *Violence Against Women, 11*(7), 876–911.

Logan, T. K., Cole, J., Shannon, L., & Walker, R. (2007). Relationship characteristics and protective orders among a diverse sample of women. *Journal of Family Violence, 22*(4), 237–246.

Malone N., Baluja K. F., Costanzo J. M., et al. (2003). *The foreign-born population: 2000.* Washington: U.S. Census Bureau.

McFarlane, J., Parker, B., & Moran, B. (2006). *Abuse during pregnancy: A protocol for prevention and intervention (3rd edition).* White Plains, NY: March of Dimes.

Mehrotra, M. (1999). The social construction of wife abuse: Experiences of Asian Indian women in the United States. *Violence Against Women, 5*(6), 619–640.

Nolan, M. (2005). Violence and violence prevention in rural America. *Online Journal of Rural Nursing and Health Care, 5*(2), 4p.

Orloff, L. E. (2000). *Statement of NOW Legal Defense and Education Fund in support of HR 3083: The Battered Immigrant Women's Protection Act of 1999.*

Persily, C. A., & Abdulla, S. (2000). Domestic violence and pregnancy in rural West Virginia. *Online Journal of Rural Nursing and Health Care, 1*(3), 11–20.

Raj, A., & Silverman, J. (2002). Violence against immigrant women: The roles of culture, context, and legal immigrant status on partner violence. *Violence Against Women, 3*, 367–398.

Ramirez, R. R. (2004). "We the People: Hispanics in the United States." *Census 2000 Special Reports.* Washington: U.S. Census Bureau.

Reeves, T. J., & Bennett, C. (2004). We the People: Asians in the United States. *Census 2000 Special Reports.* Washington: U.S. Census Bureau, 2004.

Riddell, T., Ford-Gilboe, M., & Leipert, B. (2009). Strategies used by rural women to stop, avoid, or escape from intimate partner violence. *Health Care for Women International, 30*, 134–159.

Shiu-Thornton, S., Senturia, K., & Sullivan, M. (2005). "Like a bird in a cage": Vietnamese women survivors talk about domestic violence. *Journal of Interpersonal Violence, 8*, 959–976.

Song, Y. I. (1996). *Battered women in Korean immigrant families: The silent scream.* New York: Garland.

Teaster, P. B., Roberto, K., & Dugar, T. A. (2006). Intimate partner violence of rural aging women. *Family Relations, 55*, 636–648.

U. S. Census Bureau, (2000). *US Census.*

U.S. Census Bureau (2005). The urban and rural classifications (Ch. 12). Geographic Areas Reference Manual. Retrieved from http://www.census.gov/geo/www/garm.html.

U.S. Department of Commerce, Bureau of Census. (2004). *Current population survey.* Washignton, DC: Author.

Van Hightower, N. R., & Gorton, J. (1998). Domestic violence among patients at two rural health care clinics: Prevalence and social correlates. *Public Health Nursing, 15*(5), 355–362.

Van Hightower, N. R., & Gorton, J. (2002). A case study of community-based responses to rural woman battering. *Violence Against Women, 8,* 845–872.

Websdale, N. (1998). *Rural woman battering and the justice system: An ethnography.* Thousand Oaks, CA: Sage.

Websdale, N., Johnson B., 1998. "An ethnostatistical comparison of the forms and levels of women battering in urban and rural areas of Kentucky." *Criminal Justice Review.* Vol. 23 # 2 Autumn 1998: 161–196.

Willis, S. M. (1998). Recovering from my own little war: Women and domestic violence in rural Appalachia. *Journal of Appalachian Studies, 4,* 255–270.

World Health Organization. (2002). *World report on violence and health.* Geneva: World Health Organization.

World Health Organization. (2005). *WHO multi-country study on women's health and domestic violence against women: Summary report of initial results on prevalence, health outcomes and women's responses.* Geneva: World Health Organization.

9

Nursing Care and Teen Dating Violence: Promoting Healthy Relationship Development

Nina M. Fredland, PhD, RN, FNP
Candace Burton, PhD(c), RN

INTRODUCTION

Adolescence is a period of significant physical, cognitive, social, and emotional growth and development. Young people progress through adolescence into adulthood via similar, but not identical pathways, and at different rates of maturation. Their exposures and experiences along the way affect their responses to the developmental tasks that lead to adult role performance. Some adolescents have more difficulty than others negotiating life's paths and finding their own unique identity. Individual characteristics and demographic factors can either facilitate opportunities for successful maturation or place vulnerable adolescents at additional risk for negative health outcomes.

Interest in romantic relationships often begins in adolescence. By middle school, most adolescents admit some experience with boyfriend or girlfriend relationships. Unfortunately, some encounter negative relationship behaviors in early adolescence, either as victims or perpetrators of abuse. This phenomenon is often referred to as teen dating violence (TDV) and is a form of intimate partner violence (IPV). Adolescent patterns of relationships and relationship abuse do not necessarily parallel adult patterns, however. Therefore, it is imperative that nurse clinicians assess adolescents for TDV using developmentally appropriate approaches. Such strategies necessarily differ from approaches appropriate for assessing adult relationship behavior. In addition to the theories of family violence discussed in chapter 1, the clinician is well advised to consider adolescent developmental stages, as well as "adolescent culture."

Adolescents may be more vulnerable to relationship abuse due to the age-related combination of increased personal mobility and desire for social interaction with limited experiences upon which to base judgments about risk and safety (Finkelhor, Ormrod, & Turner, 2007; Fonagy, 2004; Wolfe, Jaffe, & Crooks, 2006). Although dating violence may have different characteristics and manifestations in the adolescent population, the issue is of no less concern and should not be trivialized. Clinicians such as advanced practice nurses, pediatric nurses, school nurses, and other health care providers who care for adolescents can positively affect adolescent relationship formation while reducing TDV.

DEFINING ADOLESCENCE

The American Academy of Pediatrics (AAP) defines adolescence as the ages between 11 and 21 years (see http://www.aap.org/topics.html). Young people between 11 and 14 years of age are in early adolescence; middle adolescence falls between 15 and 17 years; and late adolescence includes those up to age 21. Some sources further suggest that late adolescence extends into the mid-20s (Arnett, 2000; Brooks-Gunn & Petersen, 1984). For the purposes of this chapter, we will adhere to the AAP categories with a focus on the early and middle adolescence when dating is likely to begin. This represents an excellent window of opportunity for health care professionals to assess for and discuss healthy dating with teens.

The many changes and influences that come to bear on young people during adolescence make for a complex experiential climate and one which care providers must carefully account for in seeking to promote healthy relationship development. During early adolescence, males and females alike experience distinct bodily changes, which may affect both personal and socially defined perceptions of self (Foster, Hagan, & Brooks-Gunn, 2004). Although 11 to 14 or 15 years is usually the age range for the onset of puberty, it is important to note that precocious puberty can begin as early as 8 or 9 (Brooks-Gunn & Petersen, 1984). Full physical maturity is usually achieved by late adolescence. Typically, males lag behind females in pubertal as well as social development. The resulting differences between same-age gender groups have important implications for how each experiences and interacts with peers, family, and other social groups. Gender socialization may influence how friends and dating partners are selected, and how the self is valued—especially where physical maturation leads to changes in relationships. Changes in physicality can also influence self-esteem as well as body image, and physical development greater than that of peers has been correlated with increased risk of relationship abuse as well as decreased perceived social efficacy in some settings (Eccles et al., 1993; Foster et al., 2004). Physical and psychosocial experiences are thus intimately related during adolescence.

Among important psychosocial experiences in adolescence are the developmental tasks of relationship formation and achievement of greater independence from the family of origin (Wolfe et al., 2006). Particular hallmarks of this stage are the increased importance of the peer group and awareness of others' perceptions of the self (Sears, Byers, & Price, 2007). Relationships—whether romantically oriented or not—become a vehicle for evaluating social standing and ultimately self worth as young people examine themselves through the eyes of others (Guthrie, Loveland-Cherry, Frey, & Dielman, 1994; Raty, Larsson, Soderfeldt, & Larsson, 2005). Throughout adolescence, dating relationships may evolve from a group to dyadic orientation with increasing emotional and physical intimacy between partners (Wolfe et al., 2006). Most late adolescents have had at least some experience with a one-on-one caring relationship. For sexual minority (lesbian, gay, bisexual, or transgender) youth, the added dimension of sexual orientation different from heterosexual peers can complicate and even increase the social and personal risks of relationship formation (Freedner, Freed, Yang, & Austin, 2002). Conflicting demands may cause young people to feel that they must choose between risky options—for example, staying in an abusive relationship or becoming a social outcast.

To family members, the adolescent may appear newly self-absorbed and to be spending considerable time alone. Family relationships are often the first to evince the effects of changes in role performance by the adolescent and much has been written about conflict between adolescents and parents (Anthony, 1969; Eccles et al., 1993; Lawson & Brossart, 2004). Although an introspective period is not unusual, negative health symptoms associated with the traumas and growing pains of adolescence may go unnoticed. Communication between parent and adolescent may suffer, especially during the early phases of this transition, when the existing structure and function of the family unit are disrupted (Arnett, 1999; Lloyd, 2004; Petersen, 1988). Nonetheless, communication within the family—whether harmonious or acrimonious—is critical to the adolescent transition and can help to facilitate role change (Gilligan, 1987; Lloyd, 2004). Further, adolescents in many studies have indicated a desire to have open communication with family members even if they are unable to suggest a means of establishing it (Banister & Schreiber, 2001; Lloyd, 2004; Riesch, Jackson, & Chanchong, 2003). Existing relationships—such as those within the family—are critical reference points for adolescents embarking on more significant relationships outside the family. Identifying psychosocial problems and intervening early is critical to prevent negative health sequelae or behaviors associated with this process.

The complexity of adolescence stems from physical and psychosocial growth, both of which are important influences on relationships. Relationships take on new importance during adolescence, and the advent of romantic involvements is an important developmental milestone. Gender socialization, age, and maturity in both physical and psychosocial realms must all be considered in the development of prevention and intervention strategies to promote the health of this vulnerable population. Understanding these and other elements of adolescent culture will allow the clinician to engage in appropriate discussion of dating behaviors and healthy relationship markers with young people.

Adolescent Dating Culture

Many adolescents report experience with "dating" as early as middle school. Fredland, Campbell, and Han (2008) found that 88% of 7th graders stated they had a boy or girlfriend in the past year. Fifty-five percent were currently in a boy or girlfriend relationship, consistent with prevalence rates for dating in the literature. However, the term "dating," in reference to the adolescent population, is outdated or at least inaccurate especially with the early adolescent population (Brown, Puster, Vazquez, Hunter, & Lescano, 2007). Adolescents frequently have different definitions of particular phenomena than adult caregivers or researchers, leading to confusion when assumptions of shared understanding are violated (Haglund, 2003). Adolescents may use terms such as "going out," "hanging out," "hooking up," or "being together" to indicate either emotional or physical relationship interactions. Associated behaviors on a continuum of dating might mean sitting together in the school lunch room at one end of the scale and include sexual behaviors such as oral sex and intercourse at the other (Fredland, Ricardo, Campbell, Sharps, Kub, & Yonas, 2005). Clinicians must be careful not to assume the absence of such behaviors simply because an adolescent denies dating or having a boyfriend or girlfriend (Brown et al., 2007).

Among adolescents, sexual activity may occur in a variety of contexts, often before dyadic dating officially begins. At times, it occurs outside the parameters of a dating-type relationship or one in which a defined couple actually goes somewhere or shares an activity. Astute clinicians must consider the variety of experiences that may increase vulnerability to dating violence and negative health outcomes, as well as personal biases that may influence interactions with adolescents.

Adolescents' efforts to communicate may be obscured by care providers' expectations of difficulty in working with young people, and important health issues can go unresolved. As many as half of all adolescents engage in at least one health risk behavior, including tobacco or alcohol abuse, unprotected sex, or disordered eating (Kulbok & Cox, 2002). These behaviors—at times undertaken to relieve stress or as a means of gaining social status—can be off-putting to care providers, who may infer from the decision to engage in these behaviors a disregard for health and well-being (Kann, Brener, Warren, Collins, & Giovino, 2002; Pinto, 2004). Relationships with supportive health care providers may also be complicated by the difficulty adolescents and young adults face in learning to fully recognize and communicate health-related needs (Machoian, 2005; Montgomery, 2002). This increases the intensity of risks that might otherwise be alleviated by supportive care. Young women, in particular, have been shown to choose silence or evasion rather than risk violating social expectations or causing conflict when dealing with health care providers (Short, Mills, & Rosenthal, 2006). Careful and explicit wording must be used to assess this age group for risks associated with dating or sexual relationships. This assessment should be conducted in a private atmosphere after trust has been established between the adolescent and the clinician and the boundaries of confidentiality are understood.

Conceptualization of Risk and Resilience Factors

In addition to ensuring parity and trust between adolescent and clinician when assessing the health of relationship behaviors, it is also important to be aware of factors that either support or impede the development of healthy relationships among adolescents. Bronfenbrenner's description of the "ecology of human development" proposes that development is fully enmeshed in and always to some degree influenced by "the changing immediate environments in which (an individual) lives, as this process is affected by relations obtaining within and between these immediate settings, as well as the larger social contexts, both formal and informal, in which the settings are embedded" (1977, p. 514). Young people, especially older adolescents, may exhibit behaviors or outward indicators typical of adults, but still lack coping skills for managing unfamiliar situations that are not within their realm of influence. In such situations, the factors in the personal environment that either promote or lessen the potential for an adaptive response are often referred to as risk or resilience (protective) factors. Both can occur in or across multiple aspects of individual experience.

Rew (2005) discusses individual, family, and community factors that protect children and adolescents from adverse outcomes. Individual protective factors promoting healthy growth and development include easy-going temperament, sense of humor, positive self-image, using self-care strategies, internal locus of control, religiosity, intolerance of deviance, good communication skills, academic competence, participation in extracurricular activities, and experience caring for siblings or pets. Family level protective factors include caring parents who connect positively with children; are home at key times of day; expect academic success; disapprove of unhealthy behaviors; and provide a family structure adequate to support healthy family function. Additional protective influence may come from the presence of two parents in the home, fewer than four children, and no prolonged parental absences. Community-related protective factors such as prosocial peer groups and the presence of caring adults including teachers, pastors, and prosocial neighborhood figures to provide positive adult role modeling are also important. Health-promoting communities may be further characterized by the placing of value on the contributions of youth; designating resources for youth development; and creating opportunities for positive youth expression within clear and consistent boundaries. Adolescents growing up in such environments are more likely to complete the developmental tasks of adolescence without becoming derailed by those vulnerabilities and challenges inherent within the adolescent stage of development. Finkelhor et al. (2007) report data from the *Developmental Victimization Survey*, which sought to assess childhood victimization in a longitudinal and nationally representative manner. The findings of this study suggest that although a significant proportion of young people (64% in this sample; $N=1,467$) reported more than one incidence of victimization, not all of them exhibited trauma symptomatology. This implies that for some young people, protective or resilience factors in their environments supported effective coping and reduced vulnerability to particular sequelae of a traumatic experience.

Clearly not all adolescents are fortunate enough to grow up under the supportive circumstances outlined by Rew (2005). An adolescent's health and behavior may be negatively affected by their own exposures and experiences. Many struggle to establish a sense of identity and meet the normative demands of adolescence amid chaotic and dangerous circumstances, as in the study reported above. The effects of such circumstances have been conceptualized as *structural violence*. Structural or social violence refers to the persistent and powerful negative effects of divisions based on race, class, gender, socioeconomic status, or other socially constructed markers that indicate hierarchical ranking (Galtung, 2004; Hardy & Laszloffy, 2005; Scheper-Hughes, 2004). From a developmental perspective, adolescents are seeking new ways to identify themselves and to be identified within society (Wolfe et al., 2006). This often involves confronting the effects of social divisions and recognizing the implications of those divisions at the individual level. Gender, in particular, is often a central issue during this period, with rigidly enforced delineations between male and female (Wiseman, 2002; Wolfe et al., 2006). Much as the demands of multiple, changing social roles must be considered in working with adolescents, so too it is important to consider the diversity of risk for exposure to violence. Modern technological advances and increased mobility afford adolescents many choices and opportunities, some positive and others not so. Compounded by destructive violent media images and in the absence of positive adult role models, these exposures may unduly influence peer and beginning romantic relationships. Family and community violence, inadequate parenting, chaotic or inconsistent family functioning, access to firearms and devitalized, impoverished neighborhoods are risk factors associated with dating violence (Glass, Fredland, Campbell, Sharps, & Kub 2003).

TEEN DATING VIOLENCE

Dating violence in the adolescent population is commonly referred to as TDV in the literature and media; however, it should be noted that TDV encompasses more than physical battering. Adolescents who report abusive relationship experiences include emotional, social, sexual, and economically abusive experiences in their descriptions (Banister, Jakubec, & Stein, 2003; Ismail, Berman, & Ward-Griffin, 2007; Wingood et al., 2006).

An early definition described dating violence as "the use of threat of physical force or restraint that has the purpose of causing injury or pain to another individual" within a dating relationship (Sugarman & Hotaling, 1991, p. 101. Wolfe and colleagues defined dating violence as "any attempt to control or dominate another person [dating partner] physically, sexually, or psychologically, causing some level of harm" (Werkerle & Wolfe, 1999, p. 436.) The Center for Disease Control and Prevention (CDC) defines TDV as a form of IPV including physical, emotional, and sexual abuse (CDC, Understanding Teen Dating Violence Fact Sheet, 2008). Physical abuse includes behaviors such as pinching, scratching, hitting, choking, biting, burning with cigarettes, pushing, shoving, or kicking. Emotional or psychological abuse includes behaviors such as name calling, hurtful teasing, bullying, attacking one's sense of self-worth, isolating a partner from family/ friends, and making threats or engaging in physically threatening behavior. This may also include attempting to engender jealousy in a partner or open displays of infidelity (Banister & Schreiber, 2001; Foshee, Bauman, Linder, Rice, & Wilcher, 2007). Sexual abuse is defined as "forcing a partner to engage in a sex act when he or she does not or cannot consent" (CDC, 2008). Sexual coercion, manipulation, and harassment or teasing may also be present (Poitras & Lavoie, 1995). Other abusive behaviors described in studies of adolescents include damaging personal property (Foshee et al., 2007); constantly calling or texting, visiting a workplace, following a partner from school or work (Chung, 2007); and using social networking sites such as Facebook or MySpace to spread rumors (Picard, Glauber, & Randel, 2007).

Prevalence

TDV is a significant public health problem affecting adolescents of all ages. It is difficult to determine the exact prevalence of TDV due to methodological issues including inconsistent definitions, instrumentation, and time frames for victimization and perpetration. Although most dating violence studies included college age or adult samples, TDV prevalence ranged from 9% to 46% across studies of middle and high school youth, (Glass et al., 2003). Data from the national *Youth Risk Behavior Surveillance Survey* revealed in the year prior to the survey 9.2% of high school students were "hit, slapped or physically hurt on purpose by their boyfriend or girlfriend" and 7.5% were forced to have sexual intercourse without giving consent (CDC, 2008). Forty-eight percent of college-age women (*N*=863) between the ages of 18 and 25 years assessed with the *Abuse Assessment Screen* reported at least one form of dating violence (Amar, & Gennaro, 2005). If unhealthy relationship behaviors are not addressed in young adolescents either before or when they first emerge, negative relationship patterns may evolve into more serious forms of relationship aggression. Some studies report rates of physical victimization less than 10% (Ackard & Neumark-Sztainer, 2002), while others suggest that closer to one half of adolescents have experienced physical abuse in a dating relationship (Halpern, Oslak, Young, Martin, & Kupper, 2001; Hanson, 2002). An often quoted study by Silverman, Raj, Mucci, and Hathaway (2001) found that one in five adolescent girls in high school reported physical or sexual abuse in a dating relationship, and in fact, estimates of the prevalence of dating abuse among adolescent girls have ranged as high as 37% for physical violence and 96% for verbal or psychological aggression (Halpern et al., 2001; Rhatigan & Street, 2005).

Prevalence of dating violence has been shown to have a direct relationship to the age of the population studied, implying that the likelihood of a violent dating experience increases both over time and with number of dating partners (Ackard & Neumark-Sztainer, 2002; Eaton, Davis, Barrios, Brener, & Noonan, 2007). Furthermore, some studies indicate that violence is more common in longer dating relationships as well as in those that are more serious or committed (Marcus, 2004; Munoz-Rivas, Grana, O'Leary, & Gonzalez, 2007; Rhatigan & Street, 2005). This may be due to increasing personal and social investment in longer relationships, which may, in turn, lead to greater tolerance for abusive behaviors.

The study of partner abuse in adolescence usually incorporates some measure of incidents of violence, but there is considerable disagreement about what constitutes a violent incident in an adolescent dating context. Some studies have found evidence that violence in such relationships tends to be bidirectional, initiated by both partners, and committed as often by females as by males—while others have found that the violence is committed by one partner, usually male, and that females are victims more often than not (Cercone, Beach, & Arias, 2005; Foshee et al., 2007; Munoz-Rivas et al., 2007; Sears et al., 2007). Questions have arisen from this research about the incidence of injurious violence versus "play fighting," as described by some participants, as well as about gender-based acceptance of violence and abuse among teenagers in romantic relationships (Cercone et al., 2005; Foshee et al., 2007; Sears, Byers, Whelan, & Saint-Pierre, 2006; Sears et al., 2007). Further, some scholars have questioned the reliability of adolescent-related data collected through questionnaires because of the difficulty associated with establishing definitional consensus with young people (see, for example, Haglund, 2003). As noted previously, adult caregivers must take extra care to ensure that they and their adolescent patients use shared vocabulary to discuss "dating" behaviors. In addition, adolescents' heightened awareness of how they are perceived by others may factor into how and when they disclose physical abuse in response to survey methods (Kann et al., 2002). Both were suggested by the results of a multiple-method study using both questionnaires and follow-up interviews. Although the participants selected for interview were specifically those who had previously reported use of at least one type of physically aggressive behavior in a dating relationship, nearly one fifth denied physical aggression of any kind, while approximately one third described their behaviors as strictly playful in nature (Foshee et al., 2007). Here, as in other aspects of adolescent health study, the importance of accounting for psychosocial context and development is demonstrated.

Despite evidence that psychological and emotionally abusive behaviors are both more common and often the precursors to physical violence in adult relationships, little research has yet been published about the role of these issues in adolescent dating relationships. What data have been gathered indicate that these nonphysical types of abuse are extremely common, with some studies suggesting that they occur in up to 90% of dating relationships (Foshee et al., 2007; Halpern et al., 2001; Hanson, 2002; Hines & Saudino, 2003; Munoz-Rivas et al., 2007). Further, it is apparent from the extant literature on dating abuse that psychological and emotional abuse are of concern to adolescents in dating relationships (Banister et al., 2003; Sears et al., 2006). In part, the difficulty with studying psychological or emotional abuse in adolescence arises from their ubiquity among this age group, whether in the context of a dating relationship or otherwise (Munoz-Rivas et al., 2007). Since such attacks often have no immediate outward manifestations, they may continue unabated for some time (Matheson, Skomorovsky, Fiocco, & Anisman, 2007). Psychological abuse may thus be used as a means of controlling a dating partner when other types of control are not possible. This is uniquely important in the context of adolescent dating relationships, where partners usually do not live together and may even be separated from each other regularly (Lewis & Fremouw, 2001).

The issue of who has more control in the relationship is often particularly problematic with regard to sexual decision making among adolescents and complicates assessment of the prevalence of sexually abusive behaviors in adolescents' relationships. An analysis of data from the 1995 *Youth Risk Behavior Survey* (YRBS) found that forced sexual activity positively predicted violence in a date situation (Kreiter, Krowchuk, Woods, Sinal, Lawless, & DuRant 1999), illustrating the complex functions of sexual coercion in abusive dating relationships and suggesting how such coercion may combine both physical and emotional abuse. Recognizing the many ways in which abusive behaviors can affect adolescents' dating experiences will assist the clinician in providing appropriate prevention, intervention, and support resources.

HEALTH OUTCOMES AND TEEN DATING VIOLENCE

Abusive relationship experiences may occur even before the second decade of life and may set the stage for difficult relationship patterns that extend into adulthood. Recent literature suggests that traumatic experiences, such as IPV, have both immediate and long-term effects and that these effects are compounded by repeated exposure (Epel et al., 2004; Epel et al., 2006; Follette, Polusny, Bechtle, & Naugle, 1996). Current research suggests that each incidence of violence and abuse increases overall lifetime risks for additional exposures, often encompassing the development of patterns across the lifespan (Finkelhor et al., 2007; Silverman et al., 2001). The authors of the Adverse Childhood Experiences (ACE) study reported consistent and graded relationships between increasing numbers of traumatic exposures before the age of 18 and incidence of adult health problems (Dube et al., 2006). In addition, traumatic experiences prior to adulthood may contribute to the development of certain chronic illnesses later in life—including cancer, stroke, chronic bronchitis or emphysema, ischemic heart disease, and depression (Green & Kimerling, 2004; Walker, Newman, & Koss, 2004).

Relationship violence has been specifically correlated with negative health outcomes. The important work of Campbell and colleagues (2002) focused attention beyond the physical injuries associated with abuse. In a case control study of women ($N=2,535$) age 21 to 55 years of age, researchers found that the abused women reported significantly more aches, pains, sexually transmitted infections (STIs), stress, neurological and digestive symptoms when compared with nonabused women (Campbell et al., 2002). These same health problems may occur in adolescents who experience abuse. Home violence exposures and personal victimization were also found to have significant direct effects on physical, mental, and behavioral health in a sample ($N=309$) of urban African American middle school students (Fredland et al., 2008).

Dating violence is particularly associated with risky behaviors that impact health such as early sexual debut (before age 15), increased number of sexual partners, increased use of alcohol, alcohol use initiated at a younger age, increased use of illegal substances, and smoking (Eaton et al., 2007; Diaz, Simantov, & Vaughn, 2002). Adolescent female victims of dating violence (physical and/or sexual) were significantly more likely to abuse drugs, engage in unhealthy forms of weight control, begin sexual activity earlier, become pregnant, and attempt suicide (Silverman et al., 2001). Elsewhere, a sample of African American adolescent females reporting experiences of dating violence were more likely to have been pregnant, contracted a sexually transmitted infection, and had nonmonogamous relationships than peers who did not report abuse (Wingood, DiClemente, McCree, Harrington, & Davies, 2001). The same sample demonstrated negative views of their overall sexual health, ability to sustain healthy relationship dynamics, or negotiate contraception practices.

Pregnancy is a particularly important issue related to adolescent dating abuse because of the overlapping issues of adolescent pregnancy, development, and abusive relationships. Negative health outcomes related to pregnancy have been positively correlated with abuse and include low birth weight babies, uterine bleeding, anemia, and infections (McFarlane, 2004). Renker (1999) found that pregnant adolescents experiencing physical abuse had significantly lower birth weight babies than nonabused counterparts, and that the same group experienced more complications of pregnancy and had greater rates of substance use during pregnancy. Conversely, a sample of adolescent males participating in a program for perpetrators of dating violence indicated disregard for pregnancy prevention as well as a willingness to engage in risky sexual behaviors with multiple partners (Silverman et al., 2006). Similarly, a study of young women's descriptions of partners' behavior in abusive relationships indicated that pregnancy prevention was often rejected or sabotaged by the partner (Miller et al., 2007). Further, Lindhorst and Oxford (2008) showed that depressive symptoms in early adulthood and experiences of intimate partner violence among adolescent mothers were related. These findings clearly demonstrate the health risks that proceed from TDV. Further investigation is warranted related to TDV and health outcomes particularly since rates for adolescent relationship abuse are as prevalent as or higher than adult reports of IPV.

Assessing Teen Dating Violence

Nurses and other health professionals advocate for routine screening for abuse; yet, this is not widely or consistently implemented. Specific guidelines for the assessment of dating violence in adolescents are not yet available. Websites such as Guidelines. gov provide information related to incorporating sexuality education into pediatric practice, particularly for female adolescents who are sexually active. The guideline is titled "Sexuality Education for Children and Adolescents" available at http:// www. guideline.gov/summary/summary.aspx?doc_id=3084&nbr=002310&string=dating+ AND+violence. A number of agencies have resources available specific to TDV. Suggestions for important assessment topics and selected tools are detailed in the following paragraphs.

The SAFE TIMES Health Interview is a mnemonic aid to assist clinicians in organizing a comprehensive screening for adolescents. Although it is not specific for TDV, the subject of safety and abuse are part of the interview. (see Table 9.1 for the SAFE TIMES Health Interview.)

TABLE 9.1   SAFE TIMES Health Interview

SAFE TIMES Health Interview	
Topic	Focus of Assessment
Sexuality	Reproduction, sexual activity, sexual transmitted infections (STIs), and relationships
Affect/Abuse	Feelings of sadness, depression, alcohol and other drug use including
Family	Family history, adolescent living situation, family conflicts
Examination	Self breast/testicular exam, pelvic exam if sexually active
Timing of Development	Explore attitudes around rate of maturation, body image, weight
Immunizations	See www.cdc.gov for updates and recommended child and adolescent immunization schedule
Minerals	Healthy nutritional choices include calcium, iron, and cholesterol/lipid
Education/Employment	School performance, work situation, future goals
Safety	Drinking and driving, seat belt use

Another mnemonic aid, HEEADSSS, may be preferred as a clinical tool. It is more specific to the prevention of sexual violence and related negative sequelae. HEEADSSS (HEADS) prompts clinicians to assess the following:

- Home
- Education, Employment, Eating
- Activities with peers
- Drugs
- Sexuality, Suicide and depression, Safety

A full explanation of the guide and sample questions in each area is available at the American Academy of Pediatrics internet site available at http://www.aap.org/pubserv/PSVpreview/start.html.

Another brief assessment tool, *Health Survey for Adolescents*, developed as part of a collaborative initiative between the New York State Department of Health and the University of Rochester Adolescent Medicine Division, can be easily incorporated into the adolescent interview. This tool is available at http://www.adolescenthealth.org/clinicalcare.htm#ScreeningQuestionnaires. The questions in Exhibit 9.1, adapted from the *Health Survey for Adolescents*, clearly state the behaviors being assessed in language understandable to the adolescent age group and are designed to assess high-priority health areas for adolescents. Response choices are: *never, once or twice, three or more times.*

EXHIBIT 9.1 | *Adapted from Health Survey for Adolescents*

- Have you ever done something violent because you were angry?
- Have you had sex (vaginal, anal, oral)?
- If you have had sex, how often do you use condoms (rubbers)?
- Have you ever been forced to have sex you did not want or has someone touched you in a way that made you feel uncomfortable (touching of breasts, buttocks, or genitals)?
- Has anyone at home, school, or anywhere else made you feel afraid, threatened you, or hurt you?

For tips related to establishing a trust relationship and maintaining confidentiality for the adolescent during the health interview, visit the internet site: http://www.adolescenthealth. org. Health care providers can also access helpful tips for coding and billing while maintaining confidentiality at the same site sponsored by The Society for Adolescent Medicine.

EVIDENCE-BASED INTERVENTIONS TO REDUCE TEEN DATING VIOLENCE

A systematic review of scientific evidence published in the literature was conducted by the Community Preventive Services Task Force (Hahn, Fuqua-Whitley, Wethington, Lowy, Liberman, Crosby, et al., 2007). Their recommendation to implement universal school-based programs was based on strong evidence that such primary prevention strategies can prevent or reduce violent behavior. Of the studies reviewed, only one was evidence-based and specific for TDV prevention, the Safe Dates Program. *Safe Dates*, a school-based intervention designed to change normative behaviors and improve problem solving, includes both primary and secondary strategies and advocates for community participation in the program (Foshee, et al., 1996). Students (N = 957) in 8th and 9th grade in 10 rural public schools were randomly assigned by schools matched according to size to either the treatment or control condition. Students in the treatment school were exposed to a dating violence play and received a 10-session education curriculum. Students who participated in the *Safe Dates* program were significantly less likely to report physical and sexual dating violence victimization and perpetration at the 4-year follow-up assessment (Foshee et al., 2004).

Primary prevention effort should begin before dating and before the age when TDV is likely to emerge, usually between the ages of 15 and 16 years (Wekerle & Wolfe, 1999). Many adolescents engage in a coercive "playful" interactional style. When "play" becomes a pathway to dating, violence remains unclear. Adolescent girls have voiced concerns that boys use the term "play" to justify aggressive actions (Fredland et al., 2005). Frequently, adolescent intimates confuse jealousy and controlling behaviors with love and devotion (Werkerle & Wolfe, 1999). Most prevention strategies have focused on primary prevention through classroom education (Foshee et al., 1996; Jaffe, Suderman, Reitzel, & Killip, 1992; Macgowan, 1997, Avery-Leaf, Cascardi, O'Leary, & Cano, 1997). However, prevention programs have not been widely adopted. Screening for abuse has occurred in school settings in the context of research (Foshee, et al., 1996; Coker, et al., 2000). Mostly, this has been anonymous data gathered for the purpose of gathering information on TDV prevalence (Glass et al., 2003).

Secondary prevention through routine assessment of all teenagers for IPV has been advocated, since the rates of IPV reported actually have been higher in teens compared to adult women (Parker, McFarlane, Soeken, Torres, & Campbell, 1993; McFarlane & Parker, 1994). There were also no differences in the severity or frequency of the violence experienced between the groups of teens or adults. Despite the fact that victims and perpetrators of dating violence routinely visit health clinics, including school-based clinics, the practice of routine screening has not been implemented. Research findings support the screening of all women including teenagers.

Contrary to the view that women and girls might be offended by nurses and other health care professionals asking about experiences of IPV, evidence suggests that women are supportive of the practice. In a qualitative study (N = 36), Koziol-McLain and colleagues found that 35 women (97%) screened either in the emergency department or clinic setting positively endorsed IPV assessment (Koziol-McLain, Giddings, Rameka, &

Fyfe, 2008). This was true for women who had a history of IPV, women who were currently in an abusive relationship, and also for those women who stated they never were abused by an intimate partner. These women appreciated being asked about IPV. The women with abusive histories felt they now had permission to disclose the abuse experienced, and women who were not ever abused by an intimate partner thought it was an important strategy to reduce IPV for all women.

Additionally, abused women seek health services more often than nonabused women (Willson et al., 2001); therefore, it is likely that teens in abusive relationships use school health services more frequently than teens not in abusive relationships. Nurses in all settings are well positioned to initiate screening for teens (Lazzaro & Mc Farlane, 1991). Nurses and other health care professionals in school settings have a unique opportunity to access adolescents and screen for dating violence.

Sexual Coercion and Assault

Sexuality is often initially explored during adolescence. Approximately 80% of young people will have a sexual encounter sometime between puberty and the end of the transition to adulthood (Wolfe et al., 2006). Decision making about sexual issues may therefore be subject to the influences of peers, social groups, dating partners, and others who contribute to the adolescent's conceptualization of identity (Fantasia, 2008). Adolescents may, in fact, rely heavily on such external sources of evaluative criteria because they lack sufficient personal experiences to support negotiation and self-determination in making sexual decisions (Wolfe et al., 2006). This creates a situation of considerable vulnerability for many young people, in that opportunities for manipulation and victimization around sexual activity may be considerable. For adolescents and young adults experiencing abusive relationships, sexual activity may represent an additional locus of control and victimization. The issue of control as it relates to standing in the relationship is particularly problematic with regard to sexual decision making among adolescents. Banister et al. (2003) reported that among the young women in their study, a "position of disadvantage in the relationship" was evident in descriptions of sexual negotiation (p. 23). These young women referred to sex as a means of sustaining their relationships, rather than as a mutually agreed-upon aspect of romantic partnership: "The participants were so fearful of 'losing the relationship,' and thus their social status, that they subordinated their own needs to the . . . needs . . . of their boyfriend" (p. 23). Other investigators have reported similar findings with regard to the ways in which sexual coercion occurs in adolescent relationships, notably combining the dynamics of other types of abuse. For example, Foshee and colleagues (2007) describe a young man who stated that he had pushed a girl out of the car for refusing to have sex with him, and an analysis of data from the 1995 YRBS found that forced sexual activity positively predicted violence in a date situation (Kreiter et al., 1999). In another study by Banister and Schreiber (2001), young women voiced unhappiness with what they saw as their partners' disrespect for them when pressured to have sex, as well as a sense of lost self-respect in succumbing to such pressure.

Nurses, particularly those on school and college campuses, must be aware of various types of sexual coercion and assault or forced sex. Rape is often assumed to refer to an act of completed sexual penetration that is unwanted, forced, or threatened by force, but many sexually assaultive encounters do not involve penetration and some may not even involve physical contact (Banyard & Cross, 2008; Foshee et al., 2004; Fredland, 2008;

Koss et al., 2007; Sears et al., 2007). Many studies report that 16- to 24-year women are the most vulnerable to rape in the sense of forced sexual intercourse, with one in four experiencing such an assault (Sampson, 2003). Other types of sexual assault, such as unwanted sexual touching, sexual coercion—whether successful or not, sexual bullying or harassment, showing pornographic materials without consent, using technology such as social networking sites or cell phones to start sexual rumors or to send unwanted sexual messages or images, or creating sexual or pornographic images without the subject's consent are also common, with rates over 50% in some samples (Fisher, Cullen, & Turner, 2000; The National Campaign to Prevent Teen and Unplanned Pregnancy, 2008). Such insidious sexual attacks are particularly problematic among adolescents because of the complex social structures and peer interactions that are characteristic of this population (Armstrong, Hamilton, & Sweeney, 2006). The perpetrator is often known to the victim and may, in fact, be a part of the victim's social group. In such situations, adolescents may feel compelled by peers to remain silent about the assault in order to sustain group and individual relationship dynamics (Black, Tolman, Callahan, Saunders, & Weisz, 2008; Schad, Szwedo, Antonishak, Hare, & Allen, 2008).

Much effort has been made to prevent sexual assaults among adolescents and young adults. Historically, many prevention programs focused on sexual violence by a stranger. These programs emphasized self-defense, being aware of one's surroundings, not being alone in dark and lonely places, etc. Of course this is prudent; however, current statistical data indicates that many sexual assaults are not committed by unknown perpetrators (Rickert, Wiemann, & Vaughan, 2005; Tjaden & Thoennes, 2000). Moracco, Runyan, Bowling, and Earp (2007) found that known intimates were the perpetrators of sexual assaults against women three times as often as unknowns. Among adolescents, experiences of sexual assault, coercion, and bullying are likely even more often committed by someone close to the victim due to the constancy of many adolescents' involvement in social groups or peer milieus. This social context is an important consideration, and in cases of sexual coercion and bullying among adolescents, it is critical for health care providers to be aware of the psychosocial and developmental ramifications of such experiences. Nurses who are knowledgeable about the risks of sexual assaults by acquaintances or peers will have enhanced assessment skills, enabling them to provide anticipatory guidance conversations, appropriate treatment options, and counseling in preventing and treating adolescents who are at risk for or who have experienced sexually assaultive attacks.

Little research has yet addressed the use of technology as a tool of sexual bullying or coercion, and it may be that cell phones and social networking websites are often used in these ways, such that even while living at home, adolescents can incur considerable risk for these types of attacks. The increasing use of technology by young people has important implications for nursing care of this population, since it is accessible to adolescents of all ages. Although recent effort has been made to protect young people from online predation, little emphasis has been placed on peer interactions that may be abusive in nature.

Another type of sexual assault, acquaintance or date rape usually occurs at the end of a date and accounts for 13% of completed college rapes (Sampson, 2003). If attempted rape is also included in the definition, the prevalence rises to 35%. Studies suggest that the availability and consumption of alcohol plays a role in the occurrence of such assaults (Parks, Hsieh, Bradizza, & Romosz, 2008; Ullman, Karabatsos, & Koss, 1999). Further, drugs such as gamma hydroxybutyrate (GHB), ketamine, and flunitrazepam (Rohypnol) have been implicated as facilitators of sexual assault when added to drinks in social situations (Nicoletti, 2009). As such, adolescents should be made aware of the dangers of acquaintance rape, as well as the associated temporal and spatial risk factors. The role of alcohol consumption as a contributing factor cannot be denied and should be addressed; however, survivors must be supported and encouraged to not blame themselves or fail to report incidents of rape out of fear of reprisal, shame, or because they doubt their story will be perceived as a credible one. Trust is a critical element of successful relationships between adolescent and health care providers, and especially in cases where an adolescent has already experienced a sexual assault, must be preserved in order to provide effective care.

The challenges of providing preventive and intervention resources to adolescents with regard to abuse, sexual coercion, and assault in the context of relationship behaviors are considerable. As with other abusive relationship behaviors, prevention of sexual victimization among adolescents requires emphasis on healthy relationship behaviors and peer culture in combination with education on personal awareness and safety. The health consequences of sexual victimization can include disordered eating, depression, and anxiety (Krupnick et al., 2004), as well as posttraumatic stress disorder (Breslau, Wilcox, Storr, Lucia, & Anthony, 2004) and sexual risk behaviors (Senn, Carey, Vanable, Coury-Doniger, & Urban, 2007). Any of these outcomes can have severe and long-term effects on the health of an adolescent or young adult, and represents significant risk without intervention. Nurses and other health care providers must consider the potential health impact of sexual victimization among adolescents, and should be prepared to assess for symptoms as well as provide supportive care options.

Teen Dating Violence Warning Signs

Signs and symptoms of an unhealthy or abusive dating relationship may be quite subtle. Frequently, teens will not tell anyone about their concerns, or they may not recognize the behaviors as aberrant. For this reason, it is important for clinicians to be vigilant, maintain a high degree of suspicion, as well as become astute in recognizing TDV, assessing for TDV, and intervening when indicated.

Physical Signs and Symptoms

Physical evidence is most likely to be observed if it is on a part of the body that is easily observed. Opportunities to assess unusual marks are easily inquired about during the course of the physical examination. The literature has documented that patients are willing to disclose, but are often not asked about abuse or the disclosure is not recognized as disclosure (McFarlane, Groff, O'Brien, & Watson, 2006). Therefore, clinicians should maintain a high degree of suspicion and inquire about the following:

- Bruises, scratches, or injuries
- Explanations that do not seem to fit the injury

For example, a young woman in late adolescence presented to the Emergency Department with a wound to the knee requiring several stitches. She stated that in the process of cooking a knife fell off the counter and caused injury to the knee, when, in fact, she was a victim of stabbing by an abusive boyfriend. Asking a few additional questions would likely have encouraged the young woman to disclose the truth. For example, the nurse clinician could ask: Who was with you at the time of the "accident"? What other injuries have you had in the past (recent or in the more distant past)? The next natural inquiry would ask about the quality of any existing or past relationships. Remember that abuse can continue even after a relationship has ended.

Psychological Signs and Symptoms

Psychological or emotional abuse is often overlooked or not considered to be as harmful as physical abuse, but indeed, it may be the most prevalent and possibly the most devastating form of TDV. These behaviors left unchecked may escalate to physical abuse. Clues to possible emotional abuse are presented in Table 9.2.

The *Teen Equality Wheel* (available at: http://www.ncdsv.org/images/TeenEquality-wheelNOSHADING-NCDSV.pdf) developed and distributed by the National Center on Domestic and Sexual Violence is a positive approach to educating teens about nonviolent healthy relationships and is in contrast to the often used Power and Control Wheel. Both wheels can be used in practice as a primary prevention strategy to promote healthy relationships by engaging adolescents in conversations about their relationships. Eight important areas are addressed in the Teen Equality wheel: Communication, Negotiation and Fairness, Nonthreatening Behavior, Respect, Shared Power, Self-Confidence and Personal Growth, Honesty and Accountability, and Trust and Support.

The Abuse Assessment Screen (AAS), a three-item measure developed by McFarlane, Parker, Soeken, and Bullock (1992) for assessing abuse during pregnancy is widely used

TABLE 9.2   *Psychological (Emotional) Abuse*

What to look for in someone who is the recipient or perpetrator of abuse	
Recipient of the Abuse:	Perpetrator of the Abuse:
• Apologetic attitude about a boyfriend or girlfriend's behavior • Fearfulness toward a boyfriend or girlfriend • Sudden change in appearance or behavior • Loss of interest in things or activities formerly enjoyed, such as skateboarding, going to the movies with friends, and/or joining in after school activities • Change in school performance (less time for studying or attending class) • Less time spent with family members and friends • Personality or mood changes including anxiety, depression, acting out, or spending more time alone than usual • Abnormal secretive behaviors, avoidance, not making eye contact, unexplained crying, or irrational outbursts • Alcohol or other drug use • Joking about the boyfriend's or girlfriend's temper or aggressive behavior, but using the excuse of "just playing"	• Controlling behavior related to decision-making, dressing, friends or familial associations. • Jealous, possessive behavior; i.e., checking up or stalking behavior, either directly or indirectly through cell phones and other forms of media/communication • Continual criticisms or insulting put down messages • Aggressive, abusive behavior of a boyfriend or girlfriend toward other individuals or animals • Vandalism behavior toward the property of the patient or others

Adapted from the National Youth Violence Prevention Resource Center: http://www.safeyouth.org/scripts/faq/datingwarning.asp

for screening, in general, because it is brief. This tool can be used with teens although to our knowledge has not been scientifically tested in this population. Clinicians can easily incorporate the following questions into their practice regimen and alter the language so that it resonates with adolescents.

1. Have you ever been emotionally or physically abused by your partner or someone important to you?
2. Within the last year have you been hit slapped, kicked, or otherwise physically hurt by someone?
3. Within the last year, has anyone forced you to have sex?

It may also be important to include a question about pushing and shoving as that may indicate more severe forms of violence. Adolescents state that hallways and passing periods are opportunities for violence. For example, one middle school-age girl reported being slammed into the lockers during school. The assistant principal accused her of being partly to blame as she had been spotted walking home with the male perpetrator on multiple occasions. Upon further questioning, the girl disclosed that she was an unwilling participant escorted home from school by the male in question. Her mother worked three jobs and was not home at a critical time, i.e., when she returned home from school. Sometimes what seems obvious is not the reality of the situation. In reality, the young adolescent was being stalked on a daily basis. The Family Violence Prevention Fund site includes questions that can help teens decide if they are in a healthy or unhealthy relationship. Key questions specific to teens are included in Table 9.3.

Safety Planning

All teens should have a safety plan even if they are not in an unhealthy or abusive relationship. Such a plan is a safety measure, so they will be prepared if they ever find themselves in an unexpected or uncomfortable situation. If TDV is disclosed, clinicians should specifically address a safety plan. Cohabitating adolescents are most at-risk and should establish a regular routine for leaving home without drawing attention to their actions. For example, leaving for work, school, or to go to the gym on a regular basis is a good idea. Touching base with a trusted friend or adult at specific time intervals is an-

TABLE 9.3 *Healthy Versus Unhealthy Relationship*

Healthy Relationship	Unhealthy Relationship
Does a boyfriend or girlfriend: • Communicate openly with you when there are problems? • Give you space to spend time with your friends and family? • Act supportive and respectful?	Does a boyfriend or girlfriend: • Control where you go, what you wear, or what you do? • Try to stop you from seeing or talking to family or friends? • Call you derogatory names, put you down, or criticize you? • Threaten or scare you? • Hit, slap, push, or kick you? • Force you to do something sexual when you do not want to?

Adapted from: http://endabuse.org/userfiles/file/PublicCommunications/Recognizing%20Teen%20Dating%20Abuse.pdf

other safety measure recommended for all individuals regardless of age or circumstance. If the adolescent drives, he or she should keep the gas tank full and have an extra set of keys available. Hotlines such as the National Teen Dating Abuse Helpline (866-331-9474) can provide temporary shelter in an emergency. See Exhibit 9.2 for a detailed Teen Safety Plan adapted from the *Family Violence Prevention Fund* internet site: http://endabuse.org/ userfiles/file/PublicCommunications/Create%20a%20Teen%20Safety%20Plan.pdf.

The most dangerous time for an adult is usually when the abused person decides to leave their abuser. Similarly, ending an abusive teen relationship may also be the most dangerous time. Teens should seek advice from a trained expert by calling the National Teen Dating Abuse Helpline or a local resource to ensure safety after leaving the relationship. Remember, family members may not always understand what the teen is going through. Many times, they may inadvertently support ways to reconcile differences. This may be well meaning, but some blame is inappropriately placed on the victim. Family members may not realize that the violence in an abusive relationship usually escalates over time. In such situations, teens should find another trusted person to confide in such as a teacher, nurse, or coach. More information is available at www.endabuse.org under TEENS.

A compendium of IPV and sexual violence assessment tools, although not specific for adolescents, is a useful reference and includes the *Abuse Assessment Tool* as well as a school/work assessment tool and one specific for pediatric settings (Basile, Hertz, & Back, 2007). Reviewing these instruments may help nurses and other health care professionals gain knowledge about available victimization assessment tools and aid in the selection of the most appropriate screening instrument for a particular setting. Documentation can be facilitated by the use of a good instrument, and this aspect of assessment is an important consideration for clinical and legal reasons. Please refer to chapter 14 for further discussion related to documentation.

EXHIBIT 9.2 | *Teen Safety Plan*

Items to keep handy:
- Cash
- Keys
- ATM cards/checkbooks
- Driver's license/passport/official ID
- Medications, eyeglasses/contact lenses
- Medical records
- Mobile phone, jump drive, lap top
- Legal documents, such as a protection or restraining order
- A change of clothes

If a teen is a parent in custody of a child, additional child related items include:
- Bottles, formula, lactation pump
- Diapers
- Birth Certificate, custodial agreement
- Medical records, medication
- Extra clothes
- Comfort object-toy, stuffed animal, pacifier, and/or security blanket

Call a hotline or someone you trust. Keep phone numbers handy.
Choose a safety code word or action to signal immediate danger.
Have a secret meeting place where you can be picked up by friend or family.
If safety is a concern, do not end the relationship in person.

EXHIBIT 9.3 | *Case Study*

Advanced practice nurses attending a regional meeting were distressed by the report of an alleged rape of a sophomore girl in the parking lot of a local high school by her "boyfriend." The incident spawned discussion among the nurses about dating practices, alcohol consumption, and sexual activity among the students. Several of the nurses worked in school-based clinics or in health services for nearby school districts. The consensus was that the issue of dating violence needed to be addressed on all levels in developmentally appropriate ways. The nurses decided to make TDV prevention a health priority for the upcoming school year. An ad hoc committee drafted the following agenda to explore the issues:

1. Establish a core committee to develop guidelines for developmentally appropriate primary, secondary, and tertiary prevention strategies addressing TDV in middle and high schools within school districts.
2. Partner with local schools of nursing, a natural strategy since primary care sites and schools are regular sites for clinical rotations for public health student nurses, family, and pediatric nurse practitioner students.
3. Using the *School Health Personnel TDV Survey*, assist interested parties with the assessment to determine the level of education nurses and school professionals have about the topic of TDV, and their confidence in recognizing and intervening related to TDV (see *School Health Personnel TDV Survey*).

School Health Personnel TDV Survey
- Did a student report observing TDV to you in the past year?
- Did a student report a personal experience with TDV to you in the past year?
- How prepared do you feel to respond when a TDV incident is reported to you?
- Have you observed an incident of aggression between teen dating couples in the past year?
- How prepared do you feel to intervene when you observe an incident of TDV?
- Have you ever intervened in a TDV situation in school?
- Have you ever assisted a student victim of TDV?
- How prepared do you feel to address TDV with a student victim?
- Have you ever assisted a student perpetrator of TDV?
- How prepared do you feel to address aggressive behavior with student perpetrator of TDV?
- Is there a program or policy related to TDV where you work?
- How receptive would administrators, faculty/staff at your school be to implement a TDV policy?

Exhibit 9.3 presents a hypothetical scenario and a method for community assessment as a first step to determine the ability, perceptions, and willingness of nurses who work with adolescents to identify and intervene in situations of TDV.

SUMMARY

Dating abuse during adolescence has many possible impacts on young people's health and safety. This chapter provides an overview of some of the most pertinent considerations for nurses and other health care professionals seeking to intervene with adolescents in unhealthy and abusive relationships. Ensuring young people's awareness of this risk and of available resources is an important function of those serving this population. Being prepared to engage adolescents in dialogue about relationships involves cultivating understanding of the ways in which both healthy and unhealthy types of relationships occur in and affect their lives, as well as recognizing the role of the care provider in assessing for and remediating abusive experiences.

Critical changes in self-perception occur during adolescence, notably the transition from a centering on self-perception to awareness of and focus on the perceptions of others (Wolfe et al., 2006). As such, the significance of relationships of all kinds in the lives of adolescents cannot be overestimated. Social, emotional, physical, and cognitive developmental factors are critical concerns in the establishment of strategies for the prevention of and intervention in abusive adolescent relationships. An understanding of adolescent developmental issues and their role in relationship formation can help nurses and other care providers to provide care appropriate to both the age and cultural environment of the adolescent.

Adolescent patterns of formation and participation in romantic and other relationships are not always similar to those of adults, and may vary with age and physical development (Foster et al., 2004). Further, both of these factors may bear on personal self concept and self-esteem, which have been shown to affect perceptions of social efficacy and identity (Raty et al., 2005). Identity, in particular, is at issue for many adolescents, who may be newly cognizant of peer group affiliations and relationships as markers of social standing (Guthrie et al., 1994). Gender socialization is also often a significant part of peer group dynamics, influencing interactions between dating partners as well as overall group interactions. Gender norms can influence relationship behaviors in many ways, and adolescents may feel that adhering to the norms of their peers requires them to value dating and other kinds of relationships in specific ways—potentially at the expense of their own health or other needs (Wolfe et al., 2006).

In addition to the roles of developmental processes, physical changes, gender, and peer norms, environmental factors may also affect the potential for abusive dating experiences among adolescents. Both risk and resilience can be generated by elements in the adolescent's environs, ranging from individual-level elements such as self-care behaviors and communication skills to community-level elements such as contact with prosocial role models and youth resources (Rew, 2005). Where environmental risk factors are especially pernicious, and coupled with social divisions that enforce hierarchical identification, adolescents may be affected by structural violence. Structural violence conceptualizes the experience of being part of a denigrated social group as a particularly personal type of violent experience and one that can have ramifications for the health of adolescents as significant as any other type of violent exposure (Scheper-Hughes, 2004).

Commonly referred to as TDV, abusive relationships between adolescents may encompass behaviors well beyond physical violence. These include emotional and sexual victimization and may range from threats to harm self or others to forced sexual intercourse (Banister & Schreiber, 2001; Foshee et al., 2007). Among adolescents, behaviors involving social manipulation such as electronic abuse via social networking sites, text messaging, or alienation from peer groups may pose considerable threat to sense of self and identity development processes as well (Banister et al., 2003; Picard et al., 2007). Given the diversity of behaviors occurring in abusive relationships between adolescents, prevalence estimates vary wildly depending upon the definition of abuse employed and whether assessments were for a single relationship or lifetime incidences: studies have shown rates ranging from 9% to 96% (Glass et al., 2003; Halpern et al., 2001). Factors affecting these rates also include age of participants and length of relationship (Chung, 2007; Munoz-Rivas et al., 2007), commitment to the relationship (Rhatigan & Street, 2005), gender of perpetrator and victim (Cercone et al., 2005; Sears et al., 2007), definitions of violence versus flirtatious or "play" behavior (Foshee et al., 2007), and the establishment of trust and congruency between researcher and participants (Chung, 2007; Kann et al., 2002). The diversity of these considerations alone demonstrates the many considerations health care providers must have in mind when working with adolescents to establish healthy patterns of relationship behavior and to prevent TDV.

A major concern for health care providers, the ramifications of TDV for health during adolescence and into adulthood are as diverse as the issues affecting its prevalence. Although some health care providers have been reluctant to screen for relationship violence, failing to do so may have great impact on an adolescent's health and safety. Unplanned pregnancy, acquisition of sexually transmitted infection, use of alcohol and other substances, smoking, suicidal ideation and attempt, and unhealthy weight control have all been correlated with experiences of TDV (Eaton et al., 2007; Lindhorst & Oxford, 2008; Silverman et al., 2006; Silverman, Raj, & Clements, 2004; Silverman et al., 2001; Wingood et al., 2001). The immediate risks to the health of adolescents engaging in these behaviors, compounded by involvement in abusive relationships, are considerable and may affect health well into adulthood. Traumatic experiences—such as TDV—have been linked to a range of chronic health problems, as well as to increases in risk for additional victimization and to the development of patterns of violent experience across the lifespan (Campbell et al., 2002; Finkelhor et al., 2007; Follette et al., 1996; Walker et al., 2004).

Tools to identify and intervene with adolescents experiencing TDV are critical to the efforts of nurses and other care providers who seek to prevent the advent of these and other poor health outcomes. Mnemonics including "SAFE TIMES" and "HEEADSSS" offer concise means to ensure evaluation of the many ways in which adolescents may incur risk for or direct experience of TDV, and may afford the clinician the opportunity to assess responses for clarity and veracity in one-on-one interviews. Survey tools such as the *Health Survey for Adolescents* (http://www.adolescenthealth.org/clinicalcare.htm#ScreeningQues tionnaires) can also help to identify areas of concern or priority with regard to health by allowing the adolescent to indicate what kinds of experiences create uncomfortable or difficult situations. These tools may be especially helpful to clinicians in cases where signs and symptoms of TDV are also present, since it can be difficult to determine whether adolescents feel secure enough to disclose abusive experiences in full (Brown et al., 2007). Consistent screening practices and the provision of relationship education that helps adolescents learn to identify the qualities of healthy and unhealthy relationships are also important means of engendering trust and open dialogue between health care professionals and adolescents (Olson, Rickert, & Davidson, 2004. Further, information and education on safety planning may be offered to all adolescents in order to encourage thinking about these subjects. Even for those not currently in relationships, such information may be useful later in life or when shared with friends facing difficult relationship situations.

CONCLUSION

Abusive dating relationships between adolescents represent a complex problem for nurses and other health care professionals. The interactions between physical and psychosocial development, environment, and health create a dynamic and rapidly changing

---

EXHIBIT 9.4 | *Education and Web Resources*

The following resources are available for nurses and other health care providers for the sexual education and guidance of adolescents who are of dating age and likely to be in various stages of romantic relationships.

The *Choose Respect* program is a national effort to educate teens about healthy relationships, challenge them to choose to be in healthy relationships, and take a stand against behaviors that are harmful or abusive. The *Choose Respect* site has a wealth of resources available online specific for teens and their parents including videos, media clips, and materials that can be used in primary prevention school-based educational programs.
http://www.chooserespect.org/

National Youth Violence Prevention Resource Center
This federal site offers community resources related to the problem of TDV and other forms of violence committed by and against youth. It provides information on prevention programs, training opportunities, funding sources, electronic newsletters, and publications.
http://www.safeyouth.org

National Sexual Violence Resource Center
http://www.nsvrc.org

Connected Kids: Safe, Strong, Secure
An American Academy of Pediatrics site offers advice for parents including a brochure titled: *Teen Dating Violence: Tips for Parents.* This brochure can be distributed by clinicians to parents to assist them in guiding their children to sort out and choose healthy partnerships. This informative tool is a particularly helpful if parents suspect abuse in their teen's relationship.
http://www.aap.org/connectedkids/samples/datingviolence.htm

Hotlines: The following hotlines are good resources for teens.

National Teen Dating Abuse Helpline
866-331-9474
866-331-8453 TTY
www.loveisrespect.org

National Domestic Violence Hotline
800-799-SAFE (7233)
800-787-3224 TTY
www.ndvh.org

Rape, Abuse & Incest National Network (RAINN) Hotline
800-656-HOPE (4673)
www.rainn.org

---

backdrop to daily life for many young people. Experiences of TDV have the potential to cause considerable damage to the adolescent's sense of self, whether through physical injury, impact on peer interaction, or developmental effect. Many adolescents demonstrably prioritize relationships and place considerable personal focus on the maintenance of those relationships (Banister & Schreiber, 2001; Banister & Schreiber, 2001; Graves, 2005). These relationships are an important point of access for care of this population, in part, because they have not always been acknowledged or validated (Fitzgerald, 2005).

Understanding the roles of and risks associated with adolescents' relationships is fundamental to the prevention of TDV and the amelioration of its health consequences. Nurses, for whom the formation and utilization of relationships is often an important aspect of practice, are uniquely situated to generate care options appropriate to this population. See Exhibit 9.4 for education and Web resources.

REFERENCES

Ackard, D. M., & Neumark-Sztainer, D. (2002). Date violence and date rape among adolescents: Associations with disordered eating behaviors and psychological health. *Child Abuse & Neglect, 26*(5), 455–473.

Amar, A. F., & Gennaro, S. (2005). Dating violence in college women: Associated physical injury, healthcare usage, and mental health symptoms. *Nursing Research, 54*, 235–242.

American Academy of Pediatrics. Children's Health Topics. Retrieved from http:// www.aap.org/topics.html

American Academy of Pediatrics: Committee on Psychosocial Aspects of Child and Family Health and Committee on Adolescence. Sexuality education for children and adolescents. Pediatrics 2001 Aug;108(2):498–502. Retrieved from http://www.guideline.gov/summary/summary.aspx?doc_id= 3084&nbr=002310&string=dating+AND+violence

Anthony, J. (1969). The reactions of adults to adolescents and their behavior. In G. Caplan & S. Lebovici (Eds.), *Adolescence: Psychosocial perspectives* (pp. 54–78). New York: Basic Books.

Armstrong, E. A., Hamilton, L., & Sweeney, B. (2006). Sexual assault on campus: A multilevel, integrative approach to party rape. *Social Problems, 53*(4), 483–499.

Arnett, J. J. (1999). Adolescent storm and stress, reconsidered. *American Psychology, 54*(5), 317–326.

Arnett, J. J. (2000). Emerging adulthood. A theory of development from the late teens through the twenties. *American Psychology, 55*(5), 469–480.

Avery-Leaf, S., Cascardi, M., O'Leary, K. D., & Cano, A. (1997). Efficacy of a dating violence prevention program on attitudes justifying aggression. *Journal of Adolescent Health, 21*(1), 11–17.

Banister, E., Jakubec, S., & Stein, J. (2003). "Like, what am I supposed to do?": Adolescent girls' health concerns in their dating relationships. *Canadian Journal of Nursing Research, 35*(2), 17–33.

Banister, E., & Schreiber, R. (2001). Young women's health concerns: Revealing paradox. *Health Care for Women International, 22*(7), 633–647.

Banyard, V. L., & Cross, C. (2008). Consequences of teen dating violence: Understanding intervening variables in ecological context. *Violence Against Women, 14*, 998–1013.

Basile, K. C., Hertz, M. F., & Back, S. E. (2007). *Intimate partner violence and sexual violence victimization assessment instruments for use in healthcare settings: Version 1*. Atlanta (GA): Centers for Disease Control and Prevention, National Center for Injury Prevention and Control.

Black, B. M., Tolman, R. M., Callahan, M., Saunders, D. G., & Weisz, A. N. (2008). When will adolescents tell someone about dating violence victimization? *Violence Against Women, 14*(7), 741–758.

Breslau, N., Wilcox, H. C., Storr, C. L., Lucia, V. C., & Anthony, J. C. (2004). Trauma exposure and posttraumatic stress disorder: A study of youths in urban America. *J Urban Health, 81*(4), 530–544.

Bronfenbrenner, U. (1977). Toward an experimental ecology of human development. *American Psychologist, 32*(7), 513–531.

Brooks-Gunn, J., & Petersen, A. C. (1984). Problems in studying and defining pubertal events. *Journal of Youth and Adolescence, 13*(3), 181–196.

Brown, L. K., Puster, K. L., Vazquez, E. A., Hunter, H. L., & Lescano, C. M. (2007). Screening practices for adolescent dating violence. *Journal of Interpersonal Violence, 22*(4), 456–464.

Campbell, J., Jones, A. S., Dienemann, J., Kub, J., Schollenberger, J., O'Campo, P., Gielen, A. C. et al., (2002). Intimate partner violence and physical health consequences. *Archives of Internal Medicine, 162*, 1157–1163.

Centers for Disease Control and Prevention (2997). Youth Risk Behavioral Surveillance—United States. MMWR2008;57 (No.SS#4).

Centers for Disease Control and Preventionn(2008). Understanding teen dating violence fact sheet. Retrieved from http://www.cdc.gov/ViolencePrevention/pdf/DatingAbuseFactSheet-a.pdf

Cercone, J. J., Beach, S. R., & Arias, I. (2005). Gender symmetry in dating intimate partner violence: Does similar behavior imply similar constructs? *Violence and Victims, 20*(2), 207–218.

Chung, D. (2007). Making meaning of relationships: Young women's experiences and understandings of dating violence. *Violence Against Women, 13*(12), 1274–1295.

Coker, A. L., McKeown, R. E., Sanderson, M., Davis, K. E., Valois, R. F., & Huebner, S. (2000). Severe dating violence and quality of life among South Carolina high school students. *American Journal of Preventive Medicine, 19*(4), 220–227.

Diaz, A., Simantov, E., & Rickert, V. I., (2002). Effect of abuse on health. *Archives of Pediatric Adolescent Medicine, 156*, 811–817.

Dube, S. R., Miller, J. W., Brown, D. W., Giles, W. H., Felitti, V. J., Dong, M., et al. (2006). Adverse childhood experiences and the association with ever using alcohol and initiating alcohol use during adolescence. *Journal of Adolescent Health, 38*(4), 444.e1–444.e10.

Eaton, D. K., Davis, K. S., Barrios, L., Brener, N. D., & Noonan, R. K. (2007). Associations of dating violence victimization with lifetime participation, co-occurrence, and early initiation of risk behaviors among U.S. high school students. *Journal of Interpersonal Violence, 22*(5), 585–602.

Eccles, J. S., Midgley, C., Wigfield, A., Buchanan, C. M., Reuman, D., Flanagan, C., et al. (1993). Development during adolescence. The impact of stage-environment fit on young adolescents' experiences in schools and in families. *American Psychologist, 48*(2), 90–101.

Epel, E. S., Blackburn, E. H., Lin, J., Dhabhar, F. S., Adler, N. E., Morrow, J. D., et al. (2004). Accelerated telomere shortening in response to life stress. *Proceedings of the National Academy of Sciences U S A, 101*(49), 17312–17315.

Epel, E. S., Lin, J., Wilhelm, F. H., Wolkowitz, O. M., Cawthon, R., Adler, N. E., et al. (2006). Cell aging in relation to stress arousal and cardiovascular disease risk factors. *Psychoneuroendocrinology, 31*(3), 277–287.

Family Violence Prevention Fund. *Recognizing teen dating abuse.* Retrieved June 25, 2009, from http://endabuse.org/userfiles/file/PublicCommunications/Recognizing%20Teen%20Dating%20Abuse.pdf

Family Violence Prevention Fund. *Creating a teen safety plan.* Retrieved June 25, 2009, from http://endabuse.org/userfiles/file/PublicCommunications/Create%20a%20Teen%20Safety%20Plan.pdf

Finkelhor, D., Ormrod, R. K., & Turner, H. A. (2007). Polyvictimization and trauma in a national longitudinal cohort. *Development and Psychopathology, 19*(1), 149–166.

Fantasia, H. C. (2008). Concept analysis: Sexual decision-making in adolescence. *Nursing Forum, 43*(2), 80–90.

Finkelhor, D., Ormrod R. K., & Turner, H. A. (2007). Polyvictimization and trauma in a national longitudinal cohort. *Developmental Psychopathology, 19*, 149–66.

Fisher, B. S., Cullen, F. T., & Turner, M. G. (2000). *The sexual victimization of college women.* Washington, DC: U.S. Department of Justice, Office of Justice Programs.

Follette, V. M., Polusny, M. A., Bechtle, A. E., & Naugle, A. E. (1996). Cumulative trauma: The impact of child sexual abuse, adult sexual assault, and spouse abuse. *Journal of Traumatic Stress, 9*(1), 25–35.

Fonagy, P. (2004). Early-life trauma and the psychogenesis and prevention of violence. In J. Devine, J. Gilligan, K. A. Miczek, R. Shaikh, & D. Pfaff (Eds.), *Youth violence: Scientific approaches to prevention* (Vol. 1036, pp. 181–200). New York: New York Academy of Sciences.

Foshee, V. A., Linder, G. F., Bauman, K. E., Langwick, S. A., Arriaga, X. B., Heath, J. L., et al., (1996). The Safe Dates project: Theoretical basis, evaluation design, and selected baseline findings. *American Journal of Preventive Medicine, 12*(5 Suppl), 39–47.

Foshee, A., Bauman, K. E., Ennett, S. T., Linder, F., Benefield, T., & Suchindran, C. (2004). Assessing the long-term effects of the *Safe Dates* program and a booster in preventing and reducing adolescent dating violence victimization and perpetration. *American Journal of Public Health, 94*(4), 619–624.

Foshee, V. A., Bauman, K. E., Linder, F., Rice, J., & Wilcher, R. (2007). Typologies of adolescent dating violence: Identifying typologies of adolescent dating violence perpetration. *Journal of Interpersonal Violence, 22*(5), 498–519.

Foster, H., Hagan, J., & Brooks-Gunn, J. (2004). Age, puberty, and exposure to intimate partner violence in adolescence. *Annals of the New York Academy of Science, 1036*, 151–166.

Fredland, N., Ricardo, I., Campbell, J. C., Sharps, P., Kub, J., & Yonas, M. (2005). The meaning of dating violence in the lives of middle school adolescents: Results of a qualitative focus group study. *Journal of School Violence, 4*(2), 95–114.

Fredland, N. (2008). Sexual bullying: Addressing the gap between bullying and dating violence. *Advances in Nursing Science, 31*(2), 95–11.

Fredland, N., Campbell, J., & Han, H. (2008). Effect of violence exposure on health outcomes among young urban adolescents. *Nursing Research, 57*(3), 157–165.

Freedner, N., Freed, L. H., Yang, Y. W., & Austin, S. B. (2002). Dating violence among gay, lesbian, and bisexual adolescents: results from a community survey. *Journal of Adolescent Health, 31*(6), 469–474.

Galtung, J. (2004). Violence, war, and their impact on visible and invisible effects of violence [Electronic version]. Retrieved from http://them.polylog.org/5/fgj-en.htm

Gilligan, C. (1987). Adolescent development reconsidered. *New Directions in Child Development* (37), 63–92.

Glass, N., Fredland, N., Campbell, J. C., Sharps, P., & Kub, J. (2003). Adolescent dating violence: Prevalence, risk factors, health outcomes and implications for clinical practice. *Journal of Obstetric, Gynecologic and Neonatal Nursing, 32*(2), 227–238.

Graves, V. (2005). The unique health needs of young women: application of occupational health professionals. *AAOHN Journal, 53*(7). 320–325.

Green, B. L., & Kimerling, R. (2004). Trauma, posttraumatic stress disorder, and health status. In P. P. Schnurr & B. L. Green (Eds.), *Trauma and health: Physical consequences of exposure to extreme stress* (1st ed., pp. 13–42). Washington, DC: American Psychological Association.

Guthrie, B. J., Loveland-Cherry, C., Frey, M. A., & Dielman, T. E. (1994). A theoretical approach to studying health behaviors in adolescents: An at-risk population. *Family and Community Health, 17*(3), 35–48.

Haglund, K. (2003). Sexually abstinent African American adolescent females' descriptions of abstinence. *Journal of Nursing Scholarship, 35*(3), 231–236.

Hahn, R., Fuqua-Whitley, D., Wethington, H., Lowy, J., Liberman, A., Crosby, A., et al. (2007). The effectiveness of universal school-based programs for the prevention of violent and aggressive behavior: A report on recommendations of the task force on community Preventive services. *MMWR.* August 10, 2007/56(RR07); 1–12.

Halpern, C. T., Oslak, S. G., Young, M. L., Martin, S. L., & Kupper, L. L. (2001). Partner violence among adolescents in opposite-sex romantic relationships: findings from the National Longitudinal Study of Adolescent Health. *American Journal of Public Health, 91*(10), 1679–1685.

Hanson, R. F. (2002). Adolescent dating violence: prevalence and psychological outcomes. *Child Abuse and Neglect, 26*(5), 449–453.

Hardy, K. V., & Laszloffy, T. A. (2005). *Teens who hurt: Clinical interventions to break the cycle of adolescent violence.* New York: The Guilford Press.

Hines, D. A., & Saudino, K. J. (2003). Gender differences in psychological, physical, and sexual aggression among college students using the revised conflict tactics scales. *Violence and Victims, 18*(2), 197–217.

Ismail, F., Berman, H., & Ward-Griffin, C. (2007). Dating violence and the health of young women: a feminist narrative study. *Health Care for Women International, 28*(5), 453–477.

Jaffe, P. G., Sudermann, M,, Reitzel, D., & Killip, S. M. (1992). An evaluation of a secondary school primary prevention program on violence in intimate relationships. *Violence and Victims* 7(2), 129–146.

Kann, L., Brener, N. D., Warren, C. W., Collins, J. L., & Giovino, G. A. (2002). An assessment of the effect of data collection setting on the prevalence of health risk behaviors among adolescents. *Journal of Adolescent Health, 31*(4), 327–335.

Koss, M. P., Abbey, A., Campbell, R., Cook, S., Norris, J., Testa, M., et al. (2007). Revising the SES: A collaborative process to improve assessment of sexual aggression and victimization. *Psychology of Women Quarterly, 31*(2007), 357–370.

Koziol-McLain, J., Giddings, L., Rameka, M., & Fyfe, E. (2008). Intimate partner violence screening and brief intervention: experiences of women in two New Zealand health care settings. *Journal of Midwifery and Women's Health, 53*(6), 504–510.

Kreiter, S. R., Krowchuk, D. P., Woods, C. R., Sinal, S. H., Lawless, M. R., & DuRant, R. H. (1999). Gender differences in risk behaviors among adolescents who experience date fighting. *Pediatrics, 104*(6), 1286–1292.

Krupnick, J. L., Green, B. L., Stockton, P., Goodman, L., Corcoran, C., & Petty, R. (2004). Mental health effects of adolescent trauma exposure in a female college sample: exploring differential outcomes based on experiences of unique trauma types and dimensions. *Psychiatry, 67*(3), 264–279.

Kulbok, P. A., & Cox, C. L. (2002). Dimensions of adolescent health behavior. *Journal of Adolescent Health, 31*(5), 394–400.

Lazzaro, M. V., & McFarlane, J. (1991). Establishing a screening program for abused women. *JONA, 21*(10), 24–28.

Lawson, D. M., & Brossart, D. F. (2004). The developmental course of personal authority in the family system. *Family Process, 43*(3), 391–409.

Lewis, S. F., & Fremouw, W. (2001). Dating violence: A critical review of the literature. *Clinical Psychology Review, 21*(1), 105–127.

Lindhorst, T., & Oxford, M. (2008). The long-term effects of intimate partner violence on adolescent mothers' depressive symptoms. *Soc Sci Med, 66*(6), 1322–1333.

Lloyd, S. L. (2004). Pregnant adolescent reflections of parental communication. *Journal of Community Health Nursing, 21*(4), 239–251.

Machoian, L. (2005). *The disappearing girl: Learning the language of teenage depression.* New York: Dutton.

Macgowan, M. J. (1997). An evaluation of a dating violence prevention program for middle school students. *Violence and Victims, 12*(3), 223–235.

Marcus, R. F. (2004). Dating partners' responses to simulated dating conflict: Violence chronicity, expectations, and emotional quality of relationship. *Genetic, Social, and General Psychology Monographs, 130*(2), 163–188.

Matheson, K., Skomorovsky, A., Fiocco, A., & Anisman, H. (2007). The limits of adaptive coping: Well-being and mood reactions to stressors among women in abusive dating relationships. *Stress, 10*(1), 75–91.

McFarlane, J., Parker B., Soeken, K., & Bullock, L. (1992). Assessing for abuse during pregnancy. *Journal of the American Medical Association, 267,* 3176–3178.

McFarlane, J., & Parker B., (1994). Preventing abuse during pregnancy: An assessment and intervention protocol. *The American Journal of Maternal Child Nursing, 19*(6): 321–324.

McFarlane, J. (2004). Intimate partner violence and physical health consequences. *Journal of Interpersonal Violence, 19*(11), 1335–1341.

McFarlane, J. M., Groff, J. Y., O'Brien, J. A., & Watson, K. (2006). Secondary prevention of intimate partner violence: a randomized controlled trial. *Nursing Research, 55*(1), 52–61.

Miller, E., Decker, M. R., Reed, E., Raj, A., Hathaway, J. E., & Silverman, J. G. (2007). Male partner pregnancy-promoting behaviors and adolescent partner violence: Findings from a qualitative study with adolescent females. *Ambulatory Pediatrics, 7*(5), 360–366.

Montgomery, K. S. (2002). Health promotion with adolescents: Examining theoretical perspectives to guide research. *Research and Theory for Nursing Practice, 16*(2), 119–134.

Moracco, K. E., Runyan, C. W., Bowling, J. M., & Earp, J. A. (2007). Women's experiences with violence: a national study. *Women's Health Issues, 17*(1), 3–12.

Munoz-Rivas, M. J., Grana, J. L., O'Leary, K. D., & Gonzalez, M. P. (2007). Aggression in adolescent dating relationships: Prevalence, justification, and health consequences. *Journal of Adolescent Health, 40*(4), 298–304.

National Youth Violence Prevention Resource Center, Retrieved from http://www.safeyouth.org/scripts/faq/datingwarning.asp.

Nicoletti, A. (2009). Teens and drug facilitated sexual assault. *Journal of Pediatric and Adolescent Gynecology, 22*(3), 187–187.

Olson, E. C., Rickert, V. I., & Davidson, L. L. (2004). Identifying and supporting young women experiencing dating violence: what health practitioners should be doing NOW. *Journal of Pediatric and Adolescent Gynecology, 17*(2), 131–136.

Parker, B., McFarlane, J., Soeken, K., Torres, S., & Campbell, D. (1993). Physical and emotional abuse in pregnancy: A comparison of adult and teenage women. *Nursing Research, 43*(3), 190–191.

Parks, K. A., Hsieh, Y. P., Bradizza, C. M., & Romosz, A. M. (2008). Factors influencing the temporal relationship between alcohol consumption and experiences with aggression among college women. *Psychol Addict Behav, 22*(2), 210–218.

Petersen, A. C. (1988). Adolescent development. *Annual Review of Psychology, 39,* 583–607.

Picard, P., Glauber, A., & Randel, J. (2007). *Tech abuse in teen relationships study.* Northbrook: Teenage Research Unlimited for Liz Claiborne, Inc.

Pinto, K. C. (2004). Intersections of gender and age in health care: Adapting autonomy and confidentiality for the adolescent girl. *Qualitative Health Research, 14*(1), 78–99.

Poitras, M., & Lavoie, F. (1995). A study of the prevalence of sexual coercion in adolescent heterosexual dating relationships in a Quebec sample. *Violence Vict, 10*(4), 299–313.

Raty, L. K. A., Larsson, G., Soderfeldt, B. A., & Larsson, B. M. W. (2005). Psychosocial aspects of health in adolescence: The influence of gender, and general self-concept. *Journal of Adolescent Health, 36*(6), 530.e521–530.e528.

Renker, P. R. (1999). Physical abuse, social support, self-care, and pregnancy outcomes of older adolescents. *Journal of Obstetric, Gynecologic, and Neonatal Nursing, 28*(4), 377–388.

Rew, L. (2005). *Adolescent Health: A multidisciplinary approach to theory, research, and intervention.* Thousand Oaks: Sage.

Rhatigan, D. L., & Street, A. E. (2005). The impact of intimate partner violence on decisions to leave dating relationships: A test of the investment model. *Journal of Interpersonal Violence, 20*(12), 1580–1597.

Rickert, V. I., Wiemann, C. M., & Vaughan, R. D. (2005). Disclosure of date/acquaintance rape: who reports and when. *J Pediatr Adolesc Gynecol, 18*(1), 17–24.

Riesch, S. K., Jackson, N. M., & Chanchong, W. (2003). Communication approaches to parent-child conflict: young adolescence to young adult. *Journal of Pediatric Nursing, 18*(4), 244–256.

Sampson, R. (2003). *Acquaintance rape of college students.* U.S. Department of Justice, Office of Problem-Oriented Policing. Retrieved from http://www.cops.usdoj.gov/files/RIC/Publications/e07063411.pdf

Schad, M. M., Szwedo, D. E., Antonishak, J., Hare, A., & Allen, J. P. (2008). The broader context of relational aggression in adolescent romantic relationships: predictions from peer pressure and links to psychosocial functioning. *Journal of Youth and Adolescence, 37*(3), 346–358.

Scheper-Hughes, N. (2004). Dangerous and endangered youth: Social structures and determinants of violence. In J. Devine, J. Gilligan, K. A. Miczek, R. Shaikh, & D. Pfaff (Eds.), *Youth violence: Scientific approaches to prevention* (Vol. 1036, pp. 13–46). New York: New York Academy of Sciences.

Sears, H. A., Byers, E. S., Whelan, J. J., & Saint-Pierre, M. (2006). "If it hurts you, then it is not a joke": Adolescents' ideas about girls' and boys' use and experience of abusive behavior in dating relationships. *Journal of Interpersonal Violence, 21*(9), 1191–1207.

Sears, H. A., Byers, S. E., & Price, L. E. (2007). The co-occurrence of adolescent boys' and girls' use of psychologically, physically, and sexually abusive behaviours in their dating relationships. *Journal of Adolescence, 30*(3), 487–504.

Senn, T. E., Carey, M. P., Vanable, P. A., Coury-Doniger, P., & Urban, M. (2007). Characteristics of sexual abuse in childhood and adolescence influence sexual risk behavior in adulthood. *Arch Sex Behav, 36*(5), 637–645.

Short, M. B., Mills, L. C., & Rosenthal, S. L. (2006). When adolescent girls say, "I don't know". *Journal of Pediatric and Adolescent Gynecology, 19*(4), 267–270.

Silverman, J. G., Decker, M. R., Reed, E., Rothman, E. F., Hathaway, J. E., Raj, A., et al. (2006). Social norms and beliefs regarding sexual risk and pregnancy involvement among adolescent males treated for dating violence perpetration. *Journal of Urban Health, 83*(4), 723–735.

Silverman, J. G., Raj, A., & Clements, K. (2004). Dating violence and associated sexual risk and pregnancy among adolescent girls in the United Sates. *Pediatrics, 114*(2), e220–225.

Silverman, J. G., Raj, A., Mucci, L. A., & Hathaway, J. E. (2001). Dating violence against adolescent girls and associated substance use, unhealthy weight control, sexual risk behavior, pregnancy, and suicidality. *JAMA, 286*(5), 572–579.

Society of Adolescent Medicine. *Clinical care resources. Health screening questionnaires.* Retrieved from http://www.adolescenthealth.org/clinicalcare.htm#ScreeningQuestionnaires.

Society of Adolescent Medicine. *Clinical care resources. Tips for protecting your confidentiality.* Retrieved from http://www.adolescenthealth.org/clinicalcare.htm#ScreeningQuestionnaires.

Society of Adolescent Medicine. *Clinical care resources. Billing for confidential adolescent health services.* Retrieved from http://www.adolescenthealth.org/clinicalcare.htm#ScreeningQuestionnaires.

Sugarman, D. B., & Hotaling, G. T. (1991). Dating violence: A review of contextual and risk factors. In B. Levy (Ed.), *Dating violence: Young women in danger* (pp. 100–118). Seattle WA: Seal Press.

The National Campaign to Prevent Teen and Unplanned Pregnancy. (2008). *Sex and Tech: results from a survey of teen and young adults.* Washington, DC.

Tjaden, P., & Thoennes, N. (2000). *Full report of the prevalence, incidence, and consequences of violence against women.* Rockville and Atlanta: National Institute of Justice and Centers for Disease Control and Prevention.

Ullman, S. E., Karabatsos, G., & Koss, M. P. (1999). Alcohol and sexual assault in a national sample of college women. *Journal of Interpersonal Violence, 14*(6), 603–625.

Walker, E. A., Newman, E., & Koss, M. P. (2004). Costs and health care utilization associated with traumatic experiences. In P. P. Schnurr & B. L. Green (Eds.), *Trauma and health: Physical health consequences of exposure to extreme stress* (pp. 43–70). Washington, DC: American Psychological Association.

Werkerle, C., & Wolfe, D. A. (1999). Dating violence in mid-adolescence: Theory, significance, and emerging prevention initiatives. *Clinical Psychology Review, 19*(4), 435–456.

Willson, P., Cesario, S., Fredland, N., Walsh, T., McFarlane, J., Gist, J. et al. (2001). Primary healthcare provider's lost opportunity to help abused women. *Journal of the American Academy of Nurse Practitioners, 13*(12), 565–570.

Wingood, G. M., DiClemente, R. J., Harrington, K. F., Lang, D. L., Davies, S. L., Hook, E. W., et al. (2006). Efficacy of an HIV prevention program among female adolescents experiencing gender-based violence. *American Journal of Public Health, 96*(6), 1085–1090.

Wingood, G. M., DiClemente, R. J., McCree, D. H., Harrington, K., & Davies, S. L. (2001). Dating violence and the sexual health of black adolescent females. *Pediatrics, 107*(5), E72.

Wiseman, R. (2002). *Queen bees and wannabes: a parent's guide to helping your daughter survive cliques, gossip, boyfriends, and other realities of adolescence*. New York: Three Rivers Press.

Wolfe, D. A., Jaffe, P. G., & Crooks, C. V. (2006). *Adolescent risk behaviors: Why teens experiment and strategies to keep them safe*. New Haven: Yale University Press.

10

Child Maltreatment: Assessment, Practice, and Intervention

Susan J. Kelley, PhD, RN, FAAN

INTRODUCTION

Child maltreatment is a serious social, legal, and public health issue that is frequently encountered by nurses in a variety of practice settings. Research findings underscore the negative consequences of child maltreatment, both physical and psychological, during childhood and across the life span (see chapter 4). Research on the neurodevelopment of children indicates that early abuse results in altered physiological response to stressful stimuli, a response that negatively affects the child's subsequent socialization and behavior (Stirling & Amaya-Jackson, 2008). Child maltreatment is associated with increased emotional problems, including depression and posttraumatic stress disorder (PTSD), poor school performance, difficulty in relationships with peers, and behavior problems in childhood (Cicchetti, Rogosch, & Toth, 2006; Daignault & Herbert, 2009; Holbrook et al., 2005; Ward & Haskett, 2008). The long-term impact includes a significant increase in psychological and physical health problems in adulthood (Afifi, Boman, Fleisher, & Sareen, 2009; Chapman et al., 2004; Danielson et al., 2009; Schumm, Briggs-Philip, & Hobfoll, 2006; Yates, Carlson, & Egeland, 2008).

Estimates of the actual scope of the problem are difficult to ascertain for two main reasons: (1) definitions of child maltreatment and investigative procedures vary among states and (2) reported cases of child maltreatment represent only the "tip of the iceberg" as many cases of child maltreatment go unreported to officials. Nonetheless, we know that it is all too common. In a nationally representative survey of children and youth, 2–17 years old, approximately one in eight were found to be maltreated from 2002 to 2003 (Finkelhor, Ormrod, Turner, & Hamby, 2005). Self-reported histories of childhood maltreatment in a national survey reveal that 14.2% of men and 32.3% of women were sexually abused in childhood and that 22.2% of men and 19.5% of women experienced physical abuse (Briere & Elliot, 2003). This chapter will address a number of practice issues related to the abuse and neglect of children including the identification, treatment, and prevention of child maltreatment.

ASSESSMENT OF PHYSICAL ABUSE

Keeping a high, but healthy, index of suspicion of child maltreatment is important to recognizing it, as early recognition and intervention are the keys to preventing subsequent abuse and further negative sequelae.

History

It is essential to elicit and document a careful, detailed history of all injuries in cases of suspected child maltreatment, keeping in mind that the presenting history may not be one of trauma, but rather of related symptoms such as irritability, lethargy, or vomiting. Families will respond best when health care providers pose questions in a neutral, nonthreatening manner. Histories should include the periods of time before, during, and after the injury abuse occurred, as well as who witnessed the injury.

Histories can begin with simple questions such as "please tell me what happened," followed with more specific questions. It is also important to determine if the history provided is consistent with the observed injury. If a discrepancy exists between the reason given for an injury and the physical findings, abuse should be suspected. Whenever possible, the child and caretaker should be interviewed separately, as discrepancies may exist between the caretaker's and the child's accounts. Also, when interviewed alone, the child is more likely to accurately report the actual cause of an abusive injury and the identity of the perpetrator. Evoking as many details as possible helps to reveal any inconsistencies between the child's and the caregiver's account. The child's past health history, including any previous injuries, should be carefully elicited. When available, the child's health record should be reviewed for previous suspicious injuries. In cases of a fall, it is important to question the height from which the child fell, as well as the contact surface. Information in histories that should alert nurses to the possibility of child abuse is summarized in Exhibit 10.1.

A delay in seeking attention for a child's injury should raise the suspicion of abuse; some abusive parents and other caretakers ignore the seriousness of an injury in the hope that it will heal without health care attention, thereby avoiding detection and legal ac-

---

EXHIBIT 10.1 | *Features of History That Raise Suspicion of Abuse*

- A history inconsistent with an existing injury
- Injury without history of trauma
- Reluctance of the caretaker to provide information
- Caretaker blames a child for his or her own injury
- Child is developmentally incapable of incurring injury
- Delay in attention of significant injury
- Inconsistencies in the histories given
- History of repeated child injuries or hospitalizations
- Family seeks health care in many different settings that are in close proximity
- Inappropriate response to severity of injury
- Previous placement of child in foster care or other involvement with child protective services (CPS)

tion. Another important factor to consider is the distance over which the caretaker traveled to seek care for the injured child. If the caretaker has traveled an unusual distance for treatment, bypassing care facilities closer to home, the caretaker may be trying to avoid detection by staff members who have suspected him or her of abuse on previous occasions. It is important to note that abusive parents often seek health care at many different treatment facilities in order to avoid detection.

One must consider whether it is developmentally possible for a child to have injured him or herself in a particular manner. For example, if the mother of a 1-month-old infant with a skull fracture reports that the baby rolled over on the dressing table and fell to the floor, abuse should be suspected because infants are not capable of rolling over until 3 to 5 months of age. Likewise, fractures of the limbs are unusual in infants who have not yet learned to walk.

The child's appearance and behavior should be observed and documented, especially parent–child interaction. It is not unusual for a child to seek comfort from the adult who abused or neglected them. Some maltreated children will appear fearful of the adult who brought them in for health care. Other abused children may appear withdrawn and anxious or demonstrate behavioral problems that could be related to a past history of maltreatment. Thus, it is important to remember that there is no one "typical" appearance and behavior of an abused child. Exhibit 10.2 contains screening tools that may assist in identifying children and families at risk for maltreatment, as well as measures for examining the impact of child maltreatment.

PHYSICAL EXAMINATION

A complete physical assessment, without clothing, is indicated in all cases of suspected child maltreatment. It is important to be aware that many cases of abusive injury in children are identified while a child is being treated for a condition other than the injury. For example, inflicted rib fractures may be found during a chest X-ray done to rule out pneumonia in an infant who presents with an upper respiratory infection. Similarly, previously undiagnosed fractures of an extremity may be detected on X-rays made to assess a recent, unintentional injury.

Cutaneous Lesions

Cutaneous lesions are the most common manifestations of physical abuse in children, and the most easily recognized sign of abuse. Cutaneous lesions caused by maltreatment include contusions, abrasions, lacerations, burns, bite marks, and hair loss. The size, shape, location, distribution, and color of all injuries should be carefully documented.

Bruises change color with time as blood is reabsorbed from the skin. As the blood cells and hemoglobin break down, the bruise will go through a succession of colors, including red, violet, black, blue, green, and/or brown. However, there does not seem to be a predictable order or chronology of color presentation. Thus, bruise color should <u>not</u> be used to determine the age of a bruise (Jenny & Reece, 2009). Multiple bruises occurring in clusters, as well as larger bruises, are more likely to be from abuse.

There are two common characteristics separating abusive from nonabusive bruises: location and patterns. Bruises found on the shins, lower arms, under chin, forehead, hips, elbows and ankles tend to be accidental, while those located on the upper arms, upper

---

EXHIBIT 10.2 | *Screening Measures*

Parent/Caregiver Measures
Depression:
- Edinburgh Post Partum Depression Scale (EPDS) (Cox, Holden, & Sagovsky, 1987)
- Center for Epidemiological Studies Depression Scale (CES-D) (Radloff, 1977)
- Symptom Checklist-90 (SCL-90) (Derogatis, 1993), assesses for depression and psychological distress

Risk Assessment for Child Maltreatment:
- Child Abuse Potential (CAPI) (Milner, 1986)
- Parenting Stress Index (PSI) (Abidin, 1997)

Child Abuse Screening:
- Parent–Child Conflict Tactics Scales (CTSPC). (Straus, Hanby, Finkelhor, Moore, & Runyan, 1998)

Alcohol and Other Drugs (AOD):
- Shorted Michigan Alcoholism Screening Test (SMAST) (Shields, Howell, Potter, & Weiss, 2007)

Child Measures
Mental Health:
- Children's Depression Inventory (CDI) (Saylor, Finch, Spirito, & Bennett, 1984)
- Trauma Symptom Checklist for Young Children (TSCYC) (Briere, Johnson, Bissada, Damon, Crouch, Gil, Hanson, & Ernst, 2001)
- UCLA PTSD Index (Steinberg, Brymer, Decker, & Pynoos, 2004).

Developmental Screening:
- Ages & Stages Questionnaires (ASQ): A Parent-Completed, Child-Monitoring System (Bricker & Squires, 1999)

References

Abidin, R. R. (1997). Parenting stress index: A measure of the parent-child system. In Zalaquett, C. P., & Wood, R. (Eds.), *Evaluating stress: A book of resources* (pp. 277–291). Scarecrow Press, Inc: Lanham, MD.

Bricker, D. & Squires, J. (1999). *Ages & Stages Questionnaires (ASQ): A parent-completed, child-monitoring system* (2nd ed.). Paul H. Brookes Publishing CO. 800/638-3775, www.brookespublishing.com/asq.

Briere, J., Johnson, K., Bissada, A., Damon, L., Crouch, J., Gil, E., Hanson, R., & Ernst, V. (2001). The Trauma Symptom Checklist for Young Children (TSCYC): Reliability and association with abuse exposure in a multi-site study. *Child Abuse & Neglect, 25,* 1001–1014.

Cox, Holden, & Sagovsky (1987). Detection of postnatal depression: Development of the ten item Edinburgh Post Partum Depression Scale. *British Journal of Psychiatry, 150,* 782–787.

Derogatis, L. R. (1993). *SCL-90-R administration, scoring, and procedures manual-II.* Minneapolis: National Computer Systems.

Milner, J. (1986). *The Child Abuse Potential inventory: Manual,* (2nd ed.). Webster, NC: Psytec.

Radloff, L. S. (1977). The CES-D Scale: A self-report depression scale for research in the general population. *Applied Psychological Measurement, 1,* 385–401.

Saylor, C. F., Finch, A. J., Spirito, A., and Bennett, B. (1984). The Children's Depression Inventory: A systematic evaluation of psychometric properties. *Journal of Consulting and Clinical Psychology, 52,* 955–967.

Shields, A. L., Howell, R. T., Potter, J. S., & Weiss, R. D. (2007). The Michigan Alcoholism Screening Test and its shortened form: A meta-analytic inquiry into score reliability. *Substance Abuse and Misuse, 42,* 1783–1800.

Steinberg, A. M., Brymer, M. J. Decker, K. B., & Pynoos, R. S. (2004). University of California PTSD Reaction Index. *Current Psychiatric Reports, 6,* 96–100.

Straus, M. A. Hanby, S. L. Finkelhor, D. Moore, D. W. & Runyan, D. (1998). Identification of child maltreatment with the Parent–Child Conflict Tactics Scales: Development and psychometric data for a national sample of American parents. *Child Abuse and Neglect, 22,* 249–270.

anterior thighs, trunk, genitalia, buttocks, face, ears, and neck are often the result of inflicted trauma (Jenny & Reece, 2009).

The pattern of an abusive bruise often reflects the method or instrument used to inflict the abuse. Bruises consisting of straight lines are uncommon in accidental injuries. When implements are used to injure a child, they often cause marks that reflect the outline of that object. Injuries from objects should be considered when linear contusions or contusions in unusual configurations, such as those having sharp angles, are noted. Evidence of the objects frequently used to strike children include the characteristic loop-shaped mark made by a doubled overextension or lamp cord; linear marks from a belt, strap, or stick; and imprints from a spoon, buckle, paddle, spatula, or hairbrush.

Linear marks, often found over curved body surfaces, generally indicate injury with a belt or strap. In some cases, an imprint of the belt buckle is noted. If a hand is used to strike a child, especially on the face, characteristic parallel linear marks may be noted, representing the fingers and the spaces between them. The characteristic loop-shaped marks made by a doubled electrical extension or lamp cord are typically found on the back, buttocks, upper arms, and thighs. In contrast, marks from a coat hanger leave a wider loop mark, caused by the flat base of the hanger. Circular or oval marks on the upper arm may be the result of forceful grasping of a child with application of pressure to the site. Cords or rope used to bind ankles and wrists leave thin, circumferential bruises; thicker marks may indicate a child being tied up with sheets.

Infants and young children may be gagged or have clothes or objects stuffed in their mouths to stop them from crying (Mouden & Kenney, 2005). Gag marks leave downturned lesions at the corners of the mouth. Other types of oral trauma include burns caused by excessively hot food or fluids placed in the child's mouth; injuries to the labial frenulum or lingual frenulum are often caused by forcing a bottle or spoon into the child's mouth. Missing or loosened teeth and oral lacerations may be signs of direct blunt trauma to the face.

Examination for cutaneous lesions may reveal bite marks or evidence of hair pulling. Human bite marks appear most frequently on the upper extremities and may resemble a double horseshoe or have an irregular doughnut shape. They should be measured in order to determine whether they were inflicted by an adult or a child. Adult bite marks have a 3-cm or greater distance between canine teeth. Unlike dog bites, human bites typically do not leave puncture marks. Bite marks should be carefully photographed with, and without, a size standard and swabbed with sterile water or saline to recover genetic markers left behind from saliva (Jenny & Reece, 2009).

Patchy areas of hair loss or swelling of the scalp, most often on the top of the head, may be the result of child being pulled by the hair. This condition is referred to as traction or traumatic alopecia. Petechiae on the face and neck, as well as conjuctival hemorrhages, can result from compression of the chest and neck, causing increased venous pressure. Strangulation or suffocation by occlusion of the airway can cause similar lesions (Jenny & Reece, 2009).

Burns

Inflicted burns are seen in approximately 10% of substantiated cases of child abuse and are the third leading cause of death from child abuse. Between 10% and 25% of burns involving children are deliberately inflicted by adults (Johnson & French, 2005). Two thirds of these cases involve children less than 3 years of age. Abuse-related burns are generally more serious and more likely to require excision and grafting, be full-thickness, and involve longer hospital stays than accidental burns (Jenny & Reece, 2009).

Children who repeatedly suffer burns should be carefully evaluated for abuse. Suspicion should be raised when treatment of a child's burns is delayed for more than 24 hour or when the parent who was not home at the time of the injury seeks health care. Intentionally inflicted burns may involve hot liquids or objects and often leave identifiable patterns on the skin. Although burn injuries result from a wide variety of causes, most inflicted burns are caused by hot water (Jenny & Reece, 2009).

Intentional scalding is often the result of a child being immersed in hot water. The resulting injury is typically uniform, with sharp lines of demarcation. Inflicted immersion burns are typically symmetric, whereas accidental burns are usually asymmetric. Inflicted burns are often bilateral, involving feet, hands, and buttocks and often appear "sock-like" on the feet, "glove-like" on the hands, and "doughnut-like" on the buttocks or genitalia. They also tend to be uniform in depth, symmetrical, and have sharp lines of demarcation. Flexion creases are usually spared because the child flexes his or her extremities in the hot water. Immersion burns of the hands can be caused by the exploratory behavior of a child, though tap-water scald burns are often inflicted; an immersion burn of the buttocks and lower extremities of an infant is more likely, than not, to have been deliberately caused by the caretaker. Accidental hot water burns are usually not as clearly demarcated on their edges as are inflicted immersion burns. Moreover, inflicted burns tend to be full thickness burns, whereas unintentional burns are often of partial thickness.

Patterned burns result from contact with cigarettes and other hot objects. Accidental cigarette burns typically occur on or around the face of a child who walks into a lighted cigarette being held by an adult at waist height. Cigarette burns found on the soles of the feet, palms of the hands, buttocks, or back are often inflicted. Inflicted cigarette burns tend to be multiple, in various stages of healing, circular, and 7 to 10 mm in diameter, indurated at their margins, and third degree. Accidental cigarette burns are usually shallower, more irregular, and less circumscribed than deliberately inflicted burns.

Contact burns in the configuration of a heated object are often inflicted on children and tend to have sharply demarcated edges. Objects often involved in intentional contact burns include steam irons, electric stove burners, hot plates, forks, knives, curling irons, automobile cigarette lighters, conventional cigarette lighters, radiators, hair dryers, furnace grates, and candles. Caretakers have been known to place toddlers in the process of being toilet trained on radiators to dry their wet diapers, resulting in linear burns to the buttocks.

Fractures

Fractures are the second most common manifestation of physical abuse after cutaneous lesions and are usually the result from traumatic injury to bone, which causes the continuity of the bone tissues to be disrupted or broken. Age is the single most important risk factor for abuse-related skeletal injuries, with younger children being at greatest risk. Eighty percent of abuse-related fractures are found in infants younger than 18 months, whereas only 2% of accidental fractures occur in this age group (Cooperman & Merten, 2009). Whenever one or more fractures are present, there may also be associated head and abdominal trauma.

Fractures and dislocations that are inconsistent with the mechanism of injury are highly suspect of abuse. Because caretakers often delay seeking treatment in cases of inflicted injury, manifestations typically seen in the acute phase of skeletal injury, such as swelling and tenderness, may not be present in children with abuse-related bone injuries. A complete radiologic skeletal survey in children younger than age two is indicated in cases of suspected child maltreatment (American Academy of Pediatrics, 2000).

Fractures of the extremities are the most common skeletal injuries in abused children. They may be limited to a single bone, or may involve multiple bones. The mechanism of extremity fractures in abused children may be difficult to determine because the abuse is often unobserved. Transverse fractures, which are at a 90° angle to the bone, may be the result of blunt trauma, whereas spiral fractures of long bones may result from the intentional twisting of an extremity. Fractures of the humerus are particularly suspicious for such abuse. Femoral fractures in infants and toddlers, as well as fractures of the skull or facial structures, are also often the result of abuse.

Rib fractures, also common in abused children, are frequently multiple, bilateral, posterior, often reflecting a squeezing of the chest. Lung or visceral damage from fractured ribs may manifest as chest deformity or costochondral tenderness. Fractures of the sternum, vertebrae, and pelvis are uncommon in children and should, therefore, be considered suspicious. Metaphyseal fractures require biomechanical forces that are not produced by the usual accidental trauma of infancy and should also be considered suspicious. This type of fracture often involves rotational forces that often occur in the violent shaking of young children. Multiple fractures in various stages of healing are highly suspicious. Recognition of inflicted fractures in children, and especially in infants, is critical because these children are at high risk for subsequent abuse.

The possibility that multiple fractures in a child are related to an underlying disease, such as osteogenesis imperfecta, scurvy, rickets, congenital syphilis, Menke's syndrome, neoplasia, osteomyelitis, and infantile cortical hypertosis should also be considered (Cooperman & Merten, 2009). These unusual diseases can be ruled out by appropriate diagnostic procedures. Obstetric trauma, including breech deliveries, can cause certain skeletal injuries in otherwise healthy neonates, with clavicular and humeral fractures occurring most commonly. The delicate osteopenic bones of premature infants place them at increased risk for fractures from normal handling, with long-bone and rib fractures most common (Cooperman & Merten, 2009).

Abusive Head Trauma

Abusive head trauma (AHT) is the leading cause of death in abused children, with children under 1 year of age being at highest risk. Mortality is significantly higher for children with inflicted head injury compared to those with accidental injury. When comparing factors that assist in distinguishing inflicted from noninflicted head trauma, those that are found most often for AHT victims include a child less than 1 year of age, lack of history of a significant traumatic event, a changing history from the caregiver, the presence of head injury symptoms and seizures at the time of presentation, poor outcome, and the belief by the caregiver that home resuscitation caused the injury (Rorke-Adams, Duhaime, Jenny, & Smith, 2009). It is important to note that the vast majority of the literature on childhood falls indicates that short falls rarely result in serious or life-threatening head injuries (Rorke-Adams et al., 2009).

Abusive head trauma may result from direct trauma, vigorous shaking, or a combination of the two. The resulting injuries are referred to as shaken baby syndrome (SBS). SBS is a unique and prevalent form of intracranial injury that may leave no external signs of trauma. It results from acceleration–deceleration injuries due to vigorous shaking, which may, or may not, involve blunt trauma to the head. Victims of SBS may present with seizures, lethargy, vomiting, and irritability. Physical findings can include retinal hemorrhages, hemotympanum, subdural or subarachnoid bleeds, cerebral edema, grip marks to rib cage and upper arms, and fractures of the humeri or ribs. The major precursor to the occurrence of SBS is persistent infant crying, which triggers abusive behavior in a caregiver who has lost control of his or her emotions and behaviors.

Ocular Injuries

Inflicted eye injuries may leave no external evidence of trauma. A fundoscopic examination is, therefore, essential in suspected cases of abuse. Eye injuries that can result from physical abuse include periorbital hematomas, retinal hemorrhages, fractures of the orbital or facial bones, subconjunctival hemorrhage, dislocation of the lens, corneal abrasion, and optic atrophy. The vast majority of infants and young children with retinal hemorrhages have been abused, thus, a very high level of suspicion is indicated in such cases. Retinal hemorrhages are present in approximately 85% of cases of SBS (Levin & Morad, 2009). In such cases, the shearing and sudden deceleration forces cause retinal hemorrhage.

Ear Injuries

Injuries sustained from physical abuse may leave internal or external signs. The external ear may show evidence of contusions, abrasions, and swelling. Ecchymoses on the internal surface of the pinna may be the result of "boxing" the ear and crushing it against the skull. A direct blow to the ear may also cause hemotympanum and perforation of the tympanic membrane.

Abdominal Trauma

Abdominal injuries, although infrequent compared to other forms of inflicted abuse, ranks second to head trauma as the leading cause of death from child abuse. The high mortality rate associated with inflicted abdominal trauma is related to the young age of the victims, the severity of injuries sustained, delay in seeking appropriate health care, and delay in accurately diagnosing the injury due to the misleading histories given by caregivers (Nance & Cooper, 2009). Blunt abdominal trauma, the most common type of inflicted abdominal trauma in abused children, usually results from their having been punched or kicked in the abdomen. It may produce intra-abdominal hemorrhage with few external signs of trauma. The blow is usually to the mid-abdomen.

The child may present for treatment with persistent vomiting, abdominal pain or distension, fever, or signs of hypovolemic shock. Internal organs that may be injured by blunt trauma include the pancreas, duodenum, jejunum, mesentery, liver, spleen, and kidneys.

Genital Injuries

Injuries to the genitalia may be accidental or acquired as a result of child sexual abuse. Refer to chapter 12 for a full discussion of child sexual abuse.

Münchausen by Proxy

Münchausen by proxy (MBP), also known as factitious disorder by proxy, was previously considered a rare form of child maltreatment. However, it is now thought to be more common than previously recognized and can have very serious consequences, including death of a child (Ayoub et al., 2002). Roy Meadow described the first case in 1977 in England. In cases of MBP, a parent or other caregiver, deliberately falsifies a child's illness through fabrication or creation of symptoms and then seeks health care. It is important to note that 95% of all cases of MBP are perpetrated by mothers. In some cases, the motivation is a compulsive need to deceive health care providers or garner attention for herself as an ideal parent. The recidivism rate of mothers suffering from MBP is very high, with 6% of cases resulting in the death of the child victim (Schreier, 2002).

Younger children, especially infants and toddlers, are more vulnerable to this type of maltreatment than older children, most likely because they have not yet developed verbal abilities. Males and females are at equal risk of abuse involving MBP. Child victims of MBP are at significant risk of short- and long-term physical and psychological harm, and even death. In fatal cases, the perpetrator unintentionally goes too far. In the largest study of deaths related to MBP, apnea was the commonly reported symptom that preceded death (Rosenberg, 2009). Seventy-five percent of fatal cases occur in hospitals. It is crucial to note that siblings of victims of MBP tend to die in alarming numbers, often with the diagnosis of Sudden Infant Death Syndrome (Rosenberg, 2009).

In many cases of MBP, there is a long history of suspicious symptoms that do not make clinical sense and lead to multiple, unnecessary diagnostic and therapeutic procedures. The mother often appears genuinely concerned over her child's illness. For instance, when the child is hospitalized, she may rarely leave the child's bedside while continuing to induce symptoms. In fact, many cases are diagnosed when the child's symptoms disappear when separated from the mother. In many instances, the mother has trained in one of the health care professions and is, therefore, adept at making falsified information appear credible.

Perpetrators of MBP may induce physical symptoms in their children with manual suffocation, administration of drugs or toxic substances, or contaminating central lines. When drugs are used, they often involve laxatives to induce severe diarrhea, insulin to induce hypoglycemia and seizures, ipecac to induce vomiting, and drugs or alcohol to cause an alteration in level of consciousness. Salt may be added to an infant's formula to induce hypernatremia. In addition, mothers have been known to add their own blood to a child's urine, stool, or vomitus to mimic a bleeding disorder. Suffocation of an infant or child is also used to induce symptoms. Although less common, MBP may also involve falsification of psychological or developmental symptoms. In such cases, the mother may provide false descriptions of a child's behavior that are consistent with a psychological or behavioral disorder (Schreier, 2000).

Child Abuse by Poisoning

Child abuse by poisoning refers to the intentional administration of a medication or toxic substance to a child with the intention to cause harm, as well as the unintentional poisoning of a child due to severe neglect (Henretig, Paschall, & Donaruma-Kwoh, 2009). Child abuse by poisoning may involve oral ingestion, inhalation, injection, or placement on skin or mucous membranes. Caregivers may administer antihistamines, such as Benadryl, for the desired side effect of sleepiness, so that the caregiver is free of supervision of the child for several hours.

Child abuse by poisoning can also involve alcohol or illicit drugs. One common scenario is for a child to ingest alcohol or illegal drugs. It can also occur from breathing "secondhand" smoke when caregivers smoke crack cocaine, marijuana, heroin, or methamphetamine in the presence of children. Children are also exposed to toxic substances when a caregiver has a methamphetamine laboratory in the home. In some circumstances, a caregiver may give the child alcohol or other drug for entertainment purposes. Even if a child is not directly exposed to an illicit drug, it is very important for nurses to be concerned whenever it becomes known that the caregiver is involved in substance abuse, given the strong association between child maltreatment and substance abuse (Kelley, 2002).

Neglect

Although neglect receives considerably less attention in the professional literature and public media than physical abuse, it is far more prevalent (Dubowitz & Black, 2009). Child neglect generally involves acts of omission, or failure to meet the basic needs of a child that results in actual or potential harm. Neglect tends to be chronic, while abuse is often episodic.

Each child's specific situation needs to be assessed to determine whether their needs are being met. In considering neglect, several factors need to be considered: whether actual or potential harm has occurred, the severity of the harm involved, and the frequency or chronicity of the circumstances (Dubowitz & Black, 2009). Neglect is often related to poverty, lower parental educational attainment, lack of parenting skills, substance abuse, and depression. It may also include health neglect, educational neglect, and emotional neglect.

Physical indicators of neglect can include malnourishment, inadequate hygiene, and inappropriate attire, such as light weight clothing in cold weather or very soiled clothing. Neglected children may have a history of numerous accidental injuries due to inadequate supervision. A child may have evidence of inadequate health care, such as lack of immunizations and untreated health problems, including dental caries. Neglect may also involve exposure to interpersonal violence, secondhand cigarette smoke, and guns.

Behavioral indicators of neglect may include developmental delays, behavioral or school problems, apathy, and excessive quietness. Malnourished children generally do poorly in school due to low energy and inability to concentrate. Children may also underperform in school due to lack of sleep when parents fail to adequately supervise their bedtime schedules. When assessing cases of neglect, it is important to identify the circumstances that may have contributed to the neglect such as inadequate resources, lack of social support, and chaotic living arrangements, in order to effectively intervene.

Psychological Abuse

Psychological maltreatment consists of psychological abuse or neglect, occurring alone, or along with other forms of child maltreatment. It is important to recognize that there is inherently a psychological component to all forms of child maltreatment. Even when psychological maltreatment occurs in the absence of other forms of abuse, it can be as detrimental as other forms of child maltreatment. Similar to neglect, psychological abuse is often of a chronic nature. Of all forms of child maltreatment, psychological maltreatment has historically received the least amount of attention. In addition to issues of definition and identification, one major reason is that it is often assumed that the consequences of emotional abuse are not as severe as those of more obvious forms of child maltreatment (Egeland, 2009). Even though it does not leave physical signs, psychological abuse can be devastating in its consequences (Miller-Perrin, Perrin, & Kocur, 2009; Shaffer, Yates, & Egeland, 2009).

Psychological maltreatment is often characterized into the following six major types (Hart, Brassard, Binggeli, & Davidson, 2002):

1. Spurning behaviors include verbal and nonverbal caregiver acts that reject and degrade a child. Spurning includes belittling, degrading, and other nonphysical forms of overtly hostile or rejecting treatment; shaming and/or ridiculing the child for showing normal emotions such as affection, grief, or sorrow; consistently singling out one child to criticize and punish or receive fewer rewards; and more public humiliation.
2. Terrorizing behaviors include threats to physically hurt, kill, abandon, or place the child or child's loved ones in dangerous situations. Terrorizing includes placing a child in chaotic, unpredictable, or dangerous situations; and setting unrealistic expectations with the threat of loss, harm, or danger if they are not met.
3. Isolating behaviors that include caregiver acts that consistently deny children opportunities to meet their needs for interacting or communicating with peers or adults within, or outside of, the family. It includes confining the child or placing unreasonable limitations on the child's movements within his or her environment and placing unreasonable limitations or restrictions on social interactions with peers or adults in the community.
4. Exploiting and corrupting behaviors that include caregiver acts that encourage the child to develop inappropriate behaviors including self-destructive, antisocial, criminal, deviant, or other maladaptive behaviors.
5. Denying or ignoring social responsiveness, which includes caregiver acts that ignore the child's attempts for emotional engagement. It involves caregivers being detached and uninvolved through either incapacity or lack of motivation, interacting only when absolutely necessary, and failing to express affection, caring, or love for the child.
6. Mental health, physical health, and educational neglect, which includes unwarranted caregiver acts that ignore, refuse to allow, or fail to provide the necessary treatment of the mental health, physical health, and educational needs or the child.

DOCUMENTATION

Accurate and detailed documentation of the history, physical findings, behavioral observations, and laboratory assessment is critical in all cases of suspected child abuse and neglect and is of utmost importance. All questions asked by the health care professional and all answers provided by the child and caregivers should be carefully documented verbatim. Documentation of the history should include:

- how and when the injury occurred
- whether the injury was witnessed, and if so, by whom; person responsible for the child at time of injury
- general health of the child
- child's previous surgeries and hospitalizations
- child's significant health history
- whether the child was previously evaluated for the presenting symptoms or injury, and if so, where (Pierce-Weeks & Giardino, 2003)

All significant statements made by parents and children during the nursing interview should be carefully recorded, with as many direct quotations as possible. The behavior of the child and parents should be described carefully. The nurse has an important responsibility to carefully report all facts, omitting subjective opinions.

It is not enough to write "multiple bruises in various stages of healing noted." Rather, each bruise, lesion, or burn needs to be described in detail according to its size, location, color, and shape. It is important to be cognizant that the patient's health record also serves as a legal document. If courtroom testimony becomes necessary, a well-documented chart helps to refresh the clinician's memory. In cases of neglect, documentation includes charting evidence from the history and observation of the child, including how well the child's basic needs are being met such as shelter, food, clothing, school attendance, and health care issues.

Photodocumentation

Color photographs of all injuries should be taken with a 35-mm camera, whenever possible. While instant cameras may be less costly and easier to operate, they produce photographs with poor resolution. In some jurisdictions, parental permission to take a child's photograph is needed, whereas in others, photography can be taken without parental consent. Even the most severely abused children are often physically healed by the time of a court hearing. Photographs help the judge or jury understand the extent of the child's injuries. They are also helpful when seeking a second opinion or for peer review and teaching. Photographs become part of the permanent health record. It is important to also include any outline drawings of the child's body to show the area photographed. A measuring device should be positioned above, or below, the injury to depict the size of the injury.

When taking photographs, it is important to photograph all injuries with, and without, a color/measure standard, take a photo of the face to identify the patient, include a landmark such as an elbow or a knee so that the viewer can identify the location of the injury, and carefully label and store all photos (see Ricci & Shapiro, 2009 for a detailed discussion of photodocumentation in cases of suspected maltreatment).

CHILD MALTREATMENT FATALITIES

Any child fatality is tragic and particularly so when it involves maltreatment. In the vast majority of cases, the fatal incident is not the first occurrence of abuse or neglect, but is rather the culmination of a series of abusive incidents or neglectful behaviors, underscoring the need for early identification and intervention. It is estimated that 1,760 children died from either neglect or physical abuse in 2007, with neglect being the more common cause (Children's Bureau, 2009). Of these child fatalities, children younger than 4 years were at greatest risk and involved more than three quarters (75.7%) of the cases. Of children in this age group, those 1 year of age and younger were of greatest risk, with boys at the highest risk for fatalities.

The vast majority of states have multiagency, multidisciplinary child death review teams (CDRTs) at the local or state level for systematically evaluating and managing cases of suspicious child fatalities, with the purpose of preventing future fatalities. CDRT findings can help to focus local, state, and national prevention efforts. Over time, the mission of CDRTs has expanded in many jurisdictions to include nonabuse-related deaths and older children rather than simply looking at child abuse-related deaths in young children (Alexander, 2007). Between 1992 and 2001, the number of states with CDRTs has grown from 21 to 48, plus the District of Columbia (Webster & Schnitzer, 2007).

These CDRTs typically comprise representatives of the medical examiner's office, public health, law enforcement agencies, and child protective service agencies, as well as prosecutors, pediatricians, and nurses with child abuse expertise. Among the advantages of such review teams are improved communication and cooperation among agencies, increased knowledge of risk factors for child homicide, systematic evaluation of agency actions and inactions, and the identification of surviving siblings at risk for maltreatment. CDRTs in most states have mechanisms for communicating their findings and recommendations to officials and the general public (Webster & Schnitzer, 2007).

Intimate partner violence (IPV) in the home places a child at increased risk for maltreatment. This fact underscores the need to evaluate all child fatalities for the presence of IPV in the home and whether and how the IPV contributed to the deaths (Kuelbs, 2007). Children may be inadvertently fatally injured during physical violence in the home or through neglectful behaviors, such as the absence of appropriate parental supervision. Domestic violence fatality review committees are increasing across the United States. Similar to CDRTs, they seek to determine the circumstances surrounding the fatality and what could be done to prevent such deaths. Focus is at system-wide levels, rather than individual ones, in an effort to effect system changes rather than assess blame (Kuelbs, 2007).

INTERVENTION

Treatment

Although research has documented that children suffer both short- and long-term consequences of maltreatment, most abused children do not receive mental health treatment. Even when they do receive treatment, it may not be from clinicians who are well versed in evidenced-based approaches to providing effective therapy. When children are referred for therapy, it is critical that they are seen by clinicians trained in evidenced-based treatment. To date, research indicates that trauma-focused, cognitive behavioral therapy (TF-CBT) is the most effective approach to working with abused children (Cohen & Kolko, 2009; Deblinger & Runyon, 2005; Kolko, 1996). Children who have experienced any form of maltreatment should be referred for a psychological evaluation to determine whether there is a need for therapy, as not all children suffer negative sequelae from abuse. The more severely dysfunctional child victim may need residential treatment. Because child maltreatment most often occurs in the family setting, therapy should address not only the child's individual needs, but parent and family dysfunction as well.

The National Child Traumatic Stress Network (NCTSN), a national network of over 60 sites, provides community-based treatment and services across the United States to improve the standard of care for traumatized children, adolescents, and their families. The NCTSN can be accessed at www.NCTSNet.org. It provides information for professionals, including referral sources. It also provides information for parents of traumatized children.

Legal Issues

Every state has a law requiring the reporting of suspected child maltreatment to designated child protection or law enforcement authorities. Although anyone in any state may report a suspicion of child abuse, reporting laws usually mandate reporting only for professionals who have regular contact with children (Myers, 2005). In each of the 50 states, nurses are mandated reporters.

Reporting requirements provide that a report must be made if the mandated reporter suspects or has reason to believe that a child has been abused or neglected; health care professionals do not need to be absolutely certain that abuse or neglect occurred. A professional who postpones reporting until all doubt is eliminated probably will have violated the reporting law (Myers, 2005). Reporting laws deliberately leave the ultimate decision about whether abuse or neglect occurred to investigating officials, not to mandated reporters.

Nurses and other professionals reporting child maltreatment in good faith are typically immune from civil or criminal liability, while mandated reporters who knowingly, or intentionally, fail to report suspected abuse or neglect are subject to civil or criminal liability. Some states impose criminal liability even if the mandated reporter did not realize the child was abused when a reasonable professional would have suspected abuse (Myers, 2005). Deliberate failure to report suspected abuse is a considered a crime (Myers, 2005).

The disposition in cases of child abuse depends on many variables, such as the severity of the presenting injury and the circumstances under which it occurred. The most important single factor to assess is whether the child is at immediate risk of further abuse if returned home. If such a risk exists, the child may be temporarily removed from the home through admission to the hospital, placement in the home of a relative, such as a grandparent or aunt, or emergency placement in a foster home. Often, temporary removal from the home allows time for the parent to receive necessary support services.

All states provide a mechanism for protecting children in emergencies (Myers, 2005). If a parent refuses to allow a child to be admitted to the hospital or placed with a relative or in foster care, an emergency care and protection order can be obtained via telephone from a judge in most jurisdictions. This gives the hospital authority to temporarily remove the child from the home, pending further investigation into the child's safety; it also allows time for arrangement of support services for the family.

Interdisciplinary Approach

An interdisciplinary approach to child maltreatment involving nurses, physicians, therapists, attorneys, and social workers is imperative. The problem of child maltreatment is complex, and thus cannot be addressed by any single discipline or intervention. Most tertiary care settings that treat children have interdisciplinary child protection teams that work together to properly identify and intervene with children who have been maltreated.

A number of professional organizations exist to support nurses and other professionals who work with maltreated children and their families. Most disseminate research and other information to support professionals working with survivors of violence. In addition to providing information on various aspects of violence, they provide an opportunity for professionals to come together to support each other, in what is often very challenging work. Please refer to Exhibit 10.3 for a list of such organizations and referral sources.

PREVENTION

The Centers for Disease Control and Prevention's (CDC) child maltreatment prevention program seeks to prevent violence-related injuries and death through surveillance, research and development, capacity building, communication, and leadership (CDC, 2009). Surveillance allows the assessment of the magnitude and impact of public health issues and how they change over time. This public health approach to child maltreatment prevention is based on the premise that safe, stable, and nurturing relationships are the antithesis of maltreatment and other adverse exposures that occur during childhood and compromise health over the life span. The promotion of safe, stable, and nurturing relationships, if done effectively, can have synergistic effects on a broad range of health problems, as well as contribute to the development of skills that will enhance the acquisition of healthy lifestyles.

The three dimensions of safe, stable, and nurturing relationships represent important aspects of the social and physical environments that protect children and promote their optimal development. Each can be thought of as being on the positive end of a continuum that extends from safe to neglectful and violent relationships/environments, from stable to unpredictable and chaotic relationships/environments, and from nurturing to hostile/cold or rejecting relationships/environments. While these dimensions overlap, each represents important and distinct aspects of a child's relationships and environment that are crucial to healthy development. Because young children experience the world through their relationships with parents and other caregivers, these relationships are fundamental to the healthy development of the brain and the development of physical, emotional, social, behavioral, and intellectual capacities.

According to the CDC, there is substantial evidence that promoting safe, stable, and nurturing relationships can be effective in reducing child maltreatment by teaching parents positive child-rearing and management skills and strategies that are safe and

EXHIBIT 10.3 | *Professional Organizations and Resources*

American Professional Society on the Abuse of Children (APSAC)
The American Professional Society on the Abuse of Children (APSAC) is a national organization whose mission is to enhance the ability of professionals to respond to children and families affected by abuse and violence. APSAC tries to fulfill this mission in a number of ways, most notably through providing education and other sources of information to professionals who work in child maltreatment and related fields.
APSAC
350 Poplar Avenue
Elmhurst, IL 60126
Phone: (630)941.1235
Toll Free: (877) 402-7722
Fax: (630) 359-4274
E-mail: apsac@apsac.org
Website Address: http://www.apsac.org

Academy on Violence and Abuse (AVA)
The Academy on Violence and Abuse (AVA) exists to advance health education and research on the prevention, recognition, treatment, and health effects of violence and abuse. By expanding health education and research, the AVA:
 • Integrates knowledge about violence and abuse into the training of all health professionals,
 • Promotes the health of all people,
 • Protects the most vulnerable, and
 • Advances health and social policy that promotes safe families, workplaces and communities.
Academy on Violence and Abuse
14850 Scenic Heights Road, Suite 135A
Eden Prairie, MN 55344
Phone: (952) 974-3270
Fax: (952) 974-3291
Website Address: http://avahealth.org

Family Violence Prevention Fund (FVPF)
The Family Violence Prevention Fund works to prevent violence within the home, and in the community, to help those whose lives are devastated by violence because everyone has the right to live free of violence.
Mailing Address/Phone:
Family Violence Prevention Fund
383 Rhode Island St., Suite #304
San Francisco, CA 94103-5133
Phone: (415) 252-8900
Fax: (415) 252-8991
TTY: (800) 595-4889
E-mail: info@endabuse.org
Website Address: http://endabuse.org

The International Society for Prevention of Child Abuse and Neglect (ISPCAN)
The International Society for Prevention of Child Abuse and Neglect (ISPCAN)'s mission is to prevent cruelty to children in every nation, in every form: physical abuse,

sexual abuse, neglect, street children, child fatalities, child prostitution, children of war, emotional abuse and child labor. ISPCAN is committed to increasing public awareness of all forms of violence against children, developing activities to prevent such violence, and promoting the rights of children in all regions of the world.
International Society for Prevention of Child Abuse and Neglect
13123 E. 16th Ave. B390
Aurora, CO 80045 USA
Telephone: (303) 864-5220
Fax: (303) 864-5222
Email: ispcan@ispcan.org
Website Address: http://www.ispcan.org

International Association of Forensic Nurses (IAFN)
The mission of the International Association of Forensic Nurses (IAFN) is to provide leadership in forensic nursing practice by developing, promoting, and disseminating information internationally about forensic nursing science. The International Association of Forensic Nurses organizational goals are:
- To incorporate primary prevention strategies into our work at every level in an attempt to create a world without violence
- To establish and improve standards of evidence-based forensic nursing practice
- To promote and encourage the exchange of ideas and transmission of developing knowledge among its members and related disciplines
- To establish standards of ethical conduct for forensic nurses
- To create and facilitate educational opportunities for forensic nurses and related disciplines.

International Association of Forensic Nurses
1517 Ritchie Hwy, Ste 208
Arnold, MD 21012-2323
Phone: (410) 626-7805
Fax: (410) 626-7804
Website Address: http://www.iafn.org

Prevent Child Abuse America (PCA)
Since 1972, Prevent Child Abuse America (PCA America) has led the way in building awareness, providing education and inspiring hope to everyone involved in the effort to prevent the abuse and neglect of our nation's children. Prevent Child Abuse America is committed to promoting legislation, policies and programs that help to prevent child abuse and neglect, support healthy childhood development, and strengthen families.
Prevent Child Abuse America
500 North Michigan Avenue
Suite 200
Chicago, IL 60611-3703
Phone: (312) 663-3520
Fax: (312) 939-8962
E-mail: mailbox@preventchildabuse.org
Website Address: http://www.preventchildabuse.org
Information and Referral:
(800) CHILDREN
(800) 244-5373

Continued

EXHIBIT 10.3 *Continued*

National Center for Missing & Exploited Children (NCMEC)
The National Center for Missing & Exploited Children's® (NCMEC) mission is to help prevent child abduction and sexual exploitation; help find missing children; and assist victims of child abduction and sexual exploitation, their families, and the professionals who serve them.
National Center for Missing & Exploited Children
Charles B. Wang International Children's Building
699 Prince Street
Alexandria, Virginia 22314-3175
24-hour Hotline: (800) THE-LOST (800) 843-5678)
Fax: (703) 274-2200
Website Address: http://www.missingkids.com

Nursing Network on Violence Against Women, International (NNVAWI)
The mission of Nursing Network on Violence Against Women, International (NNVAWI) is to eliminate violence through advancing nursing education, practice, research, and public policy.
Nursing Network on Violence Against Women, International
PMB 165
1801 H Street B5
Modesto, CA 95354-1215
(888) 909-9993
Website Address: http://www.nnvawi.org

---

nurturing (CDC, 2009). There is ample evidence that the parent training programs and behavioral family interventions delivered in clinical settings and focusing on influencing children's behavior through positive reinforcement are effective at influencing the parenting practices of families and reducing child maltreatment. Parent–child interaction therapy (PCIT) has also been effective in reducing child maltreatment in families who have been referred to child protective services. PCIT is an intensive behavioral intervention for parents and children that involves training parents on specific skills using live coaching and dyadic parent–child sessions. Other approaches to promoting safe, stable, and nurturing relationships include providing social support to parents and families, as it can buffer the effects of chronic and situational stress. Parent education and social support can be enhanced through center-based child development programs and home visitation programs (CDC, 2009).

Child maltreatment prevention can also be achieved by addressing social determinants of child maltreatment. Social determinants that are associated with child maltreatment include neighborhood economic distress and disadvantage; housing stress, low social capital, low family income, low parental education, and inadequate social support (CDC, 2009). From a public health perspective, interventions that target prevalent and neglected risk factors such as poverty, partner violence, teenage pregnancy, and social norms tolerating violence toward children need to be developed and evaluated (Klevens & Whitaker, 2007).

While there are many theoretically sound child maltreatment prevention models, many fewer have established efficacy through rigorous scientific evaluation. There are several evidence-based child maltreatment prevention programs available for implementation in

EXHIBIT 10.4 | *Case Study*

Brief background

Isabella is a 13-month-old Caucasian female who is brought to the emergency department (ED) at the local community hospital by her mother and father. Her 20-year-old, single mother stated that when she came home from work at 6:30 P.M. that day she found her daughter "drowsy" and not "acting normal." The child had been left home all day in the care of her boyfriend, the child's father. The father denied any history of an injury. While the mother was a high school graduate, the father did not finish high school and is currently unemployed. A review of the hospital health record revealed that when 11 months old, Isabella had been brought to the same emergency department because of two bruises on the face and irritability. An X-ray revealed no fractures, and the child was discharged home. There were similar circumstances to the current ED visit in that the infant had been in the care of her father while the mother was at work, and the father denied any knowledge of a trauma.

Assessment

The nurse's history for the present visit revealed further information. When interviewed alone, the father admitted to have been smoking marijuana and drinking beer while caring for Isabella. He indicated that he smoked marijuana daily and consumed approximately six beers a day. The father stated the infant cried often and was inconsolable at times. During an interview with the mother, in the absence of the father, she indicated that he had a very bad temper and was often impatient with the baby. The mother believed that she had no other choice than to leave the baby with her boyfriend while she was at work because they could not afford a babysitter and had no family in the area. The mother indicated that the child's immunizations were up to date; the infant had no known illnesses or allergies, and was achieving normal developmental milestones. When an MRI indicated significant brain injury and confronted with the suspicion of abusive head trauma, the father admitted to violently shaking the infant in an attempt to get her to stop crying.

The nurse's physical examination include, but is not limited to the following:

An initial assessment focused on airway, breathing, circulation, and neurologic status. The infant's vital signs were stable, but she appeared lethargic and pale, and did not respond to verbal or visual stimuli. The assessment also revealed bruises to the child's upper arms that were reddish-blue in color, bilateral, and resembled grasp marks. Bruises were also found on the infant's upper chest. These bruises were also reddish-blue in color and bilateral. Each of these lesions was measured, their location noted on a diagram and photographed accordingly to recommended photdocumentation guidelines. A head-to-toe exam did not reveal any other obvious signs of trauma.

Nursing diagnoses, outcomes, interventions, and evaluation

The three nursing diagnoses identified are described in order of priority.

Nursing Diagnosis:
Risk for delayed development related to head trauma
Short-Term Client Goal:
Infant will remain safe while in the ED and upon discharge as evidenced by:
- Infant is protected from further injury while in ED
- Parents are prevented from leaving hospital against advice
- Mother's agreement to cooperate with social services, child protective services, and law enforcement
- Mother's agreement not to give access to infant's father until family intervention has occurred

Continued

EXHIBIT 10.3 *Continued*

Nursing Interventions:
- Support airway, breathing, and circulation
- Continually monitor level of consciousness using the AVPU method (*A*lert, responds to *V*erbal stimuli, responds to *P*ainful stimuli, *U*nresponsive) or Glasgow Coma Scale method
- Continually monitor vital signs
- Facilitate rapid diagnostic testing, include MRI
- Provide emotional support to parents
- Encourage mother to hold and reassure infant
- Provide discreet supervision of parents' interactions with infant

Evaluation:
Because the nursing process is still in development, no evaluation is possible.

Long-Term Client Goal:
Infant will not be abused or neglected after hospitalization and will achieve her developmental potential as evidenced by:
- Long-term neurological deficits will be minimized by participation in early intervention program
- Father will receive professional help for substance abuse and remain alcohol and drug free
- Documented participation with child protective services
- Documented participation with community agencies
- Mother receives adequate social support

Nursing Interventions:
Family is referred to public health nurse for monitoring of infant and family, as well as safety of home.
The public health nurse will:
- Provide information to mother regarding community resources, including early intervention
- Provide teaching on normal growth and development
- Coordinate services with child protective services
- Use strength-based approach to help mother develop effective parenting strategies
- Work with mother to child-proof the home

Evaluation:
Long-term evaluation will be conducted by the public health nurse.

Nursing Diagnosis:
Anxiety due to the uncertainty of the infant's prognosis.

Short-Term Client Goal:
Family will be provided with support and up-to-date information on infant's status in ED as evidenced by:
- Frequent updates on vital signs and laboratory results
- Nonjudgmental approach will be used in all interactions with parents
- Parents are informed of need to admit infant to hospital

Evaluation:
Because the nursing process is still in development, no evaluation is possible.

Long-Term Client Goal:
Mother will be supported throughout hospital stay and upon discharge as evidenced by:
- A reduction in social isolation
- Documented use high-quality child care

- Referral for counseling
- Referral for home visitation parenting program such as SafeCare, the Triple P program, etc. (refer to section on prevention)

Evaluation:
Long-term evaluation will be conducted by the public health nurse.

Nursing Diagnosis:
Altered Family Processes
This is a family-level nursing diagnosis and addresses the potential for further abuse of the infant related to lack of social support and resources, as well as father's history of substance abuse.

Short-Term Client Goal:
Family will not resort to violent behavior in hospital as evidenced by:
- Continual monitoring of infant and parents during hospitalization
- Father is never left alone with infant
- Parents do not have opportunity to remove child from hospital until discharge

Nursing Interventions:
- Work with hospital's child protection team to obtain care and emergency protection order to assure parents cannot remove child from hospital against advice
- File report of suspected abuse to child protective services
- Reassure mother that report to child protective services is meant to assure that support services are provided and is not meant as a punitive measure
- Inform mother that child protective services will determine if child is safe to be discharged to the care of the mother
- Encourage mother to seek counseling

Long-Term Goals:
Family will not resort to violent behavior and will develop more effective parenting strategies as evidenced by:
- Father will enter substance abuse treatment program
- Father will seek treatment for poor impulse control and anger management
- Child will not be left in care of father until professionals ascertain his risk to the child
- Mother is able to set limits on father's access to infant
- Parents seek counseling if mother chooses to remain with child's father

Nursing Interventions:
As noted above, referral is made to public health nursing for continued monitoring of child, family, and home.

Evaluation:
Long-term evaluation will be conducted by the public health nurse.

the community or clinical setting. Those with most well-established evidence of their effectiveness include the Triple P program (Prinz, Sanders, Shapiro, Whitaker, & Lutzker, 2009); SafeCare model (Edwards & Lutzker, 2008), Safe Environment for Every Kid (SEEK) model (Dubowitz, Feigelman, Lane, & Kim, 2009), Family Connections (DePanfilis & Dubowitz (2005), and the Nurse Family-Partnership (Olds, 2006; Zielinski, Eckenrode, & Olds, 2009).

The general public views nurses as one of the most trusted professional groups. This trust can be parlayed with high-risk families by reaching out to those who are struggling to provide nurturing and safe environments for their children. Nurses and other health professionals should make opportunities to provide information related to child safety and parenting skills to all families. This can be accomplished by providing families with referrals to resources within their community that help strengthen families and enhance child rearing. Nurses may also help to prevent abuse and neglect by assisting families in identifying sources of social support and where to obtain the resources necessary for raising children. Many communities offer telephone hotlines for parents experiencing high levels of stress. Nurses need to pay particular attention to the safety of children when there is a history of interpersonal violence or substance abuse in the family.

CULTURAL CONSIDERATIONS

Because we live in a multicultural society, it is important to recognize that there are many different approaches to parenting, including child discipline. Professionals should not judge child-rearing practices that differ from their own unless they pose harm, whether physical or psychological, to the child. Some racial and ethnic groups value the use of corporal punishment more than others. In a study examining cultural factors that influence child physical abuse reporting, researchers found that the ethnicity of the respondent was a significant predictor of reporting tendencies for African American respondents, but not Hispanics and Caucasians (Ibanez, Borrego, Pemberton, & Terao, 2006). African American participants indicated a greater acceptance of corporal punishment than did Hispanics and Caucasians and were less likely to report cases of physical abuse.

Although child maltreatment affects children of all ethnic groups, ethnic differences in the prevalence rates of child maltreatment have been reported. In 2007, the most recent year for which federal data were available, African American children, American Indian and Alaska Native children had disproportionately higher rates of substantiated cases of child maltreatment compared to Hispanics and Caucasians (Children's Bureau, 2009). African American children, American Indian, and Alaska Native children had the highest rates of victimization at 16.6, 14.2, and 14.0 per 1,000 children, respectively. Hispanic and Caucasian children had rates of 10.3 and 9.1 per 1,000 children, respectively. Asian children had the lowest rate at 2.4 per 1,000 children. Nearly one half of all victims were Caucasian (46.1%); one fifth (21.7%) were African American, and one fifth (20.8%) were Hispanic (Children's Bureau, 2009). Children of color are also disproportionately represented in the foster care system.

There are many factors that could contribute to the disproportionate reporting of child maltreatment in minority children. They include poverty, which increases the likelihood of contact with multiple public agencies, and thus greater visibility to mandated reporters. Poverty can also contribute to increased stress within the family due to crowded housing conditions and lack of available resources to raise children. Biases in reporting and case substantiation may also play a factor as professionals from minority groups are underrepresented in most professional groups.

Cultural Practices Mistaken for Child Abuse

It is important for health professionals to be aware that there are certain cultural practices that can be mistaken for child maltreatment. Coin rubbing, sometimes referred to as Cao Gio, is practiced in Southeast Asia and southern China as a healing method. It involves placing an oil or balm to the skin and then rubbing the skin with the edge of a coin that results in linear bruises and may, or may not, cause pain or discomfort. Because the bruising resolves in a short time, many communities do not consider it a form of maltreatment. A practice, referred to as cupping, is used in some Asian and European countries. Similar to coining, it is used to promote healing. A cup is heated, sometimes with hot oil or alcohol, and placed against the skin and held until the trapped air cools and contracts, forming a vacuum (Hymel & Boos, 2009). The suction can cause petechiae in the shape of the cup. Because the resulting lesions are usually nonpainful, many communities do not consider this a form of child maltreatment. Moxibustion is the Chinese healing practice of burning small amounts of an herb near acupuncture points. When it causes burns, it may be considered abuse. When assessing such cultural practices, it may be useful to consult with members of the same ethnic community to determine the norms in their culture.

CONCLUSION

Child maltreatment is an all too common phenomenon, with serious long-term physical and mental health consequences. Astute observations of child and family dynamics, knowledge of the causes of intentional and unintentional injury, and prompt recognition of abuse and neglect may help nurses decrease the morbidity and mortality associated with child maltreatment. Nurses are mandated by law to report suspected abuse and neglect. Collaborating with the hospital's child protection team is essential for facilitating the care of maltreated children. Involvement in nursing organizations concerned with abuse, as well as interdisciplinary organizations, can facilitate learning about evidence-based practice, networking, advocacy, and support from other professionals who work with maltreating families and adult survivors.

REFERENCES

Afifi, T. O., Boman, J., Fleisher, W., & Sareen, J. (2009). The relationship between child abuse, parental divorce, and lifetime mental disorders and suicidality in a nationally representative adult sample. *Child Abuse & Neglect, 33*, 139–147.

Alexander, R. (2007). Overview. In R. Alexander (Ed.), *Child fatality review: An interdisciplinary guide and photographic reference* (pp. 3–12). St. Louis: G. W. Medical Publishing.

American Academy of Pediatrics (2000). Diagnostic imaging of child abuse. *Pediatrics, 105*, 1345–1348.

Ayoub, C., Alexander, R., Beck, D., Bursch, B., Feldman, K. W., Libow, J. Sanders, M. J., Schreier, H.A. & Yorker, B. (2002). Position paper: Definitional issues in Munchausen by proxy: APSAC Taskforce on Munchausen by prosy, definitions working group. *Child Maltreatment, 7*, 105–111.

Briere, J., & Elliot, D. M. (2003). Prevalence and psychological sequelae of self-reported childhood physical and sexual abuse in a general population sample of men and women. *Child Abuse & Neglect, 27*, 1205–1222.

Centers for Disease Control and Prevention (2009). *Preventing child maltreatment through the promotion of safe, stable, and nurturing relationships between children and caregivers.* Atlanta: CDC.

Chapman, D. P., Whitfield, C. L., Felletti, V. J., Dube, S. R., Edwards, V. J., & Anda, R. F. (2004). Adverse childhood experiences and the risk of depressive disorders in adulthood. *Journal of Affective Disorders, 82*, 217–225.

Children's Bureau (2009). *Child maltreatment 2007.* Washington, DC: Administration for Children and Families, DHHS.

Cicchetti, D., Rogosch, R. A. & Tooth, S. L. (2006). Fostering secure attachment in infants in maltreating families through preventive interventions. *Development and Psychopathology, 18*, 623–649.

Cohen, J. A., & Kolko, D. J. (2009). Posttraumatic Stress Disorder (pp. 1285–1291). In T. K. McInerny, H. M. Adam, D. E. Campbell, D. M. Kamat, & K. J. Kelleher (Eds.), *American Academy of Pediatrics textbook of pediatric care*. Elk Grove Village, IL: American Academy of Pediatrics.

Cooperman, D. R., & Merten, D. F. (2009). Skeletal manifestations of child abuse. In R. M. Reece & C. W. Christian (Eds.), *Child abuse: Medical diagnosis and treatment* (3rd ed., pp. 121–166). Chicago: American Academy of Pediatrics.

Daignault, I. V., & Herbert, M. (2009). Profiles of school adaptation: Social, behavioral and academic functioning in sexually abused girls. *Child Abuse & Neglect, 33*, 102–115.

Danielson, C. K., Amstadter, A. B., Dangelmaier, R. E., Resnick, H. S., Saunders, B. E., & Kilpatrick, D. G. (2009). Trauma-related risk factors for substance abuse among male versus female young adults. *Addictive Behaviors, 34*, 395–399.

Deblinger, E., & Runyon, M. K. (2005). Understanding and treating feelings of shame in children who have experienced maltreatment. *Child Maltreatment, 10*, 364–367.

DePanfilis, D., & Dubowitz, H. (2005). Family connections: A program for preventing child neglect. *Child Maltreatment, 10*, 108–123.

Dubowitz, H., & Black, M. M. (2009). Child neglect. In R. M. Reece & C. W. Christian (Eds.), *Child abuse: Medical diagnosis and treatment* (3rd ed., pp. 427–463). Chicago: American Academy of Pediatrics.

Dubowitz, H., Feigelman, S. Lane, W., & Kim, J. (2009). Pediatric primary care to help prevent child maltreatment: The safe environment for every kid (SEEK) model. *Pediatrics, 123*, 858–864.

Edwards, A., & Lutzker, J. R. (2008). Iterations of the SafeCare model: An evidence-based child maltreatment prevention program. *Behavioral Modification, 32*, 736–757.

Egeland, B. (2009). Taking stock: Childhood emotional maltreatment and developmental psychopathology. *Child Abuse & Neglect, 22*, 22–26.

Finkelhor, D., Ormrod, R., Turner, H., & Hamby, S. L. (2005). The victimization of children and youth: A comprehensive, national survey. *Child Maltreatment, 10*, 5–25.

Hart, S. N., Brassard, M. R., Binggeli, N. J., & Davidson, H. A. (2002). Psychological maltreatment. In Myers, J. E. B. Myers, L. Berliner, J. Briere, C. T. Hendrix, C. Jenny. & Reid. (Eds.), *The APSAC handbook on child maltreatment* (2nd ed., pp. 79–103).

Henretig, F. M., Paschall, R., & Donaruma-Kwoh, M. M. (2009). Child abuse by poisoning. In R. M. Reece & C. W. Christian (Eds.), *Child abuse: Medical diagnosis and treatment* (3rd ed., pp. 549–599). Chicago: American Academy of Pediatrics.

Holbrook, T. L., Hoyt, D. B., Coimbra, R., Potenza, B., Sise, M., & Anderson, J. P. (2005). Long term trauma persists after major trauma in adolescents: New data on risk factors and functional outcome. *Journal of Trauma, 58*, 764–771.

Hymel, K., & Boos, S. (2009). Conditions mistaken for child physical abuse. In R. M. Reece & C. W. Christian (Eds.), *Child abuse: Medical diagnosis and treatment* (3rd ed., pp. 227–255). Chicago: American Academy of Pediatrics.

Ibanez, E. S., Borrego, J., Pemberton, J. R., & Terao, S. (2006). Cultural factors in decision-making about child physical abuse: Identifying reported characteristics influencing reporting tendencies. *Child Abuse & Neglect, 30*, 1365–1379.

Jenny, C., & Reece, R. M. (2009). Cutaneous manifestations of child abuse. In R. M. Reece & C. W. Christian (Eds.), *Child abuse: Medical diagnosis and treatment* (3rd ed., pp. 19–51). Chicago: American Academy of Pediatrics.

Johnson. C., & French, G. (2005). Bruises and burns in child maltreatment. In A. P. Giardino & R. Alexander (Eds.), *Child maltreatment: A clinical reference* (3rd ed., pp. 63–81). St. Louis: G.W. Medical.

Kelley, S. J. (2002). Child maltreatment in the context of substance abuse. In Myers, J. E. B. Myers, L. Berliner, J. Briere, C. T. Hendrix, C. Jenny, & Reid. (Eds.), *The APSAC Handbook on Child Maltreatment* (2nd ed., pp. 105–117).

Klevens, J., & Whitaker, D. J. (2007). Primary prevention of child physical abuse and neglect: Gaps and promising directions. *Child Maltreatment, 12*, 364–377.

Kolko, D. J. (1996). Individual cognitive behavioral treatment and family therapy for physically abused children and their offending parents: A comparison of clinical outcomes. *Child Maltreatment, 1*, 322–342.

Kuelbs, C. L. (2007). Intimate partner violence. In R. Alexander (Ed.), *Child fatality review: An interdisciplinary guide and photographic reference* (pp. 673–679). St. Louis: G.W. Medical Publishing.

Levin, A. V. & Morad, Y. (2009). Ocular manifestations of child abuse. In R. M. Reece & C. W. Christian (Eds.), *Child abuse: Medical diagnosis and treatment* (3rd ed., pp. 212–225). Chicago: American Academy of Pediatrics.

Miller-Perrin, C. L. Perrin, R. D., & Kocur, J. L. (2009). Parental physical and psychological aggression: Psychological symptoms in young adults. *Child Abuse & Neglect, 33*, 1–11.

Mouden, L., & Kenney, J. (2005), Oral injuries. In A. P. Giardino & R. Alexander (Eds.), *Child maltreatment: A clinical reference* (3rd ed., pp. 91–102). St. Louis: G.W. Medical.

Myers, J. E. B. (2005). Legal issues. In A. P. Giardino & R. Alexander (Eds.), *Child maltreatment: A clinical reference* (3rd ed., pp. 707–721). St. Louis: G.W. Medical.

Nadel, F. M. & Giardino, A. P. (2003). Differential diagnosis: Conditions that mimic child maltreatment. In E.R Giardino & A. P. Giardino (Eds.), *Nursing approach to the evaluation of child maltreatment* (pp. 215–249). St. Louis: G.W. Medical.

Nance, M. L., & Cooper, A. (2009). Visceral manifestations of child physical abuse. In R. M. Reece & C. W. Christian (Eds.), *Child abuse: Medical diagnosis and treatment* (3rd ed., pp. 167–187). Chicago: American Academy of Pediatrics.

Olds, D. (2006). The nurse-family partnership: An evidence-based preventive intervention. *Infant Mental Health Journal, 27*, 5–25.

Pierce-Weeks, J. & Giardino, E. R. (2003). Documentation of the evaluations in cases of suspected child maltreatment. In E.R Giardino & A. P. Giardino (Eds.), *Nursing approach to the evaluation of child maltreatment* (pp. 289–307). St. Louis: G.W. Medical.

Prinz, R. J., Sanders, M. R., Shapiro, C. J., Whitaker, D. J., & Lutzker, J. R. (2009). Population-based prevention of child maltreatment: The U.S. Triple P system population trial. *Prevention Science, 10*, 1–12.

Ricci, L. R., & Shapiro, R. A. (2009). Photodocumentation and other technologies. In R. M. Reece & C. W. Christian (Eds.), *Child abuse: Medical diagnosis and treatment* (3rd ed., pp. 755–792). Chicago: American Academy of Pediatrics.

Rorke-Adams, L., Duhaime, C., Jenny, C., & Smith, W. (2009). Head trauma. In R. M. Reece & C. W. Christian (Eds.), *Child abuse: Medical diagnosis and treatment* (3rd ed., pp. 53–119). Chicago: American Academy of Pediatrics.

Rosenberg, D. A. (2009). Munchausen Syndrome by Proxy. In R. M. Reece & C. W. Christian (Eds.), *Child abuse: Medical diagnosis and treatment* (3rd ed., pp. 513–547). Chicago: American Academy of Pediatrics.

Schreier, H. A. (2000). Factitious disorder by proxy in which the presenting problem is behavioral or psychiatric. *Journal of the American Academy of Child and Adolescent Psychiatry, 39*, 668–670.

Schreier, H. A. (2002). Understanding the dynamics in Munchausen by proxy: The case of Kathy Bush. *Child Abuse & Neglect, 26*, 537–549.

Schumm, J. A., Briggs-Philip, M., & Hobfoll, S. E. (2006). Cumulative interpersonal traumas and social support as risk and resiliency factors in predicting PTSD and depression among inner city women. *Journal of Traumatic Stress 19*, 825–836.

Shaffer, A., Yates, T. M., & Egeland, B. R. (2009). The relation of emotional maltreatment to early adolescent competence: Developmental processes in a prospective study. *Child Abuse & Neglect, 33*, 36–44.

Stirling, J., & Amaya-Jackson, L. (2008). Understanding the behavioral and emotional consequences of child abuse. *Pediatrics, 122*, 667–673.

Ward, C. S., & Haskett, M. E. (2008). Exploration and validation of clusters of physically abused children. *Child Abuse & Neglect, 32*, 577–588.

Webster, R. A., & Schnitzer, P. (2007). Coming of age: Child death review in America. In R. Alexander (Ed.), *Child fatality review: An interdisciplinary guide and photographic reference* (pp. 495–501). St. Louis: G.W. Medical Publishing.

Yates, T. M., Carlson, E.A, & Egeland, B. (2008). A prospective study of child maltreatment and self-injurious behavior in a community sample. *Development and Psychopathology, 20*, 651–671.

Zielinski, D. S., Eckenrode, J., & Olds, D. L. (2009). Nurse home visitation and the prevention of child maltreatment: Impact on the timing of official reports. *Development and Psychopathology, 21*, 441–453.

11

Childhood Exposure to Intimate Partner Violence

Helene Berman, PhD, RN
Jennifer L. Hardesty, PhD
Annie Lewis-O'Connor, NP-BC, MPH, PhD
Janice Humphreys, PhD, RN, NP, FAAN

Your Choice

Friendship, a feeling, a thought.
A sort of caring, a sort of concern.
It is invisible, but can be seen,
It is in you, it is in me.

Hatred, a cruelty, a wall
A sort of loathing, a sort of aversion.
It is mean, it is vicious,
It is in you, it is in me.
Your Choice.

—*Phillip, a 14-year-old boy who spent many years*
watching his father abuse his mother

INTRODUCTION

Violence is a daily occurrence for many children throughout the world. They may experience it directly or indirectly, as the intended "targets" or as witnesses, in their homes, their schools, their neighborhoods, through the media, or in the context of war. Until recently, only those who were the direct recipients of violence, and thus bore the physical scars of abuse, were deemed worthy of research or programmatic attention. During the past 20 years, a growing body of scholarly work has reversed this trend and provided ample evidence that children who witness violence endure many of the same outcomes as those who are abused directly.

Typically, children who witness violence in their homes do so during their growth years, during the phase of life when they are learning about themselves, their relationships

279

with others, and the world around them. While childhood is most commonly thought to be a time of innocence and predictability, this depiction is by no means the reality for large numbers of children who grow up amid violence. Instead, children exposed to the abuse of their mothers experience the world as a place where adults in intimate relationships hurt each other and sometimes other people around them, where women are subordinate to men and where men assert their power through physical and emotional control. For these young people, the world is experienced as a place where violence is an integral part of everyday life, where danger is commonplace and where interactions are chaotic and unpredictable. The central task for these children is to find safety in a world that feels unsafe and seek trust from people who have been untrustworthy.

Since the previous version of this chapter was published in 2003 (Berman, Hardesty, & Humphreys, 2003), much has changed. A considerable body of research has emerged, largely extending and confirming earlier findings. However, we now have a more comprehensive understanding of the multiple risks and challenges faced by children who grow up as witnesses to violence in their homes. Researchers have demonstrated that witnessing violence at home rarely occurs in isolation (Margolin et al., 2009). Instead, many of these children live in a larger social and political context whereby violence is woven into many aspects of their lives. Finally, we have a deeper grasp of the impact of gender, race, ability, and other markers of social identity on children who are exposed to intimate partner violence (IPV). This body of work has contributed to greater insights regarding the identification and treatment of children at risk for violence exposure and the development of evidence-based programs and policies aimed at the promotion of healthy and equal relationships. In this chapter, we focus on children who have been exposed to the abuse of their mothers by intimate male partners. While it is acknowledged that both mothers and fathers may be perpetrators and/or recipients of violence, available statistics continue to support the notion that women are by far the recipients, while men are most often the perpetrators of violence. Information on the estimated number of children exposed to the abuse of their mothers, theoretical frameworks that attempt to explain children's experiences, current knowledge regarding the effects of witnessing violence, and proposed nursing care are presented.

SCOPE OF THE PROBLEM

Determining how many children are exposed to violence in their homes is a complex and controversial undertaking due to a variety of conceptual and procedural challenges. Despite the increase in research, we still have only limited data in Canada and the United States that directly measure the number of children who are exposed to violence in their homes. Estimates have been projected from family violence surveys, with adjustments made for the number of families with children and the average number of children in each household. We also have data from police and child protection agencies on the presence of children during a violent incident; however, those data are not available in aggregate. In 1984, Carlson used figures from the first National Family Violence Survey to estimate that, based on an average of two children in 55% of violent households, at least 3.3 million children in the United States between the ages of 3 and 17 years were at risk for exposure to parental violence every year. This figure continues to be the most widely cited, and more recent estimates suggest that the problem has not abated in the intervening years (Fantuzzo & Fusco, 2007). McDonald, Jouriles, Tart, and Minze, (2009) reported that 15.5 million children, or approximately 30%, live in homes in which some form of marital violence has occurred. Recent statistics from Canada similarly suggest that these numbers have remained relatively constant. Although parents often believe that they have shielded their children from IPV, research shows that children see or hear about 40–80% of occurrences (Health Canada, 2007).

While these figures lend strong support to the assertion that large numbers of children are exposed to violence each year, a number of constraints remain. The lack of consensus in the literature regarding what, precisely, the problem is and how "witnessing violence" is defined has led researchers to use inconsistent parameters. Whether the focus should be on children who witness all forms of violence between intimate partners, or solely on those who witness violence against women, has been a source of contention among researchers (Jouriles, McDonald, Norwood, & Ezell, 2001). While children are likely to be affected by their exposure to any form of violence, there is compelling evidence that male-to-female violence is qualitatively different from female-to-male violence.

Another thorny area concerns the inclusion criteria for participants in prevalence surveys. More specifically, whether surveys should utilize samples of couples or samples of individuals is an area about which there is little consensus. Surveys that include data from individuals who are not part of an intimate relationship are likely to yield much lower findings of IPV than those surveys that are limited to couples.

How violence is defined presents further challenges. Much of the research to date has utilized narrow conceptualizations of violence, with physical acts of aggression as measured by the Conflict Tactics Scale (Straus, 1979) being the most commonly used indicator of violence. Other researchers have argued for the use of broader definitions that encompass physical, emotional, and sexual dimensions of violence. The use of divergent definitions of violence results in markedly inconsistent estimates, which, in turn, have enormous implications for reported estimations of the number of children who are exposed to violence in the home. Furthermore, whether children respond differently to different forms of violence exposure is not well understood. In view of the multitude of ways women are abused, and the recognition that children are affected by their exposure to multiple forms of violence, it is critical that definitions be sufficiently broad and have enough clarity to capture the full range of children's exposure.

Understanding what it means to witness violence presents additional challenges to researchers. Throughout this chapter, the notions of "witnessing violence" and "violence exposure" are used interchangeably and are defined broadly to include acts that are directly observed as well as those that are heard. Alternatively, children may neither see nor hear the violence, but will see bruises or other behavioral changes to their mothers in the aftermath of a violent episode. Consistent with the general trend in the literature, we include the many ways in which children may be exposed to the abuse of their mothers in the home in our understanding of what it means to witness violence.

A final noteworthy issue concerns the reliance on parent reports regarding what their children have seen or been exposed to. This "adultcentric" bias, or tendency to examine the worlds of children from the vantage point of the adults in their lives, may contribute to an inaccurate portrayal of children's experiences. There is some evidence that children often see or hear more than their parents think and that they are, in fact, much more aware of the violence in their homes than their parents realize or acknowledge (Edleson et al., 2007; Osofsky, 1997, 2003). The net result is that published estimates that are based solely on parent reports may not fully reflect the extent to which children are exposed to violence in their homes. Given the many challenges implicit in this focus of study, and the lack of consensus regarding relevant definitions and constructs, arriving at agreed-upon estimates is a daunting, but necessary, task.

Relationship to Other Types of Abuse

The exposure of children to the abuse of their mothers rarely occurs in isolation and is often associated with other forms of violence and aggression in their homes and communities (Margolin et al., 2009). In general, it is agreed that a supportive and nurturing family environment, in conjunction with opportunities to interact with peers and others outside the home, are necessary for children to grow and thrive. Furthermore, it is widely acknowledged that when violence and aggression are common features of family and community life, the child's capacity for growth is significantly impaired. The effects of violence are further shaped by the presence or absence of an appropriate response (Graham-Bermann & Levendosky, 1998; Graham-Bermann & Seng, 2005).

The early research on child witnesses to the abuse of their mothers offers convincing evidence that many, although not all, of these children are at risk for emotional and behavioral problems during childhood and adolescence (Jaffe, Wolfe, & Wilson, 1990; Wolfe, Wekerle, Reitzel, & Gough, 1995). As adults, several authors have stated that children who come from violent homes are likely to experience violence in future relationships. In one of the earlier studies examining this relationship, Kalmuss (1984) used survey data from adults and found that observing violence between parents was more strongly related to involvement in severe marital violence than was being a victim of abuse during adolescence. Later studies support this general pattern. According to Margolin (2005), male abusers consistently report that they had witnessed violence in their families of origin. These researchers also noted that this finding was much more apparent among men than among women.

In a comprehensive review of the long-term effects of childhood exposure to domestic violence, Rossman (2001) examined retrospective and prospective studies of children who had been exposed to violence. While many of the studies included in this review used samples of individuals who had experienced various forms of childhood abuse, not solely those who were exposed to the abuse of their mothers, findings demonstrated a clear relationship between childhood exposure to domestic violence and later participation in criminal and violent behavior. As well, witnessing violence in the home was associated with violence in later interpersonal relationships.

Few prospective studies have been conducted. However, the Adverse Childhood Experiences (ACE) study, which included over 17,000 adults, has demonstrated a reasonably strong link between victimization during childhood and subsequent aggression during adulthood (Centers for Disease Control and Prevention, 2006). Many authors have also noted a significant overlap between abuse of women and child abuse (Edleson, 2001; Gewirtz & Edleson, 2007; McDonald et al., 2009; Moffitt & Caspi, 2003; Parkinson, Adams, Emerling, & Frank, 2001). As well, there is evidence that violence in dating relationships strongly correlates with childhood exposure to violence between parents (Carr & VanDeusen, 2002; Reitzel-Jaffe & Wolfe, 2001; Tjaden & Thoennes, 2000; Wolfe et al., 1995).

Many children who grow up amid violence in their homes are routinely exposed to a multitude of other forms of violence in their communities, neighborhoods, through the media, and in their schools (Osofsky, 2003). In research on violence in the lives of girls,

Berman, McKenna, Traher, Taylor, and MacQuarrie (2000) and Berman and Jiwani (2002) documented the occurrence of sexual harassment as a common feature of everyday life for girls as young as 8 years of age. According to these researchers, sexual harassment is one of the most pervasive, pernicious, and highly public forms of violence that girls encounter. Furthermore, efforts to stop it are often met by dismissive attitudes on the part of adults in trusted positions.

Malik (2008) examined relations between children's violence exposure, at home and in the community, and symptoms of externalizing and internalizing problems. Using the Achenbach Child Behavior Checklist (CBCL), findings indicated that community violence was related to all measures of children's adjustment, whereas exposure to IPV was related to externalizing problems. Garbarino, Kostelny, and Dubrow (1991) studied the dangers that children face in the war zones throughout the world and the "smaller" war zones of the inner cities in the United States. These researchers traveled to Mozambique, Cambodia, Nicaragua, Palestine, and Chicago. Based on extensive interviews with children, Garbarino and his associates concluded that the environmental hazards confronting children in large American cities are comparable only to the dangers experienced by children living in situations of armed conflict. Untangling the unique effects of the multiple forms of violence poses a significant challenge to researchers interested in understanding the effects of violence on children, but acknowledging and studying the multiple and intersecting forms of violence are critical.

THEORETICAL PERSPECTIVES

Various theoretical and conceptual models of children's responses to the abuse of their mothers have been described in the literature. Together, these offer a contextual framework for greater understanding regarding the needs and issues faced by this population and provide some general direction for further research. The first two, social learning theory and posttraumatic stress theory, have informed much of the published research in this field and collectively provide a framework for examining individual children's responses to violence exposure. The third, critical/feminist theory has received less attention but is included because of its potential to contribute important knowledge and understandings and its insistence that individual responses to violence must be explored within their broader social, political, and cultural contexts.

Social Learning Theory

One of the widely held theories about aggressive behavior in children and adults is the belief that "violence begets violence" (Widom, 1989) and the intergenerational transmission of violence theory. Derived in part from social learning theory, the essence of the intergenerational transmission of violence perspective is that children who learn violent behavior patterns in the home are more likely to engage in similar patterns later in life (Straus, Gelles, & Steinmetz, 1980). While the belief that victims of violence grow up to become perpetrators of violence has contributed to the fears among young men that they will someday become like their abusive fathers; in fact, there are many men who grew up in violent homes who have never been abusive toward a women. Varying degrees of support for the social learning perspective have been described in the literature. The early research related to children exposed to the abuse of their mothers documented a multitude of behavioral and emotional problems (Holden & Ritchie, 1991; Hughes, 1988; Jaffe, Wolfe, Wilson, & Zak, 1986). Most of these studies used the CBCL and revealed the presence of internalizing behaviors, primarily among girls, and externalizing behaviors, more evident in boys. Although not a direct test of social learning theory, the occurrence of aggressive behaviors in children who witness violence lends support to the notion that such behaviors are learned in the home, at least in part through observations of their parents. Jouriles, Murphy, and O'Leary (1989) and Jouriles, Spiller, Stephens, McDonald, and Swank (2000) have demonstrated that marital aggression is a strong predictor of child misconduct and personality problems. Further support comes from a study of 46 preschool-age children. In this research, Graham-Bermann and Levendosky (1998) found that children who were exposed to violence at home had significantly more internalizing and externalizing problems than comparison children. Exposed children also showed more negative affect, used power, control, and bullying tactics in interactions with their peers, were more aggressive, and had more ambivalent relations with their caregivers.

While the social learning perspective has some merits as well as considerable intuitive appeal, findings from a number of studies have led researchers to question its relevance, at least as the sole explanatory framework. Kaufman and Zigler (1987) raised important criticisms of the intergenerational transmission of violence hypothesis when they drew attention to the fact that not all children who experience violence go on to become abusers themselves, as previously mentioned. These authors reviewed the research on adults who grew up amid violence but were not abusive with their own children and concluded that no more than 30% of those who experienced or witnessed violence as children were currently abusive. Kaufman and Zigler identified a variety of mitigating factors that contributed to the cluster of protective factors. These included the following: lack of parental ambivalence about their children; healthy children, few life stressors, ability to openly express anger about their own abuse, abusive behavior by only one parent, a supportive relationship with the non-abusive parent, and a determination not to perpetuate the cycle of violence. The role of protective factors and resilience are discussed later in this chapter and warrant more exploration through research.

The best conclusion that can be drawn from these findings is that a history of violence in the family of origin can, indeed, seriously affect children, but exposure to violence does not automatically result in serious behavioral problems and a certainty of violence in future relationships. More importantly, the findings of these studies imply that the trajectory from violence exposure to violence perpetration is neither simple nor linear and that a more complex constellation of factors, including type and duration of violence exposure, as well as environmental and structural factors, must be brought to bear when seeking to understand what happens when children are exposed to violence directed toward their mothers.

Posttraumatic Stress Theory

During the past 20 years, a number of investigators have examined the relevance of posttraumatic stress disorder (PTSD) for an understanding of the consequences of children's exposure to violence or trauma. The primary symptoms of PTSD are intense fear, helplessness, or horror; young children may exhibit disorganized or agitated behavior. The remaining symptoms of PTSD are (a) re-experiencing phenomena, (b) avoidant symptoms, and (c) autonomic hperarousal (APA, 1987). This body of research has included children who have grown up in various war zones around the world (Arroyo & Eth, 1985; Berman, 1999; Garbarino, et al., 1991; Kinzie, Sack, Angell, Manson, & Rath, 1986; Saigh, 1991), those who had been kidnapped (Terr, 1990), and children who had witnessed the murder of a parent (Pynoos & Eth, 1984). Although first conceptualized with respect to adults, and more specifically Vietnam veterans, the presence of PTSD symptomatology in these children suggests that it may have relevance to children and adolescents.

Building upon this literature, a growing number of studies reveal traumatic responses among children who had been exposed to violence in their homes (Berman, 1999; Graham-Bermann & Levendosky, 1998; Rossman & Ho, 2000; Silvern & Kaersvang, 1989). Silvern and Kaersvang (1989) have suggested that observing violence between parents traumatizes children and that trauma can result from perceived endangerment, even if no physical harm actually occurs. This idea is consistent with Saigh's (1991) finding with respect to children in Beirut that traumatic responses may result from direct encounters with traumatic events or the awareness that such events have occurred.

While trauma theory likely has some relevance and contributes to a general understanding of the stressful nature of early exposure to violence, the use of PTSD as an organizing construct for understanding children's responses to violence exposure has some important constraints. As first articulated by the American Psychiatric Association (1987), traumatic events were defined as those events that were "outside the range of usual human experience" (p. 247). This definition has been challenged by several writers (Brown, 1991; Herman, 1992). The essence of the criticisms is that because violence is such a common part of the everyday lives of many women and children, it cannot be construed as being outside the range of normal.

For many children who grow up amid violence in their homes, trauma is not a single, isolated event. When children are forced to confront violence repeatedly, the trauma becomes a central condition of their lives; there is no "post" trauma period. Even if they are fortunate enough to escape from immediate harm, the task goes beyond "getting over" a horrible experience. Rather, the challenge is to find ways to make sense of their lives and their families where terrifying experiences are a part of everyday reality, where traumatic stress is chronic and enduring. Herman (1992) has persuasively argued for the need to recognize "complex PTSD" to reflect this more chronic form of trauma. In response to this concern, the revised Diagnostic and Statistical Manual of Mental Disorders, fourth edition criteria no longer includes the original "outside the range of usual experience" proviso.

While this change represents a significant improvement, other limitations remain. By focusing on a set of symptoms as the primary determination of children's responses, it is easy to pathologize and individualize the problem of violence. Similarly, the current emphasis on identification of a "disorder" effectively discourages investigators from examining the strengths and resources that enable children to grow and thrive in the face of seemingly overwhelming challenges. Concerns regarding the cultural relevance of PTSD across diverse settings also warrant consideration. Although many of the same signs and symptoms may be evident among individuals exposed to trauma in differing cultural groups and societies, these do not necessarily mean the same thing across the varied contexts.

Finally, PTSD was first conceptualized in relation to adults. Whether a similar construct can capture the experience of children, or whether their responses are qualitatively different from those observed in adults, is not yet well understood. However, the early research in this area demonstrates that children's post-traumatic responses are distinctly different from those observed among adults (Pynoos & Nader, 1993; Terr, 1990). Despite limitations inherent in the conceptualization of posttraumatic stress, its potential relevance for understanding the meaning of growing up amid violence is clear and convincing. The literature discussed thus far demonstrates that many of children's responses to overwhelming life events fall under the broad category of trauma responses and can result in significant effects upon biopsychosocial health.

Critical Feminist Perspectives and Intersectionality Theory

The African American socialist and feminist writer Bell Hooks (1984) observed that violence directed against women and children is an expression of male domination, but she cogently argued that an analysis of violence must be more comprehensive than that which focuses solely on male domination over women. Instead, violence must be conceptualized as a means of social control, which is manifested in many ways, and at many different levels, throughout society. Furthermore, such an analysis must take into consideration other intersecting sources of oppression including that based on race and class (Collins, 2000).

The violence that children witness in their homes, typically perpetrated by their fathers against their mothers, is influenced and shaped by social, economic, cultural, and ideological structural processes. These processes are woven deeply into the fabric of the modern family and the larger society. Thus, the violence in children's lives is not purely spontaneous, made under conditions freely chosen. Rather, it is socially produced and experienced in situations that have been handed down from countless generations. From a critical feminist or intersectionality framework, it becomes possible to conceptualize children's exposure to violence, not as a private or individual problem but as a public issue demanding social change.

Much of the research in the broad area of violence against women has been conducted from a critical and/or feminist perspective. With respect to research related to child witnesses, this is not the case. Most of this research has been conducted using theoretical models linked to social learning, trauma, or developmental theory. While each of these perspectives has contributed to a substantial body of knowledge regarding this group of children, a number of limitations are noteworthy. The emphasis of the research on children exposed to violence has been on individual responses and patterns of behavior, devoid of gender analyses. In the context of violence against women and children, gender-neutral descriptions obscure the root causes of violence and leave the underlying gender-related dynamics unnamed and invisible. Instead, structured and systemic social problems appear as random, unpatterned, and individualized.

Beginning in the 1970s and continuing today, a number of explicitly critical and/or feminist studies have been conducted, many by nurse researchers (Berman, 1999; Berman et al., 2000; Ericksen & Henderson, 1998; Humphreys, 1995, 2001a). Berman's research was a "critical narrative analysis" designed to examine the experiences of two groups of children who had grown up amid violence, namely children of war and children of battered women. An assumption underlying this research was that the contextual dimensions of children's experiences are valued and inseparable from the way in which children strive to bring a sense of coherence into their lives. Thus, by listening to the stories children told, this research sought to give voice to individual experiences and meanings but placed them in a broader context and thereby examined the social and political connectedness of those experiences. Although the critical feminist perspectives and, in more recent years, intersectionality theory have informed much of the research on violence against women, we believe that it also holds considerable promise for those committed to an understanding of the needs of children who are exposed to violence.

HEALTH EFFECTS OF EXPOSURE TO VIOLENCE IN THE HOME

In the last decade, a growing body of research has demonstrated that children's exposure to IPV is a significant public health problem, and as a result, children of abused women have received increased attention in the literature. Approaches to studying these children have become more sophisticated, as researchers attempt to untangle the complex relationships between violence exposure and child health outcomes. Despite a variety of methodologies, instruments, and samples, the research consistently shows that exposure to violence is associated with negative health effects for children (Carlson, 2000; Holt, Buckley, & Whelan, 2008; Onyskiw, 2003; Osofsky, 2003). Still, not all children exposed to the abuse of their mothers exhibit negative effects, leading some researchers to examine factors that contribute to resiliency in this group of children.

Physical Health Effects

Physical health effects on children exposed to IPV have received limited attention in the literature (Onyskiw, 2003). However, existing knowledge suggests the need to further explore this area. Some common physical health effects include allergies, respiratory tract infections, somatic complaints (e.g., headaches and back pain), gastrointestinal disorders (e.g., nausea and diarrhea), and sleep difficulties (e.g., nightmares and bedwetting) (Berman, 1999; Campbell & Lewandowski, 1997; Graham-Bermann & Seng, 2005; Lemmey, McFarlane, Wilson, & Malecha, 2001). Attala and McSweeney (1997) reported speech, hearing, and visual problems, as well as delays in immunizations.

Growing up in a violent home also affects children's use of health services. In a health maintenance organization studied by Rath, Jaratt, and Leonardson (1989), children of abused women used health services six to eight times more often than comparison children. Onyskiw (2002) examined the health status and use of health services in children exposed to violence in a representative sample of Canadian children. Exposed children had lower general health status and more health problems than comparison children, which limited their participation in age-appropriate activities. However, exposed children had no more contact with family practitioners and less contact with pediatricians than comparison children. Instead, they reported more contact with other medical doctors, public health nurses, child welfare workers, and therapists. They also reported more use of prescription medications than non-exposed children.

Several researchers have demonstrated that child exposure to violence can result in health effects that persist adulthood. Some have observed a graded or dose–response relationship between the number of types of childhood adverse experiences (e.g., child abuse and witnessing of violence against mother) and both risk behaviors (e.g., drug use and smoking) and disease (ischemic heart disease, cancer, and skeletal fractures) in adulthood (Edwards, Holden, Felitti, & Anda, 2003; Felitti et al., 1998). The ACE survey of 17,337 adults found that greater exposure to IPV as children resulted in increased likelihood of alcoholism, illicit drug use, and intravenous drug use as adults (Dube, Anda, Felitti, Edwards, & Williamson, 2002).

Mental Health Effects

In an extensive literature review of 11 years of research on children's exposure to IPV, Holt, et al. (2008) concluded that children and adolescents living with violence are at considerable risk for emotional and behavioral problems. These children tend to have higher rates of depressive symptoms, higher levels of anxiety, worry, and frustration, lower self-esteem, and more stress-related disorders than other children (Graham-Bermann & Levendosky, 1998; Humphreys, 1991; Hurt, Malmud, Brodsky, & Giannetta, 2001; Johnson et al., 2002; Turner, Finkelhor, & Ormrod, 2006). A significant number of exposed children have scores in the clinical ranges for depression on standardized measures (Graham-Bermann, De Voe, Mattis, Lynch, & Thomas, 2006). According to the National Longitudinal Survey of Children and Youth (Dauvergne & Johnson, 2002), Canadian children exposed to physical violence at home are significantly more likely than children in nonviolent homes to exhibit hyperactivity and emotional/anxiety disorders. Exposed children also show elevated rates of posttraumatic stress symptoms (Boney-McCoy & Finklehor, 1995; McCloskey, Figueredo, & Koss, 1995), with some meeting the diagnostic criteria for PTSD (Levendosky, Huth-Bocks, Semel, & Shapiro, 2002; McCloskey & Walker, 2000; Moretti, Obsuth, Odgers, & Reebye, 2006; Silva et al., 2000). Risk factors associated with higher levels of PTSD for children include age, gender, race/ethnicity, mothers' mental health, social support, cultural context, and socioeconomic status (Graham-Bermann et al., 2006). From a public health perspective, recent meta-analyses indicate that exposure to IPV results in significant additional psychopathology among children and adolescents (Kitzmann, Gaylord, Holt, & Kenny, 2003; Wolfe, Crooks, Lee, McIntyre-Smith, & Jaffe, 2003).

Early exposure to IPV may result in long-term mental health effects. Studies indicate that exposure during childhood is associated with higher rates of depression, stress symptoms, alcohol-related problems, and low self-esteem in adulthood (Caetano, Field, & Nelson, 2003; Henning, Leitenberg, Coffey, Turner, & Bennett, 1996; Silvern et al., 1995; Straus, 1992). However, Langhinrichsen-Rohling, Monson, Meyer, Caster, & Sanders (1998) did not find a relationship between depression, hopelessness, and suicidal behaviors of college students and their childhood exposure to violence. Other factors, such as severity and frequency of the violence witnessed and the child's coping strategies, are likely to play a role in increasing or decreasing the likelihood that child witnesses will experience mental health problems in adulthood (Dube et al., 2002; Goldblatt, 2003; Maker, Kemmelmeir, & Peterson, 1998).

Social Effects

Exposure to IPV is associated with lower levels of social competence in children (Graham-Bermann & Levendosky, 1998; Moore & Pepler, 1998), lower levels of prosocial behaviors (Onyskiw & Hayduk, 2001), and less positive and less effective interactions with other children (Baldry, 2003; Dauvergne & Johnson, 2002; Lundy & Grossman, 2005). The behavioral responses of these children are likely to contribute to their social adjustment difficulties (Rossman, 2001). For example, children with high levels of externalizing behaviors may act aggressively toward peers, which may lead to rejection by peers. Exposed children tend to have greater expectations of aggressive or hostile intent in social interactions than do non-exposed children (Lundy & Grossman), which may interfere with their ability to appropriately respond to peers. On the other hand, children with high levels of internalizing problems may appear shy and withdrawn and have difficulty initiating social interactions. Exposed children also have difficulty developing empathy and perspective-taking skills necessary for forming positive peer relationships (Rossman, 2001).

Violence exposure also affects social relationships through its effect on attachment security. Greater exposure to violence is associated with less secure attachment in children, (Margolin, 2005), which, in turn, can lead to difficulty establishing close interpersonal relationships. A study of high school students found that abuse in the family of origin and early attachment problems were associated with a higher risk of dating violence (McGee, Wolfe, & Wilson, 1997), particularly for girls (McCloskey & Lichter, 2003).

Academic Effects

Research related to the effects of IPV exposure on academic performance has revealed mixed results. After controlling for socioeconomic status, Rossman (1998) found no significant differences in verbal scores between exposed and non-exposed children. However, in a study of preschool children, Huth-Bocks et al. (2001) found that exposed children had significantly poorer verbal abilities, even when controlling for socioeconomic status and child abuse. Similarly, Blackburn (2008) examined reading and phonological awareness skills in a sample of 40 children, ages 6–9 years, and found that exposure to IPV may negatively impact children's reading skills.

Others have used measures of academic performance, such as learning problems and/ or grade point average, to assess cognitive effects. A study of inner-city children found that higher exposure to family and community violence was correlated with lower grade point average and lower school competency. Child gender, child IQ, caregiver IQ, caregiver self-esteem, caregiver cocaine use, or the quality of the home environment did not account for the associations (Hurt et al., 2001). In contrast, Mathias, Mertin, & Murray (1995) found no differences in academic abilities between exposed and non-exposed children. Stalford, Baker, Beveridge, and Mckie (2003) support the view that there is a correlation between direct exposure to IPV and children's progress at school. Aitken (2001) notes that IPV affects not only academic performance but also emotional and behavioral development and interpersonal relationships with one's peer group. Byrne and Taylor (2007) report a qualitative study conducted in Northern Ireland where perceptions of education welfare officers, child protection workers and teachers were explored regarding the impact of IPV on schooling. Findings confirmed the major effect that IPV can have on children's schooling and relationships. Clearly, more research is needed to delineate the complex relationships between violence exposure, academic performance, and other risk factors.

Behavioral Responses to Intimate Partner Violence Exposure

Based on studies using the CBCL (Achenbach & Edelbrock, 1978), children exposed to IPV exhibit higher levels of internalizing and externalizing behaviors compared to non-exposed children (Jaffe et al., 1990; Kernic et al., 2003; Sternberg, Lamb, Guterman, & Abbott, 2006). For a significant number of children, scores on internalizing (Onyskiw, 2003) and externalizing (Kernic et al., 2003; Onyskiw, 2003) scales are high enough to warrant clinical intervention. Internalizing and externalizing behaviors are common initial responses to traumatic experiences. Over time, the behaviors tend to decrease if exposure to violence ends (Holden, Stein, Ritchey, Harris, & Jouriles, 1998; Rossman, 2001). Behavioral responses may vary by gender, with boys exhibiting more externalizing behaviors and girls more internalizing behaviors (Jaffe et al., 1986; Kerig, 1998). Onyskiw and Hayduk (2001) found that boys exhibited more externalizing behaviors than girls but found no sex differences for internalizing behaviors. Others have found girls to show more externalizing and internalizing problems and more depressive symptoms or more problems in the clinical range compared to boys, or they have found no significant differences in boys and girls (Grych, Jouriles, Swank, McDonald, & Norwood, 2000; Hughes, Vargo, Ito, & Skinner, 1991; Sternberg et al., 1993). No gender differences were found in outcome studies of child maltreatment and community violence (Lynch & Cicchetti, 1998) and studies of IPV and child abuse (Litrownik, Newton, Hunter, English, & Everson, 2003). According to Grych et al., the variability in children's outcomes in prior studies reflects the diversity and complexity of children's experiences and highlights the need for further research.

Heyman and Slep (2002) systematically investigated gender differences in childhood exposure IPV. The findings indicate that women appeared more susceptible to the long-term effects of multiple and differing forms of prior violence. For men, current violence perpetration was uniquely associated with their having witnessed violence perpetrated by their fathers toward their mothers. For women, increased exposure to mother-to-father abuse elevated the likelihood of their own use of violence with their children (Herrenkohl, Sousa, Tajima, Herrenkohl, & Moylan, 2008).

Kerig's (1998) study of gender, appraisals, and children's response to violence suggests different pathways to the development of maladjustment in girls and boys. For girls, as exposure to violence increases, and as their parents' arguments become more frequent, intense, and unresolved, so does their tendency to blame themselves for their parents' arguments, which may lead to problems of internalizing such as hopelessness, anxiety, and depression. Boys feel increasingly threatened as exposure to violence increases and as the arguments become more frequent, intense, and unresolved. Kerig suggests that the pathways to maladjustment for boys may be a mismatch between their belief that they should be able to do something to stop the violence and the ineffectiveness of doing so. The resulting frustration from this situation may result in boys feeling anxiety and behaving aggressively.

Child's age or stage of development is another potential influence. Some studies indicate that young children are at greater risk of developing traumatic stress than are older children (Pynoos, Steinberg, & Wraith, 1995). Lieberman (2007) discussed the impact of exposure to IPV on infants, toddlers, and preschoolers and manifestations of posttraumatic stress in first years of life. In outcome studies of children exposed to IPV, younger age is consistently associated with greater risk of negative outcome (Fantuzzo & Mohr, 1999; Holden et al., 1998; Jouriles, McDonald, Slep, Heyman, & Garrido, 2008).

Behavioral changes in infants and preschool children include sleep disturbances, somatic complaints, and regression in toilet training and language. School-age children may demonstrate behavior problems specific to the school environment and peer relationships. Adolescents may act out with substance abuse and delinquency. Boys in particular may try to intervene in violent episodes to protect their mothers, placing themselves as risk for injury (Margolin, 2005). Mohr, Lutz, Fantuzzo, & Perry (2000) encourage researchers to use a developmental perspective in their theoretical and methodological approaches to understanding the effects of IPV exposure on children. Similarly, Margolin recommends developmentally sensitive theories and methods to better understand children's risk and resilience to violence exposure. Other factors to consider include social and economic disadvantage, parental separation, repeated moves, maternal depression, proximity to violent events, frequency and severity of violence, mothers' responses to violence, child strengths, and social and cultural supports (Campbell & Lewandowski, 1997; Onyskiw, 2003). Gewirtz and Edleson (2007) employed a development risk and resilience framework to examine the impact of exposure to IPV on young children facing economic hardship. The authors weave together two separate literatures, one on emotional and behavioral development in high-risk settings and the other on children exposed to IPV. They argue that, for any intervention to be successful, it must attend to the family's economic and cultural context and needs and build on the natural supports around the child and family.

A criticism of the research on children's behavioral responses to violence exposure is the overuse of samples from battered women's shelters. In Onyskiw's (2003) review of 47 studies, 70% included children residing with their mothers in shelters for battered women. Women who seek shelter differ from those who do not in terms of socioeconomic status, severity and duration of abuse, and access to social support. Shelter residence is typically a time of stress and crisis; thus, children's behaviors at that time may reflect the stress of change more than the effects of violence exposure. Because mothers' reports are most frequently used, reports of externalizing behaviors may be elevated or more negatively skewed due to the distress of staying at a shelter.

Ware et al. (2001) attempted to address this criticism in their study of 68 children who scored at clinical levels of conduct problems during shelter residence. Follow-up assessment indicated that, while mothers' distress levels decreased after leaving the shelter, their reports of their child's conduct problems remained high. On the other hand, mothers' reports of children's internalizing behaviors decreased over time, suggesting that mothers' distress may impact their reports of child internalizing problems. Their findings support the notion that children who reside in shelters are a high-risk group for aggressive and defiant behavior. Studies indicate that about one-third of children in shelters demonstrate such conduct problems at clinical levels, in contrast to about 2–15% in community samples. For example, Spilsbury et al. (2008) studied a community-program-based sample of 175 school-aged children exposed to IPV. They reported that 69% of children were below clinical thresholds for any internalizing or externalizing problem, 18% were characterized as having externalizing problems with or without internalizing problems, and 13% consisted of children with internalizing problems only.

Intimate partner violence may indirectly affect children's adjustment through its effect on mothers' parenting abilities, frequently eroding their mental health and coping capacity (Arias & Pape 1999; Lindhorst, Evans-Campbell, Huang, Walters, 2006). Abused women experience high levels of psychological distress, including heightened levels of fear, anxiety, and depression, and lower self-esteem. Each of these conditions can negatively affect parenting by decreasing emotional availability and responsiveness (Levendosky, Leahy, Bogat, Davidson, & von Eye, 2006). For example, Onyskiw and Hayduk (2001) found that exposure to IPV increased preschool and young school-age children's use of physical and indirect aggression through its disruption of maternal responsiveness. In addition, maternal depression directly increased children's internalizing behaviors (e.g., depression), which in turn influenced externalizing behaviors (e.g., aggression). In contrast, Levendosky and Graham-Bermann (2001) found that mothers' psychological functioning had direct effects on children not solely mediated through its effects on parenting. Thus, even if abused mothers are able to effectively parent, their depressed mood may still affect children, particularly because children worry about their mothers and may be sensitive to variability in parental functioning. Some women experience long-term physical and emotional health consequences, including higher rates of substance abuse, which will continue to affect their parenting. Kelleher et al. (2008) examined the association between physical violence victimization and self-reported disciplinary practices among female parents/caregivers in a national sample of families referred to child welfare. The findings indicate that IPV is associated with more self-reported aggressive and neglectful disciplinary behaviors among female caregivers.

Several researchers have challenged the assumption that abuse compromises mothers' parenting abilities (Edleson, Mbilinyi, & Shetty, 2003). According to Wuest, Berman, Ford-Gilboe and Merrit-Gray (2002), both mothers and children reported that abused women are nurturing parents who are emotionally available to their children and who care for their children in diverse and creative ways. According to adult daughters of abused women, mothers are essential to the ability to overcome the challenges of growing up in a violent home (Humphreys, 2001a). Furthermore, Sullivan, Juras, Bybee, Nguyen, and Allen (2000) found no evidence that abuse increased mothers' parenting stress or use of discipline. Instead, abuse directly affected children's adjustment, and, in turn, children's heightened adjustment problems affected mothers' parenting stress.

In response to the abuse of their mothers, children may exhibit caring and protective behaviors. Humphreys (1989, 1990) found that children of abused women demonstrated deliberate, creative, and diverse caring behaviors. Through these behaviors, children attempted to protect (e.g., intervening to stop abuse and calling the police) and support their mothers. Supportive behaviors included instrumental assistance in the home to alleviate the general burden to the mothers. Children's supportive behaviors also served to enhance the relationship between the abused mother and child, a relationship that may mediate the long-term effects of violence on the child. Although children take protective and supportive actions, exposure to violence cannot be viewed as beneficial to children.

Noticeably absent from the literature is attention to the influence of fathers on children's adjustment (Guille, 2004; Levendosky & Graham-Bermann, 2001). In one of the earlier studies, Ericksen and Henderson (1998) reported the strong connection children feel to their fathers despite the violence; thus, children are likely to be sensitive to the quality of their fathers' parenting. The abuser's relationship to the child is important to consider. In the study of Sullivan et al. (2000), children's reports of their competency and self-worth were related to their relationship to the mother's abuser. Children of biological and stepfather abusers scored lower on all measures of child adjustment (behavior problems, self-perception, and depression) compared to children of non-father figures (i.e., partners or former partners who did not play a significant role in the child's life). Stepfathers and non-father figures were more emotionally abusive to children and created more fear for the children. Although biological fathers were more available, children were more likely to witness abuse from biological fathers. Witnessing this violence may be particularly painful for children and may contribute to more negative effects.

Considerations of Race, Ethnicity, and Other Markers of Difference

In recent years, several leading scholars have identified the need to research into multiple and intersecting forms of violence in the lives of children (Berman & Jiwani, 2002; Daro, Edleson, & Pinderhughes, 2004; Finkelhor, Ormrod, & Turner, 2007; Sanders-Phillips, 2009). The argument put forward is that exposure to violence in the home rarely occurs in isolation and that these children often face racism, classism, and other types of systemic violence that are often condoned in subtle and not-so-subtle ways. In a review of the literature related to the impact of racial discrimination on children of color, Sanders-Phillips asserted that racism should be recognized as a form of violence with significant negative impacts on the health of children, parents, and communities. Sullivan (2009) similarly drew attention to the particular challenges and risks faced by children with disabilities who are exposed to violence in their homes and communities. Overall, however, this body of literature remains quite limited.

Much of what is known about race and ethnicity in children exposed to traumatic events is derived from research on children exposed to war in other parts of the world (Allwood, Bell-Dolan, & Hussain, 2002). Few researchers have examined the cultural effects on responses to IPV in a North American context. O'Keefe (1994) examined white, Latina, and African American abused women's reports of their children's adjustment and noted that their children had serious behavioral and emotional problems; however, African American mothers rated their children more competent as compared to the other mothers. In recent years, a growing literature has emerged that explores the role of race and ethnicity in IPV among ethnic minority populations, including immigrants and refugees (Shiu-Thornton, Senturia, & Sullivan, 2005). Graham-Bermann et al. (2006) report a study where traumatic stress symptoms were assessed for 218 children, ages 5–13, following exposure to IPV. It was found that 33% of White and 17% of minority children were diagnosed with PTSD. White children were more likely to have a PTSD diagnosis following exposure to IPV. In addition, their probable risk and protective factors were centered on mother's well-being (Graham-Bermann et al., 2006). On the other hand, some studies suggest that the relationship between violence exposure and PTSD symptoms appear to be independent of ethnicity (Griffing et al., 2006; McGruder-Johnson, Davidson, Gleaves, Stock, & Finch, 2000; Vogel & Marshall, 2001). Similarly, Grych et al. (2000), who sampled African American, Hispanic, and European American children and calculated their profiles of adjustment following IPV exposure, found no significant differences in adjustment outcomes associated with the ethnicity of the child. It is possible, however, that differences across ethnic groups may play a role in the prevalence of IPV, family members' perceptions of violence, and their willingness to disclose or report abuse. Kasturirangan, Krishnan, and Riger (2004) reviewed the literature on the impact of culture on minority women's experiences of IPV and found that family structure, acculturation, immigrant status, community response, and histories of oppression affect their experiences of and responses to violence. For example, racial and ethnic minority women "may be unwilling to disclose their experience . . . for fear of bringing shame to their families and communities or of reinforcing stereotypes" (p. 321).

Resiliency of Children Exposed to Violence

Although exposure to IPV is associated with a myriad of negative health effects, some reports indicate that 50–70% of children go on to lead productive lives and successful relationships as adults (Wolfe & Korsch, 1994). Resilience, a pattern of successful adaptation in individuals despite challenging or threatening circumstances, is thought to explain this phenomenon (Garmezy, 1981). Resilience is increasingly described as a pattern (Masten, 2001) or a developmental progression in which new strengths and vulnerabilities emerge over time and under changing circumstances (Luthar, Cicchetti, & Becker, 2000). Gewirtz and Edleson (2007) note that while some children's functioning may become compromised during stressful circumstances (e.g., while witnessing violence and leaving home for shelter), they may quickly recover when they return to permanent safe living arrangements with their mothers.

Using the life history method, Humphreys (2001a,b) conducted in-depth interviews with 10 resilient adult daughters who had grown up in violent homes. The process that contributed to resiliency for these women was dynamic and involved characteristics of the child, supportive aspects of the family, and external forces. Child characteristics included physical attractiveness, intelligence, and a cognitive style that allowed them to remain optimistic and persevere as a child. Family factors included supportive relationships with a caring adult, especially a mother or grandmother. External support came from friends, school, and the media. Through external relationships, the women learned that the violence in their homes was not a normal part of family life. Despite being resilient, the women were not completely protected from suffering. In young adulthood, some experienced weight problems and periods of depression. Nonetheless, the combination of risk and protective factors in these women's lives contributed to successful and productive adult lives. Minimizing the number of risk factors to which children are exposed while simultaneously encouraging protective processes can be highly effective in reducing negative outcomes (Gewirtz & Edleson, 2007).

CASE FINDING AND EARLY IDENTIFICATION

Every child should be assessed for her/his exposure to violence. With respect to children who are potentially witnesses to violence, the imperative to assess is particularly important because the signs are often subtle and easy to overlook. One challenge of identifying these children in adult health care settings is that the focus is often on the individual adult, so children's needs often remain unidentified or unmet. Recognition that the family may be the more appropriate unit of care would facilitate the inclusion of children in the assessment process. With increasing awareness of children's responses to violence, health care professionals are recognizing the need to also assess children (Socolar, 2000).

Until recently, assessing for violence exposure was not a routine part of child health care visits. Although pediatricians received training on the identification of child abuse and neglect, they often were not trained on the identification of IPV nor did they consider it part of their role (Culross, 1999). The American Academy of Pediatrics (AAP) (1998) now recognizes the profound effects of IPV exposure on children. Pediatricians, in collaboration with nurses and nurse practitioners, are in a position to identify abused women and intervention on their behalf is an effective way to prevent negative child outcomes.

Efforts to assess for IPV must extend beyond primary health care settings. According to Onyskiw (2002), children of abused women may be more likely to visit other health care providers, which may include providers in walk-in clinics or emergency departments. Abused women may be reluctant to take their children to a family practitioner or pediatrician where abuse may be more likely detected. This is problematic because nurses in these other settings may have less opportunity to become familiar with the family's situation and thus may not attribute children's health problems to violence exposure.

Interventions are as follows:

Primary prevention—responding proactively:

- Prevention of violence against women and children
- Decreased societal tolerance for violence (within families, communities, and the media)
- Community-based interventions and programs
- Family life classes in schools that provide experience with child-rearing and adult relationship dilemmas
- Big Brothers and Big Sisters programs
- Education in schools on family violence and violence in dating relationships
- Nonviolent conflict resolution programs for children

Secondary prevention—responding to violence that has occurred:

- Development and implementation of protocols to routinely identify, treat, and refer survivors of family violence
- Programs for women and children at battered women's shelters

   (a) Developmentally appropriate support and encouragement to discuss worries and concerns
   (b) Health screening for women and children on entry
   (c) Crisis intervention
   (d) Academic programs for shelter children
   (e) Structured, developmentally appropriate daily programs for children
   (f) Therapy and counseling as needed
   (g) Parent–child programs that enhance child-rearing
   (h) Follow-up to evaluate the effectiveness of programs and services

Tertiary prevention—intervention for children who have been exposed:

- Public health or visiting nurse referrals for rehabilitation services
- Support and services to assist in marital and/or child custody disputes.

Assessment

Currently, there are no reliable and valid tools that can be used to ascertain with any degree of certainty whether or not children have been exposed to IPV. However, one way to assess the safety of the child is to assess the safety of the mother (see chapter 5). In this discussion, we focus on strategies that can be used by nurses to identify children who may be at risk for violence exposure and offer suggestions for intervention at the primary, secondary, and tertiary levels.

Indicators from History and Physical Examination

An opportunity to assess children for violence exposure exists in child health care settings during routine child health examinations. Although the indicators that children are witnessing abuse in their homes are often subtle and difficult to detect, there are a number of behavioral and developmental cues that may suggest that a child is at risk. These are summarized in Exhibit 11.1.

If any of these changes are noted, further investigation is warranted. Other signs of distress may include unexplained somatic complaints. Even in the absence of any signs, children of any age may be asked a question such as, "What happens in your house when people get angry?" (Zink, 2000). Humphreys (2001a) suggests that a simple question like

---

EXHIBIT 11.1 | *Nursing Assessment: Impact of Exposure to Abuse on Child Development and Behavior*

Infants & Toddlers
- Easily startled by loud noises
- Lethargic, apathetic
- Prolonged distress, inconsolable
- Vivid visual images associated with violence can be distressing
- Disturbed parent-infant attachment with lack of attentiveness to infant's physical and/or emotional needs
- Inhibited exploration and play due to fear and instability

Pre-schoolers
- Unhealthy expressions of anger and aggression
- Confusion regarding conflicting messages
- Egocentrically attribute violence to something they did
- Regression in developmental milestones
- Learn gender roles associated with violence and victimization

School-age children
- Greater awareness of impact of violence on others (mother's safety, father being charged)
- More susceptible to rationalizations used to justify violence (alcohol as a cause, victim did something to deserve it)
- Guilt or self-blame that they somehow caused the violence
- Learning/academic performance may be compromised (difficulty concentrating, easily distracted)
- Increased risk for bullying and other hostile attitudes and behaviors
- May learn gender roles associated with partner abuse

Adolescents
- Parent-child conflict may result in poorly developed communication skills
- Increased risk for early home leaving, dropping out of school
- Shame about family dynamics
- High risk behaviors as a way to impress peers
- Use of aggression
- Distorted view of self due to abuser's degradation of mother and/or child maltreatment

- Disordered eating patterns
- Avoidance of intimacy, or premature seeking of intimacy and child-bearing
- Difficulty establishing healthy relationships
- Highly susceptible to negative media messages regarding violent behavior and gender role stereotypes.

Adapted from Cunningham, A. & Baker, L. (2007). *Little eyes, little ears: How violence against a mother shapes children as they grow.* London, ON: The Centre for Children and Families in the Justice System.

"What is dinnertime like at your house?" may elicit information about the day-to-day life of children. When asking children these questions, nurses need to be aware of children's fear of reprisals if they disclose information about abuse. She recommends prefacing questions with: "Because violence in families is so common, I routinely ask everyone I see about it."

The most effective approaches are those that are individualized and based on an understanding of each child's situation. In particular, the nurse should assess and document the nature, frequency, severity, and harm inflicted. As well, the current safety of the child and her/his mother needs to be assessed. Because children who are exposed to the abuse of their mothers are also at risk for direct maltreatment, they should simultaneously be assessed for the occurrence of multiple types of adversity.

How the child's problems manifest themselves may warrant different types of responses. For example, it may be more appropriate to respond to the child's symptoms while these are particularly intense, and to respond to the underlying root cause of the problem after the symptoms have subsided. Frequently, children may use coping mechanisms, such as numbing of emotions or blocking disturbing thoughts, which appear initially to be helpful and adaptive for the short term. However, when these are prolonged, they may be difficult to change and result in long-term harm.

Thus, an important role of the nurse is to understand the developmental and behavioral changes that may occur at different stages of childhood and adolescence and to assess the impact of these changes. How does the child feel about what she/he has witnessed? What strategies have been used to "ake it better"? Does the child consider these strategies to be effective in minimizing the pain or otherwise ameliorating the situation?

Intervention

Interventions with children who have been exposed to the abuse of their mothers cover a broad spectrum. The nurse is concerned about the inadvertently injured child of an abused woman as well as the adolescent who has questions about violence in adult relationships. The following discussion describes general areas of intervention according to the level of prevention. The box above summarizes primary, secondary, and tertiary interventions.

Primary Prevention

Primary prevention includes all interventions that prevent violence against women and children (for the primary prevention strategies discussed for child abuse see chapter 10). Prevention of woman abuse is discussed at length in chapter 5, and readers are referred to those earlier sections in the text. Primary prevention includes child and family health promotion activities with both well and "at-risk" populations. The type of nursing intervention at this level varies with the location and nature of practice. We begin this section by presenting a framework, or guiding principles, for the development and implementation of primary prevention programs. We then describe primary prevention initiatives that may be implemented in a wide array of settings including schools, health settings, or community organizations.

In a review of the research related to antiviolence programs, Haskell (1998) identified four key elements necessary for an effective framework. These are as follows: that the framework explicitly states the normative assumptions informing policies and programs; that violence be examined using both individual and social explanations; that a gendered analysis be used to situate violence in social relations of inequality; and that it assist young people to address, and end, violence and sexism in their personal lives.

There are many examples of exemplary educational programs that have been developed. Based on the collective knowledge that has been gleaned from these programs, and building upon Haskell's framework, we suggest five interrelated principles as necessary core components of effective school-based antiviolence education. *First*, programs need to be appropriately tailored to the unique developmental needs of each age group. *Second*, effective antiviolence programs must incorporate a recognition of the multiple realities and positions of privilege that influence how violence is understood and experienced. In particular, attention to social identities based on age, race, class, ability, or sexual orientation are essential aspects of any effective programming initiative. Programs must address not only how to act as individuals but as groups witnessing or participating in violence. Furthermore, programming must incorporate a recognition of the multiple ways that violence is enacted, including physical, emotional, verbal, or sexual, and provide personal and hypothetical examples of the various forms of violence.

Third, prevention programs are needed that address the root causes of violence and that are sufficiently broad in scope and analysis. Too often, programs are directly aimed at increasing individual awareness and assertiveness, self-esteem, or focus on conflict resolution. According to Olweus (1993), however, most bullies score average or above-average on standard self-esteem measures. The implicit assumption of assertiveness programs is that violence occurs because of problems in self-esteem, communication, or conflicts "gone awry." It is further assumed that it is the responsibility of the individual on the receiving end of violence to stop it. The fundamental problem with such programs is that they tend to ignore unequal power relations and imply a level playing field. In effect, this approach fosters a "blame-the-victim" attitude and decreases the transparency surrounding how gendered violence is experienced. Instead of becoming more visible, the manifestations of violence are camouflaged, further obscuring the potential for children to name, negotiate, and resist, the violence in their lives.

Closely related to the third principle, we propose a *fourth* principle, that gender-neutral teaching strategies, which ignore the social context in which violence is perpetuated, be eliminated. Gender neutral strategies overlook or minimize the importance of deconstructing traditional notions of femininity. As a result, conflict resolution and empathy-building programs based on gender neutral policies fail to recognize that girls are likely to be over-socialized toward an empathic role in relationships and, thus, tend to reinforce this role.

The *fifth* principle is that the relevance of content in anti-violence programs be increased and that a gender analysis becomes the organizing principle for all support programs for children and youth. This approach will encourage *girls and boys* to think critically about gender and to examine the effects of gender socialization on their lives. Such programming should begin with elementary school children. We recommend that a gender-based curriculum be located within a primary prevention framework with committed government funding and attention focused on the function, which sexual aggression serves for men. The goal is to establish interventions that build male and female self-esteem without invoking perpetrator/victim identification.

Community-Based Interventions

All types of abuse of family members occur in a society that condones violence within the context of the family. Implicit and explicit approval for the use of violence contributes to its occurrence within families. Frequently, such approval is manifested in the perpetuation of unequal power relationships based on gender inequality. Therefore, interventions at the societal level that diminish tolerance for violence and that challenge gender inequality as a root cause of violence serve as primary prevention for all types of violence. When violence against family members, including corporal punishment as a means of discipline for children, is no longer tolerated under any circumstances, much will have been accomplished toward diminishing the incidence of violence of all kinds.

Because violence in the home does not occur in isolation, efforts aimed at the prevention of violence in the lives of children must simultaneously focus on the home and the community and should ideally involve every realm of social and cultural life. It is therefore critical that primary prevention programs be conceptualized as collaborative initiatives and that such programs be developed in partnership with schools, parents, counselors, community agencies, and health professionals. Although not generally mentioned in the literature, we believe that children and youth should also have a voice in the development of programs intended to be of benefit to them.

In order for programs to be effective, they need to be appropriate to the child's developmental needs. At the level of primary prevention, programs for infants and preschool children should include provisions for home visitation by public health nurses or specially trained paraprofessionals for all new parents. Because of the large number of women who have experienced violence, it is important that such initiatives be geared to all new families, not only those traditionally considered to be "at risk." Consistent with this notion, a growing number of programs have incorporated screening for woman abuse as a routine, universal component of the family assessment. Although the mandate of home visitation programs varies considerably, most afford excellent opportunities for public health nurses to engage in dialogue about the child's developmental needs and the challenges of parenting faced by new mothers. At the same time, home visits are an ideal way to gain insight into family relationships and the potential for violence. Despite the effectiveness of home visitation programs, current political and economic priorities in Canada and the United States have resulted in a reduction in many excellent programs and those that are offered tend to be limited to designated "at risk" groups (Olds et al., 1998; Wolfe & Jaffe, 2001).

Programs such as Big Brothers and Big Sisters can assist school-age children and adolescents to develop significant, supportive relationships outside their immediate families. When children lack frequent contact with one parent, most often fathers, such community-based programs can provide positive experiences and role modeling that can enhance children's resilience to potential and actual stressors.

The adolescent years represent a critical phase in the life cycle during which young people experiment with different roles develop an expanded repertoire of problem-solving skills, become increasingly able to think abstractly, begin to comprehend more fully the consequences of their actions, and contemplate possibilities for the future (see also chapter 9 on "Teen Dating Violence"). The influence of parents is at least partially replaced by influence from peers. For many youth, adolescence represents a time for experimentation with, and initiation of, intimate relationships. Primary prevention programs that are most likely to succeed are those that incorporate a recognition of the issues that are of importance to this group and that are presented in a non-judgmental manner.

Adolescent programs that afford youth opportunities to discuss social relationships, what it means to engage in healthy relationships, and the varied forms of violence that might occur, have many potential benefits. Providing a safe space in which teens can openly share their thoughts regarding relationships, discuss the choices and responsibilities that accompany dating, and the multiple meanings that abuse has for young men and women are all critical in raising awareness regarding the potential for dating violence (Gray & Foshee, 1997).

School-Based Interventions

Anti-violence education should be an integral component of the curriculum in every primary and secondary educational institution. Gamache and Snapp (1995) have described five strategies for violence prevention that are applicable at the elementary school level. The first, called "peacemakers," encourages young children to think globally about world issues or about individuals who have helped to make the world a better place. This exercise provides a means for children to discuss values and responsibility but is most relevant when combined with other antiviolence approaches.

Affective education programs build on self-esteem. Several limitations to this approach were noted above, but they are appropriate when conducted in conjunction with other efforts. One example of an effective school-based antiviolence curriculum is the Fourth R, a grade 9 program that was developed and tested in Canada and is currently being implemented in several states in the United States (Wolfe, Crooks, Hughes, & Jaffe (2008)). In general, this program entails a combination of assertiveness training, self-control, problem solving, and conflict resolution.

Family life classes in schools provide school-age children and adolescents with opportunities to experiment with various child-rearing and adult relationship dilemmas under the supervision of experienced nurses, counselors, and teachers. Parental involvement in such programs further allows parents to become more knowledgeable and to guide their children toward greater understanding of the difficulties of adult relationships and parenting.

Secondary Prevention

When children are exposed to the abuse of their mothers, nursing interventions are termed "secondary prevention." The goals of secondary prevention are early identification and intervention to prevent recurrence of violence. Nursing interventions are aimed at limiting the impact of battering on mothers and their children. Nurses clearly have an important role in identifying abused women and their children and are in a unique position to provide treatment and support services, document abuse, and advocate for their clients.

ASSESSMENT. Before assessing women for IPV, nurses should inform their clients of any legal obligation to report abuse. Nurses are mandated reporters of child abuse. In states and provinces where witnessing domestic violence is considered child abuse, nurses are mandated reporters of this form of abuse. Except in those states or provinces and in cases where child abuse is occurring, nurses will keep information about violence in the home confidential. Edleson (2004) warns against defining all exposure to domestic violence as child maltreatment because it denies that the majority of children in these situations show no negative development problems and show strong coping abilities, and it denies the women's efforts to provide safe environments for their children.

When children exposed to domestic violence are not identified in the health care system, they have increased health problems that result in more frequent emergency department visits, other hospitalizations, and increased use of outpatient health care facilities (Campbell & Lewandowski, 1997). Abused women and their children most often visit the emergency department for medical complaints, not trauma, suggesting the need to intervene in other health care settings. Primary care settings are ideal for identification of and intervention with abused women and their children. A significant number of abused women have indicated they prefer to receive help in a health care setting rather than in a shelter for battered women (Hadley, Short, Lesin, & Zook, 1995). Women in the early stages of battering may not identify themselves as abused and may not associate their children's physical and mental health problems with IPV. Thus, a health care setting may be a viable alternative for early identification and intervention.

According to McFarlane, Parker, Soeken, and Bullock (1992), pregnancy offers a window of opportunity in which abused women are most regularly seen by their health care providers and can receive assessment and intervention. Abuse during pregnancy can have serious consequences (e.g., low birthweight and lethality) for the mother and the fetus. The implications of abuse are as serious as any other potential problems during pregnancy and thus should be part of a routine assessment. Pregnancy can be a point of early intervention for some women and may have the potential to prevent children's exposure to violence in the future (see chapter 6 for further discussion).

A challenge of identifying children of abused women in adult health care settings, however, is that the focus is often on treating the individual (the adult) so children's needs often remain unidentified or unmet. Greater recognition that the family may be the more appropriate unit of care would facilitate the inclusion of children in the screening process. Nonetheless, intervening on behalf of abused women has the potential to also help children. For example, when screening women for abuse, nurses should also ask about their children's exposure to violence and their responses. With increasing evidence of children's responses to violence, health care professionals are recognizing the need to also screen and assess on behalf of children (Socolar, 2000). The American Medical Association's recommended IPV screening questions could be asked with children ages 2–3 or younger in the room. More general questions (e.g., "What happens in your house when people get angry?") could be asked with children of any age in the room (Zink, 2000).

An opportunity to screen children for violence exposure exists in child health care settings during routine child health examinations. Depending on the child's age, nurses may directly screen children for exposure to abuse. Humphreys (2001a) suggests that a simple question like "What is dinnertime like at your house?" may elicit information about the day-to-day life of children. When screening children, nurses need to be aware of children's fear of reprisals if they disclose information about abuse. She recommends prefacing questions with: "Because violence in families is so common, I routinely ask everyone I see about it." Nurses also can routinely screen mothers during child health visits to give them an additional opportunity to disclose abuse. In contrast to direct screening, nurses can also detect possible exposure to domestic violence by recognizing signs of distress, such as aggressive behavior, running away, or unexplained somatic complaints.

Until recently, screening for violence exposure was not a routine part of child health care visits. Although pediatricians received training on the identification of child abuse and neglect, they often were not trained on the identification of adult domestic violence nor did they consider it part of their role (Culross, 1999). The American Academy of Pediatrics (1998) now recognizes the profound effects of IPV exposure on children. Pediatricians are in a position to identify abused women, and intervention on their behalf is an effective way to prevent negative child outcomes. The AAP encourages pediatricians to be aware of the signs of abuse (e.g., facial bruising, depression, anxiety, failure to keep appointments and reluctance to answer questions about discipline) in the mothers of children they see and to intervene in a sympathetic way that assures confidentiality and prioritizes safety. Pediatricians can call on nurses to assist in screening and assisting abused women and their children.

Efforts to screen for IPV must extend beyond primary health care settings. According to Onyskiw (2003), children of abused women may be more likely to visit other health care providers, which may include providers in walk-in clinics or emergency departments. Abused women may be reluctant to take their children to a family practitioner or pediatrician where abuse may be more likely detected. This is problematic because nurses in these other settings may have less opportunity to become familiar with the family's situation and thus may not attribute children's health problems to violence exposure.

When children of abused women are identified, nurses should conduct a thorough history (abuse history and psychosocial history), assess the mental and physical health effects, taking into account the total situation including the psychosocial context, and instigate suitable interventions including appropriate referrals and long-term follow-up. The safety of the children and their mothers, the mothers' desires and motivations to change or leave the abusive partner, and children's attachment to the abuser should be assessed. Even in the case of mandated reporting, a careful assessment of risk and protective factors is necessary before drawing conclusions about risk and harm to children (Edleson, 2004).

In addition to assessing danger, nurses should assess for mothers' perceptions of the children's involvement in and responses to violence. Frequently, mothers are unaware of, or underestimate, their children's perceptions of IPV. In one study, neither parents nor teachers recognized the high anxiety in children exposed to family and community violence (Hurt et al., 2001). Ericksen and Henderson (1998) suggest that abused women and their children have diverging realities in terms of their perceptions of violence in the home and the children's needs. Through in-depth interviews, they discovered that while mothers gave very vague descriptions of abuse and minimized the abuse their children were exposed to, children provided very explicit and clear descriptions of the violence they witnessed. For this reason, nurses should directly assess children in addition to assessing their mothers.

Nurses in primary care should continue to assess children over time, as the health effects of violence exposure may persist over time or surface later (Humphreys, 2001b). In Berman's (1999) study, children described numerous ways in which witnessing violence compromised their health (e.g., loss of sleep, eating disturbances, difficulty carrying on with daily routine, and lack of energy), effects that persisted over time. Assessment should continue even if children have been removed from the violent situation. Abuse does not typically end when women leave abusive partners, and children often witness violence that occurs after separation. In one study, children were more likely to witness abuse if incidents occurred after separation (Hotton, 2002), possibly because violence occurs in the context of shared custody tasks, such as exchanging the children for visitation. Several researchers have reported that women who shared custody with their abusers after divorce face continued abuse and ongoing efforts to ensure their own and their children's safety (Hardesty & Ganong, 2006; Hardesty, Khaw, Chung, & Martin, 2008; Wuest et al., 2002). By assessing abused women and their children over time, nurses can identify ways in which domestic violence continues to affect children's health and safety.

PLANNING. After a thorough assessment, nurses can develop short- and long-term interventions. Planning for interventions should take into account personal, family, cultural, and environmental factors as well as the potential risk to abused women and their children. Interventions should include appropriate referrals to community resources for safety, advocacy, and support.

Safety planning should be predicated on the degree of danger (Campbell, 1995; Hardesty & Campbell, 2004) and should be a part of all interventions regardless of whether the mother is returning to or leaving the abusive partner. The risk of danger is particularly high when the woman has left or is planning to leave the abuser. For some, safety concerns continue long after leaving because they remain in contact with their abusers through shared custody arrangements (Ericksen & Henderson, 1998; Hardesty & Ganong, 2006). A key risk factor after separation is the abuser's access to the woman, making unsupervised visitations and exchanges a risky time for severe or lethal violence to the woman and/or her children (Sheeran & Hampton, 1999).

Many abused women want their children to maintain a relationship with their fathers after separation. They face a dilemma of balancing safety needs with the desire for their children to have contact with both parents (Hardesty & Ganong, 2006). They may also feel guilty for "breaking up" a two-parent family, and they may worry about their children's adjustment to separation or divorce. Nurses can acknowledge this dilemma and normalize mothers' worries. Some abused mothers are required by courts to maintain contact through shared custody arrangements, thereby allowing the abuser to continue their pattern of control and further abuse (Hardesty, 2002; Wuest et al., 2002). Nurses can encourage abused women to prioritize safety when making decisions about father/child contact after separation/divorce. For example, nurses can suggest to women that they create a parenting plan to be approved by the court that includes specific safety strategies (e.g., use of a third party to exchange children for visitation; Hardesty & Campbell, 2004).

In many cases, the best way to protect the child is to protect the mother from the abuser. Safety planning with the mother will help the child, as the child's safety is intricately related to and dependent on the mother's safety (Culross, 1999). However, when possible, safety planning with mothers should include specific strategies for children (see Box 2) (Hardesty & Campbell, 2004). With the help of the mother, nurses can facilitate safety planning with children. Safety planning can help empower children to identify safety issues and problem solve in ways that will afford protection. It also can minimize risk and help reduce children's anxiety and fears. Nurses can encourage critical thinking by working collaboratively with children in the identification of appropriate strategies (Hart, 2001).

Specific safety strategies for children should be age appropriate and the child must be capable of and competent enough to carry them out. Development also should be considered both in terms of understanding and responding to violence. For example, in planning for what to do if things get dangerous, an older child may be more able to dial 911 whereas it may be safer to instruct a younger child to go to the neighbors. Also it may be more necessary to advise older children to escape and not intervene than younger children who are less likely to intervene. It is also necessary to take into account the degree of attachment the child has to the abuser. It may be unreasonable to expect a boy strongly attached to his father to call the police on his "dad." Nurses can also assess the availability of social supports to assist the child in safety planning. A caring and trusted adult can provide the child with a safe place to go when necessary.

Direct interventions with children depend on the timing of the encounter, age and responses of the child, and family circumstances. Even children in battered women's shelters require different interventions. If the child is returning to the violent home, interventions may need to focus on the most basic safety needs. If the family is relocating, the nurse may have the opportunity to help the mother and child to learn new ways of living and responding. Interventions in battered women's shelters that address a variety of potential times and experiences are presented below.

SHELTER-BASED PROGRAMS. Although there is some variability, battered women's shelters are generally emergency shelters for women and their children, where they are provided temporary safe haven within a communal shelter setting. Abused women and their children are allowed to stay at the shelter for a relatively short period of time (usually a maximum of 30–60 days), during which they are assisted in assessing their situation, gaining knowledge and insight about woman abuse, and obtaining social services. The women and their children may leave the shelter to relocate with family or friends, or to their own new residence. Many women and their children also return to their homes with the hope and belief that their leaving and their new information and insight will help to stop the violence.

In recent years, attention to the needs of children who accompany their mothers to shelters has increased. Because of limited funds, however, resources have generally been directed toward assisting the mothers with counseling, social, and potential relocation services, all of which indirectly benefit children. Even with limited funds, many shelters have always offered specialized services to children. Nurses involved with shelters can contribute to those services or assist in their development when such services are unavailable. As with every practice setting, certain aspects constrain practice. For example, abused women and their children are often a transient population (length of shelter stay varies from a few days to months) and children represent a wide age range (infants to teenagers) and a variety of developmental stages. Shelters face challenges such as limited availability of staff and limited privacy, space, and accessibility to provide services and treatment.

All children admitted to shelters for abused women should have access to health screening and treatment. An individual health history and assessment of each child should be conducted to identify his or her experience and response. Health problems should receive immediate attention through nursing staff or community referral. Clinical experience with abused women and their children in shelters has revealed many more commonalities to the provision of maternal-child care in these and other settings than might be expected. In addition, children of abused women may have difficulties that are unique to their experience. Some children have been physically injured in the attack on their mothers immediately preceding admission to the shelter. These injuries require the same attention as any other injury, with particular attention to preventing infection, maintaining alignment with fractures, and facilitating suture removal.

Mothers also have needs for information regarding their children's growth, development, state of health, and anticipatory guidance. Nursing staff can develop with the mother and children a health plan with health-related goals to achieve while at the shelter. Nursing involvement is an obvious benefit and can provide an excellent opportunity for nursing student clinical experiences (Urbancic, Campbell, & Humphreys, 1993).

Children commonly experience a variety of stress-related symptoms during their stays at shelters. They may return to behaviors such as bedwetting, thumb sucking, and bottle-feeding that previously had been abandoned. Nurses can assess children's stress and coping and discuss them with mothers. Mothers may lack knowledge of children's responses and are reassured to know that these are normal and generally disappear once order has been established. Preliminary evaluation studies also suggest that the therapeutic environment of the battered women's shelter can help to reduce children's symptoms (Graham-Bermann, 2001).

Battered women's shelters with children's services usually offer some structured programs to children. The form of these programs varies greatly. They generally include all or part of the following components: crisis intervention activities, academic program, daily program, therapy/counseling, parent-child program, and/or advocacy program. These components are not mutually exclusive. Various approaches to these components have been reported and are presented in the following discussion.

ACADEMIC PROGRAMMING. Children in shelters frequently are unable to attend their regular schools for safety (fathers may attempt to find them through school attendance) and other reasons (teasing or harassment by peers). Some shelters send children to local schools where the circumstances of children's attendance are understood. Others provide on-site educational services.

School nurses can make important contributions to specialized academic programs for children exposed to violence. Previously discussed approaches that encourage children and mothers to disclose their worries and fears help children in school settings as well. Often nurses who are initially approached with some physical problem will be sought out in the future for other less tangible difficulties after they have been perceived as helpful by children. School nurses also can help teachers and other staff members understand why children sometimes return to the security of habits (i.e., thumb sucking, special toys, nail biting) during times of stress. Nursing assessments of children's physical complaints (e.g., stomach pains,) can serve to reassure everyone that the problem can be "cured" with attention, quiet time, and reassurance rather than a visit to the emergency room.

DAILY STRUCTURE AND CONSISTENCY. Daily programs for children in shelters vary greatly. Generally programs are structured to ensure that a similar schedule is followed most weekdays. At a minimum, routine childcare allows mothers to attend to the many obligations associated with obtaining social services, hunting for an apartment, and finding employment. For children in shelters, structured time and activities provide organization and security in strange environments. If sufficiently qualified staff is available, routine play sessions can be used for additional educational and therapeutic group sessions that enhance individual counseling.

It is important for children of abused women to be exposed to adults, both female and male, who respect each other and work together. Early in the women's shelter movement, men were rarely seen inside shelters. Fortunately, many male staff and volunteers now provide positive role models for children.

THERAPY/COUNSELING. Children need to talk about their experiences and their feelings. They may blame themselves for the violence in their homes, especially if abusive episodes were associated with parental conflicts over childrearing. Children may also feel that they are responsible for their mother's decision to leave the home, to return, or to get a divorce. What appears to be an egocentric perception by children of abused women may be reality. The best interests of children are frequently central to women's decisions about the future. A mother may stay in an abusive relationship because she believes that her children will benefit from the ongoing presence of an adult male. Alternatively, women may ultimately decide to leave an abusive situation because the violence is affecting the children (Hardesty, 2001; Humphreys, 1998). In either case, children may feel responsible, not just for themselves, but also for the entire family.

Children may have spent an inordinate amount of time trying to be "good" to prevent future episodes of violence. If children have intervened in attempts to stop violence between adults, they may have a false sense of confidence in their abilities to keep batterers from abusing again. If they were successful in the past at stopping abuse, children may feel personal failure if subsequent interventions were unsuccessful.

Many authors have described the valuable role of therapy for children. Therapy approaches vary and can include individualized approaches, such as trauma-focused therapy, or small group therapy to help children express their emotions and feelings. Approaches may vary from Big Brother/Sister recreational-type approaches to play therapy to longer-term, more intensive contacts that more closely resemble traditional psychotherapy. Therapy with children can include the whole family, sibling groups, or the mother/child dyad. The type of intervention depends on the ages, developmental levels, and needs of the children. Individualized therapy can be particularly useful when cultural background or other characteristics are likely to influence children's responses to domestic violence.

PARENT–CHILD PROGRAMS. Some shelters provide services to abused women intended to enhance their relationships with their children and, if necessary, learn nonviolent methods of childrearing. Shelters do not allow the use of violent conflict resolution tactics, including corporal punishment, by anyone. For some mothers this necessitates learning new ways of disciplining their children. Nurses can take an active role in helping mothers develop a repertoire of disciplinary approaches, considering the most appropriate approaches for their children and circumstances, and role modeling the use of the different strategies. The goal is to improve children's adjustment by improving mothers' parenting competence.

Sullivan et al. (2000) warn against assuming that all abused women are impaired in their ability to parent or that they are responsible for their children's adjustment problems. As these authors aptly note, it is men's use of violence that increases children's behavioral problems, which in turn increases mothers' parenting stress and need to use discipline. To reduce the negative effects of violence exposure on children, parenting classes must be mandated for abusive fathers, not the mothers whom they have abused. Women who want or need parenting classes should be able to access them, but should not be required to attend classes just because they have been abused. Most mothers will want help understanding their children's behavioral problems and how they can appropriately respond to them. However, we should not assume that all abused mothers want or need help. Women are active agents who, despite abuse, nurture their children in diverse and creative ways. Any assistance should be driven by what these women request and should acknowledge their strengths and capabilities.

ADVOCACY PROGRAM. Finally, abused women and their children need follow-up services after they leave shelters. At a minimum, shelter staff can connect women and children to appropriate community services. Nurses can help them develop goals and objectives for maintaining and improving their well-being after leaving the shelter. Some shelters provide outreach services, such as therapy/counseling, information, or education programs, that women and their children can take advantage of after leaving the shelter.

Children of abused women are often victimized by prolonged legal disputes over custody and visitation issues. The legal battle can be a prolonged affair, involving years of threats and conflicts, which many children discover continues long after the separation and any court decisions. Some shelters provide legal advocacy programs that provide information and support related to custody and visitation.

TERTIARY PREVENTION. Ideally, abuse of women is never allowed to progress to this stage of intervention; however, this is often the case. Tertiary prevention is required when children of abused women have experienced irreversible effects from the violence. The goal of tertiary prevention is rehabilitation and healing of the children to the maximum level of functioning possible with the limitations of any negative effects. Many of the secondary prevention strategies apply to tertiary prevention. One difference is that a goal of tertiary prevention is to establish long-term comprehensive services for women and children.

Home visitation programs are one option for long-term services. When physical injuries have resulted in disability, women and their children may be eligible for a visiting nurse program. Home visiting nurses can provide assistance with actively finding social support, and they can advocate for women and children as they negotiate community resources. Home visiting programs also can be educational interventions. For example, in Sullivan and colleagues' (1998) home visitation advocacy program, advocates provide instrumental support to help mothers solve problems. Instrumental problems include finding jobs, arranging transportation, getting information about educational opportunities, and helping mothers communicate with the school system. The goal is to reduce mothers' frustrations and improve parenting.

A coordinated community response (CCR) involving the health care system, legal system (including those who work with divorce and custody issues), domestic violence advocates, and child welfare worker is important at any level of intervention but may be particularly useful at the tertiary level. A CCR seeks to integrate the variety of resources from which abused women and their children are likely to require services (Sullivan & Allen, 2001). An integrated effort increases the availability and accessibility of resources, advocacy, and support to women and their children. A CCR also increases the communication within and among organizations, exchange of resources, and development of shared goals. In addition, a CCR may decrease revictimization, duration of families involved in the system, families who return to system, and encourage batterer accountability. Unfortunately, child welfare workers and abused women's advocates often find themselves at odds with each other while working with families. They share similar interests in stopping violence; however their perspectives and approaches differ. Nurses are in an excellent position to collaborate with both groups of professionals to work toward a common goal.

Implementation

Most abused women care about their children's safety and want to protect them. Their worries and the energy they spend worrying affects how they respond to battering, which in turn affects their children (Humphreys, 1995). Nurses can help battered women and indirectly help their children by easing the work of worrying. One way to do this is by encouraging a discussion of worries. Clients may benefit by actively discussing their thinking and responses. Nurses can tell battered women that by helping themselves they are helping their children. This may free battered women to focus on themselves without feeling that they are neglecting their children. Humphreys (1995) indicates that nurses should use both "worry" and "fears" when initiating such discussions, as these terms mean different things to battered women. She also suggests open discussion of worries and fears in both private and group settings so that women can share their common experiences, learn and critique responses, and be reassured that they are not alone in their work of worrying.

Nurses also can help women recognize their children's needs and the ways in which they might support them. For example, the women in Ericksen and Henderson's (1998) study indicated that they did not know how to talk to their children or what questions to ask them. They reported that their children had enormous unmet needs and that they felt inadequate in helping their children. Nurses can educate mothers about the health effects of exposure to domestic violence to help them understand their children's reactions and how to respond to them.

Particularly during separation/divorce, mothers may have difficulty being emotionally available to their children, as much of their energy is expended negotiating helping systems (e.g., legal system), making custody and visitation decisions, and, for many, managing continued harassment and control (Ericksen & Henderson, 1998; Wuest, Berman, Ford-Gilbe, Merritt-Gray, 2002; Hardesty, 2002). Mothers may be concerned about the pragmatics of day day-to-day survival after separation/divorce and unaware of their children's emotional needs. They also may feel ambivalent about what is best for themselves and their children because, while they want to move on, they are tied to their former partners through the children.

During this time, children need their mothers (Ericksen & Henderson, 1998). They are likely to feel sad over their parents' separation and concerned about the uncertainty of the future, and they are likely to miss their fathers. They may worry that their mothers will leave them, too. Children of abused women, like all children, need to express their worries and concerns, but because children are often protective of their mothers, they may be reluctant to express their own feelings. They also may feel loyalty conflicts, wanting to meet the emotional needs of both parents. Nurses can ask children about their worries or fears and, with their permission, share with them with their mothers. Nurses also can educate children about domestic violence and dispel any beliefs that violence is a routine part of normal family life (Humphreys, 2001a). Finally, nurses can assess the availability of social supports that can provide valuable opportunities for children to share their conflicting feelings without getting "caught in the middle" by confiding in a parent.

From research with children of domestic violence and children of war, Berman (1999) offers several guiding principles that should apply to all interventions with children exposed to violence: (a) willingness to listen to children in a sincere and non-judgmental manner, (b) respect for the child and recognition of his or her strengths, (c) willingness to try non-traditional approaches with children from diverse cultural backgrounds, (d) awareness of the political dimension of violence, with a view to enabling the child to develop age-appropriate understandings of political and social contexts, and (e) development of strategies to help children find health in a world that often appears to be an unhealthy place.

Evaluation

Evaluation is an ongoing process through which the nurse reviews the changes made in terms of the identified goals. Long-term follow-up is necessary as situations and needs change. In terms of evaluating the effectiveness of intervention programs, existing research is in its early stages (Graham-Bermann, 2001). At present, intervention programs tend to use a "one size fits all" approach, and thus, they work for some children but not others. Children have different responses to witnessing domestic violence; some are negatively affected, while others appear to manage well. Different responses to violence exposure require intervention programs targeted to children's specific needs. Controlled outcome studies comparing the effectiveness of different interventions are clearly needed to guide nurses in choosing programs that work.

Evaluation studies with abused women and their children are challenging for several reasons. Abused women may not stay in shelters long enough to complete an evaluation. Furthermore, while evaluations with women and children residing in shelters are convenient, they are limited because only a small number of women seek shelter. Tracking is a problem when doing evaluations with women and children in the community. Women may relocate, or batterers may keep women and children isolated. Furthermore, evaluations of children after they leave shelters must account for where they go. Some children return to the home with the abuser, others relocate, and some children have continued contact with abusers through custody or visitation arrangements. These children are likely to demonstrate different outcomes after leaving the shelter.

Based on a review of existing evaluation research, Graham-Bermann offers the following suggestions for designing more effective interventions:

1. Target intervention efforts to groups of children with similar profiles, violence experiences, and exposures
2. Compare the same program with different populations of exposed children (e.g., shelter vs. community population)
3. Compare different treatment approaches in systematically controlled studies
4. Evaluate interventions designed for children with different symptoms (e.g., internalizing vs. externalizing symptoms)

EXHIBIT 11.2 | *Safety Planning With Children*

Questions to consider when developing a child safety plan:
1. What is the degree of risk to the mother?
2. What is degree of risk to the child (child abuse or lethality)?
3. What are the child's individual needs (e.g., what is the child afraid of or worried about)?
4. What are the child's abilities (e.g., age/developmental status, mental/physical health)?
5. What are the child's feelings toward the abuser (e.g., conflicted, angry, ambivalent)?

Possible safety strategies:
- Avoid places, times, or circumstances that have associated with prior violent incidences.
- Never intervene in a violent incident but instead escape to safety and call 911.
- Learn how to use the phone, including how to call long distance and practice making calls.
- Know a way to reach your mother or a trusted adult at all times and know how to call 911.
- Be familiar with any protective orders in place that may influence police response.
- Identify all ways of escape (windows, doors) and identify where all phones are located.
- Locate a safe place (e.g., church) or a trusted adult to go to if necessary.
- Create a contract to be approved by the court that outlines your rights, your father's responsibilities, and any consequences if the order is violated.

Children must understand that a safety plan is not a guarantee for safety. Just as the child is not responsible for the violence, the child is also not responsible for the failure of any safety strategy.

Based on Hart (2001). *Safety planning for children: Strategizing for unsupervised visits with batterers* [Online]. Available: http://www.mincava.umn.edu/documents/hart/hart.html.

---

5. Identify features of interventions that are effective (e.g., therapist characteristics, setting, techniques)
6. Extend the follow-up period to track program effects over time and identify which children improve, worsen, or stay the same
7. Adopt minimum standards and criteria for evaluating the effectiveness of interventions.

SUMMARY

Children exposed to the abuse of their mothers are at risk for a variety of emotional, cognitive, and behavioral difficulties. However, research has described the important mediating effects on children of even one positive relationship with a significant person. Nurses should be aware of family violence and assess every client and family for this problem. Early identification and intervention can stem detrimental effects and help individuals and families toward recovery.

REFERENCES

Achenbach, T. M., & Edelbrock, C. S. (1978). The classification of child psychopathology: A review and analysis of empirical efforts. *Psychological Bulletin, 85,* 1275–1301.

Aitken, R. (2001). *Domestic violence and the impact on children. Results of a survey into the knowledge and experience of education personnel within two European countries.* London: Refuge.

Allwood, M. A., Bell-Dolan, D., & Hussain, S. A. (2002). Children's trauma and adjustment reactions to violent and nonviolent war experiences. *Journal of the American Academy of Child and Adolescent Psychiatry, 41,* 450–457.

American Academy of Pediatrics. (1998). The role of the pediatrician in recognizing and intervening on behalf of abused women. *Pediatrics, 101*(6), 1091–1092.

American Psychiatric Association. (1987). *Diagnostic and statistical manual of mental disorders* (Rev. ed.). Washington, DC: Author.

Arias, I., & Pape, K. T. (1999). Psychological abuse: Implications for adjustment and commitment to leave violent partners. *Violence and Victims, 14*(1), 55–68.

Arroyo, W., & Eth, S. (1985). Children traumatized by Central American warfare. In S. Eth & R. S. Pynoos (Eds.), *Post-traumatic stress disorder in children* (pp. 103–120). Washington, DC: American Psychiatric Press.

Attala, J., & McSweeney, M. (1997). Preschool children of battered women identified in a community setting. *Issues in Comprehensive Pediatric Nursing, 20,* 217–225.

Baldry, A. C. (2003). Bullying in schools and exposure to domestic violence. *Child Abuse and Neglect, 27,* 713–732.

Berman, H. (1999). Health in the aftermath of violence: A critical narrative study of children of war and children of battered women. *Canadian Journal of Nursing Research, 31,* 89–109.

Berman, H., Hardesty, J., & Humphreys, J. (2003). Children of abused women. In J. Humphreys & J. Campbell (Eds), *Family violence and nursing practice* (pp. 150–187). Philadelphia, PA: Lippincott.

Berman, H., McKenna, K., Traher, C., Taylor, G., & MacQuarrie, B. (2000). Sexual harassment: Everyday violence in the lives of girls and women. *Advances in Nursing Science, 22*(4), 32–46.

Berman, H., & Jiwani, Y. (Eds.) (2002). *In the best interests of the girl child.* Ottawa, Ontario, Canada: Status of Women Canada.

Blackburn, J. F. (2008). Reading and phonological awareness skills in children exposed to domestic violence. *Journal of Aggression, Maltreatment & Trauma, 17*(4), 415–438.

Boney-McCoy, S., & Finklehor, D. (1995). Psychosocial sequelae of violent victimization in a national youth sample. *Journal of Consulting and Clinical Psychology, 63,* 726–736.

Brown, L. S. (1991). Not outside the range: One feminist perspective on psychic trauma. *American Imago, 46,* 119–133.

Byrne, D., & Taylor, B. (2007). Children at risk from domestic violence and their educational attainment: Perspectives of education welfare officers, social workers and teachers, *Child Care in Practice, 13*(3), 185–201.

Caetano, R., Field, C. A., & Nelson, S. (2003). Association between childhood physical abuse, exposure to parental violence, and alcohol problems in adulthood. *Journal of Interpersonal Violence, 18*(3).

Campbell, J. C. (1995). *Assessing dangerousness.* Newbury Park, CA: Sage.

Campbell, J. C., & Lewandowski, L. A. (1997). Mental and physical health effects of intimate partner violence on women and children. *Anger, Aggression, and Violence, 20*(2), 353–374.

Carlson, B. E. (2000). Children exposed to domestic violence: Research findings and implications. *Trauma, Violence, and Abuse, 1*(4), 321–342.

Carr, J. L., & VanDeusen, K. M. (2002). The relationship between family of origin violence and dating violence in college men. *Journal of Interpersonal Violence, 17,* 630–646.

Centers for Disease Control and Prevention (2006). Atlanta: CDC; 2006. Adverse childhood experiences study. Available from: http://www.cdc.gov/nccdphp/ace/index.htm

Collins, P. H. (2000). *Black feminist thought: Knowledge, consciousness, and the politics of empowerment* (2nd ed.). New York: Routledge.

Culross, P. L. (1999). Health care system responses to children exposed to domestic violence. *The future of children: Domestic violence and children, 9*(3), 111–121.

Daro, D., Edleson, J. L., & Pinderhughes, H. (2004) Finding common ground in the study of child maltreatment, youth violence and adult domestic violence. *Journal of Interpersonal Violence, 19*(3), 282–298.

Dauvergne, M., & Johnson, H. (2002). Children witnessing family violence. *Juristat: Canadian Centre for Justice Statistics (Statistics Canada, Catalogue No. 85-002-XPE), 21*(6), 1–13.

Dube, S. R., Anda, R. F., Felitti, V. J., Edwards, V. J., & Williamson, D. F. (2002). Exposure to abuse, neglect, and household dysfunction among adults who witnessed intimate partner violence as children: Implications for health and social services. *Violence and Victims, 17*(1), 3–17.

Edleson, J. L., Ellerton, A. L., Seagren, E. A., Kirchberg, S. L., Schmidt, S. O., & Ambrose, A. T. (2007). Assessing child exposure to adult domestic violence. *Children and Youth Services Review, 29*, 961–971.

Edleson, J. L. (2004). Should childhood exposure to adult domestic violence be defined as child maltreatment under the law? In P.G. Jaffe, L.L. Baker, & A. Cunningham. (2004). (Eds.). *Protecting children from domestic violence: Strategies for community intervention*. New York: Guilford Press.

Edleson, J. L., Mbilinyi, L. F., & Shetty, S. (2003). *Parenting in the context of domestic violence*. San Francisco: Judicial Council of California.

Edleson, J. L. (2001). Studying the co-occurrence of child maltreatment and domestic violence in families. In S. A. Graham-Bermann & J. L. Edleson (Eds.), *Domestic violence in the lives of children: The future of research, intervention, and social policy* (pp. 91–110). Washington, DC: American Psychological Association.

Edwards, V. J., Holden, G. W., Felitti, V. J., & Anda, R. F. (2003). Relationship between multiple forms of childhood maltreatment and adult mental health in community respondents: Results from the Adverse Childhood Experiences Study. *American Journal of Psychiatry, 160*, 1453–1460.

Ericksen, J. R., & Henderson, A. D. (1998). Diverging realities: Abused women and their children. In J. C. Campbell (Ed.), *Empowering survivors of abuse: Health care for battered women and their children* (pp. 138–155). Thousand Oaks, CA: Sage.

Fantuzzo, J. W., & Fusco, R. A. (2007). Children's direct exposure to types of domestic violence crime: A population-based investigation. *Journal of Family Violence, 22*, 543–552.

Fantuzzo, J. W., & Mohr, W. K. (1999). Prevalence and effects of child exposure to domesticviolence. *Future of Children: Domestic Violence and Children, 9*(3), 21–32.

Felitti, V. J., Anda, R. F., Nordenberg, D., Williamson, D. F., Spitz, A. M., & Edwards, V., et al. (1998). Relationship of childhood abuse and household dysfunction to many of the leading causes of death in adults: The adverse childhood experiences study. *American Journal of Preventive Medicine, 14*, 245–258.

Finkelhor, D., Ormrod, R., & Turner, H. (2007). Polyvictimization and trauma in a national longitudinal cohort. *Development and Psychopathology, 19*, 149–166.

Gamache, D., & Snapp, S. (1995). Teach your children well: Elementary schools and violence prevention. In E. Peled, P. Jaffe, & J. Edelson (Eds.), *Ending the cycle of violence: Community responses to children of battered women* (pp. 209–231). Thousand Oaks, CA: Sage.

Garbarino, J., Kostelny, K., & Dubrow, N. (1991). *No place to be a child: Growing up in a war zone*. Lexington, MA: D. C. Heath & Co.

Garmezy, N. (1981). Children under stress: Perspectives on antecedents and correlates of vulnerability and resistance to psychopathology. In A. I. Rabin, J. Arnoff, A. M. Barclay, & R. A. Zucker (Eds), *Further explorations in personality* (pp. 70–81). New York: Wiley Interscience.

Gerwirtz, A. H., & Edleson, J. L. (2007). Young children's exposure to intimate partner violence: Towards a developmental risk and resilience framework for research and intervention. *Journal of Family Violence, 22*, 151–163.

Goldblatt, H. (2003). Strategies of coping among adolescents experiencing interparental violence. *Journal of Interpersonal Violence, 18*(5), 532–552.

Graham-Bermann, S. A. (2001). Designing intervention evaluations for children exposed to domestic violence: Applications of research and theory. In S. A. Graham-Bermann & J. L. Edleson (Eds.) *Domestic violence in the lives of children: The future of research, intervention, and social policy* (pp. 237–267). Washington, DC: American Psychological Association.

Graham-Bermann, S. A., De Voe, E. R., Mattis, J. S., Lynch, S., & Thomas, S. A. (2006). Ecological predictors of traumatic stress symptoms in caucasian and ethnic minority children exposed to intimate partner violence. *Violence Against Women, 12*(7), 663–692.

Graham-Bermann, S. A., & Seng, J. (2005). Violence exposure and traumatic stress symptoms as additional predictors of health problems in high risk children. *Journal of Pediatrics, 147*, 349–354.

Graham-Bermann, S. A., & Levendosky, A. A. (1998). Traumatic stress symptoms in children of battered women. *Journal of Interpersonal Violence, 14*, 111–128.

Graham-Bermann, S.A., & Levendosky (1994). *Empowering battered women as mothers.* Unpublished manuscript, University of Michigan, Department of Psychology, Ann Arbor, MI, USA.

Gray, H., & Foshee, V. (1997). Adolescent dating violence: Differences between one-sided and mutually violence profiles. *Journal of Interpersonal Violence, 12,* 126–141.

Griffing, S., Lewis, C. S., Chu, M., Sage, R. E., Madry, L., & Primm, B. J. (2006). Exposure to interpersonal violence as a predictor of PTSD symptomatology in domestic violence survivors. *Journal of Interpersonal Violence, 21(7),* 936–954.

Grych, J. H., Jouriles, E. N., Swank, P. R., McDonald, R., & Norwood, W. D. (2000). Patterns of adjustment among children of battered women. *Journal of Consulting and Clinical Psychology, 68, (1),* 84–94.

Guille, L. (2004). Men who batter and their children: An integrated review. *Aggression and Violent Behavior, 9(2),* 129–163.

Hadley, S., Short, L., Lesin, N., & Zook, E. (1995). Women kind: An innovative model of health care response to domestic abuse. *Women's Health Issues, 5,* 189–198.

Hardesty, J. L, Khaw, L., Chung, G. H., & Martin, J. M. (2008). Coparenting relationships after divorce: Variations by type of marital violence and fathers' role differentiation. *Family Relations, 57(4),* 479–491.

Hardesty, J. L., & Ganong, L. H. (2006). How women make custody decisions and manage co-parenting with abusive former husbands. *Journal of Social and Personal Relationships, 23(4),* 543–563.

Hardesty, J. L., & Campbell, J. C. (2004). Safety planning for abused women and their children. In P. G. Jaffe, L. L. Baker, & A. J. Cunningham (Eds.), *Protecting children from domestic violence: Strategies for community intervention* (pp. 89–100). New York: Guilford.

Hardesty, J. L. (2002). Separation assault in the context of post-divorce parenting: An integrative review of the literature. *Violence Against Women, 8(5),* 593–621.

Hardesty, J. L. (2001). *"I just can't get him out of my life!" Co-parenting after divorce with an abusive former husband.* Doctoral dissertation, University of Missouri-Columbia.

Hart, B. J. (2001). *Safety planning for children: Strategizing for unsupervised visits with batterers.* Retrieved August 23, 2002, from http://www.mincava.umn.edu/hart/safetyp.htm

Haskell, L. (1998). *Violence prevention education in schools: A critical literature review.* Unpublished manuscript.

Health Canada (2007). Retrieved August 9, 2009, from http://www.phac-aspc.gc.ca/ncfv-cnivf/publications/rcmp-grc/fem-vioeffects-eng.php

Henning, K., Leitenberg, H., Coffey, P., Turner, T., & Bennett, R. T. (1996). Long-term psychological and social impact of witnessing physical conflict between parents. *Journal of Interpersonal Violence, 11,* 35–51.

Herman, J. L. (1992). *Trauma and recovery.* New York: Basic Books.

Herrenkohl, T. I., Sousa, C., Tajima, E. A., Herrenkohl, R. C., & Molyan, C. A. (2008). Intersection of child abuse and children's exposure to domestic violence. *Trauma, Violence, & Abuse, 9(2),* 84–99.

Heyman, R. E., & Slep, A. M. (2002). Do child abuse and interparental violence lead to adulthood family violence? *Journal of Marriage and Family, 64,* 864–870.

Holden, G. W., & Ritchie, K. (1991). Linking extreme marital discord, child rearing, and child behavior problems: Evidence from battered women. *Child Development, 62,* 311–327.

Holden, G. W., Stein, J. D., Ritchie, K. L., Harris, S. D., & Jouriles, E. N. (1998). Parenting behaviors and beliefs of battered women. In G. W. Holden, R. Geffner, & E. N. Jouriles (Eds.), *Children exposed to marital violence: Theory, research, and applied issues* (pp. 289–334). Washington, DC: American Psychological Association.

Holt, S., Buckley, H., & Whelan, S. (2008). The impact of exposure to domestic violence on children and young people: A review of the literature. *Child Abuse and Neglect, 32,* 797–810.

Hooks, B. (1984). *Feminist theory from margin to center.* Boston, MA: South End Press.

Hotton, T. (2002). Spousal violence after marital separation. *Juristat Service Bulletin: Canadian Centre for Justice Statistics* (Catalogue 85-002 ISSN 0715-271X). Ottawa: Statistics Canada.

Hughes, H. M. (1988). Psychological and behavioral correlates of family violence in child witness and victims. *American Journal of Orthopsychiatry, 58,* 77–90.

Hughes, H. M., Vargo, M. C., Ito, E. S., & Skinner, L. K. (1991). Psychological adjustment of children of battered women: Influences of gender. *Family Violence Bulletin, 7,* 15–17.

Humphreys, J. C. (1989). *Dependent-care directed toward the prevention of hazards to life, health, and well-being in mothers and children who experience family violence.* Doctoral dissertation, Wayne State University, Detroit, MI, USA.

Humphreys, J. C. (1990). Dependent-care directed toward the prevention of hazards to life, health, and well-being in mothers and children who experience family violence. *MAINlines, 11*(1), 6–7.

Humphreys, J. C. (1991). Children of battered women: Worries about their mothers. *Pediatric Nursing, 17*, 342–345.

Humphreys, J. C. (1995). The work of worrying: Battered women and their children. *Scholarly Inquiry for Nursing Practice: An International Journal, 9*(2), 127–145.

Humphreys, J. C. (2001a). Growing up in a violent home: The lived experience of daughters of battered women. *Journal of Family Nursing, 7(3),* 244–260.

Humphreys, J. C. (2001b). Turnings and adaptations in resilient daughters of battered women. *Journal of Nursing Scholarship, 33*(3), 245–251.

Hurt, H., Malmud, E., Brodsky, N. L., & Giannetta, J. (2001). Exposure to violence: Psychological and academic correlates in child witnesses. *Archives of Pediatric Adolescent Medicine, 155*(12), 1351–1356.

Huth-Bocks, A. C., Levendosky, A. A., & Semel, M. A. (2001). The direct and indirect effects of domestic violence on young children's intellectual functioning. *Journal of Family Violence, 16*(3), 269–290.

Jaffe, P. G., Wolfe, D. A., Wilson, S. K., & Zak, L. (1986). Family violence and child adjustment: A comparative analysis of girls' and boys' behavioral symptoms. *American Journal of Psychiatry, 143*(1), 74–77.

Jaffe, P. G., Wolfe, D. A., & Wilson, S. K. (1990). *Children of battered women.* Newbury Park, CA: Sage.

Johnson, R. M., Kotch, J. B., Catellier, D. J., Winsor, J. R., Dufort, V., Hunter, W., et al. (2002). Adverse behavioral and emotional outcomes from child abuse and witnessed violence. *Child Maltreatment, 7*(3), 179–186.

Jouriles, E., McDonald, R., Slep, A., Heyman, R., & Garrido, E. (2008). Child abuse in the context of domestic violence: Prevalence, explanations, and practice implications. *Violence and Victims, 23,* 221–235.

Jouriles, E. N., McDonald, R., Norwood, W. D., & Ezell, E. (2001). Issues and controversies in documenting the prevalence of children's exposure to domestic violence. In S. A. Graham-Bermann & J. L. Edleson (Eds.), *Domestic violence in the lives of children: The future of research, intervention, and social policy* (pp. 13–34). Washington, DC: American Psychological Association.

Jouriles, E. N., Spiller, L. C., Stephens, N., McDonald, R., & Swank, P. (2000). Variability in adjustment of children of battered women: The role of child appraisals of interparent conflict. *Cognitive Therapy and Research, 24,* 233–249.

Jouriles, E. N., Murphy, C. M., & O'Leary (1989). Interspousal aggression, marital discord, and child problems. *Journal of Consulting and Clinical Psychology, 57,* 453–455.

Kalmuss, D. (1984). The intergenerational transmission of marital aggression. *Journal of Marriage and the Family, 46,* 11–19.

Kasturirangan, A., Krishnan, S., & Riger, S. (2004). The impact of culture and minority status on women's experiences of domestic violence. *Trauma, Violence, and Abuse, 5*(4), 318–332.

Kaufman, J., & Zigler, E. (1987). Do abused children become abusive parents? *American Journal of Orthopsychiatry, 57,* 186–193.

Kelleher, K. J., Hazen, A. L., Coben, J. H., Wang, Y., McGeehan, J. , Kohl, P. L., et al. (2008). Self-reported disciplinary practices among women in the child welfare system: Association with domestic violence victimization. *Child Abuse & Neglect, 32*(8), 811–818.

Kernic, M. A., Wolf, M. E., Holt, V. L., McKnight, B., Huebner, C. E., & Rivara, F. P. (2003). Behavioral problems among children whose mothers are abused by an intimate partner. *Child Abuse & Neglect, 27*(11), 1231–1246.

Kerig, P. K. (1998). Gender and appraisals as mediators of adjustment in children exposed to interparental violence. *Developmental Psychology, 29*(6), 931–939.

Kinzie, J. D., Sack, W. H., Angell, R., Manson, S. M., & Rath, B. (1986). The psychiatric effects of massive trauma on Cambodian children: I. The children. *Journal of the American Academy of Child Psychiatry, 25,* 370–376.

Kitzmann, K.M., Gaylord, N. K., Holt, A. R., & Kenny, E.D. (2003). Child witnesses to domestic violence: A meta-analytic review. *Journal of Consulting and Clinical Psychology, 71*(2), 339–352.

Langhinrichsen-Rohling, J., Monson, C. M., Meyer, K. A., Caster, J., & Sanders, A. (1998). The associations among family-of-origin violence and young adults' current depressed, hopeless, suicidal, and life-threatening behavior. *Journal of Family Violence, 13,* 243–261.

Lemmey, D., McFarlane, J., Wilson, P., & Malecha, A. (2001). Intimate partner violence: Mother's perspective of effects on their children. *MCN, 26*(2), 98–103.

Levendosky, A. A., & Graham-Bermann, S. A. (2001). Parenting in battered women: The effects of domestic violence on women and their children. *Journal of Family Violence, 16*(2), 171–192.

Levendosky, A. A., Leahy, K. L., Bogat, G. A., Davidson, W. S., & von Eye, A. (2006). Domestic violence, maternal parenting, maternal mental health, and infant externalizing behavior. *Journal of Family Psychology, 20*(4), 544–552.

Levendosky, A. A., Huth-Bocks, A. C., Semel, M. A., & Shapiro, D. L. (2002). Trauma symptoms in preschool-age children exposed to domestic violence. *Journal of Interpersonal Violence, 17*, 150–164.

Lieberman, A. F. (2007). Ghosts and Angels: Intergenerational patterns in the transmission and treatment of the traumatic sequelae of domestic violence. *Infant Mental Health Journal, 28*, 422–239.

Lindhorst, T., Evans-Campbell, T., Huang, B., & Walters, K. L. (2006). Interpersonal violence in the lives of urban American Indian and Alaska native women: Implications for health, mental health, and help-seeking. *American Journal of Public Health, 96*, 1416–1423.

Litrownik, A. J., Newton, R., Hunter, W. M., English, D., & Everson, M. D. (2003). Exposure to family violence in young at-risk children: A longitudinal look at the effects of victimization and witnessed physical and psychological aggression. *Journal of Family Violence, 18*(1), 59–73.

Lundy, M., & Grossman, S. F. (2005). The mental health and service needs of young children exposed to domestic violence: Supportive data. *Families in Society, 86*(1), 17–29.

Luthar, S. S., Cicchetti, D., & Becker, B. (2000). The construct of resilience: A critical evaluation and guidelines for future work. *Child Development, 71*(3), 543–562.

Lynch, M., & Cicchetti, D. (1998). An ecological-transactional analysis of children and contexts: The longitudinal interplay among child maltreatment, community violence, and children's symptomatology. *Developmental Psychopathology, 10*, 235–257.

Maker, A. H., Kemmelmeier, M., & Peterson, C. (1998). Long-term psychological consequences in women of witnessing parental physical conflict and experiencing abuse in childhood. *Journal of Interpersonal Violence, 13*, 574–589.

Malik, N. M. (2008). Exposure to domestic and community violence in a nonrisk sample: Associations with child functioning. *Journal of Interpersonal Violence. 23*(4), 490–504.

Margolin, G., Vickerman, K., Ramos, M., Serrano, S., Gordis, E., Iturralde, E., et al. (2009). Youth exposed to violence: Stability, co-occurrence, and context. *Clinical Child and Family Psychological Review, 12*, 39–54.

Margolin, G. (2005) Children's exposure to violence: Exploring developmental pathways to diverse outcomes. *Journal of Interpersonal Violence, 20*(1), 72–81.

Masten, A. S. (2001). Ordinary magic: Resilience processes in development. *American Psychologist, 53*, 227–238.

Mathias, J. L., Mertin, P., & Murray, A. (1995). The psychological functioning of children from backgrounds of domestic violence. *Australian Psychologist, 30*, 47–56.

McCloskey, L. A., & Lichter, E. L. (2003). The contribution of marital violence to adolescent aggression across different relationships. *Journal of Interpersonal Violence, 18*(4), 390–412.

McCloskey, L. A., Figueredo, A. J., & Koss, M. P. (1995). The effects of systematic family violence on children's mental health. *Child Development, 66*, 1239–1261.

McCloskey, L. A., & Walker, M. (2000). Posttraumatic stress in children exposed to family violence and single-event trauma. *Journal of the American Academy of Child and Adolescent Psychiatry, 38*(1), 108–115.

McDonald, R., Jouriles, E. N., Tart, C. D., & Minze, L. C. (2009). Children's adjustment problems in families characterized by men's severe violence toward women: Does other family violence matter? *Child Abuse & Neglect, 33*(2), 94–101.

McFarlane, J., Parker, B. Soeken, L., & Bullock, L. (1992). Assessing for abuse during pregnancy: Severity and frequency of injuries and associated entry into prenatal care. *Journal of the American Medical Association, 267*, 2370–2372.

McGee, R. A., Wolfe, D. A., & Wilson, S. K. (1997) Multiple maltreatment experiences and adolescent behavior problems: Adolescents' perspectives. *Development and Psychopathology, 9*, 131–149.

McGruder-Johnson, A. K., Davidson, E. S., Gleaves, D. H., Stock, W., & Finch, J. F. (2000). Interpersonal violence and posttraumatic symptomatology: The role of ethnicity, gender, and exposure to violent events. *Journal of Interpersonal Violence, 15*(2), 205–221.

Mohr, W. K., Lutz, M. J. N., Fantuzzo, J. W., & Perry, M. A. (2000). Children exposed to family violence: A review of empirical research from a developmental-ecological perspective. *Trauma, Violence, & Abuse, 1*(3), 264–283.

Moore, T. E., & Pepler, D. J. (1998). Correlates of adjustment in children at risk. In G. W. Holden, R. Geffner, & E. Jouriles (Eds.), *Children exposed to marital violence: Theory, research, and intervention* (pp. 157–184). Washington, DC: American Psychological Association.

Moffitt, T. E., & Capsi, A. (2003). Preventing the intergenerational continuity of antisocial behaviour: Implications of partner violence. In D.P. Farrington & J. W. Coid (Eds.), *Early prevention of adult antisocial behaviour* (pp. 109–129). Cambridge, UK: Cambridge University Press.

Moretti, M. M., Obsuth, I., Odgers, C. L., & Reebye, P. (2006). Exposure to maternal vs. paternal partner violence, PTSD, and aggression in adolescent girls and boys. *Aggressive Behavior, 32*(4), 385–395.

O'Keefe, M. (1994). Racial/ethnic differences among battered women and their children. *Journal of Child and Family Studies, 3*, 285–305.

Olds, D., Henderson, C., Cole, R., Eckenrode, J., Kitzman, H., Luckey, D., et al. (1998). Long-term effects of nurse home visitation on children's criminal and antisocial behavior: 15-year follow-up of a randomized trial. *Journal of the American Medical Association, 280*, 1238–1244.

Olweus, D. (1993). *Bullying at school: What we know and what we can do.* Cambridge, MA: Blackwell.

Onyskiw, J. E., & Hayduk, L. A. (2001). Processes underlying children's adjustment in families characterized by physical aggression. *Family Relations, 50*, 376–385.

Onyskiw, J. E. (2002). Health and use of health services of children exposed to violence in their families. *Canadian Journal of Public Health, 93*, 416–420.

Onyskiw, J. E. (2003). Domestic violence and children's adjustment: A review of research. *Journal of Emotional Abuse, 3*, 11–45.

Osofsky, J. D. (2003). Prevalence of children's exposure to domestic violence and child maltreatment: Implications for prevention and intervention. *Clinical Child and Family Psychology Review, 6*(3), 161–170.

Osofsky, J. D. (1997). The violence intervention project for children and families. In J. D. Osofsky (Ed.), *Children in a violent society* (pp. 256–260). New York: Guilford Press.

Parkinson, G. W., Adams, B., Emerling, C., & Frank, G. (2001). Maternal domestic violence screening in an office-based pediatric practice. *Pediatrics, 108*, 43.

Pynoos, R. S., & Eth, S. (1984). The child as witness to homicide. *Journal of Social Issues, 40*, 269–290.

Pynoos, R. S., & Nader, K. (1993). Issues in the treatment of post-traumatic stress in children and adolescents. In J. P. Wilson & B. Raphael (Eds.), *The international handbook of traumatic stress syndromes* (pp. 535–549). New York: Plenum.

Pynoos, R. S., Steinberg, A. M., & Wraith, R. (1995). A developmental model of childhood traumatic stress. In D. Cicchetti & D. J. Cohen (Eds.), *Developmental psychopathology* (Vol. 2, pp. 72–95). New York: John Wiley.

Rath, G. D., Jaratt, L. G., & Leonardson, G. (1989). Rates of domestic violence against adult women by men partners. *Journal of American Board of Family Practitioners, 227*, 227–233.

Reitzel-Jaffe, D., & Wolfe, D. A. (2001). Predictors of relationship abuse among young men. *Journal of Interpersonal Violence, 16*(2), 99–115.

Rossman, B. B. R. (1998). Descartes' error and posttraumatic stress disorder: Cognition and emotion in children who are exposed to parental violence. In G. W. Holden, R. Geffner, & E. Jouriles (Eds.), *Children exposed to marital violence: Theory, research, and intervention* (pp. 223–256). Washington, DC: American Psychological Association.

Rossman, B. B. R. (2001). Longer term effects of children's exposure to domestic violence. In S.A. Graham-Bermann & J. L. Edleson (Eds.), *Domestic violence in the lives of children: The future of research, intervention, and social policy* (pp. 35–65). Washington, DC: American Psychological Association.

Rossman, B. B. R., & Ho, J. (2000). Posttraumatic stress response and children exposed to parental violence. In R. Geffner, P. Jaffe, & M. Sudermann (Eds.). *Children Exposed to Domestic Violence: Current Issues in Research, Intervention & Prevention, & Policy Development* (pp. 85–106). Binghamton, NY: Howarth Press.

Saigh, P. A. (1991). The development of posttraumatic stress disorder following four different types of traumatization. *Behavioral Research Therapy, 29*, 213–216.

Sanders-Phillips, K. (2009). Racial discrimination: A continuum of violence exposure for children of color. *Clinical Child and Family Psychological Review, 12*, 174–195.

Sheeran, M., & Hampton, S. (1999, Spring). Supervised visitation in cases of domestic violence. *Juvenile and Family Court Journal, 50*(2), 13–26.

Shiu-Thornton, S., Senturia, K., & Sullivan, M. (2005). "Like a bird in a cage": Vietnamese women survivors talk about domestic violence. *Journal of Interpersonal Violence. 20*(8), 959–976.

Silva, R. R., Alpert, M., Munoz, D. M., Singh, S., Matzner, F., & Dummit, S. (2000). Stress and vulnerability to posttraumatic stress disorder in children and adolescents. *American Journal of Psychiatry, 157*(8), 1229–1235.

Silvern, L., & Kaersvang, L. (1989). The traumatized children of violent marriages. *Child Welfare, 68,* 421–436.

Silvern, L., Karyl, J., Waelde, L., Hodges, W. F., Starek, J., Heidt, E., & Min, K. (1995). Retrospective reports of parental partner abuse: Relationships to depression, trauma symptoms and self-esteem among college students. *Journal of Family Violence, 10,* 177–202.

Socolar, R. R. S. (2000, September/October). Domestic violence and children: A review. *NCMJ, 61*(5), 279–283.

Spilsbury, J., C., Kahana, S., Drotar, D., Creeden, R., Flannery, D. J. & Friedman, S. (2008). Profiles of behavioral problems in children who witness domestic violence. *Violence and Victims, 23*(1), 3–17.

Stalford, H., Baker, H., Beveridge, F., & Mckie, L. (2003). *Children and domestic violence in rural areas: A child-focused assessment of service provision.* London: Save the Children.

Sternberg, K. J., Lamb, M. E., Guterman, E., & Abbott, C. B. (2006). Effects of early and later family violence on children's behavior problems and depression: A longitudinal, multi-informant perspective. *Child Abuse & Neglect, 30*(3), 283–306.

Sternberg, K. J., Lamb, M. E., Greenbaum, C., Cicchetti, D., Dawud, S., Cortes, R. M., et al. (1993). Effects of domestic violence on children's behavior problems and depression. *Developmental Psychology, 29,* 44–52.

Straus, M. A. (1979). Measuring intrafamily conflict and violence: The Conflict Tactics (CT) Scales. *Journal of Marriage and the Family, 41,* 75–88.

Straus, M. A. (1992). Children as witnesses to marital violence: A risk factor for lifelong problems among a nationally representative sample of American men and women. In D. F. Scwarz (Ed.), *Children and violence: Report on the 23rd Ross roundtable on critical approaches to common pediatric problems* (pp. 98–104). Columbus, OH: Ross Laboratories.

Straus, M. A., Gelles, R. J., & Steinmetz, S. K. (1980). *Behind closed doors: A survey of family violence in America.* New York: Doubleday.

Sullivan, C. M., Juras, J. Bybee, D. Nguyen, H., & Allen, N. (2000). How children's adjustment is affected by their relationships to their mothers' abusers. *Journal of Interpersonal Violence, 15,* 587–602.

Sullivan, C. M., & Allen, N. E. (2001). Evaluating coordinated community responses for abused women and their children. In S. A. Graham-Bermann & J. L. Edleson (Eds.) *Domestic violence in the lives of children: The future of research, intervention, and social policy* (pp. 269–282). Washington, DC: American Psychological Association.

Sullivan, P. (2009). Violence exposure among children with disabilities. *Clinical Child and Family Psychological Review, 12,* 196–216.

Terr, L. (1990). *Too scared to cry.* New York: Harper Collins.

Tjaden, P., & Thoennes, N. (2000). *Extent, nature, and consequences of intimate partner violence: Findings from the National Violence Against Women Survey* [Research in brief]. Washington, DC: National Institutes of Justice and Centers for Disease Control and Prevention.

Turner, H. A., Finkelhor, D., & Ormrod, R. (2006). The effect of lifetime victimization on the mental health of children and adolescents. *Social Science & Medicine, 62*(1), 13–27.

Urbancic, J., Campbell, J. C., & Humphreys, J. (1993). Student clinical experiences in shelters for battered women. *Journal of Nursing Education, 32,* 341–346.

Vogel, L. C., & Marshall, L. L. (1995). Distress and symptoms of posttraumatic stress disorder in abused women. *Violence and Victims, 10,* 23–34.

Ware, H. S., Jouriles, E. N., Spiller, L. C., McDonald, R. Swank, P. R., & Norwood, W. D. (2001). Conduct problems among children at battered women's shelters: Prevalence and stability of maternal reports. *Journal of Family Violence, 16*(3), 291–307.

Widom, C. S. (1989). Does violence beget violence? A critical examination of the literature. *Psychological Bulletin, 106,* 3–28.

Wolfe, D. A., & Korsch, B. (1994). Witnessing domestic violence during childhood and adolescence: Implications for pediatric practice. *Pediatrics, 94,* 594–599.

Wolfe, D. A., Wekerle C., Reitzel, D., & Gough, R. (1995). Strategies to address violence in the lives of high-risk youth. In E. Peled, P. G. Jaffe, & J. Edleson (Eds.), *Ending the cycle of violence: Community response to children of battered women* (pp. 255–274). Newbury Park, CA: Sage.

Wolfe, D.A., & Jaffe, P. (2001). Prevention of domestic violence: Emerging initiatives. In S. Graham-Bermann & J. L. Edelson (Eds.), *Domestic violence in the lives of children: The future of research, intervention, and social policy* (pp. 283–298). Washington, DC: American Psychological Association.

Wolfe, D. A., Crooks, C. V., Lee, V., McIntyre-Smith, A., & Jaffe, P. G. (2003). The effects of children's exposure to domestic violence: A meta-analysis and critique, *Clinical Child and Family Psychology Review, 6*(3), 171–187.

Wolfe, D. A., Crooks, C. V., Hughes, R., & Jaffe, P. J. (2008). The Fourth R: A school-based program to reduce violence and risk behaviors among youth. In D. Pepler & W. Craig (Eds), *Understanding and addressing bullying: An international perspective* (pp. 184–197). Bloomington, IN: AuthorHouse.

Wuest, J., Berman, H., Ford-Gilboe, M., & Merritt-Gray, M. (2002). Illuminating social determinants of women's health using grounded theory. *Health Care for Women International, 23,* 794–809.

Zink, T. (2000). Should children be in the room when the mother is screened for partner violence? *The Journal of Family Practice, 49*(2), 130–136.

12

Childhood Sexual Abuse

Jessica E. Draughon, PhD(c), RN
Joan C. Urbancic, PhD, RN

INTRODUCTION

Research in the area of child sexual abuse (CSA), as in so many other violence and trauma research areas, suffers from a plethora of definitions. The Child Abuse Prevention and Treatment Act defines CSA as:

> "The employment, use, persuasion, inducement, enticement, or coercion of any child to engage in, or assist any other person to engage in, any sexually explicit conduct or simulation of such conduct for the purpose of producing a visual depiction of such conduct or the rape, and in cases of caretaker or inter-familial relationships, statutory rape, molestation, prostitution, or other for of sexual exploitation of children or incest with children." (United States Department of Health and Human Services [USDHHS]; 2003, p. 44)

In layperson's terms, CSA includes incest, rape, sodomy, exhibitionism, pornography, and attempted or actual fondling occurring without consent (D'Amora, Brandhurst, & Wallace, 2006). Although any form of sexual intercourse between a child and an adolescent or adult is considered abusive, it is less clear when making a determination about same-age peers (DiGorgio-Miller, 1998). Some define CSA as any sexualized contact between children with five or more years of age difference (Johnson, 2004; Russell, 1986). However, others define any sexual contact between children regardless of age as abusive due to the likelihood that one or both have been sexually abused in another setting (Berrien, 2007; Child Welfare Information Gateway, 2006). Urbancic (1992), in clinical practice and research, identified frequent cases of female victims who were coerced into sexual activity by brothers of age similar to the victim.

Regardless of age, there is a power imbalance between the child and the offender, so the victim is unable to give consent because of physical, cognitive, and/or psychological immaturity. This is the case even though the child may believe she or he consented and may have sought the sexual activity. It is widely accepted that the child *is* always a "victim" in CSA because a child is never in a position to give informed consent. The adult is always in a power position and pressures or forces the child in various ways to cooperate. The child may fear punishment, rejection, or abandonment by the adult or, alternatively, may look forward to material rewards or special privileges. Because the sexual activity usually begins with fondling and rarely involves violence, it may be pleasurable and sexually stimulating for the child.

There are many different acts that constitute CSA. Although the most publicized and well known are arguably cases of children who have been abducted by strangers, sexually abused, and brutally murdered, this is the rare exception. Sadly, the child who is sexually abused by someone he or she knows and trusts is relatively common (Finkelhor, 2009). This is illustrated by sexual abuse of children by Catholic priests. These sensationalized cases unfortunately have more in common with the more frequent trauma and suffering caused by incestuous sexual abuse from a child's relative or close family caregiver. The abuse is characterized by betrayal of trust by a person who is expected to protect, teach, and guide children.

This chapter provides an overview of CSA, theories of causation, and effects CSA has on the child and his or her family, as well as nursing care with a specific focus on incestuous relationships. Because of the betrayal of trust, confusion, sense of helplessness, and secrecy associated with the abuse, the potential for psychological trauma is greater than if the perpetrator were a stranger (Kendall-Tackett, Williams, & Finkelhor, 1993). For more information on sexual offenders and child sexual exploitation, please refer to Table 12.1.

The National Clearinghouse on Child Abuse and Neglect found that, in 2003, there were 2.9 million referrals to Child Protective Services (CPS; Lichenstein & Suggs, 2007). In 2005, this number increased to over 3.3 million referrals for all types of abuse regarding 6 million children (USDHHS, 2007). Less than 10% of cases in 2005 were for sexual abuse; however, that still amounts to 60,000 reported cases of CSA in the United States in a single year (USDHHS, 2007). Research indicates that approximately only 10% of cases are reported (Berliner & Elliott, 2002; Hornor, 2002). Theodore et al. (2005) found a rate 15 times higher than official reports of CSA through maternal self-report of their children's

TABLE 12.1 Web Resources

Resource	Internet Link
American Academy of Child and Adolescent Psychiatry	http://www.aacap.org/cs/root/facts_for_families/child_sexual_abuse
Enough.org Internet Safety Site	http://www.protectkids.com/abuse/
Pandora's Box	http://www/prevent-abuse-now.com/index-detailed.htm
National Library of Medicine: Gateway to Information on CSA	http://www.nlm.nih.gov/medlineplus/childsexualabuse.html
Child Welfare Information Gateway	http://www.childwelfare.gov/index.cfm
Rape and Incest National Network	http://www.rainn.org 1-800-656-HOPE
International Association of Forensic Nurses	http://www.iafn.org http://www.safeta.org/
Child and Woman Abuse Studies Unit	http://www.cwasu.org/
OVC CSA Treatment Guidelines	http://www.musc.edu/cvc
National Sex Offender Public Registry	http://www.nsopr.gov
American Professional Society on the Abuse of Children	http://www.apsac.org

victimization. Menard and Ruback (2003) found that areas with higher levels of poverty and higher rates of stranger assaults were more likely to report CSA.

Although there is agreement that reports of CSA are increasing, incidence and prevalence studies with adults have reported a range of figures, primarily due to differences in definition and methodology (Finkelhor, 1994; Pereda, et al., 2009; Russell, 1986). In determining the prevalence rates of CSA, data are derived either from official records of child abuse reports or from surveys conducted with adults who disclose their abuse retrospectively. A recent review of incidence and prevalence studies built upon Finkelhor's (1994) classic prevalence study and confirmed prior rates, finding that, internationally, up to 10% of male children and 10–20% of female children experienced CSA (Pereda, et al., 2009). Male children are increasingly being recognized as victims of CSA, and research is beginning to show that male CSA is underreported and more prevalent than statistics indicate. Nevertheless, female children are sexually abused more frequently than male children, and most of the literature relates to the female child victim (Finkelhor, 1994; Herman, 2000; Pereda et al., 2009).

The best figures based on official reports are derived from the Third National Incidence Study of Child Abuse and Neglect, or NIS-3 (Sedlak & Broadhurst, 1996). Congress mandated three such studies with results published in 1981, 1988, and 1996. The NIS-4 project is scheduled to conclude in 2009, yet at the time of this writing, the updated data have not been published. Data for the NIS-4 were collected in 122 countries between 2004 and 2006 (USDHHS, 2008). The purpose of these studies was to provide updated estimates of child abuse and neglect for Congress and the nation. All three of the NIS studies used two standards of abuse, and data were gathered according to both standards.

Under the more stringent, harm standard, the incidence of CSA increased by 83% from 119,200 cases in 1988 to 217,700 in 1996. The second, and less stringent, endangerment standard indicated a 125% increase in incidence of sexual abuse from 133,600 in 1988 to 300,200 in 1996. Most authorities believe the increase in incidence is due, in part, to professionals becoming more adept at identifying and reporting abuse. Across the three published NIS studies, female children were sexually abused three times more often than male children.

HISTORICAL PERSPECTIVES

Although the theme of child sexual exploitation and incest has been prevalent in art and literature since ancient times (Cooper, 2005), research has not been extensive until the last 20 years. The earliest research focused primarily on the characteristics of the offender and the family dynamics. Few studies examined the effects of CSA on the child, and those that did were limited by sample size, control, and methodology. Nevertheless, early researchers claimed that the child often initiated and enjoyed the sexual relationship and that trauma to the child was rare (Bender & Blau, 1937). In addition, many clinicians did not think CSA was a significant issue because of its rare occurrence. As late as 1972, the prominent psychiatrist Henderson insisted that incest was an uncommon event and therefore of little concern (Henderson, 1972). Historically, victims of CSA have been discredited, disbelieved, or rendered invisible. This phenomenon is clearly illustrated in the false-memory movement of the 1900s in which alleged sexual offenders claimed they were unjustly accused of abuse and that victims' memories were implanted by incompetent therapists.

Acceptance of the reality of CSA has not been a smooth road. Because of increased child abuse reporting in the 1980s, criminal prosecution of offenders by adult victims also increased. Many court cases involved adult victims with delayed or recovered memories of their childhood abuse. Consequently, most states passed legislation to extend time limits for which a victim could prosecute their offender. In response, the False Memory Syndrome Foundation (FMSF) was mobilized to support alleged and convicted perpetrators. Composed mainly of offenders, a few academics, and defense attorneys, the FMSF conducted a highly publicized campaign in the media and courts to fight incest allegations. FMSF Executive Director Pamela Freyd led the organization in an effort to clear her husband who was accused of incest by his daughters. The FMSF concluded that their daughters' memories were false and implanted by feminist therapists determined to destroy the sanctity of the family. The FMSF was successful in mobilizing the press, garnering public support, and won several court cases. Again, victims of CSA were revictimized by a society that doubted the validity of their claims and by therapists afraid to inquire about CSA for fear of being sued.

Since that time, a growing body of research has emerged about the validity of recovered or delayed memories. The American Psychiatric Association (APA) and the American Medical Association have issued formal documents recognizing the existence of "traumatic amnesia." The Diagnostic and Statistical Manual of Mental Disorders, fourth edition, also recognizes the possibility of such memories. Research studies indicate that many women who report CSA also report having only partial memories for their abuse. Although total repression happens less often, it does occur in a small percentage of women. In one study, out of 147 women, 10% ($n=14$) reported totally forgetting their abuse memories (Urbancic, 1992). In a recent study of college women (Epstein & Bottoms, 2002), 15% ($n=14$) of the 104 women who identified themselves as experiencing CSA reported that they had a period of time in their lives when they could not remember the abuse. However, Epstein and Bottoms used multiple questions about the memories and concluded that only 4% of the sample really qualified for complete repression according to the Freudian definition. Elliott and Briere (1995), in their nationally representative general population study, reported that 30% of women and 14% of men who identified themselves as having CSA experiences reported a period of memory loss of their abuse. Other researchers have also documented that forgetting and then subsequently remembering abuse is not uncommon among women who report CSA (Chu, Frey, Ganzel, & Matthews, 1999; Williams, 1994; Wilsnack, Wonderlich, Kristhanson, Vogeltanz-Holm, & Wilsnack, 2002). Women who, only with the help of a therapist, remembered CSA ranged from 1.8% of women in the study by Wilsnack, et al. (2002) to 3% of women in a study by Polusny and Follette (1996).

Researchers have recognized that overzealously attempting to uncover abuse can be as harmful as failing to identify its occurrence (Briere, 1996; Chu et al., 1999; Courtois, 1999). A subset of adults who were severely abused as children may be more apt to dissociate, be highly imaginable, and be suggestible to false memories during psychotherapy. Briere points out that some therapists are guilty of bad therapy by being too authoritarian and trying to convince clients that they have been abused when there is no basis. However, Briere notes that bad therapy is not the same as recovering bad memories. He also asserts that those who have been falsely accused of being abusers are also victims, and thus, they have a right to legal and personal redress. However, these writers emphasize that the overwhelming majority of people who claim to have been sexually abused as children have, indeed, suffered those experiences.

THEORETICAL PERSPECTIVES

The child victim in the incestuous family is usually the oldest daughter, with the average age of approximately 9 years (Berliner & Elliott, 2002) and with a range of infancy to 17 years. In Russell's (1986) study, 11% of abuse occurred before age 5, 19% from 6 to 9 years, 41% from 10 to 13 years, and 29% 14 years of age and later. The incestuous relationship may extend over a period of many years; the average length of time is approximately 3 years. It is common for the severity of incest to increase as the abusive activity continues over the years.

Parents have the roles of teachers and protectors, not exploiters, and although all parents may experience some sexual feelings toward their children at times, the incestuous parent acts on those feelings. The majority of CSA victims never disclose, but some are able to extricate themselves from the situation in a variety of ways. If the child is able to escape the abuse, often the next youngest child is forced to assume their role in the sexual relationship. Sometimes, it is the victimization of a younger sibling that motivates the oldest to disclose CSA. CSA may cease as the child matures and becomes more assertive and better able to protect him or herself from further abuse. If the child begins dating, it often leads to conflict with the abuser due to jealousy. Escalating tension and anger may lead to acting out in terms of drug use and promiscuity. It is not unusual for the victim to accuse the offender of CSA during a family argument over delinquent behavior. The child may choose to disclose the CSA to a friend or teacher, who then reports the abuse to protective services. Running away from home is another frequent way of coping; therefore, anyone working with runaway teenagers should assess them for CSA.

The following section begins with an overview of theories of children's response to CSA, progressing to theories of causation, characteristics of offenders, and finishing with theories of the family dynamic involved in perpetuating an incestuous relationship. For a more comprehensive discussion of etiology of family violence, cycles of violence, revictimization, and child abuse please refer to the first four chapters of this text.

Psychological Theories of Children's Responses

Many frameworks attempt to explain the traumatic effects of CSA. One belief common to all current frameworks is that a child is always a victim in incestuous relationships. Flirtatious behavior is an attempt for nurturance, not sexual gratification. If the child is seductive, it is because she or he has been taught that sexual contact is an effective means to gain attention, affection, and special favors. As the sexually abusive relationship continues, it is common to progress to oral sex, mutual masturbation, and penetrative intercourse. Pressures on the child to cooperate and maintain the relationship are a crucial issue to assess. Many children have severe guilt, feelings of helplessness, and shame but continue to maintain secrecy because of fear that disclosure will lead to punishment, greater shame, rejection, or disbelief by the social network. Although a variety of psychological and physical symptoms are likely to develop as the abusive relationship continues, a minority of children self-disclose (Faller, 2002; Smith et al., 2000).

Wilson, Friedman, and Lindy (2001) used a constructionist approach to explain the psychological trauma of CSA. According to these researchers, victims "construct and construe" an individual meaning of abuse. Therapists must enter the survivor's world to understand how CSA affected her or him and what aspects were most troubling. Several researchers advocate a cognitive model to explain how children process the abuse and try to make sense out of the world (Burgess, Hartman, Wolbert, & Grant, 1987; Carmen & Rieker, 1989). A cognitive model maintains that when a traumatic experience is appropriately processed, it will be neutralized, resolved, and stored in distant memory. When traumatic experiences are not resolved, they remain in active memory or are defended by cognitive mechanisms, such as dissociation, repression, splitting, suppression, and compartmentalization. Because the abuser demands secrecy, the child is forced to establish these defenses to prevent disclosure, and the child develops under the burden of trauma encapsulation. These researchers assert that CSA results in long-term effects of low self-worth, self-blame, a lack of self-efficacy, self-fragmentation, dissociations, and self-destructive behaviors.

Finkelhor and Browne (1986) explained the effects of incest with their four trauma-causing factors called traumagenic dynamics. They maintained that some of these four factors occur in all types of psychologically traumatic situations, but only in incest do all four occur together. The four factors are the following:

1. Traumatic sexualization: an example is rewarding a child for sexual behavior, teaching that sexual behavior can be used as a means to meet one's needs.
2. Betrayal: the child may experience betrayal by the actions of the abuser, as well as from the non-offending parent and other adults from whom they seek protection.
3. Powerlessness: occurs when a child is repeatedly used sexually against her or his will and is unable to disclose the activity because of fear of the consequences.
4. Stigmatization: negative connotations of the abuse, which are integrated into the child's self image. Stigmatization may develop during the abuse itself or after disclosure when adults react with shock, horror, and blame of the child.

Psychobiological Theories of Children's Responses

The most recent and dramatic shift in theoretical explanations for effects of CSA, and incest in particular, came with the explosion of studies on traumatic stress and the psychobiological model. Awareness emerged that many survivors of childhood trauma are similar to others who experienced long-term severe trauma, such as concentration-camp survivors or political prisoners. The common presentations of these survivors led to the new diagnostic category of complex PTSD. Wilson et al. (2001) assert that PTSD is a shift in the steady state of an organism that has profound and often permanent psychobiological effects. Researchers and clinicians are expressing increased concern about PTSD because of its significance for human evolution and the survival of the species.

Today, most researchers and clinicians recognize a spectrum of PTSD, with chronic and severe childhood trauma, such as CSA, often diagnosed as complex PTSD. Wilson, et al. (2001) described the psychobiology of stress relating to the process allostasis. It refers to the body's ability to remain stable under various stressors on normal levels of adaptive biological functioning. Under typical stress, the hypothalamic–pituitary–adrenal (HPA) axis produces catecholamines and cortisol, which return to baseline once the threat is gone (McCollum, 2006). However, with chronic severe stressors such as CSA, these hormones remain elevated and increase allostatic load with pathophysiologic consequences (McEwen, 1998). In their review of 29 articles, Grassi-Oliviera, Ashy, and Stein (2008) found support for CSA causing an increase in a child's allostatic load resulting in a range of neuronal, and hormonal dysregulation during a critical period of development, with lifetime consequences.

Thus, a critical challenge for therapists working with CSA survivors with elevated allostatic loads is to assist in normalizing their stress response and reducing their hyperarousal, mood instability, cognitive distortions, anger, and other maladaptive psychobiological functioning. Research is currently underway to discern key points for intervention in the lives of these children (Grassi-Oliviera et al., 2008). Because many traumatized children have been diagnosed with PTSD or some of its components, it is helpful to examine the treatment model of Wilson et al. (2001). These researchers view PTSD as a psychobiological stress-response syndrome and assert that traumatic life events impact coping and may produce acute, chronic, delayed, and complex forms of PTSD. The foundation of the Wilson model is the relationship between core PTSD symptoms and their effect on ego states, self-structure, and identity configuration. The core triad of PTSD symptoms are the target of treatment for both adults and children: (a) re-experiencing of memories, (b) avoidance of re-experiencing traumatic events; behavior that includes numbing, depression, and coping adaptations, and (c) psychobiological changes often resulting in hypervigilance and other alterations in behavior. Besides the symptom clusters, PTSD affects interpersonal relations (i.e., attachment and intimacy) and self (i.e., identity and life-course development). When trauma occurs in childhood, such as with CSA, then personality may be affected, and features of PTSD may become part of the person's character structure. Such features can include self-destructive tendencies, shame, self-doubt, guilt, loss of self-esteem, narcissism, depression, and a sense of futility (Wilson et al., 2001). These three PTSD symptom clusters and the two symptoms relating to intimacy and self comprise the five portals to treatment for persons with PTSD (Wilson et al., 2001).

In recent years, with the advent of noninvasive technology, research on early brain development and the effects of abuse, and neglect in infancy and early childhood has become possible. By the time normal children are 3 years old, their brains have achieved 90% of their size. The development of the brain is dependent on the child receiving ongoing stimulation. Stimulation results in the process of learning: the development of brain connections called synapses. These first 3 years are critical, establishing trillions of neuronal pathways (Shore, 1997). Researchers believe that this time of rapid neurobiological development establishes the foundation for future functioning (National Clearinghouse on Child Abuse & Neglect, 2001).

Perry (2001) maintains that childhood memories are the organizing framework for brain development, and repeated stimulation of neuronal pathways establishes memories. These memories create a child's lasting impression of the world. Therefore, sexual or physical abuse or neglect creates neuronal pathways and traumatic memories potentially impacting the child's perception of the world forever. In addition, the abused child will also have oversensitized regions of the brain, and other regions will be undersensitized or undeveloped (Grassi-Oliveira, Ashy, & Stein, 2008; McCollum, 2006). For example, a child victim of ongoing sexual abuse may need to concentrate on using her brain's resources to survive by adapting to a negative environment. Other neuronal pathways, in which the child learns to respond to loving caregivers, will not be stimulated, and therefore, pathways for healthy human functioning may not develop.

Chronic abuse also causes a variety of neurochemical changes in the brain. Perry (2001) explained that chronic fear causes an overstimulation of the HPA axis, which then impairs the development of the subcortical and limbic systems (Grassi-Oliveira et al., 2008).

The impairment can be expressed as hyperactivity, aggressiveness, anxiety, sleep problems, or depression. Overstimulation of the HPA axis may also result in hyperarousal or hypervigilance so the child interprets the world as a threatening place. Although some children become aggressive as a way to survive, others learn to dissociate and withdraw. Many of these children are unable to realize their own feelings or empathize with others. Children do not just "get over it"; as they strive to survive, their brains adapt to the abusive environment, and their potential for emotional, behavioral, cognitive, and social growth is significantly lessened (Perry, 2001).

Integrated Frameworks

Briere (2002) integrated most of the previously described theories. His theory, the self-trauma model, combines trauma theories with cognitive psychology, behavioral psychology, and self-psychology. In particular, Briere incorporated the most recent neurophysiological research with early attachment and memory work and emphasizes that implicit memories and emotions are critical components in understanding and treating the traumas of childhood. He maintains that postabuse symptoms reflect an effort by the survivor to process and integrate overwhelming past trauma. The therapist's responsibility is "to help the client to do better what he or she is already attempting to do" (p. 200). This involves assisting clients to develop new resources as they repeatedly experience exposure and reprocessing of their trauma.

THEORIES OF CAUSATION

Incestuous families are characterized by closed boundaries to the outside world and lack of boundaries within the family (Hornor, 2002). Because they are physically, socially, and psychologically isolated, they become dependent on each other for physical, social, and psychological needs (DiGorgio-Miller, 1998). Courtois (1988) noted that despite excessive dependence between family members, emotional and physical deprivation prevail. The only source of love and affection for children in these families may be through sexual contact.

Many researchers have claimed that incestuous behaviors become generational patterns. Some abused girls grow into mothers who fail to protect their own children. Summit (1989) reported that 90% of mothers seeking help for child abuse had a history of CSA. Lack of self-esteem, unresolved anger, and a sense of powerlessness all cause CSA survivors difficulty in maintaining healthy relationships, and consequently, many are unable to protect themselves or their children. Although a person has been victimized as a child, she or he will not necessarily fail to protect or become an abuser. Statistics on mothers who fail to protect and of fathers who abuse are drawn from sexual abuse treatment programs and are not representative of all CSA survivors. The majority of abuse survivors do not grow up to be abusers.

Glasser et al. (2001) examined the link between CSA victimization and later perpetration. Their retrospective clinical review consisted of 843 predominantly male antisocial and sexually deviant subjects (*n*=747) attending an outpatient forensic psychotherapy center in London, UK. Among male subjects, 18% were victims and 30% were perpetrators, and the greatest predictor for becoming a perpetrator was an abusive sister or mother. Among female subjects, although 43% had been sexually abused, only one became a perpetrator. Thus, a third of men and 2% of women sexually victimized in childhood became perpetrators. Glasser et al. (2001) concluded that, although their data did not provide strong support for a "cycle of sexual abuse," prior victimization might have an effect on male subjects. Although the sample for the study was not representative of abusers, other studies and meta-analyses support their conclusions (Jespersen, Lalumiere, & Seto, 2009; Murphy & Smith, 1996; Whitaker et al., 2008).

Offenders

Research on CSA offenders is slowly evolving, as the majority of studies still recruit subjects (adult men) from the criminal justice system representing a small percentage of all abusers. In Russell's (1986) classic study, only 2% of the offenders were reported to police. Among the offenders reported, only a few are apprehended and go to trial. The even smaller number convicted probably represents the most severe and repetitive offenders (Chaffin, Letourneau, & Silovsky, 2002; Finkelhor, 1986). In addition to samples from the criminal justice system, these studies often only look at male offenders in father–daughter relationships. It is clear that criminal justice samples are not representative of all offenders. However, attempts are still underway to typify offenders to better protect against them.

Groth's (1978) pioneering description of offenders as either fixated or regressed is no longer accepted. More recently, Conte (1990) reported that most offenders are a mixture of both types: in a sample of 159 incest offenders who abused their daughters, 12% also abused nonrelated male children, 49% abused nonrelated female children, and 19% raped adult women. The American Psychiatric Association Task Force (1999) on sex offenders uses the Federal Bureau of Investigation typology for sexual abusers:

1. The regressed, immature abuser who interacts with children on a peer level
2. The morally indiscriminate (antisocial) abuser who targets anyone vulnerable when provided with the opportunity
3. The sexually indiscriminant abuser who will experiment with any type of sexual behavior
4. The inadequate abuser who may be developmentally disabled, psychotic, or senile, who takes advantage of children's vulnerability to satisfy his own curiosity.

Herman (2000) and Chaffin et al. (2002) summarized the literature on incest offenders, reporting that as abusers are so varied and appear normal, there is no appropriate psychological profile. Most offenders do not qualify for any psychiatric diagnosis and are successful in life, hiding sexually abusive behaviors over which they must continually exert control. Herman (2000) described offenders as sexual fantasy addicts fed with pornography. They are also typified by denial, rationalizations, and lack of remorse. Offenders offer a variety of complex and multifactorial explanations for their abusive behavior. Finkelhor (1986) reported preconditions for CSA: (a) the offender is motivated to sexually abuse, (b) overcomes internal inhibitions and external barriers, and (c) overcomes the child's resistance. The offender makes a conscious decision to abuse, and responsibility for CSA is always the offender's.

Although CSA offender research is limited and methodologically weak, recent studies report success with reducing recidivism (Chaffin et al., 2002). Across studies, 3–39% of

CSA offenders re-offend after treatment compared to 12.5–57% recidivism rates for CSA offenders without treatment. Treated incest offenders have lower recidivism rates than extrafamilial offenders (Levenson & Morin, 2006; Proulx, Tardif, Lamoureux, & Lussier, 2000). Biomedical treatments, such as surgical castration, antiandrogens, and antidepressants, successfully reduce recidivism rates as do cognitive–behavioral therapies (CBTs) (American Psychiatric Association, 1999). These successes contradict traditional beliefs that sex offenders always fail treatment. Hudson, Ward, and Laws (2000) asserted that the public is unaware of successful interventions for offenders, as most receive their education from media, which focuses on 1% of all sex crimes. Effective interventions match offender risk level, use cognitive–behavioral modalities, focus on criminogenic need, and promote prosocial skills. Hudson and colleagues cautioned that high-risk offenders most in need of treatment are least likely to receive it. Currently, all states have publicly available sex offend registries for sex offenders (please see Table12.1).

In recent years, researchers have directed more attention to the significantly underreported juvenile sexual offender (Barnett, Miller-Perrin, & Perrin, 1997). In the NIS-3, 22% of children were sexually abused by a perpetrator less than 26 years old (Sedlak & Broadhurst, 1996). Ryan and Lane (1991) reported that approximately one-third of CSA offenders are less than 18 years old. Sexual abuse treatment centers are also seeing greater numbers of adolescents, whose victims are mostly the same age or younger than the abuser (Gerardin & Thibaut, 2004). Similar to adult offenders, adolescent offenders are primarily male from all ethnic, racial, and socioeconomic levels, however there are increasing reports of female juvenile offenders (Gerardin & Thibaut, 2004; Ryan & Lane, 1991). In Adler and Schultz's (1995) Caucasian, middle-income sample of intact families, 92% of sibling-incest offenders had been physically abused, and 8% were sexually victimized.

There are few reports specifically on female offenders. Finkelhor (1986) claimed that males perpetrate 95% of female child abuse and 80% of male child abuse. Russell's (1986) probability sample of 930 community women found only 10 cases of female perpetrated incestuous abuse providing support for the argument that female abuse of female children represents a small portion of all CSA cases. The data from NIS-3 (Sedlak & Broadhurst, 1996) supported these statistics: 89% of all CSA perpetrated by males, 12% by females. However, in Denov's (2003) more recent 15 study review, approximately 58% of women self-reported potentially sexually abusive behaviors.

Controversy centers on the true prevalence of female CSA offenders, and whether abuse by females is less severe than that perpetrated by male counterparts (Bunting, 2007; Finkelhor, 1986; Russell, 1986). Many argue that female sex offending is underreported for similar reasons as underreporting of male rape; namely there are cultural norms precluding the existence of female sex offenders (Bunting, 2007; Denov, 2003). Furthermore, there are difficulties in case identification as female offenders often perpetrate abuse disguised as childcare (Barnett et al., 1997). Some claim that women abuse male children more frequently than female (Berliner & Elliott, 2002). However, these suspicions have not borne out in self-report surveys such as the one Finkelhor (1994) conducted with college students. Both Finkelhor and Russell assert that the evidence that women abuse male more commonly than female children is lacking.

Others reported that women are accomplices to male perpetrators in families with multiple-partner CSA (Bunting, 2007; Elliott, 1993; Urbancic, 1992). In Urbancic's (1993) convenience sample of 147 female incest survivors, 6.6% (*n*=16) of the offenders (*n*=243) were women. All 16 were part of a multiple family-abuse system, and none acted in isolation. Research suggests that women most often sexually abuse children at the instigation of male family members (Elliott, 1993; Urbancic, 1993).

Non-Offending Mothers

Despite evidence that both men and women perpetrate CSA, the majority of offenders are male. Investigators insist that the key to the incestuous family is the mother. Although the mother sometimes may be physically or mentally incapacitated, early researchers (Henderson, 1972; Justice & Justice, 1979) reported that she imposed the mother–wife role on her daughter expecting the daughter to provide nurturance. These writers also maintained that mother–daughter role reversal holds the dysfunctional family together: the father's needs are satisfied, the mother is relieved of responsibilities, and the daughter assumes a position of power. Some suggested that father and daughter unite to gain revenge on a rejecting mother. In Herman and Hirschman's study (1977), daughters viewed their mothers as weak, downtrodden, and unable to provide protection. Blaming the mother for CSA was common, instead of blaming the offender.

Today, researchers and clinicians contest assertions placing all blame and responsibility on the mother (Elliott & Carnes, 2001; Herman, 2000), maintaining that she is often depressed or physically incapacitated and unable to care for herself or her family. Although mother blaming is sometimes appropriate, it is an unreasonable assumption that she consciously or unconsciously arranges/encourages the father–daughter relationship. Some mothers tolerate physical abuse and humiliation because of their socioeconomic status. Deblinger, Hathaway, Lippman, and Steer (1993) found that mothers of children sexually abused by an intimate partner were more likely to be IPV victims than mothers of children abused by other relatives or nonrelatives.

Incest is less likely in families where the mother possesses power. This can be explained by Finkelhor's (1986) disinhibition factor: If the father believes the child will disclose to the mother and the mother will take steps against the offender, internal inhibitions to incest will be strengthened rather than weakened. Until recently, little information was available about non-offending mothers as incest literature focuses on victim and offender. Traditionally; CPS, social service, and law enforcement maintained that most mothers in CSA cases did not believe or protect their children. In Urbancic's clinical work with non-offending mothers, initially, many did not know whom to believe. If the woman believes that her partner loves her and the relationship has been successful, the revelation of an incestuous relationship is overwhelming and distressing. No one can be trusted. Nothing makes sense. Her partner has betrayed her with her own daughter. It is less devastating to believe that it did not happen.

Pintello and Zuravin (2001) described four factors that predict whether mothers believed their child's CSA allegations: the mother (a) was not the abuser's current partner; (b) was an adult, not a teenager; (c) had no knowledge of the CSA before the child disclosed; and (d) the child did not display sexualized behaviors before disclosure. Current research shows that most mothers believe their children after CSA disclosure (Elliott & Carnes, 2001; Strand, 2000). In Elliott and Carnes review, mothers believed their children 69–78% of the time. Urbancic (1993) stated that parent's initial disbelief and ambivalence should be expected given the shock of disclosure. However, Elliot and Carnes emphasized that belief does not guarantee subsequent protection of the child. No research exists examining patterns of belief in non-offending fathers.

In clinical practice, many mothers come to therapy groups feeling angry, confused, and ambivalent. However, most eventually believe their daughters, understand the situational dynamics, place blame and responsibility with the offender, and accept that they must learn how to protect their children (Cammaert, 1988; Deblinger, et al., 1993). For many, belief of a victimized child involves a crisis, followed by a grief process, feelings of shock, disbelief, ambivalence, eventual acceptance, and resulting support for the child. However, the mother must also address her child's experience: postabuse trauma, rage and blaming the mother for not believing and protecting her. Blaming the mother more than the offender is not unusual.

Social service agencies that do not follow the mother long enough may only remember her denial and shock and miss the gradual acceptance process. Certainly, some mothers consistently deny daughters' claims of CSA and join their partners in accusing the daughter of lying. Relatives and friends may see both parents as conscientious caretakers victimized by their own daughter. Some clinicians suggest that a mother's denial and failure to protect may be unconscious coping through dissociation relating to the fact that many were victims of CSA. When environmental cues threaten to trigger memories of her own abuse, the mother psychologically separates herself from the threat (Dolan, 1991; Fredrickson, 1991). These researchers maintain that offenders, non-offending parents, and child victims all use some degree of dissociation to cope with abuse.

CASE FINDING, SCREENING, AND ASSESSMENT OF CHILD SEXUAL ABUSE

Strategies for Case Finding

Professionals must be prepared to quickly and effectively intervene in cases of CSA. Nurses are positioned to intervene due to their frequent interactions in various settings with children, adolescents, and adults with a history of CSA. As mandated reporters, all nurses should become familiar with the CSA literature and screening and assessment techniques. Currently, there is no evidence based screening tool for CSA; however, tools are available for trauma assessment (Strand, Sarmiento, & Pasquale, 2005). Asking children in a private setting and in an age appropriate manner about their experience with family violence and sexual behaviors is appropriate. Both child and adult victims are more likely to disclose if asked directly about abuse. Briere and Zaidi (1989) found an increase in the rate of CSA among female psychiatric patients from 6% to 70% when clinicians began to ask directly. It is important to thank patients for sharing their experience. Nurses should temper their reaction with compassion and understand the rarity of child disclosure of CSA, which, even as an adult, is fraught with emotion and ambivalence (London, Bruck, Wright, & Ceci, 2007; Ullman, 2003). The nurse's initial reaction will directly influence their ability to elicit information and intervene in an abusive relationship.

The child's story is the most crucial information for identifying CSA (Savell, 2005). In the rare instances when children discuss their abuse, they are often confused, and unconvincing (Levenson & Morin, 2006). This does not mean their story is false. Care should be taken when interviewing children. It is prudent to defer in-depth questioning until an especially trained forensic interviewer is available. Persons trained in child interviewing techniques are able to garner more reliable and consistent information (Kuehnle &

Kirkpatrick, 2005). The nurse should refrain from questioning the child multiple times, as the more often they tell their story, the more apt it is to change which may impact later litigation. This is true for both children and adult victims.

Indicators of Child Sexual Abuse

Although adequately trained specialists should conduct investigative interviews, the nurse should still obtain a medical history and appropriate review of systems (Kellogg & the Committee on Child Abuse and Neglect, 2005). Despite multiple articles dedicated to CSA identification methods (see Table 12.2 for common indicators), providers are often misinformed regarding signs and symptoms of CSA. The American Academy of Pediatrics, Committee on Child Abuse and Neglect (Kellogg & the Committee on Child Abuse and Neglect, 2005) and the American Professional Society on Abuse of Children (1998) both maintain guidelines for case finding. Adams (2001) further systematized CSA identification melding current research with these organizations' recommendations.

In synthesizing the literature, Berliner and Elliott (2002) reported that sexually abused children are more depressed, anxious, and have lower self-esteem than nonabused children. According to Briere (1992), abused children develop an internal framework, viewing their world as hostile and dangerous. Because they were forced into helplessness and powerlessness, they overestimate danger and adversity, predisposing themselves to depression and emotional distress. Many CSA victims have interpersonal difficulties because of shame, guilt, and a perception of being different. Sexually abused children are more likely to experience PTSD symptoms, and about 30% qualify for diagnosis. In addition, these children have more cognitive deficits in school achievement than non-abused counterparts. Adolescent victims exhibit many of the same problems and others: hypersexuality in teenage girls and sexual exposure or coercion in teenage boys (Kendall-Tackett et al., 1993). Berliner and Elliott (2002) report that 10–24% of the sexually abused children do not improve over time and some decline even further.

TABLE 12.2 *History and Physical Exam Indicators of Child Sexual Abuse*

Psychosocial indicators	
Depression	PTSD
Anxiety	Anorexia and other eating disorders
Low self-esteem	School phobias
Aggression	Learning problems
Poor relationship with same sex parent	Nightmares

Developmental indicators	
Open masturbation	Dysuria
Exposure of genitalia	Self-mutilation
Sexual relationships with other children	Drug and alcohol abuse
Encopresis and/or enuresis	Pregnancy

Physical indicators	
Reddened genitalia	Absent or minimal hymen
Hymenal tears or notches	Anal tears or scars

A few additional points to consider in case identification are as follows. Although a serious concern, sexually transmitted infections (STIs) in children are not diagnostic for CSA. For example, a recent systematic review found evidence that towels and linens may be a vehicle for *Neisseria gonorrhoeae*, which, contrary to prior belief, is not solely transmitted through sexual contact in pre-pubertal children (Goodyear-Smith, 2007). Furthermore, the skin condition *Lichen sclerosis* that affects approximately 10–15% of children is often misdiagnosed as CSA, as it presents with genital/anal pain and itching (Poindexter & Morrell, 2007). However, these symptoms should not be ignored. STIs must be carefully evaluated, vertical transmission explored, contacts traced, and if no other method of transmission is identified, STIs in a pre-pubertal child are highly suspicious.

A related belief is that children displaying inappropriate sexualized behavior are CSA victims (Berrien, 2007; Child Welfare Information Gateway, 2006). Documented premature sexual behaviors include open masturbation, frequent exposure of genitalia, and becoming sexually involved with other children. This may be especially pertinent to preschool children not yet socialized to sexual taboos (Brilleslijper-Kater, Friedrich, & Corwin, 2004). Berliner and Elliott (2002) cited several studies that found more of these behaviors among sexually abused children than among neglected, physically abused, or psychiatrically disturbed counterparts. Recent research shows that nonabused children's sexual behaviors may be attributable to poor family boundaries, for example, family nudity, sexual activities among family members or on TV, and/or family stress (Johnson, 2005). While it is true that these factors may put a family at risk for CSA, as with STIs, age-inappropriate sexual behaviors are not conclusive indicators of CSA.

In order to be effective, nurses must examine their feelings and educate themselves. Many nurses and other professionals are uncomfortable discussing CSA and incest, often responding in an evasive manner and failing to report suspicions. Nurses and other professionals who do not identify and report CSA support its proliferation. In addition, not asking patients about abuse may make them think their secret is too terrible to discuss, increasing their shame, guilt, and sense of helplessness. Every state requires both physicians and nurses to report suspected cases of CSA. The American Academy of Pediatrics (1999) has guidelines to assist professionals in reporting cases of CSA.

Identifying abused children has not been easy because they do not fit the textbook picture of an abused child and often do not self-disclose. A child's ability to disclose depends on cognitive, behavioral, and emotional development. A child may be able to give a spontaneous, clear, and detailed report of abuse. Jenny (2002) recommended establishing rapport with the child, asking open-ended, non-leading questions, and inquiring about pain, bleeding, or other problems. Children should be able to ask questions with answers given at a level they understand. The majority of sexually abused children will have no physical evidence of CSA. Even with severe abuse, tissue may heal without significant changes (Berenson et al. 2000; Kellogg, & the Committee on Child Abuse and Neglect, 2005). Therefore, the child's history is the most critical component in establishing CSA (Giardino, Darner, Asher, Faugno, & Spencer, 2002).

In-Depth Assessment

A complete physical examination should be performed when CSA is suspected. The child's trust and cooperation must be gained before the sexual abuse examination to prevent retraumatization. A frightened child will tighten their pelvic floor muscles making it difficult to evaluate the vaginal canal, hymen, or anus. Although many sexually abused children do not present with physical findings (Kellogg & the Committee on Child Abuse and Neglect, 2005), each child should be examined for bruises on the entire body as well as for evidence of trauma to the external genitalia, vagina, and rectum. Cultures of the pharynx, urethra, vagina, penis, and rectum for STIs need to be obtained.

The position of the child during a genital examination depends on their age. Children younger than 3 may be most comfortable sitting on their parent's lap. Children older than three will usually cooperate and lie on an exam table (Berrien, 2007). Dolls can be used to demonstrate desired positions to the child. Jenny (2002) recommended either a supine (frog-leg) or prone (knee–chest) position. Sometimes, findings may appear abnormal in the supine position but normalize in the prone position. Colposcopy for magnification is more common today and is well tolerated in adolescents (Mears et al., 2003). Jenny (2002) reported that the typical examination is noninvasive and without pain. If instruments are needed, the child may need sedation.

Research indicates that notches or clefts in the posterior rim of the hymen are not necessarily positive for CSA in female children. Berenson et al. (2000) reported that both abused and nonabused female children may have shallow posterior notches, but only abused females have deep notches penetrating more than 50% of the hymen's posterior rim. CSA of males typically involves trauma to the anus rather than the genitals (Frasier, 2002; Jenny, 2002).

Even when data strongly indicate CSA, she or he may deny it and do so because of the relationship to the offender. Disclosure by the child is easier if the offender is not a close, trusted person to whom the child feels loyal. The child may be ambivalent due to threats that the offender made regarding disclosure, provoking anxiety about physical harm to self or other family members. The child may also fear breaking up the family: the offender going to prison and the rest of the family blaming the child. In addition, the victim may fear removal from the family and foster care placement. These fears motivate nondisclosure or later retraction. Some children choose self-sacrifice rather than destroy their family, whereas others feel the positives of the abusive relationship outweigh the abuse. To make sense of the child's denials, retractions, and vacillations, it is essential to consider the child's concerns, fears, and perceptions.

Ideally, only a professional who specializes in these evaluations should perform assessment and evaluation for CSA. It is possible that a child evaluated by a non-specialist will receive inappropriate diagnostic care, or key findings may be missed. There are providers focused solely on the acute (within 72 hours) CSA exam, and others focused solely on chronic CSA evaluation. These professionals have completed at minimum 40 hours didactic learning, 40 hours fieldwork, and required certification exams. Information on training and certification may be found in the resources section of this chapter.

Nursing Diagnosis

Appropriate nursing diagnosis will vary depending on the situation and presentation of the patient and family. Below are suggestions from the North American Nursing Diagnosis Association (Carpenito-Moyet, 2004) and the fourth edition of Nursing Interventions Classification (Dochterman, & Bulechek, 2004). These nursing diagnoses may be appropriate for the child victim, adult survivor, and non-offending family members and interchangeable among the three groups (see Table 12.3).

TABLE 12.3   Nursing Assessments and Diagnoses

North American Nursing Diagnosis Association	
Diagnosis:	**Related to:**
Ineffective coping Defensive coping	• Disruption of emotional bonds • Inadequate psychological resources
Disabled family coping	• Disclosure or discovery of CSA
Adult failure to thrive	• Diminished coping abilities • Loss of social relatedness
Parental role conflict	• Change in ability to parent secondary to disclosure or discovery of CSA
Posttrauma syndrome[a]	• Traumatic events such as sexual abuse
Powerlessness	• Long-term abusive relationship
Disturbed body image	• Physical trauma secondary to sexual abuse

Nursing Intervention Classification		
Child victims	**Adult survivors**	**Non-offending family**
Abuse Protection support	Assertiveness training	Crisis intervention
Behavior management: sexual	Body image enhancement	Emotional support
Coping enhancement	Calming technique	Family integrity promotion
Health education	Cognitive restructuring	Parenting promotion
Trauma therapy: child	Forgiveness facilitation	
	Self-esteem enhancement	

[a]May affect parents of victims as well as the child victims themselves
Source: Carpenito-Moyet, 2004; Dochterman & Bulecheck, 2004.

Documentation

To reiterate, the most crucial information is the child's report of CSA. It is imperative to document the child's story as close to verbatim as possible. It is inappropriate to "medicalize" or censor the conversation transcript (Sheridan, Nash, Hawkins, Makely & Campbell, 2006). Aside from identifying medical problems, which should be addressed, the priority of a CSA evaluation is to document findings that may be useful in litigation and subsequent protection of the child. As such, documentation must be accurate. Photographic documentation of injuries should be obtained with parent consent and patient assent. For further information on documentation, please see chapter 14.

INTERVENTIONS

Primary Prevention

Primary prevention interventions for CSA proliferated in the 1980s. As most victims do not disclose and receive treatment, there is great potential for short-and long-term effects. CSA educational programs for children, parents, and professionals are the first step in eliminating sexual abuse. It is essential that nurses value the importance of CSA educational programs and support them in schools and communities. Nurses, in promoting health and well-being should advocate for balancing themes of violence and abuse with healthy touch and intimacy.

Many agencies and institutions provide sexual abuse primary prevention programs for children, parents, and health professionals. Storybooks, coloring books, and videos on CSA are available for children, as are workshops that incorporate art and role plays (Rubenzahl & Gilbert, 2002). Past programs focused on the abusive "stranger," but the current message emphasizes that someone known and trusted may try to involve the child in sexual behavior. Children are taught to inform another known and trusted adult and to try to resist the offender in whatever manner possible. The nurse should consider the developmental level and cultural background of the children when developing or selecting materials.

CSA educational programs may help both nonabused and CSA victimized children through improving self-esteem and a sense of control in their lives (Rubenzahl & Gilbert, 2002). In Daro and Connelly's (2002) review, they report that CSA primary prevention programs effectively increase children's self-protective knowledge and create a disclosure friendly environment. Finkelhor (2007) found evidence that primary prevention educational programs effectively reduce the prevalence and effects of victimization. Although program outcomes vary, results can be maximized by individualizing content, providing practice and feedback, teaching basic assertiveness and communication skills, emphasizing the need to tell someone, and including parents (Daro & Connelly, 2002; Thakkar-Kolar, Ryan, & Runyon, 2008).

Primary prevention programs solely targeting children will not stem the tide of CSA without also educating parents. Unfortunately, studies indicate that parents are often not involved. Only 29% of parents reported discussing CSA with their children, although a majority warned against the possibility of kidnapping (Finkelhor, 1984). Parents who discussed CSA with their child started when the child was too old (older than 9 years) and often omitted crucial facts about CSA. It is common across socioeconomic, religious, and educational levels for parents to have difficulty addressing sexual issues with their children. Parents must be taught that CSA crosses all socioeconomic, ethnic, and religious groups and should be assisted in how to discuss sexual abuse with their children. Lowering parental anxiety about CSA may be more important than the actual materials presented.

Families at high risk for CSA require concentrated attention, those with (a) non-biological caregivers, (b) parents with a history of child physical or sexual abuse, or (c) developmentally or emotionally challenged children. Nurses teaching parenting classes should emphasize both parents' role in taking care of their children. In addition to involving both parents, participation of older siblings and other caretakers may be appropriate. Research suggests that parents involved in early childcare are more likely to bond with their children and less likely to sexually abuse them. Too often, only the primary parent attends parenting classes or CSA workshops. Nurses conducting classes must devise methods for involving both parents.

Professionals also need training about how to educate the public and become advocates in CSA prevention. Nurses should lobby for incorporation of sexual abuse content into nursing school curricula and places of employment through periodic in-service training. Daro and Connelly (2002) also encourage community involvement in prevention to reduce the effects of stress and isolation both strong predictors for all types of child abuse and neglect.

Secondary Prevention

When abuse is identified during health care interactions, it is crucial to determine the safety of the child's home. Nurses are legally obligated as mandatory reporters to notify authorities of their suspicions. However, as previously discussed, identification of CSA without the child's story is difficult. When a child is not willing or able to disclose, notification of CPS may be the extent of effective nursing intervention. If, however, the child discloses abuse or abuse was witnessed, initial interventions should focus on defusing the resultant crisis. Nurses working with incestuous families should focus care on the child's needs, but all family members require help. Support groups for all family members are needed for effective treatment. Such groups are developing nationally. The non-offending parent especially needs support because of their critical role in the child's recovery. Literature (Deblinger, et al., 1993; Elliott & Carnes, 2001; Strand, 2000) indicates that the non-offending parent may suffer from PTSD symptoms and depression. Periodic assessment of the parent is warranted as symptoms emerge over time and should be treated as indicated (Cohen & Mannarino, 1998; Elliott & Carnes, 2001).

Resources are becoming available for non-offending parents and professionals working with them (Levenson & Morin, 2001a,b; Strand, 2000). Initially, the parent may be so overwhelmed by the disclosure, threatened loss of children, partner, and economic security that, without assistance, he or she will side with the offender against the child. Therefore, the parent needs immediate help processing implications of abuse and to address potential denial. Levenson and Morin's (2001a) workbook is an excellent resource for non-offending parents. It addresses these issues and assists the parent to process grief and loss as well as to understand the child and create a safety plan if and when family reunification is feasible and therapeutic.

Researchers report significant improvement in outcomes with non-offending parents using CBT in individual and group modalities, compared to supportive therapy (Deblinger, Stauffer, & Steer, 2001). These researchers found a variety of CBTs effectively assisted non-offending parents to address and process the child's CSA. Exposure techniques facilitate the parent's ability to discuss the abuse. Eventually, joint sessions with the child and parent can be conducted using cognitive restructuring to correct distorted beliefs about the abuse. The parent may benefit from stress management as well as CSA education (Berliner & Cohen, 2000; Deblinger et al., 2001; Wilson et al., 2001).

Intervention with incestuous families requires direct and swift action to ensure abuse cessation and protection of the child. It also requires coordination between protective services, law enforcement, and counselors. Usually, the court orders the offender to leave the home. If the offender continues to abuse and the non-offending parent cannot or will not protect the child, the child may be removed from home. Because this is traumatic for the child, it is to be avoided if at all possible. The nurse must realize, when addressing the sexually abused child's needs, that all damaging effects are not immediately obvious. Therefore, physical and psychological assessment and intervention are necessary whether or not the child appears traumatized. Child age and developmental level are determining factors when choosing the type of therapy.

Most studies indicate that best outcomes for CSA patients involve extending and modifying existing clinical child psychology treatment models. Several meta-analytic studies examined controlled research on effective treatments with child and adolescent CSA victims (Fonagy, 1998; Kasdin & Weisz, 1998; Saywitz, Mannarino, Berliner, & Cohen,

2000). CBT methods are the most researched and well-supported (Macdonald, Higgins, & Ramchandani, 2006; Shipman & Taussig, 2009). Studies indicate that CBT is more effective than other methods, especially for depressed or anxious children or those with behavior problems. Typically, CBT is combined with gradual exposure, education, stress management, safety skill, and parent management training. These modalities can be used individually, with parent and child, or groups. Since PTSD is one of the main detrimental outcomes of CSA, child focused PTSD interventions also may be useful (Carr, 2004; Stovall-McClough, 2004).

Saywitz et al. (2000) categorized CSA victims into four groups when choosing interventions. Children without discernible symptoms of abuse are the first group, accounting for 30% of CSA victims. Approximately 70% of these children remain asymptomatic, probably because the event was not traumatic even if it was exploitive and illegal. However, 30% will develop subsequent symptoms. Because there is no reliable way to predict evolution of symptoms, all abused children should have basic treatment including educational interventions to prevent future abuse and mitigate sleeper effects. The second group of children will present with mild symptoms not exceeding symptoms seen in a general clinical population. The third group presents with serious psychiatric problems, including depression, anxiety, sexualized behaviors, aggression, and PTSD components. The fourth group meets full criteria for PTSD and comorbid depression, anxiety, and/or sleep disorders. Treatment must be individualized and target-specific symptoms. Pharmacotherapy may also be indicated.

Group therapy for sexually abused children can be a powerful modality for assisting all children three and older (Deblinger, Stauffer, & Steer, 2001). Using CBT, the group can effectively correct many traumatic sexualization behaviors exhibited by abused children. In addition, the group can address misconceptions about the child's role and the roles of others in the abuse. A major goal of therapy is decreasing abuse-related anxiety and fear. As the child addresses various aspects of abuse, learns to express anger, sadness, and grief about them, the traumatic memories lose their power. In addition, age-appropriate sex education should be provided, including cues indicating that a situation is becoming sexually threatening (Finkelhor, 2007; Thakkar-Kolar, et al., 2008).

Although an offender may complete treatment, develop coping skills, and admit full responsibility, the non-offending parent and children must be on guard for resumption of sexual abuse. Family therapy is never appropriate until the family reaches a level of stability. Nurses should be aware of community resources to make family referrals to appropriate agencies.

Tertiary Prevention With the Adult Sexually Abused as a Child

The word "survivor" replaces "victim" when describing adults abused in childhood. The terminology shift focuses on the recovery process rather than on helplessness and injury. Researchers found that up to 50% of adult survivors never disclosed (London et al., 2007). As with sexually abused children, nurses in a variety of settings have opportunities to assist adult survivors. Nurses do not need to be expert therapists to help because survivors require different levels of support. Briere (1996) emphasized the most important aspect of psychotherapy with survivors is a caring, reliable, nonexploitative therapist creating a therapeutic environment, facilitating self-awareness, and processing of traumatic experiences.

There are three stages in trauma-based treatment for adult survivors (Chu, 1998; Courtois, 1999; Draucker, 2000; Herman, 1997). The first stage establishes safety by stabilizing, containing, and reducing symptoms and learning self-care skills; the second stage is processing and resolution of traumatic memories; and the third stage focuses on personality integration and relational development. Because incest is an abuse of power, secrecy, betrayal, and disregard for the child's needs, there is increased potential for developing feelings of helplessness, shame, guilt, and confusion. Therefore, CSA interventions for resolving trauma focus on survivor empowerment, developing self-worth, mastery, competence, and control. To empower survivors, effective nursing interventions must involve collaborative effort.

The therapeutic relationship should be a partnership between nurse and patient establishing objectives to resolve incest trauma. Survivors should be encouraged to believe that they are their own expert and can therefore make decisions to promote health and well-being. In addition, the nurse and client should identify and develop strategies that will build on client's strengths and increase a sense of control while supporting actions to change their life. The following discussion covers empowerment–support nursing interventions for use with adult survivors: a basic level of intervention followed by an advanced level.

The survivor's first step is to disclose the abuse to someone trusted. The nurse should support the survivor discussing CSA whenever and however they choose. Too often, the nurse is uncomfortable with disclosure, and discomfort is communicated to the client nonverbally and discussion of CSA is interpreted as unwelcome. The survivor must feel they have permission to disclose and that the nurse will listen. The nurse must refrain from expressing shock or dismay, as these reactions may add to the survivor's feelings of alienation and unworthiness. Rather than asking intrusive questions, basic therapeutic communication techniques are effective when supporting disclosure including simply "being with" the survivor in silence, reflecting on comments, encouraging discussion of perceptions and expressing feelings. In addition, the nurse can assist survivors to recognize the strength and courage it takes to disclose.

Many empowerment support strategies nurses use with survivors involve teaching new behaviors and correcting myths and distortions. Because the myths and distortions shaped the survivor from childhood, corrective learning is a lengthy, ongoing process. The nurse should repeatedly reinforce that the offender is always responsible for CSA. Adults who, as a child, derived pleasure or sought the sexual activity may be especially shame and guilt-ridden. Therefore, the nurse should teach principles of normal physiology and child development, emphasizing that it is normal for children to seek things that are rewarding and feel good. Understanding traumatic sexualization (Finkelhor, 1986) can be helpful to a survivor having difficulty forgiving their childhood self. The survivor with young children must learn to protect them from abuse and be sensitive to their needs.

Advanced practice nurses working with adult survivors of CSA have opportunities to use more in-depth interventions. Outcome research for these interventions with adult survivors is appearing in the literature. Price, Hilsenroth, Petretic-Jackson, and Bonge (2001) reviewed eight studies for individual therapy outcomes in adult survivors. Studies involved four therapeutic methods: CBT, experiential, psychodynamic/interpersonal, and psychoeducational/supportive. The results indicated that, despite study limitations, all methods were successful in reducing symptoms of adult survivors. Similarly, de Jong and Gorey (1996) reviewed seven studies on group therapy effectiveness. As with individual-therapy outcomes, group modalities were also effective in reducing symptoms and improving overall functioning. Individual and group psychotherapy are concurrently recommended for many CSA survivors.

CBT is the most researched treatment modality. It includes a wide variety of interventions extensively reviewed in the literature. CBT's basic premise is that a person's self-beliefs profoundly influence their affect and behavior. Many books and publications detail treatment guidelines for using CBT in patients with partial, full, or complex PTSD (Chu, 1998; Courtois, 1999; Foa, Keane, & Friedman, 2000; Wilson et al., 2001). Foa et al. (2000) reviewed the effectiveness of eight CBT techniques to relieve PTSD symptoms including exposure therapy, systematic desensitization, stress inoculation training, cognitive processing therapy, cognitive therapy, assertiveness training, biofeedback, relaxation training, and various combinations of these. Most of these interventions require special training. They found that exposure therapy was the most effective and recommended its use in treating PTSD. Although exposure therapy has various forms, the common theme is that repeated exposure to threatening stimuli will gradually diminish anxiety with a resultant decrease in escapist or avoidant behaviors. The other seven modalities were difficult to evaluate because of mixed results or poor methodology, and combinations of therapies were not more effective than individual therapies, yet significant results were reported for all CBT interventions.

Researchers (Foa, et al., 2000; Friedman, 2001) also evaluated the effectiveness of pharmacotherapy in relieving PTSD symptoms across multiple randomized clinical trials. Despite mixed results, some patients experienced significant improvement. Across studies, selective serotonin reuptake inhibitors (SSRIs) were the most effective, diminishing PTSD, comorbid disorders, and associated symptoms interfering with daily functioning. SSRIs also produced less distressing side effects than other medications prescribed for PTSD.

Another intervention receiving attention is eye movement desensitization and reprocessing (EMDR), a unique application of exposure. EMDR involves the client imagining the trauma while using saccadic eye movements. Researchers (Foa et al., 2000; Zoellner, Fitzgibbons, & Foa, 2001) reported that studies examining efficacy of EMDR are methodologically weak, limiting conclusions about its effectiveness. However, more recent guidelines from the APA (2004) advocate its use in treatment as an efficacious modality.

Foy et al. (2001) reviewed outcomes for three types of group psychotherapy for PTSD patients: supportive, psychodynamic, and cognitive–behavioral. Group therapy promotes a sense of trust, commonality, community, and validation, as well as a safe, respectful, and therapeutic place to process pain as well as successes and growth. Although methodologically weak, research results on group therapy effectiveness have been consistently significant for positive outcomes across all three modalities against an array of symptoms (Foy et al., 2001).

Many other therapeutic modalities are used to treat adult CSA survivors. Psychodynamic psychotherapy is common in exploring unconscious meanings of trauma and other significant life events. Marital or family therapy may also be helpful. A variety of creative therapies may be helpful, including art, dance/movement, drama, music, poetry, and bibliotherapy, as well as body therapies, including relaxation and exercise. Survivors report positive results from learning assertiveness skills and anger control. Research on these modalities is limited at this time.

Suggested Nursing Care

The US Office for Victims of Crime (2003) developed recommendations and evidence based protocols for CSA treatment (see Table 12.1). As emphasized throughout this chapter, the nurse's primary concern is determining whether the child may safely return home. The nurse *must* report suspicions to the proper child protection agency and a thorough head-to-toe assessment and review of systems is warranted. Interventions should be tailored to the child's age and developmental stage as well as the degree of parental support. Furthermore, interventions should address both short- (refer to Table 12.2) and long-term sequelae (see Table 12.4) of CSA when possible. It is prudent to note that many CSA indicators are short-term sequelae to abuse. A nurse working collaboratively with the patient and non-offending family members may mitigate these short-term effects.

Most researchers agree that serious effects are not inevitable, particularly if the child and family receive support and treatment. In a review of literature, Kendall-Tackett, et al. (1993) found an absence of abuse-related problems in approximately 40% of sexually abused children. However, lack of symptoms does not mean lack of harm. Some believe the effects of discovery and consequent legal involvement to be more traumatic than the actual CSA, particularly when the family is separated. Berliner and Elliott (2002) pointed out that not only are dysfunctional families at greater risk for intrafamilial CSA, but once abuse occurs, family chaos may increase the sexual abuse trauma.

Cultural Competency

Treatment cannot be successful without consideration and integration of the patient's culture. Because culture may define what is normal and abnormal, when it is appropriate to seek help from an outsider, and what is appropriate to share with an outsider, respect for the patient's worldview is critical. Therefore, nurses and other health care professionals need to be patient and flexible with people from cultures different from their own, appreciate the strengths of the culture, and honestly and candidly negotiate common goals.

Regardless of the theoretical framework used to understand and work with the child, adult, and family, cultural competency is always important. Abney (2002) promoted use of a "culturally diverse" model combining the subjective worldview of a particular culture with a broader cross-cultural base. Because many destructive cultural practices leave children at risk for serious long-term harm, Abney rejected the concept of cultural relativism that holds behavior as acceptable if it is based on one's culture. With the diverse model, one recognizes that cultures vary and there is no single ideal. Cultural competency refers to making the best effort to understand another person's worldview and adapting one's practice to meet the person's cultural needs. Professionals need to adopt a culturally competent approach because of increasing diversity in the United States, underrepresentation of health care professionals from diverse cultures, and lack of access to quality and cost-effective health care. Abney maintains that if we do not, we will not be able to meet the needs of abused children and their families.

TABLE 12.4   *Long-Term Sequelae in Survivors of Child Sexual Abuse*

Category	Exemplars
PTSD	80% suffer classic symptoms: nightmares, flashbacks, intrusive thoughts, fear, numbing, hypervigilance, and hyperarousal (Briere, 1996)
	Dissociation may develop as a protective mechanism and may take the form of amnesia (Foa, Keane, & Friedman, 2000; Wilson et al., 2001)
Cognitive effects	Cognitive distortions reflected in survivors' beliefs about themselves as unworthy, shameful, and helpless, others as rejecting and scornful
Emotional effects	Anxiety disorders, depression, suicidal behaviors, anger regulation problems
	Subgroup of patients at especially high risk for psychiatric disorders and prolonged depression (Russell, 1986; Zlotnick, Mattia, & Zimmerman, 2001)
	Somatic symptoms from hyperarousal: headaches, gastrointestinal upset, muscle tension, pelvic and back pain (Berliner & Elliott, 2002; Kendall-Tackett, 2002)
	Alcohol/substance abuse, obesity, other eating disorders, and self-mutilation
Interpersonal effects	Physical and emotional dating aggression (Banyard, Arnold, & Smith, 2000)
	Increased likelihood of revictimization by strangers, and intimate partners (Briere, 1996; Herman, 2000; Kendall-Tackett, 2002; Russell, 1986)
	Sexual difficulties from dysfunction to promiscuity as well as an increase in HIV-risky behaviors (Parillo, Freeman, Collier, & Young, 2001)
	Increased likelihood of homelessness in women (Kendall-Tackett, 2002)
	Difficulties parenting their children, particularly in maintaining boundaries and meeting emotional needs (DiLillo, 2001)

SUMMARY

CSA is a profoundly disturbing experience for children and adults. Some carry the burden their entire life. Most sexually abused children and adults do not disclose. Failure to disclose often has serious short- and long-term effects. Because nurses work in a variety of settings and practice at different levels, they have many opportunities to assist victims and families. However, nurses will not make an impact until they understand their own experiences and feelings about CSA. Nurses also must become knowledgeable about incestuous behavior dynamics and appropriate evidence-based interventions for all levels of prevention. Kendall-Tacket (2002) stressed that "health" is dependent on multiple complex interacting factors as identified under long-term effects of CSA. However, mental and physical health cannot be separated. Each problem and symptom discussed has the potential to influence health. Nurses and other health professionals must make a concerted effort to address these factors to improve CSA survivor health outcomes. The ultimate nursing goal is rehabilitation of all family members and family reconstitution, if feasible and therapeutic. The concerned, caring, and knowledgeable nurse, willing to listen and learn from family members, collaborating to establish goals, and when necessary, taking firm action to protect weaker members, is a valuable resource for survivors and their families, as well as for society and the nursing profession.

REFERENCES

Abney, V. D. (2002). Cultural competency in the field of child maltreatment. In J. B. Myers, L. Berliner, J. Briere, C. T. Hendrix, C. Jenny, & T. A. Reid (Eds.), *The APSAC handbook on child maltreatment* (2nd ed., pp. 477–486). Thousand Oaks, CA: Sage.

Adams, J. A. (2001). Evolution of a classification scale: Medical evaluation of suspected child sexual abuse. *Child Maltreatment, 6*(1), 31–36.

Adler, N. A., & Schultz, J. (1995). Sibling incest offenders. *Child Abuse and Neglect, 19*(7), 811–819.

American Professional Society on the Abuse of Children. (1998). *Glossary of terms and interpretations of findings for child sexual abuse evidentiary examinations.* Chicago: APSAC.

American Psychiatric Association (1999). *Dangerous sex offenders. A task force report of the American Psychiatric Association.* Washington, DC: Author.

American Psychiatric Association (2004). *Practice Guideline for the treatment of patients with acute stress disorder and posttraumatic stress disorder.* Arlington, VA: American Psychiatric Association Practice Guidelines.

Banyard, V. L., Arnold, S., & Smith, J. (2000). Childhood sexual abuse and dating experiences of undergraduate women. *Child Maltreatment, 5,* 39–48.

Barnett, O. W., Miller-Perrin, C. L., & Perrin, R. D. (1997). *Family violence across the lifespan.* Thousand Oaks, CA: Sage.

Bender, L., & Blau, A. (1937). The reaction of children to sexual relations with adults. *American Journal of Orthopsychiatry, 7,* 500–518.

Berenson, A. B., Chacko, M. R., Woemann, C. M. Mishaw, C. O., Friedrich, W. N., & Grady, J. J. (2000). A case–control study of anatomical changes resulting from sexual abuse. *American Journal of Obstetrics and Gynecology, 182,* 820–834.

Berliner, L., & Cohen, J. (2000, July). *Guidelines for the treatment of trauma in child victims.* Paper presented at the Eighth Annual Colloquium of the American Professional Society on the Abuse of Children, Chicago, IL.

Berliner, L., & Elliott, D. M. (2002). Sexual abuse of children. In J. B. Myers, L. Berliner, J. Briere, C. T. Hendrix, C. Jenny & T. A. Reid (Eds.), *The APSAC handbook on child maltreatment* (2nd ed., pp. 55–78). Thousand Oaks, CA: Sage.

Berrien, F. (2007). Child and adolescent sexual abuse. In: R. M. Hammer, B. Moynihan, & E. M. Pagliaro (Eds.), *Forensic nursing: A handbook for practice* (pp. 279–303). Sudbury: Jones and Bartlett Publishers.

Briere, J. (1992). *Child abuse trauma.* Newbury Park, CA: Sage.

Briere, J. (1996). *Therapy for adults molested as children: Beyond survival.* New York: Springer.

Briere, J. (2002). Treating adult survivors of severe childhood abuse and neglect: Further development of an integrative model. In J. B. Myers, L. Berliner, J. Briere, C. T. Hendrix, C. Jenny, & T. A. Reid (Eds.), *The APSAC handbook on child maltreatment* (2nd ed., pp. 175–203). Thousand Oaks, CA: Sage.

Briere, J., & Zaidi, L. Y. (1989). Sexual abuse histories and sequelae in female psychiatric emergency room patients. *American Journal of Psychiatry, 146,* 1602–1606.

Brilleslijper-Kater, S. N., Friedrich, W. N., & Corwin, D. L. (2004). Sexual knowledge and emotional reaction as indicators of sexual abuse in young children: Theory and research challenges. *Child Abuse & Neglect, 28,* 1007–1017.

Bunting, L. (2007). Dealing with a problem that doesn't exist? Professional responses to female perpetrated child sexual abuse. *Child Abuse Review, 16,* 252–267.

Burgess, A., Hartman, C. R., Wolbert, W. W., & Grant, C. (1987). Child molestation: Assessing impact in multiple victims (part 1). *Archives of Psychiatric Nursing, 1,* 33–39.

Cammaert, L. P. (1988). Nonoffending mothers: A new conceptualization. In L. E. Walker (Ed.), *Handbook on sexual abuse of children* (pp. 309–325). New York: Springer.

Carmen, E., & Rieker, P. P. (1989). A psychosocial model of the victim-to-patient process. *Psychiatric Clinics of North America, 12,* 431–443.

Carpenito-Moyet, L. J. (2004). *Nursing Diagnosis: Application to clinical practice.* (10th edn.). Philadelphia: Lippincott.

Carr, A. (2004). Interventions for post-traumatic stress disorder in children and adolescents. *Pediatric Rehabilitation, 7*(4), 231–244.

Chaffin, M., Letourneau, W., & Silovsky, J. (2002). Adults, adolescents and chldren who sexually abuse children. In J. B. Myers, L. Berliner, J. Briere, C. T. Hendrix, C. Jenny & T. A. Reid (Eds.), *The APSAC handbook on child maltreatment* (2nd edn., pp. 205–232). Thousand Oaks, CA: Sage.

Child Welfare Information Gateway (2006). *What is child abuse and neglect?* Retrieved November 3, 2007 from http://www.childwelfare.gov/pubs/factsheets/whatiscan.pdf.

Chu, J. A. (1998). *Rebuilding shattered lives: The responsible treatment of complex-post-traumatic and dissociative disorders.* New York: Wiley.

Chu, J. A., Frey, L. M., Ganzel, B. L., & Matthews, J. A. (1999). Memories of childhood abuse: Dissociation, amnesia and corroboration. *American Journal of Psychiatry, 156,* 749–755.

Cohen, J. R. & Mannarino, A. P. (1998). Interventions for sexually abused children: Initial treatment outcome findings. *Child Maltreatment, 3,* 17–26.

Conte, J. R. (1990). The incest offender: An overview and introduction. In A. L. Horton, B. L. Johnson, L. M. Roundy & D. Williams (Eds.), *The incest perpetrator: A family member no one wants to treat* (pp. 19–28). Newbury Park, CA: Sage.

Cooper, S. W. (2005). In: S. W. Cooper, R. J. Estes, A. P. Giardino, N. D. Kellogg, & V. I. Vieth (Eds.), *Medical, legal, & social science aspects of child sexual exploitation: A comprehensive review of pornography, prostitution, and internet crimes* (pp. 1–24). St. Louis: G. W. Medical Publishing, Inc.

Courtois, C. (1988). *Healing the incest wound.* New York: W. W. Norton.

Courtois, C. (1999). *Recollections of sexual abuse: Treatment principles and guidelines.* New York: Norton.

D'Amora, D. A., Brandhurst, T., & Wallace, R. (2006). Sexual offenders: Who are they and why do they commit sexual abuse? In R. M. Hammer, B. Moynihan, & E. M. Pagliaro (Eds.), *Forensic Nursing: A Handbook for Practice* (pp. 233–254). Sudbury: Jones and Bartlett Publishers.

Daro, D., & Connelly, A. C. (2002). Child abuse prevention: Accomplishments and challenges. In J. B. Myers, L. Berliner, J. Briere, C. T. Hendrix, C. Jenny, & T. A. Reid (Eds.), *The APSAC handbook on child maltreatment* (2nd ed., pp. 431–448). Thousand Oaks, CA: Sage.

Deblinger, E., Hathaway, C., Lippman, J., & Steer, R. (1993). Psychosocial characteristics and correlates of symptom distress in nonoffending mothers of sexually abused children. *Journal of Interpersonal Violence, 8*(2), 155–168.

Deblinger, E., Stauffer, L. B., & Steer, R. A. (2001). Comparative efficacies of supportive and cognitive behavioral group therapies for young children who have been sexually abused and their nonoffending mothers. *Child Maltreatment, 6*(4), 332–343.

De Jong, T., & Gorey, K. (1996). Short-term versus long-term group work with female survivors of childhood sexual abuse: A brief meta-analytic review. *Social Work with Groups, 19,* 19–27.

Denov, M. S. (2003). The myth of innocence: Sexual scripts and the recognition of child sexual abuse by female perpetrators. *The Journal of Sex Research, 40*(3), 303–314.

DiGorgio-Miller, J. (1998). Sibling incest: Treatment of the family and the offender. *Child Welfare, 77*(3), 335–346.

DiLillo, D. (2001). Interpersonal functioning among women reporting a history of childhood sexual abuse: Empirical findings and methodological issues. *Clinical Psychology Review, 21,* 553–576.

Dochterman, J. C., & Bulechek, G. M. (Eds.). (2004). *Nursing Intervention Classification (NIC)*(4th ed.). St. Louis, MO: Mosby.

Dolan, Y. M. (1991). *Resolving sexual abuse: Solution focused therapy and Eriksonian hypnosis.* New York: W. W. Norton.

Draucker, C. (2000). Counseling survivors of childhood sexual abuse. Thosand Oaks, CA: Sage.

Elliott, D. M. (1993). *Female sexual abuse of children.* New York: Guilford.

Elliott, D. M., & Briere, J. (1995). Posttraumatic stress associated with delayed recall of sexual abuse: A general population study. *Journal of Traumatic Stress, 8*(4), 629–647.

Elliott, D. M., & Carnes, C. N. (2001). Reactions of nonoffending parents to the sexual abuse of their child. A review of the literature. *Child Maltreatment, 6,* 341–331.

Epstein, M. A., & Bottoms, B. L. (2002). Explaining the forgetting and recovery of abuse and trauma memories: Possible mechanisms. *Child Maltreatment, 7*(3), 210–225.

Faller, K. C. (2002). Disclosure in cases of child sexual abuse. *Newsletter of the Michigan Professional Society on the Abuse of Children, Inc., 7,* 3–6.

Finkelhor, D. (1984). *Child sexual abuse: New theory and research.* New York: Free Press.

Finkelhor, D. (1986). A sourcebook on child sexual abuse. Beverly Hills, CA: Sage.

Finkelhor, D. (1994). Current information on the scope and nature of child sexual abuse. *The Future of Children, 4*(2), 21–53.

Finkelhor, D. (2007). Prevention of sexual abuse through educational programs directed toward children. *Pediatrics, 120*(3), 640–645.

Finkelhor, D. (2009). The prevention of child sexual abuse. *Future of Children, 19*(2), 169–194.

Finkelhor, D., & Browne, A. (1986). The traumatic impact of child sexual abuse: A conceptualization. *American Journal of Orthopsychiatry, 55,* 530–541.

Foa, E. B., Keane, T. M., & Friedman, M. J. (2000). *Effective treatments for PTSD: Practice guidelines from the International Society for Traumatic Stress Studies.* New York: Guilford Press.

Fonagy, P. (1998). Prevention, the appropriate target of infant psychotherapy. *Infant Mental Health, 19,* 124–150.

Foy, D. W., Schnurr, P., Weiss, D., Wattenberg, M. S., Glynn, S. M., Marmar, C. R., et al. (2001). Group psychotherapy for PTSD. In J. P. Wilson, M. J. Friedman, & J. D. Lindy (Eds.), *Treating psychological trauma and PTSD.* New York: Guilford Press.

Frasier, L. (2002). Child Abuse or mimic? *Consultant, 769–771.*

Frederickson, R. M. (1991, October). Advanced clinical skills in the treatment of sexual abuse. Paper presented at a workshop held at Wayne State University, Detroit, MI.

Friedman, M. J. (2001). Allostatic versus empirical perspectives on pharmacotherapy for PTSD. In J. P. Wilson, M. J. Friedman, & J. D. Lindy (Eds.), *Treating psychological trauma & PTSD* (pp. 94–124). New York: Guilford Press.

Gerardin, P., & Thibaut, F. (2004). Epidemiology and treatment of juvenile sex offending. *Pediatric Drugs, 6*(2), 79–91.

Giardino, A., Datner, E., Asher, J., Faugno, D., & Spencer, M. (2002). *Sexual assault: Victimization across the lifespan.* Maryland Heights, MO: G. W. Medical Publishing.

Glasser, M., Kolvin, I., Campbell, D., Glasser, A., Leitch, I., & Farrelly, S. (2001). Cycle of child sexual abuse: Links between being a victim and becoming a perpetrator. *British Journal of Psychiatry, 179,* 482–494.

Goodyear-Smith, F. (2007). What is the evidence for non-sexual transmission of gonorrhoea in children after the neonatal period? A systematic review. *Journal of Forensic and Legal Medicine, 14,* 489–502.

Grassi-Oliveira, R., Ashy, M., & Stein, L. M. (2008). Psychobiology of child maltreatment: Effects of allostatic load? *Revista Brasileira de Psiquiatria, 30*(1), 60–68.

Groth, N. A. (1978). Guidelines for assessment and management of the offender. In A. Burgess, N. A. Groth, L. Holstrom, & S. Sgroi (Eds.), *Sexual assault of children and adolescents* (pp. 25–42). Lexington, MA: Lexington Books.

Henderson, D. J. (1972). Incest: A synthesis of data. *Psychiatric Association Journal, 17,* 299–313.

Herman, J. (1997). *Trauma and recovery.* New York: Basic Books.

Herman, J. (2000). *Father–daughter incest.* Cambridge: Harvard University Press.

Herman, M., & Hirschman, L. (1977). Father-daughter incest: Signs. *Journal of Women in Culture and Society, 2,* 735–756.

Hornor, G. (2002). Child sexual abuse: Psychosocial risk factors. *Journal of Pediatric Health Care, 16*(4), 187–192.

Hudson, S. M., Ward, T., & Laws, D. R. (2000). Whither relapse prevention? In D. R. Laws, S. M. Hudson, & T. Ward (Eds.), *Remaking relapse prevention with sex offenders* (pp. 503–522). Thousand Oaks, CA: Sage.

Jenny, C. (2002). Medical issues in child sexual abuse. In J. B. Myers, L. Berliner, J. Briere, C. T. Hendrix, C. Jenny, & T. A. Reid (Eds.), *The APSAC handbook on child maltreatment* (2nd edn., pp. 235–237). Thousand Oaks, CA: Sage.

Jespersen, A. F., Lalumiere, M. L., & Seto, M. C. (2009). Sexual abuse history among adult sex offenders and non-sex offenders: A meta-analysis. *Child Abuse & Neglect, 33,* 179–192.

Johnson, C. F. (2004). Child sexual abuse. *Lancet, 364,* 462–470.

Johnson, T. C. (2005). Young children's problematic sexual behaviors, unsubstantiated allegations of child sexual abuse, and family boundaries in child custody disputes. *Journal of Child Custody, 2*(4), 111–126.

Justice, B., & Justice, R. (1979). *The broken taboo: Sex in the family.* New York: Human Sciences Press.

Kasdin, A. E., & Weisz, J. R. (1998). Identifying and developing empirically supported child and adolescent treatments. *Journal of Consulting and Clinical Psychology, 66,* 19–36.

Kellogg, N., & the Committee on Child Abuse and Neglect (2005). The evaluation of sexual abuse in children. *Pediatrics, 116*(2), 506–512.

Kendall-Tackett, K. (2002). The health effects of childhood abuse: Four pathways by which abuse can influence health. *Child Abuse & Neglect, 26,* 715–729.

Kendall-Tackett, K., Williams, L. M., & Finkelhor, D. (1993). Impact of sexual abuse on children: A review and synthesis of recent empirical studies. *Psychological Bulletin, 113,* 164–180.

Kuehnle, K., & Kirkpatrick, H. D. (2005). Evaluating allegations of child sexual abuse within complex child custody cases. *Journal of Child Custody, 2*(3), 3–39.

Levenson, J. S., & Morin, J. W. (2001a). *Connections workbook.* Thousand Oaks, CA: Sage.

Levenson, J. S., & Morin, J. W. (2001b). *Treating nonoffending parents in child sexual abuse cases.* Thousand Oaks, CA: Sage.

Levenson, J. S., & Morin, J. W. (2006). Risk assessment in child sexual abuse cases. *Child Welfare, 85*(1), 59–82.

Lichenstein, R., & Suggs, A. H. (2007). Child abuse/assault. In: J. S. Olshaker, M. C. Jackson, & W. S. Smock (Eds.) *Forensic emergency medicine* (pp. 156–173). Philadelphia: Lippincott Williams & Wilkins.

London, K., Bruck, M., Wright, D. B., & Ceci, S. J. (2007). Review of the contemporary literature on how children report sexual abuse to others: Findings, methodological issues, and implications for forensic interviewers. *Memory, 16*(1), 29–47.

MacDonald, G., Higgins, J. P. T., & Ramchandani, P. (2006). Cognitive-behavioural interventions for children who have been sexually abused. *Cochrane Database of Systematic Reviews, 4,* art. no.: CD001930. DOI: 10.1002/14651858.CD001930.pub2.

Mears, C. J., Heflin, A. H., Finkel, M. A., Deblinger, E., & Steer, R. A. (2003). Adolescents' responses to sexual abuse evaluation including the use of video colposcopy. *Journal of Adolescent Health, 33*(1), 18–24.

McCollum, D. (March 2006). Child maltreatment and brain development. *Minnesota Medicine* [online]. Available from: http://www.minnesotamedicine.com/.

Macdonald, G., Higgins, J. P. T., & Ramchandani, P. (2006). Cognitive-behavioral interventions for children who have been sexually abused. Cochrane Database of Systematic Reviews, Issue 4. Art No.: CD001930. doi: 10.1002/14651858.CD001930.pub2.

McEwen, B. S. (1998). Protective and damaging effects of stress mediators. *Seminars in Medicine of the Beth Israel Deaconess Medical Center, 338*(3), 171–179.

Menard, K. S., & Ruback, R. B. (2003). Prevalence and processing of child sexual abuse: A multi-data-set analysis of urban and rural counties. *Law and Human Behavior, 27*(4), 385–402.

Murphy, W. D., & Smith, T. A. (1996). Sex offenders against children. Empirical and clinical issues. In J. Briere, L. Berliner, & A. Bulkley (Eds.), *The APSAC handbook on child maltreatment* (pp. 175–92). Thousand Oaks, CA: Sage.

National Clearinghouse on Child Abuse and Neglect. (2001). Understanding the effects of maltreatment on early brain development [online]. Available: http://www.calib.com/nccanch/pubs/focus/earlybrain.cfm.

Parillo, K. M., Freeman, R. C., Collier, K., & Young, P. (2001). Association between early sexual abuse and adult HIV-risky sexual behavrios among community-recruited women. *Child Abuse & Neglect, 25,* 335–346.

Pereda, N., Guilera, G., Forns, M., & Gomez-Benito, J. (2009). The international epidemiology of child sexual abuse: A continuation of Finkelhor (1994). *Child Abuse & Neglect, 33*(6), 331–342.

Perry, B. D. (2001). The neurodevelopmental impact of violence in childhood. In D. Schetky & E. Benedek (Eds.), *Textbook of child and adolescent forensic psychiatry.* Washington, DC: American Psychiatric Press.

Pintello, D., & Zuravin, S. (2001). Intrafamilial child sexual abuse: Predictors of postdisclosure maternal belief and protective action. *Child Maltreatment, 6*(4), 344–352.

Poindexter, G., & Morrell, D. S. (2007). Anogenital pruritis: Lichen schlerosus in children. *Pediatric Annals, 36*(12), 785–791.

Polusny, M. A., & Follette, V. M. (1996). Remembering childhood sexual abuse: A national survey of psychologists' clinical practices, beliefs, and personal experiences. *Professional Psychology: Research and Practice, 27,* 41–52.

Price, J. L., Hilsenroth, M. J., Petretic-Jackson, P. A., & Bonge, D. (2001). A review of individual psychotherapy outcomes for adult survivors of childhood sexual abuse. *Clinical Psychology Review, 21,* 1095–1121.

Proulx, J., Tardif, M., Lamoureaux, B., & Lussier, P. (2000). How does recidivism risk assessment predict survival? In J. R. Laws, S. M. Hudson, & T. Ward (Eds.), *Remaking relapse prevention with sex offenders: A sourcebook.* Thousand Oaks, CA: Sage.

Rubenzahl, S. A., & Gilbert, B. O. (2002). Providing sexual education to victims of child sexual abuse: What is a clinician to do? *Journal of Child Sexual Abuse, 11*(1), 1–25.

Russell, D. (1986). *The secret trauma.* New York: Basic Books.

Ryan, G., & Lane, S. (1991). *Juvenile sexual offenders.* Lexington, MA: Lexington Books.

Savell, S. (2005). Child sexual abuse: Are health care providers looking the other way? *Journal of Forensic Nursing, 1*(2), 78–81.

Saywitz, K. J., Mannarino, A. P., Berliner, L., & Cohen, J. A. (2000). Treatment of sexually abused children and adolescents. *American Psychologist, 55,* 1040–1049.

Sedlak, A., & Broadhurst, B. (1996). *Executive summary of the third national incidence study of child abuse and neglect.* Retrieved November 13, 2007, from http://www.childwelfare.gov/pubs/statsinfo/nis3.cfm

Sheridan, D. S., Nash, C. R., Hawkins, S. L., Makely, J. L., & Campbell, J. C. (2006). Forensic implications of intimate partner violence. In R. M. Hammer, B. Moynihan, & E. M. Pagliaro (Eds.), *Forensic Nursing a Handbook for Practice.* Sudbury, MA: Jones and Bartlett Publishers.

Shipman, K., & Taussig, H. (2009). Mental health treatment of child abuse and neglect: The promise of evidence based practice. *Pediatric Clinics of North America, 56,* 417–428. doi:10.1016/j.pcl.2009.02.002.

Shore, R. (1997). *Rethinking the brain.* New York: Families and Work Institute.

Smith, D. W., Letourneau, E. J., Saunders, B. E., Kilpatrick, D. G., Resnick, H. S., & Best, C. L. (2000). Delay in disclosure of childhood rape: Results from a national survey. *Child Abuse and Neglect, 24,* 273–287.

Stovall-McClough, C. (2004). Trauma focused cognitive behavioural therapy reduces PTSD more effectively than child centred therapy in children who have been sexually abused. *Evidence-Based Mental Health, 7,* 113.

Strand, V. C. (2000). *Treating secondary victims: Intervention with the nonoffending mother in the incest family.* Thousand Oaks, CA: Sage.

Strand, V. C., Sarmiento, T. L., & Pasquale, L. E. (2005). Assessment and screening tools for trauma in children and adolescents: A review. *Trauma Violence Abuse, 6*(1), 55–78.

Summit, R. C. (1989). *Treating secondary victims: Intervention with the nonoffending mother in the incest family.* Thousand Oaks, CA: Sage.

Thakkar-Kolar, R. R., Ryan, E. E., & Runyon, M. K. (2008). Child sexual abuse: From prevention to self-protection. *Child Abuse Review, 17,* 36–54.

Theodore, A. D., Chang, J. J., Runyan, D. K., Hunter, W. M., Bangdiwala, S. I., & Agans, R. (2005). Epidemiologic features of the physical and sexual maltreatment of children in the Carolinas. *Pediatrics, 115*(3), e331–e337.

Ullman, S. E. (2003). Social reactions to child sexual abuse disclosures: A critical review. *Journal of Child Sexual Abuse, 12*(1), 89–121.

United States Department of Health and Human Services (2003). *The child abuse prevention and treatment act including adoption opportunities and the abandoned infants assistance act as amended by the keeping children and families safe act of 2003.* Retrieved September 14, 2009 from http://www.acf.hhs.gov/programs/cb/laws_policies/cblaws/capta03/capta_manual.pdf.

United States Department of Health and Human Services (2008). *Fourth national incidence study of child abuse and neglect: Project Summary.* Retrieved June 13, 2009, from https://www.nis4.org/nishome.asp.

United States Department of Health and Human Services Administration for Children, Youth & Families (2007). *Child maltreatment 2005.* Washington DC: US.Government Printing Office.

Urbancic, J. C. (1992). *The relationship between empowerment support, mental health self-care, incest trauma resolution, and subjective well-being.* Doctoral dissertation, Wayne State University, Detroit, MI.

Urbancic, J. C. (1993). Intrafamilial sexual abuse. In J. Campbell & J. Humphries (Eds.), *Nursing care of survivors of family violence.* St. Louis, MO: Mosby.

Whitaker, D. J., Le, B., Hanson, R. K., Baker, C. K., McMahon, P. M., Ryan G, et al. (2008). Risk factors for the perpetration of child sexual abuse: A review and meta-analysis. *Child Abuse & Neglect, 32,* 529–548.

Williams, L. M. (1994). Recall of child trauma: A prospective study of women's memories of childhood sexual abuse. *Journal of Counseling and Clinical Psychology, 62,* 1167–1176.

Wilsnack, S. C., Wonderlich, S. A., Kristhanson, A. J., Vogeltanz-Holm, N. D., & Wilsnack, R. W. (2002). Self reports of forgetting and remember childhood sexual abuse in a nationally representative sample of U.S. women. *Child Abuse and Neglect, 26,* 139–147.

Wilson, J. P., Friedman, M. J., & Lindy, J. D. (2001). *Treating psychological trauma & PTSD.* New York: Guildford Press.

Wyatt, G. E., & Powell, G. J. (1988). *Lasting effects of child sexual abuse.* Beverly Hills: Sage.

Zlotnick, C., Mattia, J., & Zimmerman, M. (2001). Clinical features of survivors of sexual abuse with major depression. *Child Abuse and Neglect, 25,* 357–367.

Zoellner, L. A., Fitzgibbons, L. A., & Foa, E. B. (2001). Cognitive-behavioral approaches to PTSD. In J. P. Wilson, M. J. Friedman, & J. D. Lindy (Eds.), *Treating psychological trauma and PTSD* (pp. 159–182). New York: Guilford Press.

13

Elder Mistreatment

Terry Fulmer, PhD, RN, FAAN
Mary C. Sengstock, PhD, CCS
Jamie Blankenship, BSN, RN
Billy Caceres, BSN, RN
Angela Chandracomar, BSN, RN
Nina Ng, BSN, RN
Heather Wopat, BSN, RN

INTRODUCTION

Nurses care for mistreated elders every day, but sadly, in many instances, do so unaware. It is estimated that over two million older adults suffer from some form of elder mistreatment (EM) annually at the hands of both formal and informal caregivers (National Research Council, 2003). The purpose of this chapter is to provide nurses and other health care providers with the current state of best practices in the prevention and treatment of elder abuse and neglect in order to provide the highest quality care for older adults. With nearly 12% of the population over the age of 65 years, and with projections that the proportion of older adults will reach 20% in the next decade, we can anticipate an epidemic of EM unless all health care providers become better educated about EM prevention, early detection strategies, care planning, and follow up. A review of the literature indicates that there is a growing body of knowledge to guide practice in the areas of EM and every effort should be made to ensure that content is integrated into daily clinical practice. Some textbooks on geriatric nursing have chapters on EM or a section on EM including practice frameworks to guide nursing care for these older adults. Of the 18 leading gerontological nursing textbooks published over the past 5 years, only 38% have a chapter on EM. This is unacceptable for such a serious and prevalent health problem and suggests that EM is not being given the attention that it deserves.

Historically, courts and practice settings have used distinctly different lenses in framing and defining EM. However, in a seminal report, the National Research Council (NRC) (2003) defined EM as:

a. Intentional actions that cause harm or create serious risk of harm (whether or not harm is intended) to a vulnerable elder by a caregiver or other person who is in a trust relationship to the elder, or

b. Failure by a caregiver to satisfy the elder's basic needs or to protect himself or herself from harm (p. 40).

In that same report, there was a call for substantial improvements in the scope and depth, and volume of research to guide practice. While such an appeal harkens back to the 1960s when the field was emerging, it is anticipated that the current pace of EM research will accelerate, not only because of scholarly reports but also because of the growing need of practitioners. There has been a long-standing debate among professionals working with the elderly as to whether EM should be viewed as a special type of family violence or as a particular problem of old age.

PREVALENCE AND INCIDENCE OF ELDER MISTREATMENT

The best data to date indicates that between 700,000 and 1.2 million cases of EM occur annually. Using a systematic sample in their classic study, Pillemer and Finkelhor (1988) interviewed 2,020 community-dwelling older persons in Boston in person or by proxy and established that EM occurred at a rate of 3.2%, or 32 cases of EM per 1,000 older persons. Three types of EM were included: physical abuse, physical neglect, and psychological abuse. Using a similar approach, a more recent study published in the UK indicated that the national prevalence of EM occurs at a rate of 2.6% (Biggs, Manthorpe, Tinker, Doyle, & Erens, 2009).

The National Elder Abuse Incidence Study (NEAIS) estimated that there are 550,000 new cases of EM annually (The National Center on Elder Abuse at The American Public Human Services Association in Collaboration with Westat, 1998; Mixon, 2000; Thomas, 2000). This study, which obtained data from a "sentinel" sample of 20 counties in 15 states, defines EM as including physical abuse, physical neglect, and psychological abuse in persons 60 years of age and older. The NEAIS documented an estimated rate of 1.2%, or approximately 12 cases per 1,000 older persons each year (Thomas, 2000). The 1.2% figure represents the best estimate of the incidence of EM to date as no other national incidence study has since been conducted. However, in all studies of EM, the figures only represent mistreatment that has been observed and reported. Even when special care is taken, it is unknown how many cases go unobserved and unreported (National Institute of Justice, 2007). Indeed, the NEAIS cautions that as much as five times as many cases of EM may exist as are reported to Adult Protective Services (APS); this reference to the large number of unreported cases of EM has been referred to as the "iceberg theory" (The National Center on Elder Abuse at The American Public Human Services Association in Collaboration with Westat, 1998).

The most often used types of EM include abuse, neglect, exploitation, and abandonment. However, EM can be further substratified to address, for example, EM by self or by other; intentional versus unintentional. EM cases can also be multifactorial, with multiple subtypes in a single case, and may involve a substantial number of separate incidents occurring over several months or even years.

Forty-five states have EM reporting laws. The remaining five states (i.e., Colorado, New Jersey, New York, North Dakota, and South Dakota) are still considering legislation

---

EXHIBIT 13.1 | *Examples of EM Subtypes in State Reporting Laws*

- Psychological or emotional neglect includes isolating or ignoring the older person.
- Psychological or emotional abuse involves assault or the infliction of pain through verbal or emotional rather than physical means. Examples are verbal assault (screaming, yelling, and berating) and threats that induce fear, but do not involve use of a weapon.
- Violation of personal rights includes acts that deprive an older adult of the right to make his or her own choices and to act on his or her own behalf. Examples include forcing a person to move into a nursing home against his or her will, prohibiting him or her from marrying, or preventing free use of the older person's own money. Violation of personal rights, together with financial abuse (listed next), are often characterized as "exploitation" of older adults.
- Financial abuse includes the theft or misuse of an aged individual's money or property. Examples include taking money from a bank account without the older person's consent, selling a home without knowledge or permission, cashing a Social Security check and not returning the money to the recipient, and failure to use financial resources for the older person's benefit. The AMA guidelines single out this last type, financial neglect, as a separate category (American Medical Association, 1992).
- Physical neglect (National Center on Elder Abuse, 2007) includes the failure to provide an aged and dependent individual with the necessities of life: food, shelter, clothing, and medical care. In fact, such neglect may be as injurious and life-threatening as a direct attack. Abandonment, an extreme form of neglect in which a caregiver simply leaves and refuses to provide care any longer, is also included here, although some states consider it a separate category (National Research Council, 2003; Neale, Hwalek, Goodrich, & Quinn,1997; Thomas, 2000; Wolf, 1996).
- Physical abuse means apparently deliberate direct attacks that can cause physical injury. Included in this category are slaps, punches, beatings, and pushes, as well as threats in which a weapon, such as a knife or gun, is directly involved. Sexual assault is also included here, although it is often viewed as a separate category (Brandl, 2007; National Center on Elder Abuse, 2007).

Some categorizations distinguish between "active neglect" and "passive neglect," with the former being a deliberate act, and the latter resulting from inadequate knowledge of the older person's needs or the stresses of long-term caregiving (Douglass, 1988; Wolf, 1996; Wolf, 1996).

(National Center on Elder Abuse, 2006). Inconsistencies in state laws and requirements limit access to national estimates through these data.

Several investigators have documented that the majority of EM cases are neglect or self-neglect (Lachs, 2008; Pickens, Burnett, Naik, Holmes, & Dyer, 2006). This suggests that most elders are not injured by deliberate physical assaults but by the outcomes of inadequate care (Dyer, Pickens, & Burnett, 2007; National Center on Elder Abuse, 2007). Financial exploitation of older persons is also a serious problem with an estimated prevalence of 30.2% in substantiated APS reports (Rabiner, O'Keeffe, & Brown, 2006). Regardless of the type of mistreatment, careful analysis and attention to the older persons' caregiving situation, as well as their expressed wishes, are required.

THEORIES FOR UNDERSTANDING NURSING CARE FOR ELDER MISTREATMENT

Theories and conceptual frameworks provide professionals with valuable indicators for assessment and planning of care. There are several theories that attempt to address family violence and EM. The NRC report reviewed the theoretical literature related to EM and concluded that viewing EM in the sociocultural context with an analysis of constructs, such as social embeddedness, status, and equality, and power and exchange dynamics, are important (National Research Council, 2003).

ABUSER THEORIES. EM has been explained in relation to the psychopathological state of the abuser, which is related to power and exchange dynamics. This theory proposes that the abusive individual may have mental illness and that the abusive behavior is the result of this mental illness. A closely related theory associates EM with substance abuse or addiction. Others have suggested that alcohol is not the basic cause of the abusive behavior; rather, the abuser uses substance abuse as a "cover-up" for abusive tendencies that are already present (Straus & Gelles, 1992). Cases of EM where mental illness or substance abuse are present are particularly serious and difficult to manage (Schonfeld, Larsen, & Stiles, 2006).

ENVIRONMENTAL/SITUATIONAL STRESS THEORIES. Another theory relates to the presence of environmental or situational stress. Situational factors, such as poverty, isolation, or occupational stress, may trigger EM. Child abuse and intimate partner violence consistently occur more frequently (although not exclusively) in lower socioeconomic groups, which are presumed to experience greater stress because of economic deprivation, and this seems true for older adults as well (Lachs, Berkman, Fulmer, & Horwitz, 1994). It has also been documented that abusive families are socially isolated and unlikely to have social resources on which to rely when stressful situations occur. Caregiver burden may create stress and promote EM. Therefore, treatment of the entire family in EM cases is essential (Straus, 2006). One notable limitation of this stress model, however, is that it does not explain why some families are more resourceful and resilient than others despite the stress.

EXPLOITATION THEORIES. Exploitation may be provoked by financial difficulties on the part of one or more members of the family (Quinn & Zielke, 2005). The high profile court case of Brooke Astor and the confirmation of EM against her son brought the issue to the nation's attention (Eligon, 2009). The underpinnings of exploitation theories range from greed to "getting what was owed" to a caregiver. Exploitation is one of the more clear-cut EM categories, since it is consistent with other forms of theft and fraud and is punishable by law.

PATTERNS OF FAMILY VIOLENCE THEORIES. When attitudes and behaviors that support the use of violence and force are firmly established in a family, they are hard to change. It is posited that long-term abusive patterns in the family may continue for a lifetime. Such behavior, like non-violent behavior, can be learned early in life (Renner & Slack, 2006). This is consistent with the individual continuity theory. To date, there have been no longitudinal prospective cohort studies to document patterns of family violence (National Research Council, 2003).

NORMATIVE VIOLENCE THEORIES. It has been suggested by some authors that EM is part of a general pattern of "normative violence," in which violent behavior is accepted, even approved, as a normal part of family life (Straus, 2006). Several studies use the Conflict Tactic Scale, which asks respondents if they were ever punched or hit or threatened with a knife or gun (Straus, 1998). One study found that evidence of childhood trauma was associated with the outcome of EM, suggesting that older adults who experience trauma in childhood grow up to expect less quality interactions from people and have poor self-esteem, which leads to the acceptance of neglect by caregivers (Fulmer et al., 2005).

VICTIM THEORIES. Another set of explanations for EM is focused on the older adult. That is, through his or her own behavior or goading, the victim is believed to have elicited the EM behavior. This perspective comes from the domestic violence literature. However, there are limited studies related to caregiver reactions to disruptive behaviors (Fulmer et al., 1999) specifically related to EM. Nevertheless, according to these victim focused theories, family dynamics are complex for most families, and when age-related diseases and disorders add to the functional decline and dependency of the older adult, EM can ensue.

HEALTH/SOCIOECONOMIC THEORIES. Advances in health care science and technology have increased life span dramatically. While this is attributed to the new scientific breakthroughs of the twentieth century, the proportion of older adults who require formal and informal assistance has also grown dramatically (National Research Council, 2003). Assisted living facilities and home health care are expensive. Care is usually provided by spouses, relatives and even neighbors as care needs increase with age and illness. Some researchers believe that there is a dependency continuum, which can easily overwhelm the caregiver resulting in EM (Fulmer & Gurland, 1997).

DEPENDENCY THEORIES. Older adults often find that the activities they were formerly able to perform for themselves such as personal care, care of the home and meal preparation are now beyond their capacity. The social roles they formerly filled, such as caring for children or grandchildren, or holding valued positions in business or community, are no longer theirs. Older adults may become increasingly dependent on their children, not only for personal care and assistance with normal household tasks but also for most of their social needs.

PROBLEMS OF INTERGENERATIONAL LIVING. When older persons are no longer able to live alone, they may relocate to the home of an offspring or relative. Adult offspring and grandchildren may be forced to give up their privacy and alter their lifestyles to accommodate an aged person's needs. Power and control conflicts are possible. More research is needed to understand the evolution of parent–child relationships and EM (Usita, 2006).

ISOLATION THEORIES. Isolation can lead to self-neglect, and there is a growing body of knowledge specific to self-neglect (Dong et al., 2009). The evidence from these recent studies indicates that self-neglect in older adults is widespread. Research reports suggest that over 70% of all EM referrals to APS are for self-neglect. These findings provide compelling evidence that self-neglect is widespread among elders and that further study is needed in this area. In summary, theories for EM provide a way for nurses to conceptualize their approach to assessment and management of EM.

Practice Protocols Derived from Theories and Conceptual Frameworks

For over three decades, the theories and conceptual models discussed here have helped guide practice. Clinical screening protocols for EM reflect the constructs of dependency patterns of family violence, substance abuse, psychopathology of abusers, learned behavior, acculturation, and illegal behavior. Fulmer, Guadagno, Bitondo Dyer, and Connolly (2004a) documented clinical practice protocols for screening and assessment of EM and note that there are intake protocols in all APS offices that try to collect the most appropriate information to make the diagnosis of EM. The risk and vulnerability framework is an example of a framework that can guide practice protocols. Based on Rose and Killien's (1983) "Risk and Vulnerability Model" as applied to elder abuse by Frost and Willette (1994), risk refers to hazards or stressors external to the older adult, while vulnerability relates to characteristics of the elder. This model defines two latent factors as being responsible for the occurrence of EM: risk and vulnerability. Risk refers to hazards or stressors in the environment, while vulnerability refers to the characteristics of the individual. Risk might include a caregiver who is depressed or has inadequate economic support for appropriate shelter, food, and/or clothing. Vulnerability refers to characteristics of the individual elder, which might include poor health, cognitive decline, disturbing behaviors, or an inability to conduct one's own activities of daily living (ADLs) or instrumental ADLs (IADLs) and a lack of empowerment. This model corresponds well with a previous model proposed by Fulmer entitled, "the stability/options model for abuse and neglect" (Fulmer et al., 2005).

Elder Mistreatment in Diverse Communities

It is important to use culturally sensitive approaches to EM practices (Yeo, 2009). In the Hispanic population, for example, little is known about caregiving and interpersonal violence. However, the life expectancy of Hispanics is shorter, with earlier onset of the chronic diseases of old age, so caregiving may be required for persons at younger ages. It has also been found that Hispanic caregivers may have less social support than Anglo caregivers—contrary to the often-heard assumption that ethnic groups take care of their own (Phillips, 2000). Power imbalance in families has also been associated with caregiving problems (specifically abuse directed toward the caregiver); since power imbalance is more common in Hispanic families, this suggests that family caregiving may be more problematic in this group (Phillips, 2000). Older adults in this community also define EM differently; for example, some define the refusal of children to provide a home for their parents as EM (Sanchez, 1996).

According to a limited number of studies, EM in African American older adults is experienced differently than among other groups. In one study, spiritual sources, rather than physicians, were cited as a preferable approach to health in EM cases (Paranjape, Tucker, McKenzie-Mack, Thompson, & Kaslow, 2007). African Americans are particularly reticent to bring their problems to the attention of health care professionals due to a long-standing distrust of institutions in the Caucasian community (Hines, 2005). Furthermore, it has been documented that physical EM of older adults is unacceptable among African Americans; however, financial and material EM are commonplace and, in many cases, felt to be acceptable.

The special problems of working with African American elders and their families have lead to the development of a new identification measure adapted to their needs (Paranjape, Corbie-Smith, Thompson, & Kaslow, 2009). With African Americans, as with other ethnic groups, care should be taken not to assume that all members of the group are alike.

Native American populations also exhibit patterns that suggest the possibility of higher rates of mistreatment. For example, researchers have found Native Americans to have higher rates of prior abuse, such as having been abused as children (Hudson, Armachain, Beasley, & Carlson, 1998). If, as some suggest, prior abuse makes one more likely to abuse or be abused later in life, then the possibility of EM in Native American communities may be high. Native Americans also have the poorest health of any group in the United States and higher rates of numerous chronic diseases; consequently, they too may require caregiving assistance at younger ages (Hooyman & Kiyak, 2005). As a result, the risk of EM in Native American communities may be quite serious.

Conclusions and generalization based solely on ethnic origins are inappropriate. Health care professionals should be aware that communities exhibit cultural differences. For example, according to selected research, some Irish Americans tend to be secretive about their emotions and reluctant to discuss any type of problem with outsiders (McGoldrick, 2005), while persons of German origin have a tendency to see all such problems as an indication of the victim's personal failure (Windawer, 2005). In the Polish community, seeking help for any type of problem is considered a great embarrassment to the family and must be avoided (Folwarski, 2005).

There is a great need for further study of the special manifestations of EM in different segments of the population. The most important conclusion to be drawn from available data is that EM can occur with all types of older persons, including different racial and ethnic groups, income levels, and religions, and that special efforts are necessary to identify and assist these older victims.

Challenges in Identifying Elder Mistreatment

When EM does occur, the first challenge is the identification of EM victims. Services cannot be provided until professionals become aware of how to reach people who need help. It has long been recognized that abuse of older adults is probably greatly underreported (O'Brien, Thibault, Turner, & Laird-Fick, 1999). Like other survivors of family violence, victims are often reluctant to report their EM. Conversely, healthcare and social service agencies are reluctant to invade the privacy of the older adults. Older adults are often embarrassed to admit EM in the family and wish to maintain the family's reputation (American Psychological Association Office of Aging, 2009). Older victims may fail to report out of fear of the abuser, who may threaten further violence, loss of support, or other reprisals. Older victims are also reluctant to turn to professional agencies because they lack knowledge, are too embarrassed, or have fear of the agencies themselves (Chihowski & Hughes, 2008; O'Connor, 2005).

In some instances, the problem will be even more complicated by language barriers. While such cases will involve the necessity of providing translation, this adds another layer of complexity. Health care providers should not have a family member translate. A general practice is that it is preferable to obtain translation assistance from a professional or someone else who knows the language and culture but is sufficiently detached from the community so that the elder need not be concerned about a breach of confidentiality.

Researchers also suggest that the identification of such groups is complicated by a strong belief that such problems should remain within the family, as well as by community members' reluctance to confide such information to outsiders, to accept outside intervention, or to even speak openly about problems of any kind (Dong, 2005). Dementia, cognitive impairment, or a simple lack of knowledge concerning available services may also render a victim incapable of reporting EM. Those victims who are aware of available resources may still resist reporting EM because they feel incapable of coping with the responsibilities that may ensue if they do report. Possible court appearances or conversations with the police can also be difficult and fear provoking experiences (Dong, 2005).

There is great variability among agencies and professionals in their ability and capacity to identify EM. This situation occurs in part because agencies and institutions are more likely to observe EM in the areas that they are accustomed to treating (Kennedy, 2005; O'Connor, 2005). However, even within the same institution, there is likely to be variability among professionals in knowledge and concern about EM.

Many agencies and institutions have developed their own techniques for the identification of older victims of EM. These include clinical approaches for use in hospitals, procedures for use in state protective service departments, and measures for use in research (Daly & Jogerst, 2006). Common flaws, such as the inclusion of items that measure more than one type of EM, requiring observers to make multiple judgments (such as determining both the presence and deliberateness of EM), and omitting some types of abuse (particularly sexual assault), are problematic. The validity and effectiveness of measures are still under study (Fulmer, Guadagno, Bitondo Dyer, & Connolly, 2004b).

Mistreatment of older adults in institutions, such as nursing homes and long-term care facilities is also an area of concern (Jogerst, Daly, Dawson, Peek-Asa, & Schmuch, 2006). Empirical research on the subject is limited and frequently of poor quality (Quinn & Zielke, 2005). However, mandatory data collection in long-term care, such as the Minimum Data Set, provides insight into trigger events that may lead to the suspicion of EM. Identification is a particularly critical problem with this population because they often are fearful of retaliation if they report EM. They may also be unaware of their rights or physically or mentally incapable of protecting themselves (Abbey, 2009). Pay for performance measures will further improve the way care is monitored and evaluated. Victims of EM require a wide variety of services, and these should be integrated into a comprehensive, unified whole.

There is no substitute for careful and conscientious care on the part of individual professionals dealing with the complex problems of EM. All professionals must be knowledgeable about the problem of EM and aware of the types and definitions of abuse in their particular state.

NURSING CARE FOR ELDER MISTREATMENT VICTIMS

Nursing interventions and care of EM survivors needs a stronger evidence base to provide care that has the hallmarks of quality and safety. Over the past two decades, very few studies of EM have been published in the nursing literature, and it is imperative that we engage new investigators in this important topic to ensure that we are generating knowledge that can guide expert practice. At the same time, abused elders and their families need care, and there are certain principles that can guide practice as the scientific evidence and literature develops more fully. Most recently, the *Journal of the American Medical Association* (Cole & Flanagin, 2009) published a "Violence and Human Rights" theme issue that addressed elder self-neglect, abuse, and mortality, as well as intimate partner violence, and sexual abuse. It is a promising signal when a journal of such importance reminds all of the seriousness of these issues. Dong et al. (2009) documents that both elder self-neglect and abuse lead to higher mortality in older adults. Nursing service departments need to have protocols to follow when nurses are concerned or suspect any form of EM. New graduate nurses need to know who to turn to for practice guidance and that practice will vary depending on geography and type of setting.

More experienced nurses need the same type of guidance but likely have a better sense of normal and abnormal presentations in older adults, with a better sense of resources in their community and practice setting. In general, all nurses should know the expectations for their state reporting of EM, which can vary significantly. Hospital and community-based practices need to have administrators who can assist in getting this information for clinicians. At a minimum, every practice setting should have a protocol for referring suspected cases of EM. In some settings, there may be expert victimology teams that address all forms of family violence. In other settings, there may be interdisciplinary geriatric consult teams that can be called upon for expert guidance. The following sections address the nursing process with what we currently know from the literature and best practices.

Assessment

Assessment for EM should be done with a systematic and methodical approach guided by current assessment instruments. Both the National Research Council (2003) and a report by Fulmer et al. (2004a) provide assessment instruments that have been examined for their psychometric properties and adopted in different clinical settings. EM screens are a first level of assessment that broadly review signs and symptoms of EM and serve largely to help alert practitioners to the possibility of EM. Screens that are positive will then lead to more intensive assessment and evaluation, often by family violence experts or geriatric experts. Ultimately, a "positive" case is one that is argued in a court of law. However, state reporting agencies have metrics for determining screen positives and screen negatives based on extensive experience and expertise. The practicing nurse should understand that any referral made in good faith is an appropriate practice procedure. The alternative (i.e., non-reporting of a potentially positive case) could lead to the death of an older person. There have been concerns raised about false-positive reporting that can disrupt family caregiving systems. For example, if a well-intentioned daughter is providing care to frail older parents and is then "suspected" of EM, she could decide that nursing home placement is the option of last resort. More needs to be done to understand the balance between appropriate and inadequate care, as well as intentional and unintentional mistreatment.

An additional point of contention is the elder's right to self-determination. Older persons may choose to stay in an abusive or neglectful environment. This can be extremely difficult for clinicians who encounter the situation, and the tendency can be to label the older person as cognitively impaired or not fully understanding the ramifications of their decisions. As is the case with battered women, older adults with cognitive capacity have the right to self-determination, and practicing nurses will likely need support when they are engaged in these difficult moral and ethical dilemmas. The principles of autonomy, beneficence, non-maleficence, and justice all come into play in complex EM cases, and an ethics consult can be an extremely important approach to determining an appropriate nursing plan of care.

Care Planning

Once an initial screening and assessment have been conducted, the plan of care should center on the rights of the older adult and the potential safety concerns involved in the care planning. If the older adult has the cognitive capacity, their wishes for discharge planning must be honored, even if it means sending the older adult back to a potentially harmful setting. When this happens, the older adult needs a set of written instructions regarding who to contact in an emergency. This must be done with great discretion in order to avoid alerting a spouse or caregiver to the suspicion of EM. Such an alert could trigger an abusive event or increase the degree of neglect for the older person. Regular and systematic communication with a member of the health care team or health care system is very important in these situations. In rural areas, there may be fewer social service agencies and more distance required for in-person assessments. Police departments, emergency medical technicians, and fire departments may be a first line of communication and assessment. In urban areas, there may be plentiful resources, but the older person can feel equally or more isolated if they have not had careful instruction on how to access discreet services that can help in dangerous situations. The elder most at risk is the cognitively impaired older adult who still has some capacity and therefore is not appropriate for institutionalization, but has less ability to discern threatening situations or exploitative situations. Nursing care for this group requires careful interdisciplinary care planning with the physician and social worker engaged with the older adult so that every opportunity for ongoing assessment is captured.

Identifying at Risk Older Adults

In the identification of an at-risk population, the nurse should take a systematic approach to avoid eliminating possible victims. The Elder Assessment Instrument is an excellent example of a comprehensive clinical screen tool for EM (Fulmer, 2008).

The "Hwalek–Sengstock Elder Abuse Screening Test" (H–S/EAST) has been developed to assist in screening older adults for at-risk responses (Hwalek & Sengstock, 1986). This instrument is valuable in settings where a full clinical examination and disrobing are not appropriate. The complete H-S/EAST consists of 15 items, with two subsets, consisting of nine and six items respectively, being tested separately. These items may serve as an indication of questions that might be used in interviewing older adults to determine their risk for EM.

It is imperative that the nurse obtain a thorough case history of a client when EM is a possibility. Once a patient or client has had a positive screen, referral should be made to a clinical expert, expert team, administrator, or state agency.

DIFFERENTIATING EM FROM THE NORMAL AGING PROCESS. The physiological processes that govern normal aging lead to physiological changes, such as increased cap-

TABLE 13.1   *The Elder Assessment Instrument (Fulmer, 2008)*

I. General Assessment	Very Good	Good	Poor	Very Poor	Unable to Assess
1. Clothing	1	2	3	4	9999
2. Hygiene	1	2	3	4	9999
3. Nutrition	1	2	3	4	9999
4. Skin integrity	1	2	3	4	9999
5. Additional comments:					

II. Possible Abuse Indicators	No Evidence	Possible Evidence	Probable Evidence	Definite Evidence	Unable to Assess
6. Bruising	1	2	3	4	9999
7. Lacerations	1	2	3	4	9999
8. Fractures	1	2	3	4	9999
9. Various stages of healing of any bruises or fractures	1	2	3	4	9999
10. Evidence of sexual abuse	1	2	3	4	9999
11. Statement by elder re: abuse	1	2	3	4	9999
12. Additional comments:					

III. Possible Neglect Indicators	No Evidence	Probably no Evidence	Probably Evidence	Evidence	Unable to Assess
13. Contractures	1	2	3	4	9999
14. Decubiti	1	2	3	4	9999
15. Dehydration	1	2	3	4	9999
16. Diarrhea	1	2	3	4	9999
17. Depression	1	2	3	4	9999
18. Impaction	1	2	3	4	9999
19. Malnutrition	1	2	3	4	9999
20. Urine burns	1	2	3	4	9999
21. Poor hygiene	1	2	3	4	9999
22. Failure to respond to warning of obvious disease	1	2	3	4	9999
23. Inappropriate medications (under/over)	1	2	3	4	9999
24. Repetitive hospital admissions due to probable failure of health care surveillance	1	2	3	4	9999
25. Statement by elder re: neglect	1	2	3	4	9999
26. Additional comments:					

IV. Possible Exploitation Indicators	No Evidence	Possible Evidence	Probably Evidence	Definite Evidence	Unable to Assess
27. Misuse of money	1	2	3	4	9999
28. Evidence of financial exploitation	1	2	3	4	9999

Continued

TABLE 13.1 *Continued*

IV. Possible Exploitation Indicators	No Evidence	Possible Evidence	Probably Evidence	Definite Evidence	Unable to Assess
29. Reports of demands for goods in exchange for services	1	2	3	4	9999
30. Inability to account for money/property	1	2	3	4	9999
31. Statement by elder re: exploitation	1	2	3	4	9999
32. Additional comments:					

V. Possible Abandonment Indicators	No Evidence	Possible Evidence	Probable Evidence	Definite Evidence	Unable to Assess
33. Evidence that a caretaker has withdrawn care precipitously without alternate arrangements	1	2	3	4	9999
34. Evidence that elder is left alone in an unsafe environment for extended periods of time without adequate support	1	2	3	4	9999
35. Statement by elder re: abandonment	1	2	3	4	9999
36. Additional comments:					

VI. Summary Assessments	No Evidence	Possible Evidence	Probable Evidence	Definite Evidence	Unable to Assess
37. Evidence of abuse	1	2	3	4	9999
38. Evidence of neglect	1	2	3	4	9999
39. Evidence of exploitation	1	2	3	4	9999
40. Evidence of abandonment	1	2	3	4	9999
41. Additional comments:					

VII. Comments and Follow-up

illary fragility, osteoporosis, poor balance, poor vision, and musculoskeletal changes. Older adults may be more likely to lose their balance and fall, and a relatively minor fall may result in fractures and extensive bruising, subdural hematomas, and hemorrhages that may be fatal. Chronic diseases and disorders may mask or mimic EM.

Results of a physical examination should be documented and interpreted in conjunction with the history, as noted in Tables 13.2 and 13.3. Careful questioning by the nurse may determine such factors as whether a client who complains of mistreatment is exhibiting symptoms of cognitive impairment or dementia or is in fact expressing a valid complaint of EM. Thus, the importance of obtaining a thorough, objective history on older adults cannot be overemphasized.

EXHIBIT 13.2 | *Sample Questions from the Six-Item Hwalek–Sengstock Elder Abuse Screening Test (H–S/EAST)*

H-S/EAST ITEM	AT-RISK RESPONSE
4. "Decisions" Who makes decisions about your life, for example how you should live or where you should live?	"Someone else"
5. "Uncomfortable" Do you feel uncomfortable with anyone in your family?	"Yes"
7. "Unwanted" Do you feel that nobody wants you around?	"Yes"
10. "Being Forced" Has anyone forced you to do things you didn't want to do?	"Yes"
13. "Annoyance" Does anyone tell you that you give them too much trouble?	"Yes"
15. "Hurt/Harmed" Has anyone close to you tried to hurt you or harm you recently?	"Yes"

Hwalek, M.A. and Sengstock, M.C. (1986) Assessing the probability of abuse of the elderly: Toward the development of a clinical screening instrument. *Journal of Applied Gerontology*, 5, 169; and Neale, A.V., Hwalek, M., Scott, R.O., Sengstock, M.C., & Stahl, C. (1991). Validation of the Hwalek-Sengstock Elder Abuse Screening Test, *Journal of Applied Gerontology*, 10 (4), 409, 415.

An older client may be reluctant to admit the existence of EM even though physical findings point to its presence. The nurse should discuss concerns with the health care team first, then a plan should be made as to whom will ask the older person about the suspected EM. Every patient should have the benefit of a screening question related to family violence (Wasson et al., 2000), and in settings where it is possible, a family violence team or EM team can be an exemplary way to draw attention to the issue and address it rapidly. Exemplary leadership from organizations, as in the case of the Hebrew Home for the Aged in Riverdale, New York, where there is a protective shelter program (i.e., the Weinberg Center for the Prevention of Elder Abuse at http://www.elderserve. org/details.asp?ID=10), is a way to signal to people that EM will not be tolerated.

If there has been an EM event, crisis intervention might be necessary. Protective service programs can be contacted for assistance, and shelters may further be needed for the older adult. It may be important to get a geropsychiatric nursing consult, or social service consult, to assist in helping the older person cope with the stress and trauma of the event. Follow-up for evaluation of the effectiveness of the programs and services put in place is also very important. Finally, it may be important to have a plan for surveillance in place for the older person who has been a victim of EM to prevent any repeated events.

Gatekeepers in the form of volunteers, such as interfaith volunteer caregiver services (established by the Robert Wood Johnson Foundation in the 1980s), use of the faith community established in churches, and, in certain circumstances, visiting nurse services and public health nurse services, may be the most appropriate model for intervention and care. Safety is an issue for victims of EM. If there has been an event, the older person has already been in an unsafe situation, but in any intervention with EM cases, it is important to anticipate what the ramifications and reactions may be of family caregivers or volunteer caregivers. For example, will there be retribution toward the older person for having

TABLE 13.2 *Physical Examination of the Elderly: Indicators of Potential or Actual Elder Abuse or Neglect*

Area of Assessment	Symptoms of Possible Abuse/Neglect[a]
General appearance	Fearful, anxious
	Marked passivity
	Appears malnourished
	Poor hygiene
	Inappropriate dress in relation to weather conditions
	Physical handicap
	Antagonism and/or detachment between elder and caregiver
Vital statistics	
Height	
Weight	Underweight
Skin	Excessive or unexplainable bruises, welts, or scars, possibly in various stages of healing
	Decubitus ulcers
	Burns
	Infected or untreated wound
Head	
Eyes	No prosthetic device to accommodate poor eyesight
Ears	No prosthetic device to accommodate poor hearing
Nose	
Neck	
Chest	
Abdomen	Abdominal distention
Genital/urinary	Vaginal lacerations
	Vaginal infection
	Urinary tract infection
Rectal	
Musculoskeletal	Skull/facial fractures
	Fractured femur
	Fractures of other parts of the body
	Limited motion of extremities
Neurological	Difficulty with speech
	Difficulty with swallowing

[a]Symptoms listed may be symptoms of disease. Therefore, physical symptoms must be assessed in conjunction with the patient's history.

spoken to a healthcare professional about mistreatment? Is there a safety plan and strategy so the older person can avoid harm? Are hotline numbers readily available to the older person? In the event that the individual suffers cognitive impairment, is there an appropriate safety plan that can be instituted to prevent mistreatment? In the latter case, the Alzheimer's Foundation can be an essential service to help create a plan of care.

TABLE 13.3 *History of Elder: Possible Indicators of Potential or Actual Elder Abuse*

Area of Assessment	At-Risk Responses or Indicators of Possible Abuse/Neglect
Primary concern/reason for visit	Historical data that conflict with physical findings
	Acute or chronic psychological and/or physical disability
	Inability to participate independently in activities of daily living
	Inappropriate delay in bringing elder to health-care facility
	Reluctance on the part of caregiver to give information on elder's condition
	Inappropriate caregiver reaction to nurse's concern (overreacts, underreacts)
Family health	
Older adult	Substance abuse
	Grew up in a violent home (abused as child, spouse; abused children)
	Excessive dependence of elder on child(ren)
Child(ren) of elder	Were abused by parents
	Antagonistic relationship with elder
	Excessive dependence on elder
	Substance abuse
	History of violent relationship with other siblings and/or spouse
Siblings	Antagonistic relationship between siblings
	Excessive dependence of one or more siblings on another or each other
Other family members and family relations	Other history of abuse and/or neglect or violent death
Household	Violence and aggression used to resolve conflicts and solve problems
	Past history of abuse and/or neglect among family members
	Poverty
	Few or no friends or neighbors or other support systems available
	Excessive number of stressful situations encountered during a short period of time (such as unemployment, death of a relative or significant other)
Health history of elder	
Childhood	History of chronic physical and/or psychological disability
Midlife	History of chronic physical and/or psychological disability
Nutrition	History of feeding problems (GI disease, food preference idiosyncrasies)
	Inappropriate food or drink
	Dietary intake that does not fit with findings
	Inadequate food or fluid intake
Drugs/medications	Drugs/medications not indicated by physical condition
	Overdose of drugs or medications (prescribed or over-the-counter)
	Medications not taken as prescribed
Personal/social	Caregiver has unrealistic expectations of elder
	Social isolation (little or no contact with friends, neighbors, or relatives; lack of outside activity)
	Substance abuse

Continued

TABLE 13.3 *Continued*

Area of Assessment	*At-Risk Responses or Indicators of Possible Abuse/Neglect*
	History of spouse abuse (as victim and/or abuser)
	History of antagonistic relationships among family members (between family members in general, including elder)
	Large age difference between elder and spouse
	Large number of family problems
	Excessive dependence on spouse, children, or significant others
Discipline	
Physical	Belief that the use of physical punishment is appropriate
	Threats with an instrument as a means to punish
	Use of an instrument to administer physical punishment
	History of caregiver and/or others "losing control" and/or "hitting too hard"
Emotional/violation of rights	Fear-provoking threats
	Infantilization
	Berating
	Screaming
	Forced move out of home
	Forced institutionalization
	Prohibiting marriage and/or friendships
	Prevention of free use of money
	Isolation
Sleep	
Elimination	Denial of needed assistance with elimination
Illness	Chronic illness or handicap
	Disability requiring special treatment from caregiver and others
Operations/hospitalizations	Operations or illness that required extended and/or repeated hospitalizations
	Caregiver's refusal to have elder hospitalized
	Caregiver overanxious to have elder hospitalized
Diagnostic tests	Caregiver's refusal for further diagnostic tests
	Caregiver's overreaction or underreaction to diagnostic findings
Accidents	Repeated
	History of preceding events that do not support injuries
Safety	Appropriate safety precautions not taken, especially those for elders known to be confused, disoriented, and/or with physical disabilities restricting mobility
Health care utilization	Infrequent
	Caregiver overanxious to have elder hospitalized
	Health-care "shopping"
Review of systems	

Finally, the older person will need rehabilitation depending on the nature of the event. In some cases, it may be rehabilitation from a fracture or it could be rehabilitation from an emotional trauma. Nursing practice should include a careful follow-through plan with ways to monitor progress until there is resolution. In the absence of resolution, the plan will be kept indefinitely.

Evaluation of Nursing Intervention

Evaluating the effectiveness of nursing intervention in EM cases is another challenging area. Particularly in cases in which nursing intervention is short term in nature, nurses may be unable to ascertain whether they had an enduring effect on the well-being of an abused older patient. However, the nurse may use some clues to help determine whether the assistance has been of value. These include the client's acknowledgment of the abuse; willingness of the victim, the abuser, and the family to accept outside help; and/or removal of the victim from the abusive situation.

SUMMARY

Practicing nurses can have a profound positive effect on the well-being of their older patients by staying vigilant to the possibility of EM. There can be no quality of life for those who are victims of abuse, neglect, exploitation, abandonment, or any form of family violence. Every nurse has the capacity and responsibility to assess for EM and create a responsible plan of care that can address the mistreatment and create a better life for the older person. Interdisciplinary teaming, careful transitional planning, and patient education that allows for an older person to contact support services in their community or healthcare network are essential. Nurses have traditionally taken a lead in the generation of new knowledge related to EM, as well as the development of programmatic planning for the same. The next decade promises to be an important one for an improvement of strategies for the detection and treatment of EM.

REFERENCES

Abbey, L. (2009). Elder abuse and neglect: When home is not safe. *Clinical Geriatric Medicine, 25*(1), 47–60, vi.

American Medical Association. (1992). *Diagnostic and treatment guidelines on elder abuse and neglect.* Chicago: American Medical Association.

American Psychological Association Office of Aging. *Elder abuse and neglect: In search of solutions* [Web Page]. URL http://www.apa.org/pi/aging/eldabuse.html [2009, August 23].

Biggs, S., Manthorpe, J., Tinker, A., Doyle, M., & Erens, B. (2009). Mistreatment of older people in the United Kingdom: Findings from the first National Prevalence Study. *Journal of Elder Abuse Neglect, 21*(1), 1–14.

Brandl, B., Dyer, C. B., Otto, J. M., Stiegel, L. A., Thomas, R. W. (2007). *Elder abuse detection and intervention.* New York: Springer Publishing Company, LLC.

Chihowski, K., & Hughes, S. (2008). Clinical issues in responding to alleged elder sexual abuse. *Journal of Elder Abuse Neglect, 20*(4), 377–400.

Cole, T. B., & Flanagin, A. (Eds.). (2009). Violence and human rights. *JAMA, 302*(5).

Daly, J. M., & Jogerst, G. J. (2006). Nursing home statutes: Mistreatment definitions. *Journal of Elder Abuse Neglect, 18*(1), 19–39.

Dong, X. (2005). Medical implications of elder abuse and neglect. *Clinical Geriatric Medicine, 21*(2), 293–313.

Dong, X., Simon, M., Mendes de Leon, C., Fulmer, T., Beck, T., Hebert, L., et al. (2009). Elder self-neglect and abuse and mortality risk in a community-dwelling population. *JAMA, 302*(5), 517–526.

Douglass, R. L. (1988). *Domestic mistreatment of the elderly: Toward prevention*. Washington, DC: American Association of Retired Persons.

Dyer, C. B., Pickens, S., & Burnett, J. (2007). Vulnerable elders: when it is no longer safe to live alone. *JAMA, 298*(12), 1448–1450.

ElderServe. *The Harry & Jeanette Weinberg center for elder abuse prevention at The Hebrew Home for the Aged at Riverdale* [Web Page]. URL http://www.elderserve.org/details.asp?ID=10 [2009, August 23].

Eligon, J. (2009 August). Prosecution finally rests in the Brooke Astor case. *The New York Times.*, p. A21.

Folwarski, J. &. S. Jr. J. (2005). Polish families. In J. M. McGoldrick, J. Giordano, & N. Garcia-Preto (Eds.), *Ethnicity & family therapy* (3rd ed., pp. 741–755). New York: Guilford Press.

Fulmer, T. (2008). Screening for mistreatment of older adults. *American Journal of Nursing, 108*(12), 52–59; quiz 59–60.

Fulmer, T., Guadagno, L., Bitondo Dyer, C., & Connolly, M. T. (2004a). Progress in elder abuse screening and assessment instruments. *Journal of American Geriatric Society, 52*(2), 297–304.

Fulmer, T., Guadagno, L., Bitondo Dyer, C., & Connolly, M. T. (2004b). Progress in elder abuse screening and assessment instruments. *Journal of American Geriatric Society, 52*(2), 297–304.

Fulmer, T., & Gurland, B. (1997). Evaluating the caregiver's intervention in the elder's task performance: capacity versus actual behavior. *International Journal of Geriatric Psychiatry, 12*(9), 920–925.

Fulmer, T., Paveza, G., Vandeweerd, C., Fairchild, S., Guadagno, L., Bolton-Blatt, M., et al. (2005). Dyadic vulnerability and risk profiling for elder neglect. *The Gerontologist, 45*(4), 525–535.

Fulmer, T., Ramirez, M., Fairchild, S., Holmes, D., Koren, M. J., & Teresi, J. (1999). Prevalence of elder mistreatment as reported by social workers in a probability sample of adult day health care clients. *Journal of Elder Abuse & Neglect, 11*(3), 25–36.

Hines, P. M., & Boyd-Franklin, N. (2005). African American families. In M. McGoldrick, J. Giordano, & N. Garcia-Preto (Eds.), *Ethnicity & family therapy* (3rd ed., pp. 87–100). New York: Guilford Press.

Hudson, M. F., Armachain, W. D., Beasley, C. M., & Carlson, J. R. (1998). Elder abuse: Two Native American views. *Gerontologist, 38*(5), 538–548.

Hwalek, M., & Sengstock, M. (1986). Assessing the probability of abuse of the elderly: Towards the development of a clinical screening instrument. *Journal of Applied Gerontology, 5*, 153–173.

Jogerst, G. J., Daly, J. M., Dawson, J. D., Peek-Asa, C., & Schmuch, G. (2006). Iowa nursing home characteristics associated with reported abuse. *Journal of the American Medical Directors Association, 7*(4), 203–207.

Kennedy, R. (2005). Elder abuse and neglect: the experience, knowledge, and attitudes of primary care physicians. *Family Medicine, 37*(7), 481–485.

Lachs, M. (2008). What does "self-neglect" in older adults really cost? *Journal of the American Geriatrics Society, 56*(4), 757.

Lachs, M. S., Berkman, L., Fulmer, T., & Horwitz, R. (1994). A prospective community-based pilot study of risk factors for the investigation of elder mistreatment. *Journal of the American Geriatrics Society, 42*(2), 169–173.

McGoldrick, M. (2005). Irish families. In J. M. McGoldrick, J. Giordano, & N. Garcia-Preto (Eds.), *Ethnicity & family therapy* (3rd ed., pp. 596–615). New York: Guilford Press.

Mixon, P. M. (2000). Counterparts across time: Comparing the National Elder Abuse Incidence Study and the National Incidence Study of Child Abuse and Neglect. *Journal of Elder Abuse and Neglect, 12*(3/4), 19–27.

National Center on Elder Abuse. (2006). *Information about laws related to elder abuse* [Web Page]. URL http://www.ncea.aoa.gov/NCEAroot/Main_Site/Library/Laws/InfoAboutLaws_08_08.aspx [2009, August 26].

National Center on Elder Abuse. (2007). *Major types of elder abuse* [Web Page]. URL http://www.ncea.aoa.gov/ncearoot/Main_Site/FAQ/Basics/Types_Of_Abuse.aspx [2009, August 8].

National Institute of Justice. (2007). *Elder abuse as a criminal problem* [Web Page]. URL http://www.ojp.usdoj.gov/nij/topics/crime/elder-abuse/criminal-problem.htm [2009, August 4].

National Research Council. (2003). Elder mistreatment: Abuse, neglect, and exploitation in an aging America. R. J. Panel to Review Risk and Prevalence of Elder Abuse and Neglect. Bonnie, & R. B.

Wallace (Eds.). Committee on National Statistics and Committee on Law and Justice, Division of Behavioral and Social Sciences and Education. Washington, DC: The National Academies Press.

Neale, A., Hwalek, M., Goodrich, C., & Quinn, K. (1997). Reason for case closure among substantiated reports of elder abuse. *Journal of Applied Gerontology, 16*(4), 442–458.

O'Brien, J. G., Thibault, J. M., Turner, L. C., & Laird-Fick, H. S. (1999). Self-neglect: an overview and Self-neglect: challenges for helping professionals. *Journal of Elder Abuse & Neglect. II*(2), 1–19.

O'Connor, K., & Rowe, J. (2005). Elder abuse. *Reviews in Clinical Gerontology, 15,* 47–54.

Paranjape, A., Corbie-Smith, G., Thompson, N., & Kaslow, N. J. (2009). When older African American women are affected by violence in the home: a qualitative investigation of risk and protective factors. *Violence Against Women, 15*(8), 977–990.

Paranjape, A., Tucker, A., McKenzie-Mack, L., Thompson, N., & Kaslow, N. (2007). Family violence and associated help-seeking behavior among older African American women. *Patient Education and Counseling, 68*(2), 167–172.

Phillips, L., deArdon, E. T., & Briones, G. S. (2000). Abuse of female caregivers by care recipients: another form of elder abuse. *Journal of Elder Abuse and Neglect, 12*(3/4), 123–143.

Pickens, S., Burnett, J., Naik, A. D., Holmes, H. M., & Dyer, C. B. (2006). Is pain a significant factor in elder self-neglect? *Journal of Elder Abuse and Neglect, 18*(4), 51–61.

Quinn, K., & Zielke, H. (2005). Elder abuse, neglect, and exploitation: Policy issues. *Clinical Geriatric Medicine, 21*(2), 449–457.

Rabiner, D. J., O'Keeffe, J., & Brown, D. (2006). Financial exploitation of older persons: Challenges and opportunities to identify, prevent, and address it in the United States. *Journal of Aging and Social Policy, 18*(2), 47–68.

Renner, L. M., & Slack, K. S. (2006). Intimate partner violence and child maltreatment: understanding intra- and intergenerational connections. *Child Abuse and Neglect, 30*(6), 599–617.

Sanchez, Y. M. (1996). Distinguishing cultural expectations in assessment of financial exploitation. *Journal of Elder Abuse and Neglect, 8*(2), 49–59.

Schonfeld, L., Larsen, R. G., & Stiles, P. G. (2006). Behavioral health services utilization among older adults identified within a state abuse hotline database. *Gerontologist,46*(2), 193–199.

Straus, M. A. (1998). Conflict tactics scales: A short domestic violence screening tool for use in a family practice setting. In K. M. Sherin, J. M. Sinacore, Z. Q. Li, R. E Zitter, & A. Shakil (Eds.), *Family Medicine, 30,* 508–512.

Straus, M. A., & Gelles, R. (1992). National Family Violence Survey: Wife battering and violence outside the family. *Journal of Interpersonal Violence, 7,* 462–470.

Straus, M. A., Gelles, R. J., & Steinmetz, S. K. (2006). *Behind closed doors: Violence in the American family.* New Brunswick, NJ: Transaction Publishers.

The National Center on Elder Abuse at The American Public Human Services Association in Collaboration with Westat, I. (1998). *The National Elder Abuse Incidence Study: Final report.* Washington, DC: National Aging Information Center.

Thomas, C. (2000). The first national study of elder abuse and neglect: Contrast with results from other studies. *Journal of Elder Abuse and Neglect, 12*(3/4), 1–14.

Usita, P. M., Davis, J. C., & Hall, S. S. (2006). Caregiving conflict and relationship strategies of aging parents and adult children. In D. M. Devore (Ed.), *Parent–child relations: New research* (pp. 143–156). New York: Nova Science Publishers, Inc.

Wasson, J. H., Jette, A. M., Anderson, J., Johnson, D. J., Nelson, E. C., & Kilo, C. M. (2000). Routine, single-item screening to identify abusive relationships in women. *Jounal of Family Practice, 49*(11), 1017–1022.

Windawer, H., & Wetzel, N.A. (2005). German families. In M. McGoldrick, J. Giordano, & N. Garcia-Preto (Eds.), *Ethnicity & family therapy* (3rd ed., pp. 555–572). New York: Guilford Press.

Yeo, G. (2009). How will the U.S. healthcare system meet the challenge of the ethnogeriatric imperative? *Journal of the American Geriatrics Society, 57*(7), 1278–1285.

14

Legal and Forensic Nursing Responses
to Family Violence

Kathryn Laughon, PhD, RN
Angela Frederick Amar, PhD, RN
Daniel J. Sheridan, PhD, RN, FNE-A, FAAN
Sarah Anderson, PhD, RN, CEN, SANE-A

INTRODUCTION

Family violence, in all its forms, is a crime in every state in the United States. Regardless of whether it is child abuse, dating violence, intimate partner violence, elder abuse, or the abuse of vulnerable people with cognitive, mental health, or physical disabilities, it is a crime to push, slap, punch, kick, or injure anyone. Many forms of familial or institutional neglect are also potentially criminal in nature. Nurses encounter individuals who have experienced family violence. Some of these acts of violence may be investigated by law enforcement.

Forensic nurses address health care issues with a legal component. Forensic practice is part of holistic care by adding the legal issues that surround victims, perpetrators, and their families and significant others. Forensics pertains to the law and the courts; however, it is not limited to the criminal courts. While not every nurse is a trained forensic nurse, many nurses routinely encounter forensic issues in their practices. Nurses who work with survivors of family violence throughout the life cycle may be asked to collect evidence for and testify in a variety of courts, including criminal, family, guardianship, juvenile, and probate courts. This chapter introduces basic abuse-related legal definitions and provides an overview of the types of abuse commonly seen by forensic nurses and practice issues faced by nurses.

Overview of the Role of the Forensic Nurse

The role of the forensic nurse includes three broad areas: (1) provide thorough, competent, and compassionate care to patients who have experienced violence; (2) collect evidence and document findings in a manner that that allows for the use of the evidence and findings in the investigation and adjudication of a criminal case; and (3) testify about the facts

367

of the case and as an expert (Campbell, Patterson, & Lichty, 2005). To some extent, these aspects of the forensic role can be in conflict with each other. For example, the nurse's role as patient advocate could impair the nurse's ability to provide unbiased testimony in a criminal trial. Forensic nurses can best address the possibility of conflict in these roles by providing high-quality, patient-centered care and remaining as objective as possible. Forensic nurses should not think of themselves as "victim advocates" and should refer to the person for whom they are providing care as a patient, not a victim or survivor of violence. Competent nursing care always requires that nurses act in the best interests of their patients (not just forensic patients), so serving as a patient advocate does not present any conflict with other aspects of the nurses' role. Canaff (2009) makes the point that this sort of patient advocacy should be differentiated from victim advocacy. Nurses must collect evidence with the knowledge that this evidence will serve the criminal justice system, not just the prosecutors, remaining as objective and neutral as possible in their handling of the evidence and documentation of the findings. Finally, forensic nurses with a history of providing objective testimony in court, whether their testimony benefits the prosecution or defense in a particular case, will be seen as more credible than nurses biased in favor of the prosecution. Carefully objective, thoughtful forensic nursing care at all stages will ultimately provide the greatest benefit to survivors of violence.

The forensic role by definition implies interdisciplinary cooperation. In order to function effectively, forensic nurses work best within a coordinated community response team that includes representatives from the variety of legal, social service and health care agencies that serve victims of violence. Many communities have at least two different teams. Child abuse teams often examine policy issues as well as discussing specific open cases of suspected child abuse and neglect. Similar teams exist to assess for and intervene with abuse of disabled persons and elders. Sexual assault response teams work to provide a coordinated response among first responders. Membership in those teams by nurses is critical. Forensic nurses offer expertise in correctly interpreting the physical findings from forensic exams and ensure that the forensic nursing practices are meeting the legal and procedural standards of their community.

DEFINITIONS OF AND NURSING RESPONSES TO ABUSE AND NEGLECT

Child Maltreatment

Child maltreatment is the overarching category that includes all types of abuse and neglect (see chapters 4 and 10 for more detailed discussion of child maltreatment and chapter 9 for discussion of teen dating violence.) There are generally four categories: physical abuse, sexual abuse, emotional abuse, and neglect. Although Caffey first described child abuse in 1946, Kempe, Silverman, Steele, Droegmuuller, and Silver (1962) are credited with coining the phrase "battered child syndrome." In the 40 years since the salient work of Kempe et al. recognized abuse of children as a major public-health problem, in every state, laws have been enacted that not only make abuse of children illegal but also mandate health professionals, social-service workers, and teachers, to name a few, to report suspected abuse to county or state child protective agencies.

Despite efforts to drastically reduce child abuse, it is still endemic. There are more than three million referrals to child protective agencies annually with nearly a quarter of these cases substantiated (Administration of Children, Youth and Families, 2007). An estimated 1,760 children nationally died from abuse or neglect in 2006. (Administration of Children, Youth, and Families, 2007). It is generally believed that child abuse and neglect are grossly underreported.

Legal definitions of child abuse vary from state to state. However, the definitions are based on standard set by Federal and State laws so that there are enough similarities between states to discuss more generic, clinically useful definitions. For example, child abuse could be defined as physical injury of a child (under the age of 18) by a parent, household member, or other person who has permanent or temporary custody or responsibility for supervision of the child (Suggs, Lichenstein, McCarthy, & Jackson, 2001).

The Federal Child Abuse Prevention and Treatment Act defines child abuse and neglect as any recent act or failure to act on the part of a parent or caretaker that results in death, serious physical, or emotional harm, sexual abuse or exploitation, or that presents an imminent risk of serious harm.

Child Neglect

Although child abuse is much easier to identify because of visible trauma to the body, the Administrations of Children, Youth, and Families of the US Department of Health and Human Services (2007) indicates that child neglect is the most common form of child maltreatment. Underdiagnosis and underreporting of possible neglect is common because providers often attribute the neglectful behaviors to parental lack of resources or ignorance. It is much more difficult to measure neglect, especially of what appears to be minor neglect. Usually, only severe or life-threatening forms of neglect get reported to child protective services because overworked and short-staffed protective-service response systems only act immediately on the most severe of neglect cases.

Neglect, which can be physical, social, or emotional, often is defined in deprivational terms and involves actual or potential harm. Providers are often accused of failing to provide a needed item or service, or an act was omitted that resulted in actual or potential harm and that a parent or parent figure would reasonably have provided.

Neglect is reportable to child protective services anytime there is a failure on the part of the parent or person acting as parent to provide basic emotional support, food, clothing, shelter, or medical care. Actual harm does not need to have occurred for neglect to be reported (Suggs et al., 2001). Missing one pediatric appointment is usually not grounds for calling the protective-service hotline. However, a pattern of missed appointments without reasonable explanations can be an indication of a child at risk of harm.

Seldom is it clear which cases of possible neglect should be reported to protective services and which should not (Suggs et al., 2001). Most hospitals have created multidisciplinary teams, sometimes called Suspected Child Abuse and Neglect (SCAN) teams that meet on a regular basis to discuss reported cases of abuse and neglect and to review, as a group, possible neglect cases (Berkowitz, 2008). In-house SCAN team membership will vary among institutions; however, it is common to have at the table a pediatrician, registered nurse, social worker, therapists, hospital attorney, chaplain, and security officer. Representatives from local law enforcement, criminal prosecutors, and protective-service providers may also participate in the SCAN meetings. Community-based multidisciplinary teams that include forensic nurses exist in many communities as well.

Some examples of reportable medical neglect include but are not limited to failing to provide reasonable dental case, immunizations, ordered prescriptions or over-the-counter medication, needed eyeglasses, hearing aids, and assistive devices, such as a wheelchair. The most common perpetrators of child maltreatment are parents, most often women (Administration of Children, Youth, and Families, 2007). Maternal characteristics associated with child neglect include mother's age, mental illness, alcohol and drug use/abuse, and a severe lack of resources. Leaving a vulnerable child unattended or in an area where the child is at risk of harm is also neglect. This may include unintentionally leaving a 5-year-old home alone all day or having one's children living in a home where illegal drugs are manufactured or sold.

As with child abuse, the nurse does not need to prove that neglect has occurred before making a report to child protective services. Despite the less-than-clear guidelines that determine what constitutes neglect, it would be prudent for the nurse to report all cases of suspected neglect in accordance with their institutional guidelines. It is also important to consider all forms of child maltreatment as interrelated events.

Child and Adult Sexual Assault

Known or suspected child sexual assault is reportable as child abuse and usually receives a high-priority response from child protective services, especially if there are injuries or physical evidence consistent with sexual abuse. Sexual assault is not limited to penetration of body cavities. It also includes any form of sexual contact or behavior by an adult or sibling toward a child. Each legal jurisdiction has specific laws that define all the different types of child sexual abuse, from acts that are criminal misdemeanors to different levels of felonies. In general, sexual abuse includes any completed or attempted (non-completed) sexual act, sexual contact with, or exploitation (i.e., noncontact sexual interaction) of a child by a caregiver (Leeb, Paulozzi, Melanson, Simon, & Arias, 2008). In adults, sexual assault is any unwanted sexual contact obtained through force or threat (A National Protocol for Forensic Medical Exams, 2004). Different jurisdictions use a variety of terms and specific legal definitions, so nurses need to be familiar with their local laws.

Trained sexual assault nurse examiners (SANEs) can provide specialized medical forensic examinations of adults and children suspected of being sexually assaulted. The International Association of Forensic Nurses has an examination/certification examination for Adult and Pediatric Sexual Assault Examiners.

Many conditions mimic physical and child abuse, child neglect, and especially child sexual assault. Bays (2001) has written one of the most comprehensive chapters about conditions mistaken for child physical abuse that should be a must-read for any nurse who is part of the team assessing and documenting possible child abuse, child neglect, and child sexual assault. Girardin, Faugno, Seneski, Slaughter, and Whelan (1997) compiled an extensive collection of images of sexual assault-related trauma to adult patients.

Intimate Partner Violence

Intimate partner violence (IPV) is often described as physical, sexual, or psychological harm inflicted by a current or former partner or spouse (Basile, Hertz, & Back, 2007) (see chapter 3 for discussion of theories of IPV and chapter 5 for discussion of nursing practice with abused women; additional chapters in the book also address IPV with special groups, i.e., pregnant women, women with disabilities, etc.). This type of violence can occur among heterosexual or same-sex couples and does not require sexual intimacy (Sheridan, 2001). IPV is an all too common occurrence. In a recent report of over 70,000 respondents in over 18 US states and territories one in four women and one in seven men reported some form of IPV in their lifetimes. Women were not only significantly more likely to report abuse than were men, but they also were significantly more likely to report injury from IPV (Breiding, Black, & Ryan, 2009).

IPV or domestic violence, as it was first termed and is still referred to in the legal and law enforcement system, has existed for quite a long time; however, it came into public awareness during the women's movement. In 1967, the first shelter opened in Maine, and over the next decade, grassroots efforts spurred the development of many more shelters and programs in other parts of the country. Whereas emotional and financial abuse of an intimate partner is significant, it is usually not part of a forensic response. It is not illegal to call your partner degrading names. It is not against the law to control all assets within a family. It is, however, illegal to verbally threaten someone with bodily harm. It is a forensic matter when, during a divorce proceeding, one person fraudulently hides assets to keep the soon-to-be ex-partner from getting an equitable portion of the joint assets.

State laws determine how IPV is defined and legal recourse. Federal law, the Violence against Women Act, provides funds to states to augment investigation and prosecution efforts regarding violence against women and to increase pretrial detention of offenders. When domestic violence legislation was first written in the late 1970s and 1980s, most states adopted a series of civil protective orders designed to provide various legal safeguards to abused partners. These legal remedies are frequently called Domestic Restraining Orders or Orders of Protection. In many states, violating one of these civil protective orders can put the violator at risk of being arrested and charged with a crime. The protective orders can grant a variety of remedies to the abused person. In addition, for example, protective orders can give the victim temporary custody of the children, require the reported perpetrator to leave the home (temporarily), require the reported perpetrator to stay hundreds of feet away from the victim's home, workplace, or school, prohibit the reported perpetrator from harassing or interfering with the personal liberty of the victim, or any combination thereof. Over the past 25 years, the concept of protective orders has been expanded to provide additional legal protection to children and the elderly.

Nurses do not have to be expert in issues related to protective orders but should know how to refer patients for assistance in obtaining them. In addition, institutional policies should address how to manage patient-care issues related to protective orders (for example, when both parties are being treated in the same emergency department). Domestic violence advocates can accompany victims to court, provide education on the legal process, and assist with obtaining a protective order and safety planning. Nurses can have a role in working with experts in local laws and with their institutional administration to ensure that these policies are carefully crafted to ensure that both the safety and autonomy of patients, staff, and others are protected.

Elder Abuse

Definitions of what constitutes elder abuse and at what age one is considered elderly vary from state to state and from study to study (Geroff & Olshaker, 2001). In many states, "elders" are aged 65 and greater. It is important however for the nurse to become familiar with the specifics of the relevant state statutes. The terms elder "abuse" and elder "maltreatment" are often used interchangeably (see chapter 13 for more detailed discussion of elder mistreatment).

In 2002, the World Health Organization, in its report on violence and health, identified a variety of abuses and neglects inflicted on the elderly (Krug, Dahlberg, Mercy, Zwi, & Lozano, 2002). In general, elder abuse is divided into three categories:

- Elder physical and emotional abuse
- Neglect
- Financial exploitation

The plight of abused elders was first brought to the medical community's attention in the mid-1970s when two British medical journals published practice-based articles on "granny battering" (Baker, 1975; Burston, 1975). Elder abuse disproportionately affects women for two reasons. First, women live longer than men; thus, there are more women available to be abused. Second, a significant proportion of elder abuse is IPV grown older. Women battered by intimate partners in their 20s, 30s, 40s, and 50s become elder-abuse survivors in their 60s and older.

Elder abuse patients present with a variety of physical abuse and neglect symptoms, with many of the physical symptoms similar to naturally occurring underlying changes related to aging. Fractures that look traumatic in nature could be from underlying disease. What may appear, at a glance, to be severe (traumatic) bruising may in fact be a form of ecchymoses called senile purpura.

Anytime one suspects family violence in any of its forms, however, especially for possible elder abuse patients, it is prudent to ask the provider to obtain baseline lab values. Relatively common tests, such as a complete blood count with platelets, basic chemistry profile, coagulation panel, liver profile, and urinalysis, may provide evidence of malnutrition and dehydration. Grossly abnormal hematological findings may detract from a finding of abuse and support an underlying medical condition. As with the evaluation of suspected child abuse, the suspected elder abuse patient should receive a thorough radiographic evaluation to look for a pattern of multiple fractures in various stages of healing (Geroff & Olshaker, 2001). Pertinent findings on history and physical examination are shown in Exhibit 14.1.

Abuse of Vulnerable People With Disabilities

In recent years, states have begun to pass legislation making abuse and neglect against people with physical, cognitive, and mental health disabilities reportable to protective-service agencies. Many elder abuse reporting acts were expanded to include vulnerable people, or specific statutes were developed to address the abuse and neglect of vulnerable people (see chapter 7 for more detailed discussion on nursing care of women with disabilities who experience abuse).

The plight of these abused and neglected patients is often hidden behind closed doors of family homes, private homes, group homes, and institutions. In assessing for family violence throughout the life cycle, verbal histories from the victims are a key part of

EXHIBIT 14.1 | *Pertinent Findings on the History and Physical Examination*

PHYSICAL ABUSE AND NEGLECT
Patterned Injuries: Slap marks, fingertip-pressure bruises, rope, or ligature marks on wrists/ankles, bite marks, and immersion line
Bruises: Especially on areas of the body not over bony prominences, multiple stages of healing
Wounds: Laceration, abrasion, and puncture, especially if untreated or in various stages of healing; decubiti
Head injury: Traumatic alopecia and scalp swelling
Burns: Cigarette marks, scald burns with an immersion line, and absent satellite splash burns
Fractures: Spiral/oblique orientation without a given twisting mechanism, multiple fractures of difference ages, and mechanism not consistent with history
Subdural hematoma: From violent shaking with cerebral atrophy, as well as from direct blow
Nutrition: Dehydration, cachexia, weight loss, electrolyte abnormalities, and fecal impaction
Drug levels: Subtherapeutic or toxic, or presence of a drug not prescribed
Disease patterns: Untreated chronic disorders, excessive exacerbations of chronic disease
Poor hygiene: Filth, soiled with excrement, infestation, and dental caries
Personal effects: Inadequate clothing, shoes, glasses, hearing aid, and dentures
Living conditions: Fire hazard; infestation; inadequate heating, air conditioning, or plumbing

PSYCHOLOGICAL ABUSE AND NEGLECT
Communication: Ambivalence, withdrawal, poor eye contact, and cowering noncommunicative
Mood/affect: Agitation, depression, passivity, anxiety, and hopelessness
Behavior: Fear, apprehensiveness, shame, paranoia, and infantile behavior
Motor: Involuntary movement, rocking, sucking, and trembling
Psychosomatic: Poor appetite, disturbed sleep patterns, and posttraumatic stress disorder (may result from physical abuse as well)
Interactions: Caregiver insists on remaining with patient at all times and elder fearful of caregiver

SEXUAL ABUSE
Wounds: Located over breasts or genitalia
Infection: New sexually transmitted disease without reported sexual activity
Bleeding: Unexplained vaginal or anal bleeding
Pain/tenderness: Noticed during pelvic or rectal exam

ABANDONMENT
Institutional desertion: Leaving an elder at a hospital without means of return
Public desertion: Leaving an elder at a public location to be picked up by police or emergency medical service; homelessness

SELF-NEGLECT
Many of the above

most investigations. Very young children and the confused or comatose elderly are not able to verbalize what happened. Either most patients with cognitive and mental health disabilities are not verbal or their verbalizations are not necessarily credible from a legal perspective.

Evaluation of possible abuse and neglect is often based on a thorough review of care records, interviews with direct care givers, and, when available, a forensic review of injuries to help determine if the injuries are consistent (or not consistent) with the history of occurrence provided by the caretaker(s). A growing number of forensically trained advanced practice nurses provide abuse and neglect forensic consultation services to investigators of else and vulnerable person abuse.

MANDATORY REPORTING OF ABUSE

Children

All states have some form of mandatory reporting of suspected child abuse or neglect by a variety of people such as health professionals, police officers, social workers, and educators. Most of the reporting statutes protect the mandated reporter from being successfully sued if the report to child protective services was made in good faith and without malice. Failing to report child abuse can result in fines, notification of one's professional licensing board, or both.

Much controversy exists about reporting child abuse and neglect, especially when significant medical evidence supports the need to report. While critics argue that it produces many unsubstantiated reports, increasing workload for child protective services, wasting resources, and reducing the quality of service given to known deserving children and families, others feel that we should strengthen the mandate that suspicion of child abuse be reported by threatening prosecution for those who fail to report their concerns to the state child protective service agency (Berkowitz, 2008). Unfortunately, it is not unusual for providers to delay a call until they have more proof that abuse or neglect has taken place. However, the amount of evidence needed for mandatory reporting can vary from state to state. Some statutes indicate that one must call if there is reasonable cause to believe or a reasonable suspicion. Other statutes require the reporter to know that abuse has occurred, which requires a higher degree of knowledge. Most reporting statutes clearly state that one most call the child protective service hotline if one has reasonable cause to suspect abuse may have occurred. Any consideration about whether one should call signifies reasonable cause to report.

Child protective services hotlines vary by location. Many states have established a county-by-county notification system, whereas others have a statewide, central hotline that prioritizes all calls before forwarding approved cases to the appropriate county investigative system. In such systems, children who are deemed at greatest risk are seen and evaluated before those deemed at lower risk. However, children considered at great risk but hospitalized in a controlled environment may be deemed less at risk than the child's siblings who are still in the home.

Hotline numbers should be prominently posted somewhere in the treatment area of every healthcare setting and in the child abuse/neglect policy and procedure. Notification of the child protective services hotline can be delegated to a designated person. The designated individual then investigates further and makes the appropriate report, eliminating duplicate reporting from multiple individuals within the system. The original reporter is always available to provide additional information, if needed. It is, of course, always possible for a nurse to directly report to the outside agency as well, if he or she deems that necessary.

Anytime the nurse calls the hotline or notifies the designated person, he or she should document the following in the progress note:

• The reason for the call
• The time of the call
• The full name of the person who took the call
• The response of the child-protective service worker to the call if known to the nurse (i.e. accepted or not accepted)

The telephone report is usually to be made within 24 hours and the written report filed within 72 hours. Despite the laws, many nurses feel uncomfortable with mandatory reporting fearing that it disrupts the nurse–client relationship or otherwise have concerns about engendering anger and mistrust. It is important that providers view mandatory reporting as the first step to assisting victims and their families to get help, resources, and support. In addition, many states have penalties for failing to report suspected child abuse or neglect. Nurses can make the report in a collaborative way with the family member if circumstances allow. In that case, the nurse would let the family member know that he or she felt that a report was necessary and would explain that this is a way for the family to get needed support. The report can be made by the family member with the nurse present, and the nurse can provide additional information, or the nurse can make the report directly after discussing it with the family. Although this is not always an appropriate procedure, this collaborative approach can be helpful in maintaining the family's trust and in framing the family's response to the ensuing investigation.

When suspected abused and neglected children are in the treatment area, some states allow certain professionals to take emergency, temporary protective custody. In some states, only the child protective service worker can take temporary custody; in others, a police officer can also take custody of the child. In addition, some states allow physicians to take emergency, temporary custody of children, especially if it is thought that the child will be removed from the health facility by possibly abusive or neglectful parents before the police or child protective services arrive.

When the decision has been made to call child protective services, it is recommended that the parents be notified of the decision if it is believed that notifying them does not place the child, mandated reporter, or other staff and patients at risk. While not all states have mandated reporting of elder abuse, all states have legislation that allows for protection of the elderly from harm. The first agency to respond to a report of elderly abuse, in most states, is Adult Protective Services (APS). The role of APS is to investigate abuse cases, intervene, and offer services and advice. As with mandatory reporting of child abuse, the reporter does not have to have proof that elder maltreatment occurred before one's mandate to report is triggered. All that is needed to report elder maltreatment is reasonable cause to suspect abuse or neglect (physical, emotional, or financial) might have occurred. Most elder abuse mandatory reporting statutes provide immunity from being sued as long the report was made in good faith without malice. Like child abuse, in most states, failing to report suspected or known elder abuse can result in a fine, sometimes brief jail time, and notification of one's professional licensing board.

Intimate Partner Violence

Few states mandate reporting of IPV against a competent adult; however, some do. In most states, a police notification requirement for domestic abuse is limited to patients with injuries from a weapon, such as a gun, knife, or other deadly object.

Some states have enacted mandatory reporting of IPV by health care workers. Battered women's advocates have voiced concern that mandatory reporting of domestic violence places abused women, the largest percentage of abused intimates, at further risk of harm because of possible retaliation by the abuser. In a case-controlled study of more than 200 abused women, almost 50% preferred it be the women's decision to call the police, and about 66% of the abused women voiced concerns that mandatory reporting to police by health professionals would prevent women from disclosing the true nature of the their injuries (Gielen et al., 2000). In states without mandatory reporting requirements, reporting IPV without the patient's consent is a violation of the patient's right to confidentiality in the healthcare setting. In those states, the only times a nurse would make a police report without patient consent are those that involve a minor, a vulnerable adult, or injuries involving weapons.

The nurse needs to know if he or she is practicing in a state that has mandatory reporting of all forms of IPV. The controversy over mandatory reporting should not prevent the nurse from conducting routine screening for abuse using reliable and valid assessment tools. Not screening and documenting IPV in the health record may place the nurse and the healthcare institution at risk of civil suit for failing to provide a minimal standard of care. Effective tools such as the Abuse Assessment Screen and the Danger Assessment may be useful in screening for abuse (Soeken, McFarlane, Parker, & Lominack, 1998; Campbell, 1995).

EXAMINATION OF THE FORENSIC PATIENT

Before beginning the examination of the patient, the nurse should first ensure that patient's needs for comfort and safety are addressed. Patients may wish to have an advocate present, either in the form of a friend or family member who provides support and/or a trained advocate from a local service agency. The assailant may have accompanied the patient, so safety assessments should first be conducted without friends or family members present.

The first part of any examination is to explain to the patient all of the steps in the process. In the case of very young children, the detailed explanation is better directed toward the adult who accompanies the child, with brief, developmentally appropriate information given to the child. After obtaining all of the necessary consents, nurses initially obtain a basic health history and a history of the assault that will be used to guide the examination and evidence collection. Assessment of injuries should follow a head-to-toe procedure, with the genital exam, if necessary, occurring last. The nurse collects evidence in a similarly systematic manner to ensure that no steps are omitted. Nurses should follow their local protocols to ensure that documentation of injuries and collection and preservation of evidence occur in accordance with local laws and standards. There is a National Protocol for Sexual Assault Forensic Exams (2004), and many states have developed their own protocols.

Adult and adolescent patients presenting for a sexual assault examination within 72 hours of the assault should presumptively be offered prophylaxis for sexually transmitted infections (STIs) and pregnancy (emergency contraception). STI prophylaxis for children should be assessed on a case by case basis accord as should post-exposure prophylaxis (PEP) for HIV in patients of all ages. Guidance on PEP can be obtained through the National Clinicians' Post-Exposure Prophylaxis clinician's hotline: 888-448-4911. The most recent postassault prophylaxis guidelines are available at http://www.cdc.gov/std/treatment/. Testing for STIs is generally not performed at the time of the examination unless medically indicated. Patients should be instructed to follow up with their health care providers in 2 weeks for pregnancy and STI testing and instructed not to engage in sexual intercourse until treatment has been completed, and they have tested negative for infections. Patients receiving PEP will need additional follow-up. If possible, nurses can ask for permission to contact the clinic or clinician who will be providing follow-up to ensure that there is no delay in initiating follow up care.

Patients and, if appropriate, their families should be provided with information about local mental health and advocacy resources. This may include information on the local agency serving survivors of sexual assault, the local battered women's hotline and shelter, family support services, and free and low-cost legal services. As patients may find the amount of information they receive to be overwhelming, patients should also receive appropriate written materials that they can refer to at a later time.

DOCUMENTATION OF THE FORENSIC EXAM

Documentation of the forensic examination should be both written and photographic.

Written Documentation

Typically, written documentation is twofold: the forensic documentation that is specific to the forensic exam and the usual nursing documentation for the clinical site. The forensic documentation includes the health history related to the forensic exam, description of the assault and the patient's activities after the assault, the examination findings, a record of the evidence collected, and documentation of the examination findings. The usual nursing documentation will include the standard features of all nursing documentation (i.e., presenting complaint, health history, findings, treatment, and follow-up care). The standard documentation should note that a forensic examination was completed and include the referrals made.

The documentation should be as objective and complete as possible, including verbatim statements made by the patient. For example, it is better to document the specific terms used by the patient for body parts (e.g., "thing," "privates," etc.) rather than substitute the specific anatomical terms. Avoid words that can sound judgmental such as "patient claims." Use "patient states" instead. Body maps of both the full body and close-up maps of the genitalia are very useful in documenting injuries. The documentation should include labeled drawings of the injuries that provide size, location, and type of injury. Remember that forms that have not been approved by your institution will likely not be retained in medical records, so documentation should occur only on approved forms.

The nurse may be called into legal proceedings as a fact or expert witness. The fact witness has direct experience in the events that precipitated the legal case and is called to report the facts of the case. The expert witness is called into the legal proceedings due to knowledge, expertise, or skills that are consequential to one side of the case. The expert witness provides a report detailing expert testimony, provides an opinion on the case, and may be called for deposition or trial.

Use of Hearsay Evidence

Hearsay evidence is not specific to the nursing response to abuse but is important enough to merit particular attention as nurses consider how and what they document during the examination. *Hearsay* is defined as "a statement, other than one made by the declarant while testifying at the trial or hearing, offered in evidence to prove the truth of the matter asserted" (Federal Rule of Evidence 801(c). An understanding of hearsay is important to the forensic nurse, as hearsay evidence can play a role in the adjudication of abuse cases. In the case of child abuse, hearsay evidence may be introduced to avoid the need for the child to testify in court (Redlich, Myers, Goodman, & Qin, 2002). This can be because of the child's age or because it is thought that testifying is potentially too traumatizing for the child. Hearsay evidence may also be used in cases of elder abuse, sexual assault, or IPV if the victim is unavailable to testify or if the prosecution is moving forward without the active cooperation of the victim.

Hearsay is not generally admissible in court, as the actual speaker is then not available to be cross-examined in court. There are, however, exceptions to the hearsay rule. The exemptions most commonly used in forensic cases are the "excited utterance," statements made to health care professionals for diagnosis and treatment, and "residual" exceptions. In addition to meeting the criteria for the exceptions named above and described below, statements must not be "testimonial". In other words, the patient should not believe that statements are made for the purpose of investigating or prosecuting a criminal matter. For example, statements made to a detective about events resulting in injury that occurred during a sexual assault would be considered "testimonial" in almost all cases, as the patient would understand that the detective is asking these questions for the purpose of investigating a criminal matter. The same information elicited by the nurse without the detective may be admissible under one of the exceptions described below.

An "excited utterance" [Federal Rule of Evidence 803(2)] is a statement made soon after a "startling event." Statements made to health care professionals for the purpose of diagnosis and treatment can also be treated as exceptions to the hearsay rule. The residual exception (Federal Rule of Evidence 807) can be used to bring in any hearsay evidence not allowed under other exceptions if it is deemed that the evidence would be useful in understanding the facts of the case and its introduction will serve the interests of justice. This rule is particularly useful in bringing in statements made by children and elders. In all cases, the nurse should again carefully document the statements themselves and the context in which they were made, as it will be necessary to establish the trustworthiness of the testimony before it is admitted.

Nurses with forensic practice should review their local laws and procedures with local prosecutors and legal advisors. While most jurisdictions have adopted the federal rules of evidence into their codes, there are some variations.

Forensic Photography

Photographs can be taken with many different types of cameras. A high-resolution digital single lens reflex camera with a macrolens feature (or the ability to take pictures 1:1) and LCD screen provides pictures that can be viewed immediately for accuracy and technique. By reviewing digital photographs immediately, this allows the examiner to obtain additional photographs if the ones taken are not representative of the injuries seen.

In order for digital images to be admissible in court, they must be saved in the original format that the photographs were taken in. Any changes to the images in resolution, use of filters, or cropping require disclosure in order to be used. The main areas of concern that must be addressed when considering the use of forensic digital images in court are image enhancement, image restoration, and image compression.

When taking pictures, it is important to take an overview or full-body picture, an orientation or medium range shot, and then a close-up of the area emphasized. All close-up photographs should be taken with and without a scale in the picture. Care should be taken to make sure that the scale is held parallel to and in the same plane as the injury and the camera.

Since injury patterns may change over time in appearance and size, it is sometimes necessary to have the victim return 24–48 hours later to repeat photographs. Often bruises are more pronounced, and injury patterns can be easier to identify as time passes. When acute genital trauma is suspected, a repeat photographic examination can help discern whether the findings observed during the initial examination have changed or remained the same after allowing time for healing. A finding that does not change over time may indicate a non-acute injury or normal finding.

In summary, family violence is a crime that necessitates the consideration of forensic aspects of nursing care. An understanding of the legal aspects of abuse assists the nurse in planning care and referrals. As many laws are dictated by the states and may vary from state to state, nurses must identify state statutes that are relevant to practice. Careful and systematic assessment and collection of evidence coupled with documentation of the forensic evaluation are necessary for the legal aspects of patient care.

REFERENCES

Baker, A. A. (1975). Granny battering. *Modern Geriatrics, 5*(8), 20–24.

Basile, K. C., Hertz, M. F., & Back, S. E. (2007). Intimate partner violence and sexual violence victimization assessment instruments for use in healthcare settings: Version 1. Atlanta, GA: Centers for Disease Control and Prevention, National Center for Injury Prevention and Control.

Bays, J. (2001). Conditions mistaken for child physical abuse. In R. M. Reece & S. Ludwig (Eds.), *Child abuse: Medical diagnosis and management* (pp. 177–206). Philadelphia, PA: Lippincott Williams & Wilkins.

Berkowitz, C. D. (2008). Child abuse recognition and reporting: Supports and resources for changing the paradigm. *Pediatrics, 122*(Suppl. 1), 510–512.

Breiding, M. J., Black, M. C., & Ryan, G. W. (2009) Prevalence and risk factors of intimate partner violence in eighteen U.S. states/territories. *American Journal of Preventive Medicine, 34*(2), 112–118.

Burston, G. R. (1975). Granny-battering. *British Medical Journal, 3*, 592.

Campbell, J. C. (1995). Prediction of homicine of and by battered women. In J. C. Campbell (Ed.), *Assessing dangerousness: Violence by sexual offenders, batterers, and child abusers* (pp. 96–113). Thousand Oak, CA: Sage Publications.

Campbell, R., Patterson, D., & Lichty, L. F. (2005). The effectiveness of sexual assault nurse examiner (SANE) program: A review of psychological, medical, legal, and community outcomes. *Trauma, Violence, & Abuse: A Review Journal*, 6(4), 313–329.

Canaff, R. (2009). Nobility in objectivity: A prosecutor's case for neutrality in forensic nursing. *Journal of Forensic Nursing*, 5(2), 89–96.

Geroff, A. J., & Olshaker, J. S. (2001). Elder abuse. In J. S. Olshaker, M. C. Jackson, & W. S. Smock (Eds.), *Forensic emergency medicine* (pp. 173–202). Philadelphia, PA: Lippincott Williams & Wilkins.

Gielen A. C., O'Campo, P. J., Campbell, J. C., Schollenberger, J., Woods, A. B., Jones, A. S., et al. (2000). Women's opinions about domestic violence screening and mandatory reporting. *American Journal of Preventative Medicine*, 19(4):279–285.

Girardin, B. W., Faugno, D. K., Seneski, P. C., Slaughter, L., & Whelan, M. (1997). *Color atlas of sexual assault*. St. Louis, MO: Mosby.

Kempe, C. H., Silverman, F. N., Steele, B. F., Droegmueller, W., & Silver, H. K. (1962). The battered-child syndrome. *Journal of the American Medical Association*, 181(1), 17–24.

Krug, E.G., Dahlberg, L. L., Mercy, J. A., Zwi, A. B., & Lozano, R., (2002) World report on violence and health. Geneva: World Health Organization.

Leeb, R. L., Paulozzi, L. J., Melanson, C., Simon, T. R., & Arias, I. (2008). Child maltreatment surveillance: Uniform definitions for public health and recommended data elements. Atlanta: Centers for Disease Control and Prevention.

Leeb, R. T., Melanson, C., Simon, T., & Arias, I. (2008) Child maltreatment surveillance: uniform definitions for public health and recommended data elements, Version 1.0. Atlanta: Centers for Disease Control and Prevention, National Center for Injury Prevention and Control.

Redlich, A. D., Myers, J. E. B., Goodman, G. S., & Qin, J. (2002). A comparison of two forms of hearsay in child sexual abuse cases. *Child Maltreatment*, 17, 312–328.

Sheridan, D. J. (2001). Treating survivors of intimate partner abuse. In J. S. Olshaker, M.C. Jackson, & W. S. Smock (Eds.), *Forensic emergency medicine* (pp. 203–228). Philadelphia, PA: Lippincott Williams & Wilkins.

Soeken, K. L., McFarlane, J., Parker, B., & Lominack, M. C. (1998). The abuse assessment screen: A clinical instrument to measure frequency, severity and perpetrator of abuse against women. In J. C. Campbell (Ed.), *Empowering survivors of abuse: Health care for battered women and their children* (pp. 195–203). Thousand Oaks: Sage Publications.

Suggs, A., Lichenstein, R., McCarthy, C., & Jackson, M. C. (2001). Child abuse/assault-General. In J. S. Olshaker, M. C. Jackson & W. S. Smock (Eds.), *Forensic emergency medicine* (pp. 151–171). Philadelphia, PA: Lippincott Williams & Wilkins.

15

Family Violence and Ethics

Colleen Varcoe, RN, PhD
Rochelle Einboden, MN, RN

INTRODUCTION

Taking an ethical lens to the issue of family violence draws attention to individual and social values that underlie nursing and health care responses to violence. These values have implications for how violence is understood, how health care providers intervene with individuals, how health care providers participate in the wider social response to violence, and what are considered to be the morally relevant issues. In this chapter, we use a relational theoretical perspective. Drawing on a relational approach to ethics helps to analyze how power dynamics operate within broad social contexts shaped by inequities based on gender, class, racism, and other intersecting differences. This theoretical perspective also is congruent with the moral obligations of nursing, particularly with nursing's commitments to uphold autonomy, respect, confidentiality, and social justice. This chapter is designed to assist nurses to use an ethical lens to consider various forms of violence, to identify key ethical issues, and to develop ethical nursing practice in relation to violence.

Providing nursing care to people who have experienced family violence involves multiple ethical issues. How do nurses understand the "choices" that people who are victims of violence appear to make, and can nurses always respect those choices? How do nurses reconcile ethical obligations that are in conflict with organizational mandates or legal obligations? How do nurses navigate ethical obligations when these are in conflict with accepted practice norms? In the context of family violence, how do nurses balance their obligations to protect people from harm and the obligation to respect autonomy? What do nurses do when respecting the autonomy of one person may endanger another person? What are nurses' ethical obligations to perpetrators of violence? How do nurses practice ethically when they do not know who is being abused by whom? What obligations do nurses have toward ending family violence at a social and structural level?

A Relational Approach to Ethics

"Relational" refers to how people and their contexts or environments are constantly shaping one another. Nursing practice is never enacted by individual nurses making independent decisions—rather, nurses act, taking into account all the patients for whom they are providing care at any given moment (Who and what is the immediate priority?), their colleagues (Who is on lunch break? How much help does the more junior nurse need?), and the context (How busy is the practice setting? How much time do I have? What are the policies? What is "usual" practice?). Relational ethics is a form of contextual ethics that focuses on individuals in relationships with others, within specific contexts (Sherwin, 1998b; Whatmore, 1997). Moral decision making is recognized as embedded in the moral agents who deliberate and also embedded within the context of a moral environment. Using a relational approach to consider the ethics of nursing practice draws attention to the contexts within which nurses and patients live and to the relationships among people (Rodney, Brown, & Liaschenko, 2004). Nurses' ability to enact professional values will be influenced by the knowledge and attitudes of other health care providers and the "ethical climate" in the particular setting. Ethical climate is an aspect of organizational climate and refers to shared values and support for ethical decision making in an organization. McDaniel (1998), Olson (1995, 2002), and Schluter, Winch, Holzhauser, and Henderson (2008) argue that an ethical climate that is congruent with professional nursing values is required to support professional nursing practice.

A relational approach to ethics emphasizes power relations. This is of particular importance to family violence, as it involves significant abuses of power. The significance, intensity, and complexity of family relationships are not taken into account in traditional ethical approaches because they focus on individual moral actors acting independently and because they assume equal opportunity to act for all moral agents (Applebaum, 2004; Benhabib, 1992; Donchin, 1995, 2001; Sherwin, 1998a). A relational approach to moral decision making accords relevance to social and personal histories, positioning, narratives, and situated understandings. Relational ethics includes recognition that, rather than being objective and rational, ethical decision making is always influenced by varied perspectives, values, and biases, some of which dominate because of power differences. Thus, a relational approach provides ethical guidance that appreciates relative power in relationships both within families, within and among professions, and in the broader social context.

Relational ethics has important implications for nursing. Such a perspective draws attention to how nursing care is provided to people within a nexus of power relations that simultaneously constrains and enables nurses to enact professional values. A relational approach also focuses attention on the ethical aspects of the nurse–patient relationship. Bergum (2004) argues that viewing ethical action from the perspective of the nurse–patient relationship moves our thinking away from theories and problems, toward the moral space created by one's relation to oneself and to another. She claims that this relational space is the location of enacting morality and that nurses need to consider ethics in every situation, every encounter, and with every patient. If all relationships are the focus of understanding and examining moral life, she says, then, in order to practice ethically, it is important to attend to the *quality* of relationships in all nursing practices, whether with patients and their families, with other nurses, with other healthcare professionals, administrators, or politicians.

This perspective illustrates the centrality of relationships to nursing practice and how the ability to enact nursing care arises from a foundation of being in relation with another. Careful attention to the voices and narratives of patients is essential to ethical nursing practice but remains as one of the most challenging aspects of practice. Young (1997) warns that attempts to understand another person are always clouded by one's own lens; thus, even expert nurses must continuously struggle with how to authentically engage with patients in the context of multiple intersections of power. Using this perspective also directs nurses to consider the relationship between their values and actions, and how these affect their relationships with patients, whether violence is identified as an issue or not and whether nurses are caring for people who are victims or perpetrators of violence.

REFLEXIVITY. The concept of reflexivity is essential to the enactment of relational ethics. Reflexivity depends on our ability to challenge objectivity, knowledge, fact, evidence, and truth, encouraging a rigorous analysis of these both generally and in specific contexts. "Acting reflexively means that practitioners will subject their own and others' knowledge claims and practices to analysis. Knowledge, in particular, becomes not simply a resource to be deployed in practice but a topic which is worthy of scrutiny" (Taylor & White, 2001, p. 55). The process of how we have come to know or understand a situation is entirely relevant, as are the actions we take in particular contexts, as those actions effect the context, our relationships and others and their reactions, which in turn shape how we come to understand the situation, perhaps differently (Houston & Griffiths, 2000). For example, a nurse speaking to a colleague about a woman returning for care repeatedly in relation to the health consequences of abuse from her partner can speak about the woman in a judgmental way ("What an idiot, why does she keep going back?") or more respectful way ("I'm glad she felt comfortable enough to come back") with different effects on the colleague's perspective.

Dialogue is central to the process of reflexivity. Engaging in reflexive approaches requires a commitment to creating opportunities for reflection and dialogue to consider the complexity and specificity of individuals, relationships, and contexts. Furthermore, analysis of the language we use is integral to reflexive dialogue. Philosopher Habermas illustrates the complexity of language and its relationship with truth when he "argues that truth can be apprehended only through an analysis of how people communicate about truth" (Houston, 2003, p. 62). Assumptions of linguistic neutrality are rejected, and a closer analysis of discourse illustrates how language presents a particular construction or interpretation of the world, one that is heavily influenced by the relative power, understandings, and purposes of the narrator, or those engaged in dialogue (Potter, 1996; Taylor & White, 2001). The language related to family violence has been much debated, with some arguing that terms such as "family violence" and "intimate partner violence" obscure the gendered nature of such violence, whereas other terms such as "domestic violence" minimize the gravity of the problem (Marcus, 1994). Terms such as "battered woman" or "abused woman" can be used in ways that reduce people to their experiences of violence, whereas use of the term "victim" can draw attention away from a person's agency and resistance. Reflexively examining language and how it is used is critical in relation to family violence—doing so can help uncover what values are operating, including who and what are valued. In sum, reflexive approaches offer rich guidance for nurses because they encourage not only consideration of *what* one ought to do but also consideration of how one thinks and speaks and the nuances of *how* one ought to practice.

Ethical Practice and Nursing

Codes of ethics provide one source of guidance for ethical nursing practice. Although such codes have been critiqued (e.g., Bekemeier & Butterfield, 2005; Pattison, 2001; Reimer

Kirkham & Browne, 2006), they represent statements of shared values and obligations developed by professional nursing bodies and, as such, offer a starting point for considering nurses' ethical obligations. For the purposes of this chapter, we draw primarily upon the Code of Ethics published by the American Nurses Association (2001), the Canadian Nurses Association (2008), and the International Council of Nurses (ICN) (2005), and an analysis of the common moral obligations of nurses as articulated in the ICN, UK, Irish and Polish Codes of Ethics for nurses (Dobrowolska, Wronska, Fidecki, & Wysokinski, 2007).

COMPETENCE. A commonly agreed upon obligation is that nursing practice should be *competent*—that is, nursing practice should be based on knowledge, and nurses are responsible for continuously learning and maintaining their competence. In the context of family violence, achieving competence is particularly challenging because (a) family violence as a field of study is relatively new, and as previous chapters have illustrated, evidence, particularly regarding what constitutes effective intervention, is limited and (b) family violence is poorly understood in society and misunderstandings, assumptions, and myths predominate. For example, as argued in chapter 5, although there is considerable evidence regarding how social (e.g., expectations for women regarding marriage), economic (e.g., economic dependence for women), and personal historical (e.g., histories of child maltreatment) limit women's options for dealing with intimate partner violence (IPV), practice is often based on assumptions that women can choose to leave abusive partners. Nursing practice based on violence in relation to family violence requires that nurses challenge social myths and their own assumption and continuously strive to acquire the best evidence possible, including evidence derived from the growing body of literature. Seeing competence through a relational perspective draws attention to the interdependence of various health care providers. Although individuals are responsible for their own knowledge and practice, competent, ethical care arises from teams of health care providers, rather than from individuals alone.

PROMOTING HEALTH AND WELL-BEING. In general, most codes promote the idea that nursing is *oriented toward health and well-being* of people. Although most codes do not use the term "harm," there is an implicit intention for nurses to prevent or minimize harm as it interferes with the promotion of health and well-being. The idea of promoting health is central to nursing practice but is particularly challenging in relation to family violence because the dominant social responses in Western societies may eclipse concerns for health and well-being. For example, in relation to sexual assault, concern with forensic evidence may overshadow concerns for the victim's welfare; sexual assault may be equated with "stranger assault" of young women, obscuring sexual assault of elderly persons and sexual assault within intimate relationships. From a relational vantage point, promotion of health and well-being requires the involvement of patients themselves (who must have, among other things, the opportunity to describe what well-being means to them), multiple service providers, and those in the wider context of the patient's life.

AUTONOMY AND INFORMED CONSENT. *Informing* the patient and obtaining *consent for care* is also a commonly accepted value and is closely related to the idea of *autonomy*. Autonomy, also referred to as self-determination and choice, is integral to nursing practice in relation to all forms of family violence. For example, staying with an abusive intimate partner is often perceived as a *choice* and questioned by care providers and considered a *poor choice* (Dunn & Powell-Williams, 2007), particularly if the woman has dependent children. Care givers often face the challenge of wanting to protect a victim in opposition to his or her wishes. Viewing consent and autonomy from a relational perspective draws attention to how all people enact their choices in light of their relations with other people and within particular contexts, emphasizing how power operates along intersecting lines such as gender, race, and class. Analyzing the concept of autonomy from a relational perspective, Canadian feminist ethicist Susan Sherwin (1998b) illustrates how "autonomy language is often used to hide the workings of privilege and mask the barriers of oppression" (p. 25). This argument is important to nursing in relation to family violence for at least two reasons. First, if nurses see the autonomy of patients in a decontextualized manner, they fail to account for the limits to autonomy created by social position and circumstances. In the absence of an awareness of structural disadvantages and oppression, the language of autonomy encourages people to focus on individual accomplishment and, as such, can promote blaming of less-well-situated people (for example, those constrained by disability or poverty) for their circumstances. Thus, nurses and other health care providers can dismiss the plight of certain groups of people by resorting to the language of choice (women "choose" to stay with abusive partners). Second, Sherwin argues that the illusion of "choice" in the context of informed consent can operate as a mechanism to insure compliance with care providers' preferences. For example, Varcoe (2001) reported that nurses in emergency units often dismissed as "undeserving" women who had been offered help, but failed to comply with health care providers' ideas of what should be done (such as call the police, and leave the partner). Sherwin says

> "Unless we find a way of identifying in a deeper sense of autonomy than that associated with the expression of individual preference in selecting among a limited set of similar options, we run the risk of struggling to protect not patient autonomy but the very mechanisms that insure compliant medical consumers, preoccupied with the task of selecting among a narrow range of treatments." (p. 29)

DIGNITY AND RESPECT. Codes of Ethics commit nurses to attend to values of human *dignity and respect*. For example, the ICN Code of Ethics states that "Inherent in nursing is respect for human rights, including cultural rights, the right to life and choice, to dignity and to be treated with respect." While some codes specify that nursing's primary obligation is to those people requiring nursing care, or "patients," it generally is clear that nurses are expected to accord all persons with dignity and respect. Various codes specify that respect is accorded to persons regardless of particular characteristics. For example, ICN states that "nursing care is respectful of and unrestricted by considerations of age, color, creed, culture, disability or illness, gender, sexual orientation, nationality, politics, race or social status." This obligation can be particularly challenging, as we will discuss, when providing care to suspected or known perpetrators of family violence.

PRIVACY AND CONFIDENTIALITY. Closely related to dignity and respect is the obligation for nurses to maintain *privacy* and *confidentiality*. Taking a relational perspective brings into view the fact that maintaining privacy and confidentiality requires the commitment and participation of many people, and highlights that organizational contexts, including policies and processes, shape how it is possible to do so. For example, emergency nurses in one study were observed to share dramatic details regarding abused women's situations with a wide range of others, such as ambulance attendants, clerks, and physicians not involved in the women's care (Varcoe, 2001). Limits to confidentiality are usually defined in relation to decisions about patient competence and safety. In Canada, the United States, and several other nations, mandatory reporting laws override professional obligations for confidentiality when violence against a child is suspected; in some jurisdictions, there are laws that mandate the reporting of elder abuse, and in other jurisdictions, including six states in the United States (Feddock, Pursley, O'Brien, Griffith, & Wilson, 2009), reporting of IPV is mandatory. In many contexts, what is considered to be child maltreatment is extended formally under law or informally in practice to encompass witnessing violence against a parent (usually a mother). As we elaborate later, these are very complex situations because the harm that might arise from maintaining confidentiality versus breaking confidentiality is very difficult to anticipate. Humphreys (2008) identifies three problem areas related to mandatory reporting of children exposed to IPV: (a) the problem of responding to a widespread social problem through an individualized response at the tertiary end of provision rather than a focus on prevention, (b) the problem that such reporting can undermine the voluntary and empowerment model of intervention found effective for women through compulsory, statutory intervention with children, and (c) the problem of creating a mandatory pathway to an intervention system, which is not set up to work simultaneously with an adult and child victim or intervene effectively with men who use violence. A relational perspective directs critical evaluation of individuals' competence and safety contextually. Thus, in any given situation, nurses must ask how they might maintain confidentiality within the parameters of laws in particular contexts, seek to limit sharing of information without the person's permission, and disclose fully the limits to confidentiality imposed by legal obligations. Furthermore, nurses must seek the best evidence available regarding how the health and well-being of all persons might be best served and participate in wider social processes (such as legislative reform) to promote the most ethical legal approaches.

JUSTICE. Finally, many codes include a commitment to *justice*. However, as Bekemeier and Butterfield (2005) have argued in the United States, and Reimer Kirkham and Browne (2006) have argued in Canada, what is meant by justice and the extent to which professional bodies commit nurses to social justice are highly variable. In general, justice refers to fairness among groups; social justice is concerned with inequities that are due to unfair social arrangements, recognizes that all groups do not have "equal opportunity" and is concerned with inequities that are potentially remedial (Whitehead & Dahlgren, 2006; Young, 1990). The CNA Code of Ethics (Canadian Nurses Association, 2008) identifies "promoting justice" as one of seven primary nursing values, explaining that "Nurses uphold principles of justice by safeguarding human rights, equity and fairness and by promoting the public good." However, the Code separates this obligation to uphold "justice" as a notion of fairness between individuals, from "social justice" as a wider concern with social inequities, reflecting different understandings about what justice means. In societies fraught with inequalities based on income and racism (including countries such as those in the UK, Canada, and the United States), fairness is routinely undermined, including how laws are applied unfairly and unevenly by race, gender, class, and other forms of difference.

LIMITATIONS OF CODES OF ETHICS. Codes are considered a tool to support professionals in resolution of ethical dilemmas—that is, when two or more values or principles conflict, and one value or principle must be given priority to guide action and resolution. However, codes rarely advise nurses on how to balance competing values or principles. Pattison (2001) has argued that codes are inadequate and fail to offer helpful ethical guidance because they often use inexact and confusing terms, advance arbitrary values, and principles, and often exclude ordinary moral experience. Similarly, Horner and Kelly (2007) suggest that "many actual situations can fall into a grey area for which such a code must be supplemented" (p. 72). Thus, nurses can use codes as a beginning but need to critically analyze such codes in light of evolving knowledge, and engage continuously in reflection and dialogue about their values and practice. Although the problem of family violence presents nurses with numerous challenges to maintaining all of their obligations simultaneously, a relational approach to ethics can provide a theoretical basis for examining values and practices. Relational ethics also offer the opportunity to attend to context, describe the effects of different courses of action on relationships, and consider the different perspectives of those involved.

Ethical Issues and Family Violence

Ethical issues or problems encompass questions about what is right or good at individual, interpersonal, organizational, and societal levels (Storch, Rodney, & Starzomski, 2004). Ethical issues include dilemmas, but many ethical issues are much more complex than deciding which of two principles or values should prevail. While each type of family violence illustrates particular issues, dilemmas, and concepts, many ethical issues are similar across various forms of family violence.

Family violence is an ethical issue generally because it invariably involves the violation of persons' autonomy and dignity, and is in contradiction to the promotion of health and well-being. Five key ethical issues for nursing that cross forms of violence are (1) widespread tolerance for violence, (2) individualized, reactive responses, (3) lack of health care provider competence and supportive conditions for competence, (4) race, class and gender inequities and biases in responding to violence, and (5) "rescue fantasy" stances when violence is recognized.

TOLERANCE FOR FAMILY VIOLENCE. While most individuals, organizations, and societies espouse family violence as wrong or unacceptable, in practice, there is widespread tolerance for violence. Relational approaches illustrate how meanings and definitions of violence are embedded in individual experiences (whether as a child, adult, or older adult), in families, and in intimate relationships, all set within a wider context. Social and cultural norms regarding acceptable levels of violence and beliefs about the relative values of persons, are thus foundational to tolerance of violence. Among and within societies, cultures, and families, individuals differ in their understandings of what constitutes violence and this differs also with the status of the abused person.

As the World Health Organization (WHO) notes, gender-based violence, or violence against women (VAW), is a major public health and human rights problem throughout the world. Despite the profound effects of VAW, and the fact that it has been declared a human rights violation, it is a largely ignored problem. Patriarchy, racism, classism, and ageism work in ways that VAW is conceptualized as a cultural issue, rather than a global human rights issue. WHO's World Report on Violence and Health (World Health Organization, 2002) notes that the most common form, VAW by a husband or male partner, is tolerated and made invisible when legal systems and cultural norms do not treat such violence as a crime, but rather treat it as a "private" family matter or a normal part of life. For example, in Western countries, there is widespread use of violence in entertainment media, and the ways in which public media treat VAW has been shown largely to blame women for their own victimization (Meyers, 2004; Taylor, 2009; Wilcox, 2005). Specific groups of women, for example, women working in the sex trade or using illegal drugs, are often assigned lower moral status and thus are "more blamed." Again, the moral status of persons varies with their social locations, including their ages.

Despite public abhorrence of some forms of severe physical abuse and neglect, many physically violent acts against children are tolerated, and hitting, yelling, and demeaning children are common in the name of discipline. Social positioning and developmental limitations have made children vulnerable and translated to widespread acceptance of violence because discipline is often considered acceptable, ethical, and even necessary to their care. While there is considerable tolerance for acts of violence against children internationally, different social and cultural contexts dictate how much violence is accepted. The United Nations confirms that, "violence [against children] exists in every country of the world, cutting across culture, class, education, income and ethnic origin. In every region, in contradiction to human rights obligations and children's developmental needs, violence against children is socially approved, and is frequently legal and State-authorized" (Pinhero, 2006, p. 1).

The United Nations Convention of the Rights of the Child (UNCRC) (1989) has generated much international support for ending violence against children. However, despite ratification of the UNCRC by 193 countries, corporal punishment continues to be tolerated in the home in all but 23 (Durrant, Trocmé, Fallon, Milne, & Black, 2009). The United States has failed to ratify the full convention, and much of this debate relates to the issue of family rights in discipline (Browning, 2006). While Canada has ratified the UNCRC, it too has attempted to preserve parental rights to physically discipline children. Canada's Supreme Court revisited the issue of corporal punishment in 2004, and instead of abolishing violence, they developed seven limitations in an attempt to describe "reasonable force" for disciplining children. However, attempting to delineate acceptable and unacceptable levels of violence against children has proved challenging. Durrant et al. (2009) analyzed the substantiated cases of physical abuse reported in the 2003 Canadian Incidence Study on Child Abuse and Neglect and found that the majority of the substantiated cases of physical abuse actually fell within legal parameters of "reasonable force" described by the Supreme Court and were underpinned by intentions to discipline.

Some significant shifts in decreasing tolerance for violence toward children are evident, with one clear example of this being in school systems where educational theories support alternate strategies to corporal punishment for the creation of optimal learning environments, and there are far fewer schools using corporal punishment. Straus and Mathur (1996) used national surveys to demonstrate an erosion of cultural norms regarding corporal punishment in the United States. In 1968, there was near consensus in support of corporal punishment for children (94%); by 1994, only 68% approved. Even so, another American study found 94% of parents were spanking their children by the time they were 3 or 4 years old (Straus & Stewart, 1999). In spite of a substantial body of literature that provides strong evidence linking frequent corporal punishment with detrimental health effects for individuals and societies (Gershoff, 2002), support persists for parental liberty to use physical force against a child for the purpose of discipline. Along with sparse international support for ending corporal punishment in the home and important cultural differences in support of the practice, there are dilemmas for nurses working with parents. Their practice needs include communicating the evidence and helping parents find developmentally and culturally appropriate alternatives to corporal punishment without being judgemental about occasional use of the practice.

Like other forms of family violence, what is considered to be elder abuse and experiences of such abuse are shaped by changing social patterns and norms. Importantly, elder abuse encompasses both IPV that continues as people age and abuse that arises in the context of vulnerability as people age. The spectrum of abuses experienced by older persons, including physical, emotional, mental, sexual and financial abuse are shaped by changing values for the elderly, and changing family structure, and employment patterns. For example, the increasing value on individual economic productivity in Western societies often overshadows other values such as wisdom, companionship, loyalty, and so on. The increasing trend to institutionalize or "warehouse" elderly people has increased the opportunities for violence to occur in such contexts.

Tolerance for family violence can be seen in health care and nursing practice in that, in relation to the extent of the problem, very limited resources are allocated to prevention, recognition, intervention, or training for health care providers. Consequently, responses of health care systems to family violence have been shown as inadequate at best (Jones, et al., 2008; McMurray & Moore, 1994; Melton, 2005; Tower, 2007).

INDIVIDUALIZED, REACTIVE RESPONSES. Family violence is entirely preventable, unlike many other diseases or conditions that have negative impacts on health. Of considerable ethical concern then, are both the overwhelming lack of response to family violence given its magnitude and health implications and the way responses have been developed to address violence at an individual level (for both victims and perpetrators) in lieu of proactive population or social responses. This individualized response is the case for all types of family violence, although it is clear that majority of victims of violence are women, children, and elderly persons, as their relative power and status situate them socially in a more vulnerable position for abuse. Reactive responses aimed at individuals continuously will fail to adequately address problems rooted in social inequities, including inequities related to gender and age.

An ethical perspective calls attention to the failure of health care to address health and well-being of persons despite the guidance of Codes of Ethics and our professional mission. Such failure can be better understood and thus challenged, using a relational perspective to examine the historical, social, and cultural contexts in which these responses have developed. As discussed, all levels of response to family violence (individual, organizational, and social) are embedded within social contexts and shaped by assumptions, values, and beliefs. Some of these assumptions and values include: that family violence is a private matter; that different persons have different rights and values based on social positioning (age, gender, etc); that enduring violence is a "choice" and that all have equal choices; that responding to individual cases of victims and identifying perpetrators is possible and effective within the resources available; and that perpetrators of "unacceptable" violence are exceptional, and essentially either malevolent or mentally ill, and can be "characterized as . . . fundamentally different from ourselves" (Melton, 2005, p. 11).

It is important to attend more broadly to the culture of health care to further understand how individualistic approaches came to dominate responses to violence. An individual approach to health is a pervasive feature of the Western medical tradition. This creates an ethical dilemma for nursing and especially in the context of family violence, as our professional values and principles include attending to the health and well-being of populations. Sherwin (1998b) explains,

> Within the medical tradition, suffering is located and addressed in the individuals who experience it rather than in the social arrangements that may be responsible for causing the problem. Instead of exploring the cultural context that tolerates and even supports practices such as war, pollution, sexual violence and systemic unemployment—practices that contribute to much of the illness that occupies modern medicine—physicians generally respond to the symptoms troubling a particular patient in isolation from the context that produces these conditions. . . . This orientation directs the vast majority of research money and expertise toward the things that can be done to change the individual, but it often ignores key elements at the source of the problems. The [ethical issue with this approach] is that medicine, despite the limits of its expertise and focus, is the primary agent of health care activity in our society and physicians are granted significant social authority to be the arbiters of health policy. Hence, when medicine makes the treatment of individuals its primary focus, we must understand that important gaps are created in our society's ability to understand and promote good health. (pp. 29–30)

Importantly, such individualized responses overlook the circumstances of people's lives and how social and economic circumstances shape their opportunities for choice. Reactive and individualized health care responses, shaped by such contexts, are neither ethically acceptable in terms of contemporary understandings of human rights, nor based on evidence.

LACK OF HEALTH CARE PROVIDER COMPETENCE AND SUPPORTIVE CONDITIONS FOR COMPETENCE. The obligations for nurses and other health care providers to be competent is routinely challenging in relation to family violence. This obligation is challenged by three inter-related factors congruent with social tolerance for violence: inadequate educational preparation, policy directions at social and organizational levels, and provider's lack of confidence in system responses. Medical schools in the United States increasingly include IPV in curricula (Hamberger, 2007). In the United State, more than 90% of nursing programs contained IPV related content (Woodtli & Breslin, 1996), and a recent Canadian study found that 83% of colleges and university undergraduate nursing programs, and 43% of undergraduate medical programs offered at least some (mostly minimal) exposure to IPV-related content in the curriculum (Gutmanis, Beynon, Tutty, Wathen, & MacMillan, 2007). However, research has shown repeatedly that providers report that they are undereducated and underprepared to provide care related to family violence (Cann, Withnell, Shakespeare, Doll, & Thomas, 2001; Häggblom, Hallberg, & Möller, 2005). A recent survey of 1,000 physicians and 1,000 nurses (Gutmanis et al., 2007) found that over 60% of all respondents had not received any formal training regarding woman abuse, with nurses without formal training feeling less prepared than physicians to respond. Furthermore, evaluation of training programs for child abuse and neglect lack evidence to support effectiveness (Reece & Jenny, 2005).

Studies of health care responses routinely recommend better and more education. In their policy analysis of 11 national and global institutions' VAW agendas spanning 1990–2006, Koss and White (2008) found that the recommendation with greatest consensus was to train medical professionals to provide victim sensitive, non-stigmatizing health care, avoid re-victimization, and monitor responsiveness. A further high priority recommendation was to integrate violence care into emergency, reproductive, antenatal, family planning, post-abortion, mental health, HIV/AIDS, and adolescent medical services, a recommendation strongly supported by others (Cohn, Salmon, & Stobo, 2002). Similarly, reports that health care professionals feel inadequately trained to recognize and report child abuse and neglect repeatedly call for increased education to address low reporting rates (Berkowitz, 2008; Christian, 2008; Lane & Dubowitz, 2009).

Policy directions compound the effects of inadequate education by creating challenges to providing care that promotes health and upholds autonomy and dignity. Most policy effort related to family violence has been focused on mandatory reporting laws at the social level and screening for violence at the health care organizational level. Such policy directions in turn influence the education of health care providers. For example, in the case of child abuse and neglect, in Canada, although only 4% of 3,780 children who suffered from substantiated abuse had injuries that warranted medical attention (Trocmé, MacMillan, Fallon, & De Marco, 2003), training programs focus largely on recognition of patterns of physical injury. Rather than addressing family violence as a widespread social problem affecting many, if not most, families, these strategies tighten the focus on the culpability of particular individuals—individual health care providers are to identify individual victims and report individual perpetrators of abuse. From a relational ethical perspective, this approach is deeply problematic for preventing or identifying violence.

Health care providers variously resist policy directions, at least in part because of a lack of confidence about system responses following reporting (Freed & Drake, 1999; Gilbert, Kemp et al., 2009; Goad, 2008; Jones et al., 2008; Rodríguez, Wallace, Woolf, & Manigone, 2006). The fact that protection systems have not been evaluated, along with strong emerging critiques of current processes and practices, have led to erosion of health care providers' trust in the system to improve the lives of families (Gilbert, Kemp et al., 2009; Lancet, 2003; Melton, 2005; Reading et al., 2009). Despite mandatory reporting legislation in many countries around the world for various types of abuse, failure to recognize abuse and underreporting remain consistent issues (Gilbert, Kemp et al., 2009; Rodríguez et al., 2006). Lacking adequate education and support for practice and confidence in system responses, health care providers are likely to draw on their personal biases and assumptions as a basis for practice. Mirroring broader social views, health care providers have a range of views and understandings of violence. For example, Jones et al. (2008) interviewed 434 primary care clinicians in the United States regarding their decision making in regards to reporting child abuse. They found that the clinician's knowledge of and relationship with a family strongly influenced reporting and even resulted in amending initial suspicions, as did the history of and circumstances of an injury, consultation with others, and their own previous experiences with protection system. "When they did not report, clinicians planned alternative management strategies, including active or informal case follow-up management" (Jones, 2008, p. 259). Another study found that, "clinicians routinely fail to identify possible abuse, and, equally routinely, determine that reporting their suspicions to state authorities would not lead to benefit for the child or family" (Sege & Flaherty, 2008, p. 823). Similarly, Rodríguez et al. (2006) described physician decision making regarding reporting elder abuse and found that the relationship with the elderly person and family, considerations of the quality of life for the elderly person (including suitable alternatives for care), and professional judgments regarding the best interests of the client were all considered. Concerns with the quality of the services that the elderly person or family would receive if reported were significant, and one physician described services as "not always helpful; in fact, sometimes they are destructive" (Rodríguez et al., 2006, p. 406). This research demonstrates how, even with mandatory reporting policies, relationships with people involved, who is available for consultation, the contexts and circumstances of injuries, and the clinician's previous experiences defines how reporting will be handled.

Consistent with a general tolerance for violence in society, health care organizations often provide little support for nurses and other providers in their responses to family violence. Thus, while nurses themselves are faced with ethical issues in responding to individual patients, simultaneously challenges to ethical practice arise from the context of practice. Research has consistently reported that nurses are pressed for time and required to prioritize based on organizational demands rather than the needs of patients, in ways that result in responses that are inappropriate to the needs of those experiencing violence.

At the same time as health care providers are poorly educated regarding family violence and social and organizational policies provide little support and few resources for responding effectively, health care providers and other service providers are often blamed for the inadequacy of the social and health care responses—again reflecting an individualistic apportioning of responsibility. Individual professional competence is often blamed for the few tragic cases of violent murders of entire families or brutal and fatal abuse of children. Official explanations and media reports often suggest that either case managers or hospital professionals failed to appropriately recognize risks to a particular person's safety and failed protect. Recent critiques of this construction of incompetent practitioners reveal the shaky foundation on which health care practices and policies regarding family violence are built. The *Lancet* (2003) challenges such media depictions and blaming of individual practitioner competence and failure to protect children, instead questioning the lack of attention to creating a comprehensive research agenda for addressing family violence in meaningful ways. The editorial accuses health professionals of ignoring the important issue of child maltreatment, and operating programs without efforts for systematic evaluation, critique and accountability for practice. "Maltreatment is one of the biggest paediatric health challenges, yet any research activity is dwarfed by work on more established childhood ills—especially those that lend themselves to drug treatment" (*Lancet*, 2003, p. 443). The power of pharmaceutical companies to shift the focus of research calls for significant attention from an ethical perspective. The *Lancet* calls into question health care professional integrity considering the lack of knowledge and competency related to child abuse and neglect, claiming that there has been a "systematic failure of all relevant professions" (*The Lancet*, 2003, p. 443). Indeed, child protection programs have operated in many countries for almost half a century with very little done to establish the efficacy of their practices (Gilbert, Kemp, et al., 2009).

Social and political values that currently are raising the profile of child and human rights call for urgent progress in research in family violence, along with education for health care providers focusing on public health approaches to prevent ongoing abuse (Ferris, 2004; Garcia-Moreno, Jansen, Ellsberg, Heise, & Watts, 2006; Phelan, 2008; Pinhero, 2006; Reading et al., 2009; Silverman, Mesh, Cuthbert, Slote, & Bancroft, 2004). Addressing ethical issues at the level of individual providers and patients must be accompanied by attention to the ethical issues arising at organizational and systemic levels, including how structural inequities intersect with family violence.

RACE, CLASS AND GENDER INEQUITIES AND BIASES IN RESPONDING TO VIOLENCE. Race, class, and gender inequities operate in at least two key ways to create ethical issues in relation to family violence. Inequities make particular groups more vulnerable to violence, and more vulnerable to scrutiny, stereotyping, and assumptions in health care (Varcoe, 2009a). For example, the structural inequities women face, including disproportionate poverty and employment discrimination, have been shown to have a significant influence on women's possibilities for entering, staying in and leaving abusive intimate relationships (Barnett, 2000; Dunn & Powell-Williams, 2007; Lambert & Firestone, 2000). Child neglect is conflated with poverty, with disproportionate representation among those living in poverty and people of color in most Western countries (Statistics Canada, 2008; Shonkoff & Phillips, 2000).

Despite the well-known pervasiveness of family violence, and the often-cited maxim that family violence crosses every class, ethnicity, and religion, assumptions and stereotypes related to race, ethnicity, gender, class, and age operate in public and health care understandings, with some groups being stereotyped as more violent than others. Such biases have been shown to be pervasive in news media reporting of family violence (Gilchrist, 2008; Greaves et al., 2004; R. Taylor, 2009). Violence is often constructed as "cultural," confusing culture with ethnicity and masking the structural inequities particular groups face. For example, in one community, after the murder of several women from the "South Asian" immigrant community, the problem was constructed largely as a "cultural" problem (with culture being a euphemism for race or ethnicity), without considering whether the number of homicides was "proportional" to the underlying population or what structural conditions (for example, greater poverty, higher stress, greater downward mobility, and gender inequities imposed by immigration processes) characteristic of immigrant experiences might have contributed to the problem. Not surprisingly then, health care providers often hold biases regarding "who" is most likely to experience family violence.

These biases become further entrenched with mandatory reporting legislation. Biases guide the process of suspicion, and higher levels of suspicion occur for marginalized and stigmatized groups. This in turn contributes to an overrepresentation of these groups in both investigations and substantiation, therefore creating statistics that subsequently are constructed as "facts" and fed back to inform and support discriminatory practices (Freed & Drake, 1999; Varcoe, 2008, 2009b). Within these dynamics, health care providers are positioned to respond to family violence based on policy directions that contribute to ethical challenges, without adequate education to counter widespread tolerance of violence and erroneous assumptions. Individualized, reactive responses thus are often manifested in health care providers taking rescue stances in relation to those identified as the victim or the most victimized.

"RESCUE FANTASY" STANCES WHEN VIOLENCE IS RECOGNIZED. Health care and nursing practice is enacted within a complex network of power relations, so that when healthcare providers recognize violence, they are usually in a position of authority in relation to both victims and perpetrators. Without careful analysis of values and ethical obligations, nurses can slide into practices in which they "take sides" with the perceived victim (or in the case of multiple victims, the victim perceived to be most vulnerable) and indulge in rescue fantasies that can disempower victims, overriding their autonomy and imposing the health care providers' view of what constitutes an appropriate course of action. For example, a small study of experienced nurses in Finland found that without adequate preparation or guidance in dealing with VAW, nurses practiced on the basis of their emotions and personal experiences, characterizing their work in relation to women who had been battered as a "life saving mission" (Häggblom & Möller, 2006). Applying the psychoanalytic perspectives of Melanie Klein, Davis (2008) similarly takes issue with rescue fantasies. Davis argues that child protection approaches encourage a rescue orientation. Davis cautions that while "it is understandable that we might wish for the omnipotent capacity to keep children from harm, however to move forward to create more realistic and positive relations with the clients who come into contact with child protection services, we need to give up this fantasy" (p. 150). Rescue strategies aimed toward individuals who are vulnerable to violence show disregard for the underlying fundamental power inequities and reinforce rather than attempt to dismantle them on a social level. The goal of ethical practice is to uphold professional nursing values in relation to promoting respect and equity to all persons. Neither treating possible or known perpetrators with dignity and respect nor avoiding a stance of "siding with the victim" means condoning violence. Instead, these approaches build trust with all those involved and position health care professionals to support families optimally.

Tolerance for violence, lack of provider education, and policy and organizational support for competence practice, practices based on stereotypes and assumptions and disempowering practices contribute to failure to prevent harm and optimize health, failure to respect the autonomy and dignity of persons, and breaches of justice. Each of these general ethical issues plays out in specific ways in relation to particular forms of family violence.

Ethical Issues and Intimate Partner Violence

IPV can be defined as a pattern of physical, sexual, and/or emotional violence by an intimate partner in a context of coercive control (Tjaden & Thoennes, 2000). In relation to IPV, the general ethical issues common to all forms of violence manifest primarily as a discourse of choice in which women[1] are held responsible for and blamed for their own victimization. With limited education regarding IPV and often little organizational support for responding to violence, nurses often are unprepared to counter this dominant discourse and unsure how to respond, assess risk and danger, support women, and refer them to additional supports.

Very little explicit attention is paid to ethical issues in relation to partner violence in academic literature. However, although the ideas of self-determination and autonomy are not discussed as ethical concepts in relation to family violence, the notion of "choice" is repeatedly raised as a key issue. The ideas of choice and autonomy are most central in relation to the idea that women who are battered should "leave" their partners. Dunn and Powell-Williams (2007) articulate clearly the moral contradictions inherent in how victimization is understood within the culture of individualism that characterizes the United States, a culture similar to other Western countries. Based on their study of domestic violence advocates working in shelters and criminal justice settings, they show how advocates struggle to simultaneously conceive of women "as victims trapped by social, psychological and interactional forces and as agents whose choices must be

---

[1] While we acknowledge that men are also victims of intimate partner violence, and that women can be perpetrators, in this chapter we focus on women in heterosexual relationships for the purposes of illustration.

respected," in ways that overemphasize women's "choices, and thereby diminish the constraints they face" (p. 977). While advocates recognized the barriers women faced to leaving abusive partners, they did so in a way that constructed the women as "trapped" by both internal and external factors as they tried to explain battered women who stay with abusive partners. Within the context of "a powerful cultural tendency to see even the most helpless among us as freely making choices" (p. 985), the advocates were caught between constructing their clients as blameless victims and as active agents. Women who stayed with abusive partners heightened the challenge for advocates: advocates struggled to make sense of this, almost inevitably slipping into the language of choice and overlooking the contexts of women's lives. At the same time, even through advocates espoused respect for the "choice" of staying, it was not considered a fully legitimate choice. Indeed, the advocates continuously positioned themselves as revealing choices and helping women distinguish between good and bad choices. In emphasizing choice, advocates ultimately "not only fail to deflect responsibility from victims, but rather attribute it *to* them" (p. 991, emphasis in original). Dunn and Powell-Williams conclude that "in some circumstances, to speak of choice at all is to obscure and gloss" (p. 999).

Nurses and other health care providers practice within similar cultural circumstances as advocates, with individualism and the emphasis on choice pervading both nursing theory and practice (Browne, 2001), health care and society more generally (Coburn, 2004; Collins, Abelson, & Eyles, 2007). Bell and Mosher (1998) observe that the problem of health care providers being ill-equipped to detect and respond to woman abuse appropriately has been documented for as long as the problem of woman abuse has been recognized as a social problem. They argue that the health care response to woman abuse has been characterized by medicalization, which de-politicizes the issue, standardization (such as through screening), which homogenizes and de-contextualizes experience and leads to harm in the absence of adequate education, and the dichotomization of individuals into victims or agents. As Kim and Motsei (2002) note, nurses are men and women first, experiencing the same cultural values and levels of violence as their patients. Repeatedly, research has shown that the attitudes of nurses toward IPV include considerable victim-blaming (e.g., Häggblom et al., 2005; Kim & Motsei, 2002). Not surprisingly, nurses may construe women as making choices and see themselves as providing options that women can freely choose (Häggblom & Möller, 2006; Tower, 2007; Varcoe, 2001).

Understanding of the concept of "leaving" is evolving. Rather than focusing on leaving as an autonomous choice, consistent with a relational view of autonomy, leaving is increasingly understood as a complex process influenced by other people and the wider contexts of people's lives (Bostock, Plumpton, & Pratt, 2009; Martin et al., 2000). Attention is being paid increasingly to the influence of economic circumstances, racism, and social isolation (Chantler, 2006; Kim & Gray, 2008; Moore, 2003; Wilcox, 2000) with an emphasis on decreasing barriers to leaving and reducing violence regardless of whether women leave or stay. Such evolving understandings should be used as a knowledge base for more competent ethical practice in relation to woman abuse.

Ethical Issues and Child Maltreatment

Child abuse and neglect, or child maltreatment, are broadly defined in the most recent literature as "any acts of commission or omission by a parent or other caregiver that result in harm, potential for harm, or threat of harm to a child, even if harm is not the intended result" (Gilbert, Spatz Widom et al., 2009, p. 69). This definition centres responsibilities of parents and caregivers to ensure protection for children. However, a critical relational perspective suggests significant state, social, community, and family responsibility to ensure that parents are in a position to protect their children from harm. There are several ethical issues related specifically to child abuse and neglect. The two main approaches to child abuse and neglect will be compared and ethical issues arising from these explored.

Internationally, there are two main approaches to child maltreatment: the child and family welfare approach (European countries, New Zealand) and the child protection/safety approach (USA, Canada, and Australia) (Gilbert, Kemp, et al., 2009). The key difference is that "the child safety approach tends to concentrate on investigation of maltreatment and assessment of future risk of maltreatment rather than on broad welfare needs. When services are provided they are likely to be short term and to focus specifically on prevention of further maltreatment of the type reported rather than on the broader needs of the family and child" (Gilbert, Kemp, et al., 2009, p. 176).

Divergent philosophies of interventions in response to IPV and child abuse or neglect create challenges for families and health care professionals who attempt to mitigate harm, promote health and well-being, and demonstrate respect for persons. As discussed, a contemporary approach to women who suffer from abuse at home is one that attempts to support her autonomy and decision-making. However, child protection policies position professionals as being in the best position to decide what is in the best interests of the child. Mothers who stay in violent home situations are often considered incompetent parents despite evidence otherwise, and in some cases, such women have been charged with "failure to protect" their children (Lewis, 2003). In issues of child protection, women's autonomy for decision making regarding the best interests of her child is stripped from her, as "solutions generally require that the woman cooperate with CPS [child protection system], the judicial system, and law enforcement agencies by leaving the perpetrator and pressing charges against him"(Lewis, p. 358). This is often the case despite significant risks to her safety and that of her children both during the process of leaving and in the longer term depending on the woman's supports, resources, and vulnerability (Lewis, 2003). In this way, "mandatory reporting laws can inadvertently disempower the abused mother through removal of her right to determine her course of action while giving to others power over her and her children" (Lewis, p. 359). This creates an ethical dilemma for health care practitioners, as the very structure of the interventions may cause harm to women who are once again disempowered and retraumatized by this process (Lewis). Practicing ethically in the context of this law requires both an early and full disclosure to women who are abused about the professional limits of confidentiality and clarification of the processes if she were to disclose child abuse (Freed & Drake, 1999; Haggerty & Hawkins, 2000; Lewis, 2003).

A child protection system that prioritizes investigation and substantiation, and whose outcomes look to blame, punish, and criminalize acts of violence towards children, limits services to only the children for whom "adequate levels" of evidence or suspicion are developed before intervening, and interventions are implemented cautiously because of harms associated with the process (Gilbert, Kemp, et al., 2009). Of considerable ethical concern also is translation of this approach internationally, as this "singular emphasis on reporting and investigation seems to occur even in societies in which a majority of children lack adequate nutrition and shelter" (Melton, 2005, pp. 11–12). While contradictions inherent to this practice seem evident, comparison of these approaches provides a basis for the development of an international approach that emphasizes child safety within the context of child and family welfare (Gilbert, Kemp, et al., 2009). In Sweden, Belgium, and other Western European countries that use a child and family welfare approach, which is primarily assistive and does not include the substantiation component, there are increased rates of self-referral for families who are suffering from violence (Gilbert, Kemp, et al., 2009).

Melton (2005) identifies the inadequacies of social services, which emphasize investigations and substantiation of cases, rather than addressing the context of the underlying issues. A historical review shows that the child protection approach evolved with "initial misjudgments about the nature and frequency of child abuse and neglect, [and thus has resulted in]. . . a formal child protection system that is increasingly ill-matched to the needs of the children and families who enter it" (Melton, 2005, p. 12). For example, in Canada, neglect is the most prevalent type of child abuse and the most common type of neglect is "failure to supervise" (Trocmé, Fallon, et al., 2003). Examining the wider context exposes the relationship among failure to supervise, poverty (which in Canada affects approximately 1 of 10 children (Statistics Canada, 2007), and lack of accessible child care nationally. Ethical approaches to addressing issues of child abuse and neglect must consider these contexts and allocate funds toward a system that builds resources for families to be able to provide environments for optimal development of their children.

Applying a relational ethical lens illustrates how conceptualizations of harm, risk, and safety from the perspectives of the child and family need to be central to decision making about interventions and care, as do considerations of the contexts that influence safety for the child. This analysis calls into question current practice which attempts to identify risk using "an actuarial or risk-assessment approach" (Gilbert, Kemp, et al., 2009, p. 176). Predicting risk by collating either professional assessments and opinions, or identification and statistical analysis of "objective risk factors," attempts to gain clarity in the murky waters of child maltreatment (Houston & Griffiths, 2000). However, the prioritization of risk assessment strategies in decision-making processes assumes that risk can be predicted and managed to prevent harm, responds to only to children within a "high risk" category, and erases the family and child's agency and autonomy (Houston & Griffiths). A conceptualization of risk steeped in an objectivist paradigm rather than a relational one, fails to approach child maltreatment comprehensively or ethically, and, instead of bringing clarity to the situation, obscures it further. Huston and Griffiths warn that "we can no longer retreat behind an objectivist assumption that it is scientific knowledge which will provide the solutions. More research on predictive factors will provide only continuing false reassurance that we are responding effectively to the issues" (p. 8).

While a "child's welfare is paramount . . . different people hold radically disparate views about what is best for a child" (Houston, 2003, p. 62). Houston and Griffiths (Houston & Griffiths, 2000) found "the lack of congruence between professional and familial perspectives led to worse outcomes for the child" (p. 6), indicating that the processes that position professionals with power over decisions about child safety might inadvertently damage child well-being and health. Foregrounding the child, the family, and *their perspectives* about risk, harm, health, and well-being preserves autonomy and choice and recovers and prioritizes voices of those most affected by violence. This also highlights the rights of children to participate in decision making about their care at their level of developmental ability and competence. While children's participation in decisions affecting their care historically has not been honoured, the UNCRC recently has brought more attention to participatory rights for children.

In the complex practice of child maltreatment, a relational approach provides much guidance in attending closely to the context that shapes the realities and nature of a child's and family's world, and how autonomy, choice, health, and well-being, dignity and respect for persons are highly contextual and challenging to enact in the current system of care.

Ethical Issues and Elder Mistreatment

There are three features of ethical issues specific to elder mistreatment, also referred to herein as elder abuse. First is the fact that ageism underpins tolerance for elder abuse, how it is understood, and how it is perpetrated and addressed within health care. Second, of all forms of abuse, elder abuse is most likely to be perpetrated within health care contexts. Third, within both a context characterized by ageism and ideas of individuals and choice, the notion of "self-neglect" is particular to elder mistreatment.

While elder mistreatment encompasses IPV that continues into or begins as people age, as well as abuse by others, ageism, the stereotyping, discrimination, and devaluing of older persons is the central feature of elder abuse. As Phelan (2008) argues, ageism itself is abusive to older persons. As ageism infringes on dignity and respect, and often limits autonomy, ageism is inherently unethical. Ageism both contributes to systematically disadvantaging older persons and provides "a covert basis for societal tolerance of elder abuse" (Phelan, 2008, p. 320). Phelan argues that ageism coupled with the Western privileging of economic productivity both exclude older persons from full citizenship and economic participation, which in turn increases vulnerability to abuse, and has contributed to the lack of social response to limiting elder abuse.

As with any form of abuse, nurses and other health care providers are party to the same culture, stereotypes and assumptions as other members of their societies. Health care systems and nurses can perpetuate ageism in ways that affect the quality of care obscure recognition of abusive contexts and justify failure to ameliorate such situations. For example, in one recent study, an elderly woman with dementia was returned to the care of her daughter, even through physical neglect and abuse had led to her visit to emergency, because there was no hospital bed to which she could be admitted (unpublished data). Presumably, if the patient had been a small child, returning the patient to such a situation would not have been tolerated.

Finally, self-neglect is an issue that raises particular ethical concerns in relation to the elderly. The balance between respecting an older person's autonomy versus protecting the person from harm is frequently an issue in relation to elder abuse. Again, judging a person's competence to decide for him or herself must take into account the context, including how ageism shapes social and healthcare responses.

Some Principles for Ethical Practice in Relation to Family Violence

BECOME KNOWLEDGEABLE ABOUT VIOLENCE. Develop a comprehensive understanding of the prevalence of violence, the significance of it in relation to population health, and the relative lack of response from the health care professional community. Knowledge of the various forms and dynamics of violence will provide a basis for competent practice. Recognize that legal mandates and ethical obligations may conflict. Laws regarding mandatory reporting of both child and elder abuse are contentious and much debated, leaving considerable scope for interpretation, and demanding that health care providers become knowledgeable about the laws and debates, critically analyze each situation, and consider how a practitioner might best uphold both ethical and legal obligations. A knowledge base about violence will help nurses challenge their own and other's thinking in practicing within competing obligations.

DO NOT OPERATE ON ASSUMPTIONS AND STEREOTYPES. Common social understandings of violence are fraught with "victim-blaming," assumptions, and stereotypes, particularly those related to age, class, gender, race/ethnicity, and sexual orientation and gender identification. Practicing ethically always begins with self-reflective practice, which is essential to challenging stereotypes and assumptions. Dialogue with others helps to identify one's own assumptions regarding violence. In the case of family violence, dialogue often reveals many different perspectives, especially regarding "acceptable" versus "unacceptable" levels of violence. Encourage a deeper understanding of how suspicion is constructed through the multiple intersections of our positioning, our experiences, and our understanding of violence. Recognize that assumptions always underpin how we come to understand the world but that commitment to reflexivity throughout one's practice can provide opportunities that support new understandings embedded in particular contexts.

CRITICALLY EVALUATE PROCESSES AND PRACTICES. Learning about the different approaches to family violence historically and internationally provides some insights into current responses to violence. Recognition of the relative lack of evidence to support current programs and practices is an important place to begin. Asking critical questions that generate ideas for future research is essential as is engaging in discussion regarding the complexities and critique of the contradictions between legal and ethical directions for practice. Maintaining an open and curious approach to facilitate dialogue and generate contextually based knowledge to support decision making will begin to address obligations to specific clients and contribute to the development of knowledge.

FOCUS ON THE QUALITY OF ALL RELATIONSHIPS. A close examination of power relationships, which exist between family members and care providers, are foundational to nursing practice. An appreciation for the complexities in the context of relationships is important. For example, in the context of any family, an abuser is never only "an abuser"; they may also be a partner, friend, breadwinner, lover, parent, daughter, or son. Violence in family relationships occurs among other aspects of the relationship and rarely is straightforward. Similarly, each care provider's practice is shaped by the influence of others in the immediate practice context, such as colleagues, supervisors, patients, and by his or her own personal relationships, including experiences of violence. When a report of suspected violence needs to be made to a reporting agency, the report should be made with the family rather than "on" the family. In that way, it is an example of coordinating care, getting help for the family and transparency. It necessitates nurses having an existing relationship with the agencies to which they may have to report so that it is a report made with dignity and respect for all of the parties and enhances and deepens relationships with other organizations as well as with the family.

LOOK BEYOND THE IMMEDIATE INDIVIDUAL FOR WHOM YOU ARE PROVIDING CARE. Seek to practice in ways that convey respect to all persons and uphold fairness for all. Caring for clients more often includes caring for family members as well. In the case of a client who is a victim of family violence, knowing or suspecting a family member of committing violence does not absolve health care providers from their obligation and best practice by attending to the family unit. Ensuring client safety often includes demonstrating respect for their family members, and given the relative ambiguity of most situations of family violence, health care providers need to avoid being the "judge and jury." Bearing witness to and tolerating the distress of the client and family is important work of nursing. Ensuring care for all family members in a way that demonstrates respect for persons and just treatment more often is a relief for clients. From clinical experience in working with families being investigated for suspicions of child abuse or neglect, often, the priority for nursing care relates to supporting the family in a time of crisis and building trust within the context of a professional relationships, we have found that saturated with power. Developing transparency regarding practices is essential to building trust despite authority.

LEARN ABOUT THE CIRCUMSTANCES OF PATIENTS' LIVES. Attention to building a trusting professional relationship will provide the foundations to elicit the narratives of those involved and bring depth and detail to the circumstances of the client's life. Nurses need to create and hold spaces for the voices of those most vulnerable to violence to be heard and to contribute to the story in their own way. Children and elderly people need to be made aware of their right to participate in decision making regarding their care to the level of their abilities, and every effort needs to ensure their competence and abilities are maximized in the process. Nurses need to support and challenge each other to develop meaningful responses to families by listening attentively to those for whom they are caring and applying a critical lens to their practices which build on families' strengths and address the families' needs.

SEEK TO INFLUENCE THE WIDER CONTEXT. As this chapter has discussed, the hope for ending family violence lies with social change to reduce tolerance of violence and to reduce inequities. Thus, if nurses subscribe to a commitment to social justice, they need to engage in influencing change at organizational levels. While actions might include working to end poverty, to improve health care access for all, to improve child care access, or to change policies related to mandated reporting in one's community, other meaningful actions might be more modest. Cultivating a knowledgeable, ethical culture in the workplace can be a critical contribution to reducing violence.

Case Study and Analysis

BACKGROUND. Sandy, a nurse in the emergency department of a pediatric hospital, is asked to admit 5-month-old Baby Z who is being transferred by ambulance from a community hospital for investigation of "possible non-accidental head injury." She is stable, and it is unclear what the family has been told in the referring hospital. The charge nurse asks Sandy to do an admission assessment, even though she is not assigned to this family, and it is almost 11 P.M. when her shift is finished. Her colleague is busy, and the parents are "trying to leave," so it is urgent.

Baby Z is cuddled up with her father, Jeff, and is drinking hungrily from a bottle. Her parents are in their early 20s; her father is Caucasian, and her mother is Aboriginal/Native American. Sandy introduces herself to the family and asks how they are. Jeff does not look up, "shitty" he answers. Baby Z's mother, Ali, is tense, makes eye contact briefly, and turns in her seat away from the nurse, her partner, and baby; her gaze hits the wall beside her. Sandy says she understands that they are asking to leave and asks if there is something they need? Jeff replies that they have been in the hospital all afternoon and evening, and they have not eaten. He wanted Ali to go get some dinner for them, but they were told they are not allowed to leave. Sandy explains nearby stores and restaurants are closed, but offers to see what is available in the department or to bring them late night take out menus. They reply that they do not have any money. Sandy goes to the fridge, and luckily, there are still a few sandwiches and snacks left, and she brings them to the room.

PATIENT HISTORY AND PHYSICAL EXAMINATION. Sandy then explains she needs to review with them the history of Baby Z's injury and assess her. Jeff responds, "Fine. But I have no idea what happened, I was at work," as he looks to Ali. Ali again looks down and at the wall as she recounts the story. She describes how Baby Z was fussy so she was walking and bouncing her in her arms trying to settle her, just after lunch. While doing this, she tripped on a toy that had been left out from playing earlier, and Baby Z fell out of her arms, and they both fell to the floor. Baby Z cried but then settled down, and seemed okay, but tired. Ali described putting her down for a nap right after the incident. Two hours later, she woke Baby Z up and noticed her face was swollen and bruised. She called Jeff and he came home from work, and they went to their community hospital together.

On assessment, Baby Z's face is quite swollen, there is a defined line of purple bruising down the side of her face, and her eyes are red and bruised. Ali points out another small bruise on Baby Z's abdomen. Other than the facial injuries, she seems well, with a good appetite, and is smiling and cooing through her swollen face. A neurological assessment is normal, and her vital signs are as expected for her age. Sandy informs the parents of her impressions—that Baby Z looks well, but describes how, with a head injury, it is important to observe closely as it is possible that her condition could change even hours after the injury. Baby Z is giggling on Jeff's knee, and when Sandy says, "well, it's good she seems happy now," she hears Ali mutter, "yeah, she's tough, just like her mummy."

Sandy decides to ask if they understand why they have been transferred to this hospital. Jeff replies they were told it was for a special X-ray, one that the other hospital did not have. Sandy then asks if they have any concerns with being in this hospital. Jeff replies that they have no idea how they are going to get home, they do not have money for a taxi, and they have no family in town. Sandy reassures them that a social worker will help make sure they are able to get home. "No way," says Jeff. "Right, great, another social worker," Ali replies simultaneously. Sandy then asks about their experience with social workers. Ali looks up and tells Sandy that both she and Jeff have been in foster care and that she was abused in foster care. She says that she has no use for social workers. Jeff agrees and comments, "the social worker in the other hospital thought we did this, typical." After a quiet minute, Sandy says she is sorry to hear that they have had such negative experiences and says that she is aware that there have been significant problems with the child protection system. She then informs them of the obligation of health care professionals to report patterns of injuries that may have been caused by abuse and says she is sorry that they will have to go through the process of meeting with social work because of Baby Z's injury. They nod, they know. Jeff asks to see the social worker soon, to "get it over with." Sandy explains that the physician will be in next and that there will be another nurse who will be caring for them, but she will ask that social work is contacted in a timely way.

Sandy goes to the nursing station and the charge nurse asks her if the family is still trying to leave and whether or not they need to call security? Sandy reassures the charge nurse that would not be necessary, reports her assessment, and communicates the family's wishes to see social work as soon as possible, as well as their negative experiences with child protection. She struggles with what to document in the chart.

NURSING DIAGNOSIS. Nursing diagnoses for Baby Z and her family are multiple. First, it should be identified that the multiple appropriate nursing diagnoses, which relate to Baby Z's physical injuries, will not be addressed, as they are beyond the focus of this chapter (for example: potential for alterations in neurological status). The nursing diagnosis of "Potential for risks to physical, emotional and cultural safety" will be considered from the broad perspective of the needs of both Baby Z and her parents and provides a direction for meaningful nursing responses.

POTENTIAL FOR RISKS TO PHYSICAL, EMOTIONAL AND CULTURAL SAFETY. There are several issues with safety in this context—most obvious is Baby Z's physical safety, in the short and long term. While immediate threats to safety could also be conceptualized as potential deteriorations in Baby Z's neurological status, these are beyond the scope of this chapter. Physical safety in relation to Baby Z's vulnerability for further physical harm will be considered as her parents' ability to ensure her need for physical safety has been cast into question. Furthermore, there is ambiguity regarding Ali or perhaps even Jeff's physical safety. By Ali describing herself as "tough," it is unclear if she might be referring to her history of physical abuse or continued violence in her life (as the abused or even perhaps an abuser). Her comment begs further exploration. Furthermore, this family indicates a fear and mistrust of the child protection system, yet the obligation of the nurse and other health care professionals to involve the child protection in the care of Baby Z takes precedence. This suspicion might be related to the delay in seeking health care, the significance of the physical injury, and questions regarding the match between the reported mechanism of injury and the physical presentation of injury. However, there are multiple other factors that may be involved in the development of suspicion; for example, powerful stereotypical assumptions may be operating, which have not been acknowledged nor articulated. These include Ali and Jeff's age, history of abuse, socio-economic status, and Ali's ethnicity. The way health care professionals have come to understand profiles of abusers influences the development of suspicion. Ali and Jeff are all too familiar with these and anticipate that they will be suspected in causing harm to Baby Z, whether or not this was the case.

PATIENT GOALS AND NURSING INTERVENTIONS. The context of this family's access to the health care system means that they are vulnerable. While clearly Baby Z is vulnerable, her parents are also vulnerable. Attention to safety for all members of the family is the nurse's priority throughout health care encounters. While physical safety has been separated from emotional and cultural safety, this separation is somewhat artificial, as many of the interventions would be interrelated and relevant to all forms of safety. Creating as safe a space as possible will require supporting the family through the crisis of their infant's injury and in coping with the investigations of abuse. Caring for an infant with significant, obvious face and head trauma possibly attributable to abuse is difficult. However, while Baby Z is bruised and swollen, she giggles and coos as if nothing were amiss, while her parents are suffering intensely. Whether or not her injuries were accidental, what is palpable in the room is her parent's suffering. As a nurse in this situation, competent use of knowledge, respect, non-judgmental, authentic concern, and attention to the needs of the family as a unit are fundamental in providing safe and ethical care. Striving to make care more ethical will assist nurses to make care more effective. In this case, knowledge about injury patterns is important to competent care but must be supplemented by knowledge of normal infant behavior, knowledge about the effects of a history of abuse (such as Ali has shared), knowledge of nursing's ethical obligations, and, by recognizing and working on our own reactions and biases, preconceived notions. Whether or not the abuse is substantiated, they are more likely to access nursing care in the future if they are treated with dignity and respect. In the case that abuse is substantiated, they will still have a relationship with their child, and an atmosphere of respect and fostering the parent's informed consent and autonomy ultimately will enhance the relationship and relationships with future service providers. If abuse is not substantiated, then the parents will be more likely to seek care in the future with less fear if they anticipate fair and respectful treatment.

EVALUATION. The family reports feeling safe physically, emotionally, and culturally in the health care settings. No further physical harm has come to Baby Z, and this family's access to care is not inhibited by these processes. The policies and processes used by nurses and other health care professionals need to be supported by evidence, and/or research into these must begin and be informed by the voices of those most affected. A broader understanding of the complexity of the relationship among family members is developed, including a more comprehensive understanding of social support networks. Supportive structures for nursing practice reinforce best practices for care of families who are coping with violence.

Cultural Considerations in Assessment and Intervention

A relational view leads to an understanding of culture as much more than "ethnicity." Culture is more than the values, attitudes, and beliefs that particular groups hold and is an ever-changing and dynamic process in which we all participate. The first "culture" of importance to ethical practice in relation to family violence is the culture of health care. In most Western health care contexts, health care providers are encouraged to be experts and to give "orders" or at least advice to patients/clients. This stance runs contrary to the idea of "empowering victims." Furthermore, health care providers are rarely trained to consider how their social advantages (position power, education, and income level) might be quite different from those to whom they provide care, and they rarely have much education regarding family violence. Thus, health care providers, including nurses, may practice based on assumptions about both violence and the circumstances of people's lives. As we have argued, cultivating a culture in which practice is based on knowledge rather than assumptions and in which dignity and respect are accorded to all are the first steps in promoting ethical practice.

The second "culture" of importance is the broader western culture within which health care practices arise. Most importantly, as we have argued, widespread tolerance for violence is characteristic of most Western cultures, and the dominance of value for economic productivity disadvantages those who are disabled, women, children, and the elderly, increasing tolerance for violence against such groups. Furthermore, individualism places

TABLE 15.1

Short-Term Goals	Nursing Interventions—Acute Care Nurse
Ensure physical safety for family while in emergency department	Identify with family what underlies their request to leave the department. Address identified needs and concerns. Demonstrate authentic concern for entire family. Ensure family's expertise in Baby Z's care is acknowledged and support their efforts in care provision. Follow the family's lead in the provision of care. Be available and present, check in with the family frequently. Attend to family's cues, and follow up on Ali's statement about being tough (and non-verbal behaviours) at a time when you could speak privately. Provide for physical comfort: adequate privacy, seating, blankets, food and drink, orientation to unit.
Promote emotional and cultural safety for family while in emergency department	Recognize your own assumptions and reactions to Baby Z's injuries, which may be informing or affecting your responses to the family, challenge and expose these, in order to move beyond these assumptions to a place of authenticity. Avoid communicating your unwarranted disapproval. Recognizing limits of the nursing role, avoid an investigative or "rescue" orientation towards Baby Z and her family. Provide care in a way which is respectful and non-judgmental, and develop a therapeutic professional relationship with family by: <ul><li>being transparent about the care processes (including investigations) and rationales</li><li>creating space to actively listen</li><li>identifying mutual expectations during stay</li><li>being honest about your concerns</li><li>developing and verifying an understanding of the meanings of this experience to the parents</li><li>exploring individualized interventions which might help them cope</li></ul> Assist the family to identify and mobilize their resources (do they have the support of family or friends?) to ensure support and care for themselves. Advocate for family's needs and respectful care as necessary. Support other care providers in providing respectful care. Identify hospital resources that may be helpful, such as advocates, a chaplain and so on. Connect with community nurse for further support and resources that are community context dependent.

Long-Term goals	Nursing Interventions—Community/Public Health Nurse
Ensure family maintains safe access to health care services	Create a space which is attentive, supportive, respectful, non-judgmental and responsive. Ensure family's future access to health care is not compromised by assumptions/practice of yourself or colleagues.
Ensure follow up support for family which fits their needs	Identify what the family might find to be helpful in caring for Baby Z, including connections with community resources, health resources, social services.
Education for parents about injuries in childhood and strategies for prevention	Discuss injury prevention strategies especially as they relate to developmental vulnerability and achievement of developmental goals.
Promote connection for family within community	Parent and family support networks, playgroups, activities, community centres, community nurses.

Continued

TABLE 15.1 *Continued*

Long-Term Goals	Nursing Interventions—Community/Public Health Nurse
Supporting healing for family's past encounters with violence	Guided by family as to what options might be useful for them (counseling, art therapy, peer support groups, etc.)
Identify best practices for interventions when working with families who suffer from violence	Identify gaps in research regarding child abuse and neglect, and advocate for more research on which to develop best practices. Collaborate with other service providers (such as child protection services, hospital social workers) to improve practice. Seek input from those involved with the system (clients and families) as to what is not working well and what might be working well.

responsibility on particular perpetrators and victims, obscuring the fact that family violence is a social problem and drawing attention away from the need for social solutions.

Finally, the third "culture" of importance is the multiple cultures shaping each of us, providers and recipients of care alike. As we have argued, it is critical not to confuse culture with "ethnicity" or race and to understand that cultures are shaped by history, economics, and social influences. Those steeped fully in Western culture and practices have to work at developing a critical understanding of their own cultures and the influences shaping their own and others' cultures. For example, it may be easier for American-born persons to see how patriarchy shapes practices such as female genital cutting and to take a human-right lens to such an issue (rather than the less helpful idea that such practices are simply "cultural"), but more difficult to see practices within their own contexts (such as the treatment of sex trade workers) with the same critical analysis. Trying to base practice on an ethnic categorization (for example, "black," Caucasian, Latino, and Chinese) provides no useful information, given the diversity of persons who could potentially be categorized as such and given the more powerful cultural influences described above.

SUMMARY

In summary, if nurses value dignity, respect and autonomy, and justice, then in relation to family violence, we must accord these values to all persons at all times in our practice. The challenges to ethical practice arise from our own lack of knowledge, policy directions that are incongruent with ethical practice, and the wider social context characterized by individualism, tolerance for violence, and tolerance for inequities. If we value children, we should seek to work to decrease poverty, end legal sanctioning of violence against children, and promote the participation of children in decision making as it affects them. If we value women, we should seek to promote gender equity and decrease sexism. Finally, if we value elders, we should seek to combat ageism in all its guises. All of these efforts can be made in the context of day to day practice, in our personal lives, and in our participation as citizens.

EXHIBIT 15.1 | *Further Resources*

- http://www.thelancet.com/series/child-maltreatment
- http://www.phac-aspc.gc.ca/cm-vee/csca-ecve/index-eng.php (Canadian Incidence Study main Findings)

REFERENCES

American Nurses Association (2001). Code of Ethics for Nurses. Retrieved December 18, 2005, from http://www.nursingworld.org/ethics/ecode.htm

Applebaum, B. (2004). Social justice education, moral agency and the subject of resistance. *Educational Theory, 54*(1), 59–72.

Barnett, O. W. (2000). Why battered women do not leave, part 1: External inhibiting factors within society. *Trauma, Violence, & Abuse, 1*(4), 343–372.

Bekemeier, B., & Butterfield, P. (2005). Unreconciled inconsistencies: A critical review of the concept of social justice in 3 national nursing documents. [Article]. *Advances in Nursing Science, 28*(2), 152–162.

Bell, M., & Mosher, J. E. (1998). (Re)fashioning medicine's response to wife abuse. In S. Sherwin (Ed.), *The politics of women's health: Exploring agency and autonomy* (pp. 205–233). Philadelphia, PA: Temple University Press.

Benhabib, S. (1992). *Situating the self: Gender, community and postmodernism in contemporary ethics.* New York: Routledge.

Bergum, V. (2004). Relational ethics and nursing. In J. Storch, P. Rodney & R. Starzomski (Eds.), *Toward a moral horizon: Nursing ethics for leadership and practice* (pp. 485–503). Toronto, Ontario, Canada: Pearson.

Berkowitz, C. D. (2008). Child abuse recognition and reporting: supports and resource for changing the paradigm. *Pediatrics, 122*(S1), 10–12.

Bostock, J., Plumpton, M., & Pratt, R. (2009). Domestic violence against women: Understanding social processes and women's experiences. *Journal of Community & Applied Social Psychology, 19,* 95–110.

Browne, A. J. (2001). The influence of liberal political ideology on nursing science. *Nursing Inquiry, 8*(2), 118–129.

Browning, D. S. (2006). The United Nations Convention on the Rights of the Child: Should it be ratified and why? *Emory International Law Review, 20,* 157–184.

Statistics Canada (2008). *Aboriginal Children's Survey 2006: Family, Community and Child Care.* Ottawa, Ontario, Canada: Statistics Canada.

Canadian Nurses Association. (2008). CNA Code of Ethics for Registered Nurses. Ottawa, Ontario, Canada: Canadian Nurses Association.

Cann, K., Withnell, S., Shakespeare, J., Doll, H., & Thomas, J. (2001). Domestic violence: a comparative survey of levels of detection, knowledge, and attitudes in healthcare workers. *Public Health, 115,* 89.

Chantler, K. (2006). Independence, dependency and interdependence: Struggles and resistances of minoritized women within and on leaving violent relationships. *Feminist Review,* 27–49.

Christian, C. W. (2008). Professional education in child abuse and neglect. *Pediatrics, 122*(S1), 13–17.

Coburn, D. (2004). Beyond the income inequality hypothesis: Class, neo-liberalism, and health inequalities. *Social Science & Medicine, 58*(1), 41–56.

Cohn, F., Salmon, M. E., & Stobo, J. D. (2002). *Confronting chronic neglect: The education and training of health care professionals on family violence.* Washington, DC: Institute of Medicine, National Academy Press.

Collins, P. A., Abelson, J., & Eyles, J. D. (2007). Knowledge into action?: Understanding ideological barriers to addressing health inequalities at the local level. *Health Policy, 80*(1), 158–171.

Davis, L. (2008). Omnipotence in child protection: Making room for ambivalence. *Journal of Social Work Practice, 22*(2), 141–152.

Dobrowolska, B., Wrońska, I., Fidecki, W., & Wysokiński, M. (2007). Moral obligations of nurses based on the ICN, UK, Irish and Polish Codes of Ethics for nurses. [Article]. *Nursing Ethics, 14,* 171–180.

Donchin, A. (1995). Reworking autonomy: toward a feminist perspective. *Cambridge Quarterly of Healthcare Ethics: CQ—The International Journal of Healthcare Ethics Committees, 4*(1), 44–55.

Donchin, A. (2001). Understanding autonomy relationally: Toward a reconfiguration of bioethical principles. *Journal of Medical Philosophy, 26*(4), 365–386.

Dunn, J. L., & Powell-Williams, M. (2007). Everybody makes choices. *Violence Against Women, 13,* 977–1001.

Durrant, J. E., Trocmé, N., Fallon, B., Milne, C., & Black, T. (2009). Protection of children from physical maltreatment in Canada: An evaluation of the Supreme Court's definition of reasonable force. *Journal of Aggression, Maltreatment & Trauma, 18*(64–87), 1–24.

Feddock, C. A., Pursley, H. G., O'Brien, K., Griffith, C. H., 3rd, & Wilson, J. F. (2009). Attitudes of Kentucky women regarding mandatory reporting of intimate partner violence. *The Journal Of The Kentucky Medical Association, 107*(1), 17–21.

Ferris, L. E. (2004). Intimate partner violence. *BMJ: British Medical Journal, 328*(7440), 595–596.

Freed, P. E., & Drake, V. K. (1999). Mandatory reporting of abuse: Practical, moral, and legal issues for psychiatric home healthcare nurses. *Issues in Mental Health Nursing, 20*, 423–436.

Garcia-Moreno, C., Jansen, H. A. F. M., Ellsberg, M., Heise, L., & Watts, C. H. (2006). Prevalence of intimate partner violence: Findings from the WHO multi-country study on women's health and domestic violence. *Lancet, 368*, 1260–1269.

Gershoff, E. T. (2002). Corporal punishment by parents and associated child behaviour and experiences: A meta-analytic and theoretical review. *Psychological Bulletin, 128*(4), 539–579.

Gilbert, R., Kemp, A., Thoburn, J., Sidebotham, P., Radford, L., Glaser, D., et al. (2009). Child Maltreatment 2: Recognizing and responding to child maltreatment. *Lancet, 373*(9658), 167–180.

Gilbert, R., Spatz Widom, C., Browne, K., Ferguson, D., Webb, E., & Janson, S. (2009). Child Maltreatment 1: Burden and consequences of child maltreatment in high-income countries. *Lancet, 373*(9657), 68–81.

Gilchrist, K. (2008). Invisible victims: Disparity in print-news media coverage of missing/murdered aboriginal and white women. *Conference Papers—Law & Society, 1*.

Goad, J. (2008). Understanding roles and improving reporting and response relationships across professional boundaries. *Pediatrics, 122*, S6–S9.

Greaves, L., Pederson, A., Varcoe, C., Poole, N., Morrow, M., Johnson, J. L., et al. (2004). Mothering under duress: Women caught in a web of discourses. *Journal of the Association for Research on Mothering, 6*(1), 16–27.

Gutmanis, I., Beynon, C., Tutty, L., Wathen, C. N., & MacMillan, H. L. (2007). Factors influencing identification of and response to intimate partner violence: A survey of physicians and nurses. *BMC Public Health, 7*, 12.

Häggblom, A. M. E., Hallberg, L. R.-M., & Möller, A. R. (2005). Nurses' attitudes and practices towards abused women. *Nursing & Health Sciences, 7*, 235–242.

Häggblom, A. M. E., & Möller, A. R. (2006). On a life-saving mission: Nurses' willingness to encounter with intimate partner abuse. *Qualitative Health Research, 16*, 1075–1090.

Haggerty, L. A., & Hawkins, J. (2000). Informed consent and the limits of confidentiality. *Western Journal of Nursing Research, 22*(4), 508–514.

Hamberger, L. K. (2007). Preparing the next generation of physicians. *Trauma, Violence & Abuse, 8*, 214–225.

Horner, R., & Kelly, T. B. (2007). Ethical decision making in the helping profession: A contextual and caring approach. *Journal of Religion and Spirituality in Social Work, 26*(1), 71–88.

Houston, S. (2003). Moral consciousness and decision-making in child and family social work. *Adoption & Fostering, 27*(3), 61–70.

Houston, S., & Griffiths, H. (2000). Reflections on risk in child protection: Is it time for a shift in paradigms? *Child and Family Social Work, 5*, 1–10.

Humphreys, C. (2008). Problems in the system of mandatory reporting of children living with domestic violence. *Journal of Family Studies, 14*, 228–239.

International Council of Nurses. (2005). The ICN Code of Ethics for Nurses. Geneva, Switzerland: International Council of Nurses.

Jones, R., Flaherty, E. G., Binns, H. J., Price, L. L., Slora, E., Abney, D., et al. (2008). Clinicians' descriptions of factor influencing their reporting of suspected child abuse: Report of the child abuse reporting experience study research group. *Pediatrics, 122*, 259–266.

Kim, J., & Gray, K. A. (2008). Leave or stay? Battered women's decision after intimate partner violence. *Journal of Interpersonal Violence, 23*, 1465–1482.

Kim, J., & Motsei, M. (2002). 'Women enjoy punishment': Attitudes and experiences of gender-based violence among PHC nurses in rural South Africa. *Social Science & Medicine, 54*(8), 1243.

Koss, M. P., & White, J. W. (2008). National and global agendas on violence against women: Historical perspective and consensus. *American Journal of Orthopsychiatry, 78*, 386–393.

Lambert, L., & Firestone, J. M. (2000). Economic context and multiple abuse techniques. *Violence Against Women, 6*(1), 49–67.

Lancet (2003). The neglect of child neglect. *Lancet, 361*(9356), 443.

Lane, W. G., & Dubowitz, H. (2009). Primary care pediatricians' experience, comfort and competence in evaluation and management of child maltreatment: Do we need child abuse experts? *Child Abuse and Neglect, 33,* 76–83.

Lewis, N. K. (2003). Balancing the dictates of law and ethical practice: Empowerment of female survivors of domestic violence in the presence of overlapping child abuse. *Ethics & Behavior, 13*(4), 353–366.

Marcus, I. (1994). Reframing "domestic violence": Terrorism in the home. In M. Fineman & R. Mykitiuk (Eds.), *The public nature of private violence: The discovery of domestic abuse* (pp. 11–35). New York: Routledge.

Martin, A. J., Berenson, K. R., Griffing, S., Sage, R. E., Madry, L., Bingham, L. E., et al. (2000). The process of leaving an abusive relationship: The role of risk assessments and decision-certainty. *Journal of Family Violence, 15,* 109–122.

McDaniel, C. (1998). Ethical environment: Reports of practicing nurses. *Nursing Clinics of North America, 33*(2), 363–372.

McMurray, A., & Moore, K. (1994). Domestic violence: Are we listening? Do we see? *The Australian Journal of Advanced Nursing, 12*(1), 23–28.

Melton, G. B. (2005). Mandatory reporting: A policy without reason. *Child Abuse and Neglect, 29*(1), 9–18.

Meyers, M. (2004). African American women and violence: Gender, race, and class in the news. *Critical Studies in Media Communication, 21*(2), 95–118.

Moore, S. A. D. (2003). Understanding the connection between domestic violence, crime and poverty: How welfare reform may keep battered women from leaving abusive relationships. *Texas Journal of Women & the Law, 12*(2), 451–484.

Olson, L. (1995). Ethical climate in health care organization. *International Clinics of North America, 42*(3), 85–95.

Olson, L. (2002). Ethical climates as the context for nurse retention. *Chart, 99*(6), 3,7.

Pattison, S. (2001). Are nursing codes of practice ethical? *Nursing Ethics, 8,* 5–18.

Phelan, A. (2008). Elder abuse, ageism, human rights and citizenship: Implications for nursing discourse. *Nursing Inquiry, 15,* 320–329.

Pinhero, P. S. (2006). *World report on violence against the children.* Geneva, Switzerland: United Nations Publishing Services.

Potter, J. (1996). *Representing reality: Discourse, rhetoric and social construction.* London: Hutchinson.

Reading, R., Bissell, S., Goldhagen, J., Harwin, J., Masson, J., Moynihan, S., et al. (2009). Child maltreatment 4: Promotion of children's rights and prevention of child maltreatment. *Lancet, 373,* 332–343.

Reece, R. M., & Jenny, C. (2005). Medical training in child maltreatment. *American Journal of Preventative Medicine, 29*(5S2), 266–271.

Reimer Kirkham, S., & Browne, A. J. (2006). Toward a critical theoretical interpretation of social justice discourses in nursing. *Advances in Nursing Science, 29*(4), 324–339.

Rodney, P., Brown, H., & Liaschenko, J. (2004). Moral agency: Relational connection and trust. In J. L. Storch, P. Rodney, & R. Starzomski (Eds.), *Toward a moral horizon: Nursing ethics for leadership and practice* (pp. 154–177). Toronto, Ontario, Canada: Pearson Prentice Hall.

Rodríguez, M. A., Wallace, S. P., Woolf, N. H., & Manigone, C. M. (2006). Mandatory reporting of elder abuse: Between a rock and a hard place. *Annals of Family Medicine, 4*(5), 403–409.

Schluter, J., Winch, S., Holzhauser, K., & Henderson, A. (2008). Nurses' moral sensitivity and hospital ethical climate: A literature review. *Nursing Ethics, 15,* 304–321.

Sege, R. D., & Flaherty, E. G. (2008). Forty years later: Inconsistencies in reporting of child abuse. *Archives of Diesease in Childhood, 93*(10), 822–824.

Sherwin, S. (1998a). *The politics of women's health: Exploring agency and autonomy.* Philidelphia, PA: Temple University Press.

Sherwin, S. (1998b). A relational approach to autonomy in health care. In S. Sherwin (Ed.), *The politics of women's health: Exploring agency and autonomy* (pp. 19–47). Philadelphia, PA: Temple University Press.

Shonkoff, J. P., & Phillips, D. A. (2000). *From neurons to neighborhoods: The science of early child development.* Washington DC: National Academy Press.

Silverman, J. G., Mesh, C. M., Cuthbert, C. V., Slote, K., & Bancroft, L. (2004). Child custody determinations in cases involving intimate partner violence: A human rights analysis. *American Journal of Public Health, 94,* 951–957.

Statistics Canada (2007). Persons in low income after tax. Retrieved from http://www40.statcan.ca/l01/cst01/famil19a-eng.htm

Storch, J., Rodney, P., & Starzomski, R. (Eds.). (2004). *Toward a moral horizon: Nursing ethics for leadership and practice*. Toronto, Ontario, Canada: Pearson.

Straus, M. A., & Mathur, A. K. (1996). Social change and the trends in approval of corporal punishment by parents from 1968 to 1994. In D. Frehsee, W. Horn, & K. D. Bussman (Eds.), *Family violence against children: A challenge for society* (pp. 91–105). New York: Walter de Gruyter.

Straus, M. A., & Stewart, J. H. (1999). Corporal punishment by America parents: National data on prevalcnece, chronicity, severity and duration, in relation to child and family characteristics. *Clinical Child and Family Psychology Review, 2*, 55–70.

Taylor, C., & White, S. (2001). Knowledge, truth and reflexivity: The problem of judgment in social work. *Journal of Social Work, 1*, 37–59.

Taylor, R. (2009). Slain and slandered: A content analysis of the portrayal of femicide in crime news. *Homicide Studies, 13*, 21–49.

Tjaden, P., & Thoennes, N. (2000). *Full report of the prevalence, incidence, and consequences of violence against women*. Washington, DC: US Department of Justice, Office of Justice Programs, National Institute of Justice.

Tower, M. (2007). Intimate partner violence and the health care response: A postmodern critique. *Health Care for Women International, 28*(5), 438–452.

Trocmé, N., Fallon, B., MacLaurin, B., Daciuk, J., Felstiner, C., Black, T., et al. (2003). *Canadian Incidence Study of Reported Child Abuse and Neglect—2003: Major Findings*. Ottawa, Ontario, Canada: Minister of Public Works and Government Services Canada.

Trocmé, N., MacMillan, H., Fallon, B., & De Marco, R. (2003). Nature and severity of physical harm caused by child abuse and neglect: Results from the Canadian Incidence Study. *Canadian Medical Association Journal/Journal De L'association Medicale Canadienne, 169*(9), 911–915.

Varcoe, C. (2001). Abuse obscured: An ethnographic account of emergency nursing in relation to violence against women. *The Canadian Journal Of Nursing Research/Revue Canadienne De Recherche En Sciences Infirmières, 32*(4), 95–115.

Varcoe, C. (2009a). Inequality, violence and women's health. In B. S. Bolaria & H. Dickinson (Eds.), *Health, illness and health care in Canada* (4th ed., pp. 259–282). Toronto, Ontarion, Canada: Nelson.

Varcoe, C. (2009b). Interpersonal violence assessment. In C. Jarvis, A. J. Browne, J. MacDonald-Jenkins & M. Luctkar-Flude (Eds.), *Physical examination and health assessment: First Canadian edition* (pp. 119–134). Toronto, Ontarion, Canada: Elsevier.

Whatmore, S. (1997). Dissecting the autonomous self: Hybrid cartographies for a relational ethics. *Environment and Planning, 15*, 37–53.

Whitehead, M., & Dahlgren, G. (2006). *Levelling up (part 1): A discussion paper on concepts and principles for tackling social inequities in health*: WHO Collaborating Centre for Policy Research on Social Determinants of Health, University of Liverpool.

Wilcox, P. (2000). Lone motherhood: The impact on living standards of leaving a violent relationship. *Social Policy & Administration, 34*, 176–190.

Wilcox, P. (2005). Beauty and the beast: Gendered and raced discourse in the news. *Social & Legal Studies, 14*(4), 515–532.

Woodtli, M. A., & Breslin, E. (1996). Violence-related content in the nursing curriculum: A national study. *Journal of Nursing Education, 35*(8), 367–374.

World Health Organization. (2002). *World report on violence and health*. Geneva, Switzerland: World Health Organization.

Young, I. M. (1990). *Justice and the politics of difference*. Princeton, NJ: Princeton University Press.

Young, I. M. (1997). *Intersecting voices: Dilemmas of gender, political philosophy and policy*. Princeton, NJ: Princeton University Press.

16

International Perspectives on Family Violence

Sepali Guruge, PhD, RN
Agnes Tiwari, PhD, RN
Marguerite B. Lucea, PhD, MSN, MPH, RN

INTRODUCTION

Family violence is a serious global health problem. It is often considered a "private" affair, and occurrences are not always discussed with others or reported to authorities. Violence within families can occur in many forms, whether it is directed at children, intimate partners, or elders. Although both men and women can be victims of such abuse, in general, girls and women are more often the victims.

This chapter provides international perspectives on child abuse, intimate partner violence (IPV), and elder abuse. Each form of abuse is discussed in regard to definition/perception, prevalence, health consequences, and risk factors. The latter is discussed in light of how family violence can be influenced by shifts in economics, globalization, conflicts, and civil wars that can create socioeconomic inequalities within and between countries and regions that may lead to unequal production of violence among certain groups or in certain communities. Where possible, we have given examples from various studies that pertain to a variety of countries and communities. It is important to note, however, that within countries much heterogeneity exists regarding aspects of family violence and that such variations are often greater than those between countries. Thus, attention to the diversity of children, women, and the elderly, as well as their lives and experiences, is necessary to understand the complex ways in which the social, economic, gender, geographic, ethnic, cultural, and political contexts of people's lives shape their perception of and exposure to family violence and their responses to it. Discussed in each of the section are some strategies that are currently being used to address each form of abuse. We end the chapter by considering public health nursing strategies for earlier identification of family violence, awareness building about family violence and its health impacts, and creation of more supportive programs and policies that effectively respond to the needs of diverse groups and improve prevention and health-promoting initiatives.

Theoretical Approach

By far the most comprehensive approach to understanding and addressing family violence in both local and international contexts is the ecological framework. (chapter 1 in this book addresses the theoretical foundations of violence and aggression in depth). The ecological framework examines the interrelationships between individual factors, familial relationship factors, community contexts, and societal structures, and how they influence whether or not a person experiences violence in the family. In the current chapter, the risk and protective factors of familial violence in international settings are discussed using this framework. Particularly germane to examining family violence occurring within and across borders are the meaning of violence cross-culturally, the cultural positioning of violence within a society, and issues of gender inequality. What constitutes abuse and violence for some may not be perceived similarly by others, even within the same cultural group. Whether violence is seen as a "means to an end" in a given society may have an impact on how violence within families is perceived.

CHILD ABUSE AND MALTREATMENT

Definitions/Perceptions

Child maltreatment is a worldwide problem that requires the attention of clinicians. The umbrella term *child maltreatment* includes physical, sexual and emotional abuse, neglect, and exploitation of children [World Health Organization (WHO), 2008a] that results in "actual or potential harm to the child's health, survival, development or dignity in the context of a relationship of responsibility, trust or power" (WHO, 2002b, p. 3). Physical abuse involves acts that can cause actual or potential physical harm to the child. Sexual abuse refers to using a child for sexual gratification. Emotionally abusive acts include "restricting a child's movements, denigration, ridicule, threats and intimidation, discrimination, rejection and other non-physical forms of hostile treatment" (p. 60). Neglect refers to the failure of a parent to provide for the development of the child—where the parent is in a position to do so—in one or more of the following areas: "health, education, emotional development, nutrition, shelter and safe living conditions" (WHO, 2002b, p. 60).

Different cultures, communities, and societies have different norms, standards, and expectations regarding childrearing and parenting practices, and different perceptions about what acts of omission or commission might be considered child abuse and neglect (Estroff, 1997; Facchin et al., 1998; WHO, 2006a,c). Terms such as harshness, discipline, punishment, abuse, and neglect can depend on whether or not there is intent to harm, the behavior/actions of the adult, and the outcome of such actions/behavior in terms of actual or potential harm and its severity on the child (Ketsela & Kebede, 1997; Madu & Peltzer, 2000; Shumba, 2001; Straus & Hamby, 1997; Straus, Hamby, Finkelhor, Moore, & Runyan, 1998; Youssef, Attia, & Kamel, 1998). For example, non-physical disciplinary techniques such as "time out" used by parents in some countries may be regarded as "restricting a child's movement" (a form of control) and psychological abuse in other regions of the world. As Tang (2006) emphasized, parental corporal punishment is often used in combination with other disciplinary measures such as time out and withdrawal of privileges, as well as verbal abuse. However, there appears to be a general agreement across most cultures that "child abuse should not be allowed, and [virtual agreement] in this respect where very harsh disciplinary practices and sexual abuse are concerned" (WHO, 2002b, p. 60).

In the International Society for the Prevention of Child Abuse and Neglect's (ISPCAN, 2006) report based on participants from various countries ($N = 72$), the most commonly identified forms of child abuse across all or most subgroups were sexual and physical abuse by parents or caretakers. Other behaviors noted as abusive by at least 90% of the participants included failure to provide adequate food, clothing, or shelter; child prostitution; and children living on the street. Adequate food, clothing, shelter, and medical care might not be available to all children even in high-income countries and more commonly among children in countries facing extreme economic hardship or those dealing with armed conflict. At least 80% of ISPCAN's participants also identified child abandonment, physical beatings, forcing a child to beg, and infanticide as acts of child maltreatment. However, there was considerable regional variation regarding female circumcision, physical discipline, and failure to secure medical care based on religious beliefs. Physical discipline was less likely to be listed as a form of child abuse by participants from Africa and Asia, and parental substance abuse was least likely to be reported as a form of child maltreatment by participants from the Americas and Asia (ISPCAN, 2008). However, wide variations existed within these regions.

Prevalence

Global data on prevalence of child maltreatment and child deaths are limited. Even with these limitations, an estimated 57,000 fatalities of children under 15 years of age occurred in 2000 (WHO, 2002a,b), and an estimated 31,000 deaths occurred in 2002 (WHO, 2006a), with most of these occurring among children less than 4 years of age (WHO, 2002a,b, 2006a). Global rates of child deaths suggest that this risk, in general, varied according to the income level of a country and region of the world (WHO, 2002b, 2006a). For children under 5 years, the rate of homicide is 2.2 per 100,000 for boys and 1.8 per 100,000 for girls in high-income countries, and 6.1 per 100,000 for boys and 5.1 per 100,000 for girls in low- to middle-income countries. The highest homicide rates (per 100,000) for children in this age range were 17.9 for boys and 12.7 for girls in the WHO African Region. The risk of child deaths is greater in countries with considerable economic inequalities (WHO, 2006a). However, wide variations exist within regions. For example, within Europe, the child death rate in Portugal is 3.7 from maltreatment and 17.8 from all injuries per 100,000 children compared to 0.1/100,000 in Spain and 0.2/100,000 in Greece and Italy [United Nations Children's Fund (UNICEF), 2003].

Moreover, many child deaths are not investigated or autopsied, and potential homicide cases go undetected. Significant levels of misclassification in the cause of death are also evident. For example, when deaths attributed to other causes such as sudden infant death syndrome or accidents were reinvestigated in several US states, some were reclassified as homicides (Kirschner & Wilson, 2001; Reece & Krous, 2001). Thus, the prevalence rates of fatal child abuse are actually much higher.

Accurate statistics about the incidence and prevalence of non-fatal child abuse are even more difficult to obtain. This is due, in part, to a lack of globally accepted definitions of child maltreatment, substantial differences between families about what are considered suitable disciplinary measures, a nearly universal norm to keep family matters private for the sake of family honor, and fear among children to come forward and report.

Only 17 countries around the world have prohibited the use of corporal punishment in the home (Global Initiative, 2006). Globally, nearly one-third of children report being physically punished at home by the use of an implement (e.g., spoon, stick, belt, etc.; United Nations & Pinheiro, 2006). The available studies indicate that some form of physical disciplining is accepted around the world (Dubowitz & Bennett, 2007). In a study conducted in the Republic of Korea, nearly two-thirds of the parents reported whipping their children (Hahm & Guterman, 2001). Nearly half of Romanian parents admitted to beating their children "regularly" (Browne et al., 2002). Bardi and Borgognini-Tarli (2001) reported an incidence of severe violence in about 8% of Italian families. Stathopoulou (2004) found that harsh discipline tends to be common in Greece, and May-Chahal and Cawson (2005) reported that the prevalence of physical abuse ranged from 7% for severe cases (defined as regular violent actions that caused injury) to 14% for intermediate cases (occasional violent acts causing no serious injury) in the UK. In a cross-sectional survey of 3,577 high school and college/university students from six provinces in China, 54.6% of male and 32.6% of female students reported being hit or kicked very hard on the head or body by someone with an open hand, while 39.0% and 28.5% had been beaten by someone with an object during the first 16 years of their life (Chen, Dunne, & Han, 2004). In a cross-sectional survey of 1,185 secondary school students in East Jerusalem and the West Bank (Palestine), a third of the participants reported that their fathers had attacked, grabbed, or shoved them and a third reported that their mothers had slapped, pushed, or kicked them at least once during adolescence (Haj-Yahia & Abdo-Kaloti, 2003). Recently, the Global School-Based Student Health Survey asked adolescents (13–15 years old) to report on their experiences of physical abuse in the prior 12 months. As of 2007, reports of physical abuse ranged from 25% to 57%, with 43 of the 59 participating countries reporting data (WHO, 2008c).

Some international studies indicate that many children are subjected to emotional abuse as well as to neglect. However, to date, there are no accurate estimates of emotional abuse by itself. In some countries, neglect constitutes the largest proportion of reported child maltreatment cases. In a study conducted in Kenya, 21.9% of children reported that they had been neglected by their parents (Troeme & Wolfe, 2001), and in Canada, a national study of cases reported to child welfare services identified that 19% of the cases involved physical neglect, 12% abandonment, 11% educational neglect, and 48% physical harm resulting from a parent's failure to provide adequate supervision (ANPPCAN, 2002). According to the WorldSAFE study involving five countries (Chile, India, the Philippines, Egypt, and the United States), the practices of threatening children with abandonment or with being locked out of the house varied widely (WHO, 2002b). For example, the prevalence rate of threats of abandonment as a disciplinary measure reported by mothers in the Philippines was 48%; in India, 20%; in Egypt, 10%; and in Chile, 8%. The question was not asked of the participants in the United States; however, according to the Children's Bureau (2009), 59.0% of victims in the United States experienced neglect.

International studies of child sexual abuse (CSA) consistently report prevalence rates as being higher among girls than boys in both developing and developed countries. Some studies have shown that the risk was two to three times higher among girls and women (Dunne, Purdie, Cook, Boyle, & Najman, 2003; MacMillan et al., 1997; Tyler,

2002). According to WHO (2002b) estimates, more than 150 million girls and 73 million boys worldwide who are under 18 years of age have experienced sexual violence, including but not limited to forced sexual intercourse. One of the contributing factors for young girls and women experiencing sexual abuse is early marriage. In 1981, the United Nations (UN) declared the participation in and consummation of early or forced marriage of children to older adults to be a violation of human rights (UN, 1981), yet globally, over 60 million women between the ages of 20 and 24 report being married before age 18, with 31.3 million of those occurring in South Asia and 14.1 million occurring in sub-Saharan Africa (UNICEF, 2006). The contributing factors for CSA among the rest of the 90 million girls worldwide vary (see chapters 4 and 12 for a discussion of these other factors).

Variations in CSA rates exist between regions. For example, CSA rates for female and male participants appear to be similar in some areas [see Haj-Yahia and Tamish's (2001) study of Palestinian university students and Madhu and Peltzer's (2000) study of rural/ semi-urban school children in Northern province in South Africa]. Sexual harassment was found to be more common among men than women on most measures in some studies such as Zeira, Astor, and Benbenishty's (2002), conducted with Arab students in schools in Israel, where the risk was at least twice as high for Arab boys. Tang (2002) found that prevalence estimates for a range of unwanted childhood sexual experiences among a sample of Chinese university students were consistently much lower than those usually found in Western samples. Less than 1% reported sexual intercourse with an adult, compared to rates of between 6% and 10% in many Western countries. In Australia, the corresponding rates among young women in a community survey answering the same questions varied between 6.4% and 21.1% (Dunne, et al., 2003).

The previously reported rates most often cannot be compared cross-culturally or across countries because of variations in definitions and data gathering methods. For example, some studies use broad definitions, inclusive of acts such as physical contact, whereas others' definitions are narrower, focusing on specific acts such as rape. In addition, results from surveys among children cannot be accurately compared to those with adolescents or adults reporting on childhood experiences or with parents reporting on behalf of their children for clear reasons of bias and other methodological constraints. In addition, samples sizes vary significantly among studies. The rates are also constantly changing because of increased efforts by individual advocates as well as governments to educate the public about the harms of child abuse and to put measures in place to address such practices, including mandatory child abuse reporting systems.

Risk Factors

The common risks for child maltreatment around the world can be grouped according to individual, family, community, and societal factors. As with other forms of abuse, child maltreatment can be explained only by understanding the complex interaction of a number of factors at these varying levels.

Individual risk factors can be associated with the child or the parent or both. Those individual risk factors pertaining to the child include age, gender, and (dis)ability. As noted earlier, infants <4 years of age are at higher risk of fatal abuse, with those <2 years at highest risk. The range of ages for nonfatal physical abuse varies by country, peaking in China between 3 and 6, in India between 6 and 11, and in the United States between 6 and 12 (WHO, 2002b). The rates of sexual abuse tend to be higher among children after

TABLE 16.1 *Types of Abuse, Definitions, and Risk Factors*

		Child abuse and maltreatment
Definition		Includes physical, sexual, and emotional abuse, neglect, and exploitation of children (WHO, 2008a) that results in "actual or potential harm to the child's health, survival, development or dignity in the context of a relationship of responsibility, trust or power" (WHO, 2002b, p. 3).
		Gender:
		Female for infanticide, educational and nutritional neglect, forced prostitution
		Male for harsh physical punishment
		Disability:
		Higher risk for neglect and abuse
	Parents	Abused themselves as children
		Physical, cognitive problems
		Low self-esteem
		Alcohol and/or drug use
		Difficulty handling stress and anger
	Family	Limited social support for mothers working outside home
		Larger families
		Only one biological parent; step-parent
		Economic deprivation
		Marital conflicts (and other family violence)
		Rural living
	Community	Limited social support systems for families
		High levels of unemployment and overcrowding
		Social capital
	Society	Economic forces
		Gender inequalities
		Traditional cultural norms regarding gender norms, privacy of family
		Limited access to social welfare mechanisms

		Intimate partner violence
Definition		The threat of, and/or actual, physical, sexual, psychological, or verbal abuse by a current or former spouse or non-marital partner, as well as coercion or the arbitrary deprivation of liberty that can occur in public or private life (Health Canada, 1999).
Risk Factors	Individual	History of child abuse or witnessing abuse
		Alcohol use
	Relationship	Age difference between partners
		Marital status
		Alcohol/drug use
		Marital conflict and stress
		Changing gender roles
		Poverty
	Community	Presence of other types of violence in the community
		Lower social capital
		Male unemployment/underemployment
		Geographic isolation
		Limited social support networks
	Society	Migration patterns
		Armed conflict or political instability
		Gender inequalities

		Elder abuse
Definition		A single or repeated act, or lack of appropriate action, occurring within any relationship where there is an expectation of trust which causes harm or distress to an older person (WHO, 2008b). Includes physical and sexual abuse, aspects of neglect (isolation and social exclusion), violation of human, legal, and medical rights, and deprivation of choices, decisions, status, finances, and respect (WHO, 2001).

Continued

TABLE 16.1   Continued

		Elder abuse
Risk Factors	Individual	Susceptibility to illness and/or chronic conditions
		Level of dependence on others for care
	Family	Poverty, financial difficulties
		History of violence
		Alcohol and/or drug use of caretakers
		Strained relations with in-laws
	Community	Modernization, industrialization, urbanization
		Weakening of traditional social networks and support
		Socio-economic inequalities

they reach puberty and higher among girls than boys (WHO, 2002b). In most countries, girls are also at higher risk than boys for infanticide, educational and nutritional neglect, and forced prostitution. In general, boys tend to be at greater risk for harsh physical punishment (WHO, 2002b). Children with disabilities who were born prematurely are also especially vulnerable to abuse and neglect (Yen, et al., 2008). Other risk factors for abuse include disliked gender and physical attributes (Tang, 2002), poor school achievement, and behavioral problems (Alyahri & Goodman, 2008).

Some of the risk factors pertaining to parents include their having been maltreated themselves as children, believing in physical punishment of children, suffering from physical, mental, or cognitive problems, lacking self-control when angry or upset, using drugs and/or alcohol, being involved in criminal activities, and experiencing low self-esteem or feelings of inadequacy (WHO, 2002b). In addition, parental risk factors for child abuse in both developing and developed countries include low education and unemployment (WHO, 2002b). While higher education is associated with negative attitudes about abusive behavior toward children (Stephenson et al., 2006), available evidence also suggests that highly educated individuals are more likely to be employed outside the home, a factor that can lead to the potential for child neglect (Winton & Mara, 2001). Based on a study on child abuse in Fiji, Adinkrah (2003) reported that "filicidal fathers typically suffer from psychiatric problems, neurological disorders, cognitive impairment or alcoholism" (p. 559). Tang (2006) suggested that parents who are young or who have an inadequate understanding of child development, difficulty handling daily hassles and stresses, or a personality/psychiatric disorder are more likely to use violence against their children. Gender differences among abusers have also been noted. For example, in studies conducted in China, Chile, Finland, Kenya, India, and the United States, women reported using more physical discipline than men. However, it is well-known that the more severe injuries are often caused by male perpetrators, including fatal injuries (WHO, 2002b). In cases of CSA, it is far more common that the perpetrators are men, regardless of the sex of the victim. Men perpetrated the abuse in 90% of the CSA cases against girls and in 63–83% of the cases against boys (WHO, 2002b).

Family-level risk factors can include family environment and family structure, as well as parental education, employment, and substance abuse. Wong, Chen, Goggins, Tang, and Leung (2009) noted a higher risk of assault among children with mothers who work as professionals or businesswomen. In these cases, mothers are expected to be the primary caregivers to children and the elderly in addition to holding full- or part-time employment outside the home—a common situation in both developed and developing countries. In the context of loss of or limited social networks and supports, the pressure and the stress of this responsibility can increase the rates of abuse (Barnett, Miller-Perrin, & Perrin, 2005; Wong et al., 2009). Family size may also increase the likelihood of child abuse. One study in Chile found that, compared to parents with smaller families, parents of four or more children (especially those ranged closely in age) were three times more likely to hurt their children (WHO, 2002b). The risk of CSA may be higher when a girl is living with one biological parent, particularly her father, or with a stepfather (Amodeo, Griffin, Fassler, Clay, & Ellis, 2006; Bagley & Ramsay, 1986; Finkelhor, Hotaling, Lewis, & Smith, 1990).

Other family-level risk factors associated with child maltreatment include rural living, family breakdown, marital conflicts, additional family violence (such as IPV), low income and economic deprivation, and weak child–adult relationships (Alyahri, & Goodman, 2008; Doe, 2000; Haj-Yahia & Abdo-Kaloti, 2003; Stephenson et al., 2006; Tang, 2006). According to a study conducted in Yemen, rural mothers more often used harsh corporal punishment than urban mothers, even after adjusting for maternal education and family size (Alyahri, & Goodman, 2008). Family poverty (along with associated stress and increased workload) was also related to harsh corporal punishment (Alyahri, & Goodman, 2008; Cavanagh, Dobash, & Dobash, 2007; Dubowitz & Bennett, 2007). In general, increases in the quality and quantity of physical, psychological, and financial stresses create risks of child maltreatment (Cox, Kotch, & Everson, 2003).

A number of community-level risk factors have been identified with regard to child abuse. Socially isolated families with limited social support networks within the community are at higher risk for family violence, including child abuse. Those parents who are able to find support are less likely to abuse their children, even if other individual or family risk factors are present. One study in Argentina demonstrated that children in single-parent families were at higher risk for abuse when compared to children in two-parent families. Single-parent families with access to social support, however, were at decreased risk for abuse compared to similar families without support (WHO, 2002b).

In addition, communities with high unemployment, intense poverty, population turnover, and overcrowded housing report higher rates of abuse than communities without these factors (WHO, 2002b). The chronic poverty in these communities has been shown to have an impact on parental behavior which, in turn, affects the children (WHO, 2002b).

The intricate Chinese culture can provide an interesting perspective to further support findings about the influence of culture on child abuse. The enforcement since 1979 of the one-child policy has influenced Chinese social and cultural approaches to parenting (Wong et al., 2009). It has been suggested that this policy has resulted in very high parental expectations for the family's sole child, particularly in families with higher socioeconomic status (Wong et al., 2009). The relationship between socioeconomic status and physical abuse is complex and not entirely consistent between family and community. One study found that, although low familial socioeconomic status was indicative of increased risk for physical child abuse, higher community socioeconomic status may also be related to increased risk of abuse (Wong et al., 2009). The link between higher than average community-level socioeconomic status and increased risk for physical abuse may be attributed to social stress, with parents perhaps feeling the need to compete with wealthy neighbors. This is particularly true in some cultures in which parents place a high value on family pride, success, and status in their children (Wong et al., 2009). In addition, there may be a relationship between social capital and child abuse, according to WHO (2002b), such that the lack of social capital and social investment appears to have a detrimental effect on children, placing them at higher risk for abuse.

According to WHO (2002b), certain society-level factors including the following appear to have a significant impact on the well-being of children and families: economic forces, inequalities related to sex and income; cultural norms surrounding gender roles, parent–child relationships, and the privacy of the family; child and family policies; the nature and extent of preventive health care and social protection for infants and children; the strength of the social welfare system; and social conflicts and wars. As indicated by WHO (2002b), these broad societal inequalities influence parents' abilities to provide adequate care and protection for their children. For example, Lalor (2004) attributed the perceived increase in CSA in Tanzania to several factors, including erosion of traditional childcare mechanisms, increased influence of Western cultures, pervasive poverty, and the relatively low status of women and girls in Tanzanian society. The author pointed out that these factors are present in many areas of sub-Saharan Africa. This correlation implies the influence of low socioeconomic status and gender inequality on child maltreatment. The Ministry of Women and Child Development, Government of India (2007) has stated that practices such as child marriage, the caste system, discrimination against female children, and child labor can increase children's susceptibility to abuse and neglect. This situation is worsened by urban poverty or because of lack of or limited access to medicine, education, and nutrition among certain groups within the country.

Existing Strategies to Address Child Maltreatment

Several existing programs have made valuable contributions to addressing child abuse and neglect. Family support is fundamental to fostering healthy parent–child relationships. In general, programs directed toward family support are intended for families who are at high risk of abuse but programs that help parents understand child development and improve their skills in managing their children's behaviors can be beneficial to most parents (WHO, 2002a,b). In a family support program in Singapore, for example, education and coaching in parenting is introduced through classes that prepare individuals for parenthood. These begin in secondary school, where students learn about childcare and development, as well as obtain direct experience at preschool and childcare centers by working with young children (WHO, 2002b). Another promising example of preventing youth violence and child maltreatment is the implementation of home visitation programs, such as the one operated by the Parent Centre in Cape Town, South Africa (WHO, 2002b).

One of the key preventive strategies for child maltreatment is school-based programs integrated into regular school curricula to teach children to recognize violent and abusive situations as well as provide them with knowledge and skills to empower them. An example of such a program is the Stay Safe primary prevention program in Ireland, which has been incorporated in almost all primary schools (WHO, 2002b). According to Tang and Yan (2004), a CSA prevention program in Hong Kong offers children early exposure to reliable information on the issues of abuse and neglect and promotes disclosure of abuse in the case of sexual abuse.

Changing public attitudes and behaviors with respect to preventing child maltreatment is of great significance. In Zimbabwe, a program aimed at changing the community's perception of child abuse and neglect has been developed to address CSA. In this participatory and multi-sectoral program, activities such as role playing, painting, discussion groups, and drama are used to highlight the experiences of sexual abuse and the importance of detection (WHO, 2002b). In their study on child abuse in Yemen, Alyahri, and Goodman (2008) further illustrated the need to change community attitudes about child abuse in an effort to promote community and government awareness of non-physical disciplinary methods. According to ISPCAN (2006) that evaluated the usage and effectiveness of some preventive strategies for child abuse and neglect in developed and developing countries, which include regions in Africa, the Americas, Asia, Europe, and Oceania, the most commonly used strategies at individual and community levels included professional training, advocacy, media campaigns, prosecution, and increasing local services.

INTIMATE PARTNER VIOLENCE

Definitions/Perceptions

IPV occurs in most countries regardless of the social, cultural, ethnic, religious, and economic backgrounds of people. IPV is the threat of, and/or actual, physical, sexual, psychological, or verbal abuse by a current or former spouse or non-marital partner, as well as coercion or the arbitrary deprivation of liberty that can occur in public or private life (Health Canada, 1999). Such violence includes "acts of physical aggression—such as slapping, hitting, kicking and beating; psychological abuse—such as intimidation, constant belittling and humiliating; forced intercourse and other forms of sexual coercion; and various controlling behaviours—such as isolating a person from their family and friends, monitoring their movements, and restricting their access to information or assistance" (WHO, 2002e, p. 1). Although IPV is not limited to male-to-female perpetration, the majority of its victims around the world are female. Women are also far more likely to be severely injured during assaults by intimate partners than are men (Canadian Centre for Justice Statistics, 2000; Tjaden & Thonnes, 2000).

Wife abuse, in particular wife beating, results from patriarchal beliefs that provide men with authority over and the right to discipline or punish their wife. This understanding has been captured in a number of studies conducted in various countries, including Bangladesh, Cambodia, Greece, India, Sri Lanka, Mexico, Nigeria, Pakistan, Papua New Guinea, the United Republic of Tanzania, Zimbabwe, Canada, the United States, and England (Antonopoulou, 1999; Gunaratne, 2002; WHO, 2002d, 2006b). Such studies from both developed and developing countries have identified a number of justifications for IPV used by men and, at times, by women. These include not obeying the husband, arguing back or questioning the husband, not doing household work, leaving the house without the husband's permission, refusing the husband sex, and suspicion of the woman's infidelity. Although acceptance of these justifications is changing over time, such beliefs regarding IPV are still considerably condoned. In England, 50% of young men and nearly 33% of young women reported that physical or sexual violence may be acceptable under some circumstances (Donovan). In Greece, nearly 50% of the participants in a survey reported that IPV is caused by women's demands for equality and independence (Antonopoulou). Over 80% of rural women in Egypt believe that wife beating is justified in certain circumstances (El Zanaty, et al. 1995). Similar findings were noted in studies conducted in other countries (Bawah, Akweongo, Simmons, & Philips, 1999; Khan, Townsend, Sinha, & Lakhanpal, 1996; Wood & Jewkes, 1997). Some communities distinguished between "just" and "unjust" reasons for abuse and between "acceptable" and "unacceptable" levels of violence (Gunaratne, 2002; Guruge, 2007; Wijeyatilake, 2003; WHO, 2002d). In such cases, others would intervene only if the beating is judged as being too severe or without a just reason.

Prevalence

Statistics for femicide by intimate partners or other family members on a global scale are not readily available. However, those rates that are available (even though often underestimated) indicate the seriousness of the issue. A national study in South Africa estimated the rate to be 8.8 per 100,000 women (Mathews et al., 2008). Aldridge and Browne (2003) found that of the homicides in the UK, 37% of female murder victims were killed by an intimate partner, compared to 6% of the male murder victims. Similarly, in the United States, 32.7% of homicides of women were committed by an intimate partner, but only 3.1% of the men murdered were cases related to partner violence (Fox & Zawitz, 2006). Studies from Australia, Canada, Israel, South Africa, and the United States show that 40–70% of all women murdered were killed by their husbands or boyfriends (WHO, 2002b).

At a global level, non-fatal (i.e., non-femicide) IPV occurs in epidemic proportions. The rates of non-fatal IPV are comparable to those for cancer, HIV/AIDs, and cardiovascular diseases (Heise, Pitanguy, & Germain, 1994). According to the United Nations Population Fund (2000), an estimated one in three women globally has experienced some kind of sexual, physical, or psychological assault, most often inflicted by an intimate partner. Population-based surveys in developed and developing countries indicate that lifetime prevalence of IPV ranges from 26% to 42% (Fanslow & Robinson, 2004; Mirrlees-Black, 1999; Mulroney, 2003).

Physical IPV is common around the world. Taking data from 48 population-based surveys from around the world, WHO (2002d) noted that between 10% and 69% of women reported being physically assaulted by an intimate male partner at some point in their lives. The recent WHO Multi-Country Study that examined the prevalence of lifetime physical violence by male partners among women in 15 sites in 10 countries showed that prevalence ranged from 13% to 61%, with most sites reporting between 30% to 50% the prevalence of lifetime sexual violence by intimate partners ranged from 6% in Japan city to 59% in Ethiopia province, and Namibia and Tanzania had lifetime sexual violence estimates of 17% and 31%, respectively (Garcia-Moreno et al., 2006).

Most women experience multiple forms of abuse, threat, and control. A number of studies have shown that physical violence is often accompanied by psychological abuse and, in one-third to over one-half of cases, by sexual abuse (Ellsberg, Pena, Herrara, Liljestrand, & Winkvist, 2000; Koss et al., 1994; Leibrich, Paulin, & Ransom, 1995). In one study among 613 women in Japan, 57% had suffered all three types of abuse (Yoshihama & Sorenson, 1994). These findings were confirmed in the recent multi-country WHO study (2006b) where percent of women experienced more than one type of abuse.

There are numerous studies on IPV from countries around the world, and some focused on prevalence rates. However, aside from the WHO Multi-Country Study, country-to-country comparisons cannot be carried out due to differences in methodology, such as differing definitions and measures of abuse, sample sizes, sources of data, participant inclusion/exclusion criteria, and recruitment and data collection approaches, as well as socioeconomic and geographical factors and the timing and duration of abuse.

Risk and Protective Factors for Intimate Partner Violence

In many countries, the prevalence of IPV varies substantially between geographical areas, and many times, the differences between regions within countries can vary as much, if not more, than those between nations. The mechanisms behind this wide variation between communities are debatable. At the individual, familial, community, and societal levels, IPV is shaped by a complex set of interacting factors, rather than by any single cause (Guruge, 2007; WHO, 2002b, 2006b). Some of the risk factors for IPV include age differences between partners, marital status, a history of childhood abuse, and alcohol use/abuse (Barrata, McNally, Sales, & Stewart, 2005; Bui & Morash, 1999; Hyman et al., 2006; Raj & Silverman, 2002; WHO, 2006b). A history of child abuse or being a witness to IPV among parents has emerged as a risk factor in a number of studies conducted in Brazil, Cambodia, Canada, Chile, Colombia, Costa Rica, El Salvador, Venezuela, Indonesia, Nicaragua, Spain, Canada, and the U.S. (WHO, 2002a, 2002b).

One of the most influential and consistent risk factors for IPV at an interpersonal level is that of marital conflict (Black et al., 1999). Verbal conflicts between partners have been shown to be significantly related to subsequent physical violence (Jewkes, Penn-Kekana, Levin, Ratsaka, & Schrieber, 2001). This relationship remains significant, even when controlling for other risk factors such as husband's stress, socioeconomic status, and marital stability (Hoffman, Demo, & Edwards, 1994). Changing family dynamics and gender roles, as exemplified by women working outside the home or postponing marriage and children, and men being away from home for long periods due to work, may strain family relations and contribute to the abuse of women and children (deAlwis 2004; Garcia-Moreno, 2000; Hyman et al., 2004; Krug, Dahlberg, Mercy, Zwi, & Lozano, 2002; Morrison, Guruge, & Snarr, 1999; Raj & Silverman, 2002), particularly where these changes are contrary to "traditional" gender and social norms.

At the community level, higher rates of other types of violence and lower social capital seem to be positively related to IPV (WHO, 2002b). However, most of the studies conducted have been restricted in diversity with regard to culture and geography. Globalization has brought about rapid social change that sometimes results in gender, social, and economic inequalities, weak social safety nets, and societal norms condoning violence, and these, in turn, may increase women's risk of IPV at home (Maclean & Sicchia, 2004). Male unemployment and underemployment are related to increases in male alcohol use/abuse and male on male violence, as well as IPV (Guruge, 2007; Krug et al., 2002; Maclean & Sicchia, 2004). Whatever the precise mechanisms, it is probable that poverty acts as a "marker" for a variety of social conditions that, in combination, increase women's risk for IPV (Heise, 1998). Other factors associated with poverty such as overcrowding, hopelessness, frustration, sense of inadequacy, and stress need to be further explored with respect to their influence on IPV (Byrne et al., 1999; Ellsberg et al., 2000; Gonzales-de Olarte & Gavilano, 1999; Hoffman et al., 1994; Larrain, 1994; Martin et al., 1999; Moreno, 1999; Nelson & Zimmerman, 1996; Rodgers, 1994; Rosales et al., 1999; Straus et al., 1986). Stress has also been identified as an antecedent to both alcohol abuse and IPV (Barnett & Fagan, 1993; Barnett, Miller, Perrin, & Perrin, 1997; Brownridge & Halli, 2002; Heise, 1998). Other community factors, such as geographic isolation and loss of social support have been associated with women's risk of IPV (Abraham, 2000; Glodava & Onizuko, 1994; Hyman et al., 2006; Morrison et al., 1999).

It is important to note that risk and protective factors may also differ across cultures and communities. For example, migration to other countries has been identified as contributing to IPV (Fong, 2000; Guruge, Khanlou & Gastaldo, 2010; Hyman, Guruge, & Mason, 2008; Hyman et al., 2006). In addition, support for women within social networks in matrilocal communities can be a protective factor, whereas pressure on women within social networks in patrilocal communities can be a risk factor for IPV. Another community factor that influences IPV is whether or not that community is embroiled in armed conflict or political instability. More than 40 countries are presently experiencing such situations (Garcia-Moreno, 2000). Thus, attention must be paid to the influence of other violence that men and women have experienced (or perpetrated) on their perception of what constitutes IPV and the appropriateness of using violence to deal with conflict, unfairness, and injustice (Guruge, 2007).

Strategies to Address Intimate Partner Violence

The Director General of WHO (WHO, 2006b) has called for a comprehensive response to IPV, particularly in the health care sector, which takes into account the reasons why women may be reluctant to seek help. Women's responses to IPV are both individually and socially shaped, and they depend on the supports and services available to women to manage their lives within a particular community and society (Guruge & Humphreys, 2009). Extended family members, neighbors, and co-workers often have a strong influence on the couple (Abraham, 1999, 2000, 2002; Raj & Silverman, 2002). In particular, in collectivist communities where values of family ties, harmony, and order prevail, women are taught to subordinate the self to the interests of the family (Abraham, 2000; Agnew, 1998; Bui & Morash, 1999); therefore, they may feel that separation, divorce, and/or remarriage are not viable options. Women may also believe in the importance of keeping families together for the welfare of children (Ford-Gilboe, Wuest, & Merrit-Gray, 2005; Guruge, 2007; Morrison et al., 1999; Varcoe & Irwin, 2004; Wuest, Ford-Gilboe, & Merrit-Gray, 2005). Many women are reluctant to seek help for IPV due to shame, fears of being stigmatized or having their children taken away, or feeling as though they might be pressured by helpers to leave their husbands (Guruge, 2007; Varcoe & Irwin, 2004; Ford-Gilboe et al., 2005; Wuest et al., 2005). As such, women's responses to IPV must be considered within the context of the social networks that enforce gender role expectations and associated power relations.

Violence by intimate partners is an important public health problem. Resolving it requires the involvement of many sectors working together at community, national, and international levels. At each level, responses must include empowering women and girls, reaching out to men, providing for the needs of victims, and increasing the penalties for abusers. It is vital that responses should involve children and young people and focus on changing community and societal norms. The progress made in each of these areas will be key to achieving global reductions in violence against intimate partners (WHO, 2002d).

Beyond the agreement that violence against women is unacceptable and must stop, differently situated women may disagree about what constitutes violence, what causes violence, women's roles in perpetrating violence, and penalties for those who commit violent acts. IPV is socially constructed and, therefore, is shaped by cultural, religious, socioeconomic, educational, and political factors. Thus, perceptions of abuse vary widely (Mehotra, 1999; Raj & Silverman, 2002). The expression of IPV is also shaped by the context, with certain forms taking on greater prominence in specific situations. Knowing more about the ways in which IPV is expressed and perceived will help enhance the capacity of communities to respond to it and to develop culturally, linguistically, and contextually appropriate health care interventions and programs.

ELDER ABUSE

Elder abuse is a global health problem (Sherman, Rosenblatt, & Antonucci, 2008). This issue may become even more of a problem with the expected increase in the older population. Older people are the fastest growing subgroup of people worldwide (UN, 2004). The number of people over 60 years of age is expected to almost triple within the next few decades, from 672 million in 2005 to nearly 1.9 billion by 2050. The percent of increase in the elderly population is greater in the developing world (WHO, 2008a). By the year 2025, the percentage of older women living in the developing world will increase from the current 58–75% (Daichman, 2005).

Definitions/Perceptions

There is no universally accepted definition of elder abuse and maltreatment (Patterson & Malley-Morrison, 2006), but the existing definitions substantially overlap each other. *Elder mistreatment* includes physical and sexual abuse, aspects of neglect (isolation and social exclusion), violation of human, legal, and medical rights, and deprivation of choices, decisions, status, finances, and respect (WHO & International Network for the Prevention of Elder Abuse, 2001). *Elder abuse* has been defined as "the mistreatment of older people by those in a position of trust, power, or responsibility for their care" (Health Canada, 1999, p. 1). The UK's Action on Elder Abuse developed a definition that subsequently was adopted by the International Network for the Prevention of Elder Abuse (INPEA) and used by the World Health Organization (WHO, 2008b): "Elder abuse is a single, or repeated act, or lack of appropriate action, occurring within any relationship where there is an expectation of trust which causes harm or distress to an older person." The latter definition captures the frequency of abuse, omission as well as commission of acts, and the relationship between the parties and the fact that their actions might cause harm and/or distress to the older person (Daichman, 2005).

WHO (2008b) defined five types of elder abuse: physical, psychological/emotional, financial/material, sexual, and neglect. Physically abusive behavior or acts are defined as slapping, hitting, kicking, force-feeding, restraint, and striking with an object. Psychological/emotional abuse includes verbal threats or aggression, social isolation, and humiliation. Financial/material abuse includes exploitation and/or use of funds or resources that belong to the older person. Sexual abuse includes acts such as suggestive talk, forced sexual activity, touching, and fondling without consent or with a person who is not competent to consent. Examples of acts of neglect include failure to provide adequate food, clothing, shelter, medical care, and hygiene, or social stimulation.

In the WHO/INPEA (2001) ongoing study on "A Global Response to Elder Abuse" in eight developed and developing countries (Argentina, Brazil, Kenya, Lebanon, India,

Sweden, Canada, and Austria), the forms of abuse were similar across countries and included neglect (isolation, abandonment, and social exclusion); violation of human, legal, and medical rights; and deprivation of choices, decisions, status, finances, and respect. Based on a review of studies conducted in five different countries (United States, Israel, Germany, Brazil, and Japan), Patterson and Malley-Morrison (2006) concluded that physical, psychological, and economic abuse, and neglect were universally mentioned as forms of elder abuse; however, the specific examples and the severity of these forms of abuse varied across countries. Attitudes toward psychological abuse also differed considerably across countries. Interestingly, sexual abuse was rarely, if ever, mentioned.

Other studies indicate differential sensitivity to certain forms of abuse based on the age or the gender of study participants. For example, Bezerra-Flanders and Clark (2006) found that elderly women were more likely than elderly men to mention psychological abuse as a severe form of abuse. In comparison, Arai (2006) found that elderly women were more likely than men to mention psychological neglect as examples of moderate abuse. Furthernore, König and Leembruggen-Kallberg (2006) reported that (older) women were more likely than men to mention economic abuse as a form of abuse as well. In terms of the influence of age in shaping perceptions of abuse, the literature is not consistent across countries and cultures. For example, Arai (2006) found that older participants in Japan were more likely than younger ones to mention psychological abuse and neglect and less likely to mention physical aggression when considering forms of abuse. In a study in Brazil, however, the situation was reversed (Bezerra-Flanders & Clark, 2006). In terms of the gender of the abuser, evidence suggests that sons, daughters, and sons/daughters-in-law can be the abusers. Several studies have shown that considerable elder abuse is committed by daughters or daughters-in-law (Arai, 2006; Rabi, 2006; Tauriac & Scruggs, 2006), perhaps occurring in the context of their more direct roles as caregivers to elderly parents and parents-in-law.

Prevalence

There is very little data on the prevalence and incidence of elder mistreatment, and the data that do exist vary widely. According to WHO (2008a), the prevalence of elder abuse varies between 1% and 35%. These discrepancies may be related to measurement and reporting biases, differences in definitions, and variations in inclusion/exclusion criteria and survey and sampling methods.

Countrywide reporting and monitoring systems are not common in most countries, particularly in resource-limited settings. Several population-based studies in developed countries in the 1990s indicated that 4–6% of older adults have experienced abuse in the home (Comijs, Pot, Smit, Bouter & Jonker, 1998; Ogg & Bennet, 1992; Podnieks, 1992). A recent population-based survey in Britain had similar results, with 2.6% of participants reporting being abused (Biggs, Manthorpe, Tinker, Doyle, & Erens, 2009). According to the report of the World Assembly on Aging (UN, 2002), in Australia, Canada, and the UK, the proportion of abused or neglected older people ranged from 3% to 10%. A recent study in Canada found a similar range, estimating that about 4–10% of the elderly experience some kind of abuse (INPEA, 2009). In Sweden, 13% of men and 16% of women over 65 years reported experiencing some form of abuse (Eriksson, 2001). Seven percent of the women and 2.5% of the men over 65 years in Finland were noted as having experienced abuse within their families (INPEA, 2009). According to König and Leembruggen-Kallberg

(2006), elder abuse in Germany ranged from 2% for those living independently to 68% for those with dementia. Arai's (2006) study with a sample of 78 frail elders living in community settings in Japan reported an abuse rate of 17.9%. In a recent nationally representative study in Israel, over 18% of participants indicated that they had experienced at least one form of abuse (Lowenstein, Eisikovits, Band-Winterstein, & Enosh, 2009). In another recent study in Israel, 6% of the elderly participants reported being abused, while health care professionals (HCPs) believed that 21% of them had clear evidence of abuse and that 33% were at high risk of abuse (Cohen, Levin, Gagin, & Friedman, 2007).

Surveys of elderly people in South Korea found that between 30% and 38% of the participants reported some kind of abuse; emotional abuse and neglect were the most commonly reported, but physical abuse and financial abuse were also cited (Doe, Han, & McCaslin, 2009). In a recent study in China, over 35% of elders reported being mistreated or abused (Dong, Simon, & Gorbein, 2007). According to a study by Keskinoglu, et al. (2008) on the prevalence of elder abuse in two socioeconomically different districts of Izmir, Turkey, the prevalence of neglect was 27.4% for the lower socioeconomic status district and 11.2% for the higher socioeconomic status district. In a recent study in Iran (Manoochechri, Ghorbi, Hosseini, Nasiri Oskuyee, & Karbakhsh, 2009), 88% of all participants 60 years and above reported experiencing at least one type of abuse. In another recent study conducted in Croatia, Ajdukovic, Ogresta, and Rusac (2009) found that 49% of 303 elderly people were victims of partner violence, and 51% were victims of violence by other family members.

Clearly, these numbers demonstrate the enormity of the issue. Although the ranges vary and appear to be quite broad in some areas, WHO (2008a) noted that, according to some experts, "elder abuse is underreported by as much as 80%." As the world's population ages, elder abuse becomes even more of a pressing issue to address.

Risk Factors

Some of the factors that contribute to child abuse and IPV are the same for elder abuse, such as poverty and stress. Other similar, family-level risk factors have been highlighted by the Pan American Health Organization (n.d.), including the level of dependence of the older person, history of violence in the family, personal or financial difficulties in the family, caretakers' use/abuse of alcohol or other substances, social isolation, and lack of support. In addition, migration both within and between countries has been observed to affect family dynamics and structures (Guruge & Collins, 2008) and can have an impact on the treatment of elders.

Other risk factors are unique to elder abuse. Malley-Morrison, Nolido, and Chawla (2006) noted that some of these are differing systems of inheritance in some societies, normative behaviors related to caretaking of grandchildren, susceptibility of the elderly to illness and/or chronic conditions, subsequent reliance on children to care for and support them, strained relations with sons/daughters-in-law, and other issues related to multigenerational co-residence. In a WHO/INPEA qualitative study in eight developing and developed countries (Daichman, 2005), focus groups of elders identified many of the aforementioned risk factors and also included lack of information about available resources, and intergenerational conflict.

WHO (2008a) also reported that modernization, industrialization, and an aging population, coupled with urbanization and increasing numbers of women in the workforce, may explain increased reports of elder abuse and may be particularly relevant to understanding women's perpetration of abuse of elderly family members. In India, for example, older people live with their children and more often with their son than their daughter. With the increase in women engaged in education and employment, the traditional social networks and supports women had to care for their older family members have weakened (Sherman et al., 2008). Many women are now required to move to the industrial centers for employment, leaving elders without family to care for them. These situations, along with the socioeconomic inequalities faced by the considerable majority in these countries, can make the elder relatives susceptible to neglect and other kinds of maltreatment (Sherman et al., 2008). Similar findings were noted in China and Korea. Social isolation and loneliness have been identified as key risk factors in China (Dong, Simon, Gorbein, Percak, & Golden, 2007). In South Korea, shifts toward a more nuclear, rather than extended, family structure and increased participation by women in the work force have led to more neglect of elderly relatives (Oh, Kim, Martin, & Kim, 2005). The required role for daughters-in-law to care for parents-in-law was found to influence elder abuse in Japan (Arai, 2006). Sons' economic responsibility for their aging parents contributes to the potential for economic neglect by those sons (Levesque, 2002).

Strategies to Address Elder Abuse

The International Plan of Action on Ageing that was held by the UN in Vienna at the General Assembly on Ageing in 1982 (United Nations, 1991) shaped many countries' formulation of policies and programs to address elder abuse. Since then, various efforts have been devoted to develop legislation and implement programs that address elder abuse in both developing and developed countries. These efforts are in different stages in different countries (WHO, 2002c). For instance, in 2002, HelpAge International, an international not-for-profit organization, reviewed the status of national policies on aging in 79 developing countries and eastern and central European countries. Of these, 29 had national policies for older people, and 16 were in the process of developing such policies. Each country's legislation covered a variety of topics, including food and nutrition, health, employment, housing, social security, and pension provision; cultural and leisure activities; and filial piety and respect. The effectiveness of these policies in addressing elder abuse and preventing it is not well documented. However, in a number of cases, elder abuse policies were explicitly noted (Older Persons Programme, 2009). In 2000, the government of South Africa produced national guidelines for preventing, detecting/identifying, and intervening against physical elder abuse. India has a National Policy on Older Persons, which declares that the State will provide protection against abuse and exploitation. The National Plan of Action for Elderly Welfare in Indonesia emphasizes the need to protect older persons at risk for neglect. Argentina has undertaken a project to create a center for the prevention of domestic violence against older people. In South Africa, the report of any known incidences or suspicion of elder abuse is an obligation, and failure to do so is a crime.

The United States has a national system for reporting and treating cases of elder abuse. On the other hand, activities for the prevention of elder abuse in some European countries such as France, Germany, Italy, and Poland are limited mainly to individual researchers and to some local programs (INPEA, 2009). In December 2008, Norway opened a national helpline for elderly people who are exposed to violence.

In addition, the Latin American Committee for the Prevention of Elder Abuse has actively campaigned to increase awareness of the problem of elderly abuse within Latin

American and Caribbean countries (INPEA, 2009). For some countries, including Cuba, Peru, Uruguay, and Venezuela, activities have consisted mainly of professional conferences and research studies. Other countries in the region, such as Argentina, Brazil, and Chile, have moved further on the issue. For example, in Argentina, the organization Proteger was established in 1998 as one of the programs of the Department for the Promotion of Social Welfare and Old Age to work exclusively on elder abuse cases. Proteger also runs a free telephone helpline. In Chile, a law against violence in the family, including that directed at the elderly, was passed in 1994. In Brazil, the Ministry of Justice, Health, and Welfare has endorsed training HCPs about elder abuse. In other countries such as South Korea, the Older Adult Welfare Law was implemented in July 2004. As a result, a 24-hour emergency hotline was set up through which persons could report elder abuse, licensing standards for older adult protective facilities were established, and standards for caregiving professionals were instituted. In addition, 16 elder abuse prevention centers were set up with implementation manuals for effective operation (Doe et al., 2009). In June 2009, the Ministry of Human Resources and Skills Development of Canada announced the launch of a national awareness campaign on elder abuse (Government of Canada, 2009). Although, in Australia, some states have set up systems to deal with cases of elder abuse, Kurrle and Naughtin (2008) stated that Australia has not yet developed a nationally integrated system to deal with elder abuse.

With a rapid worldwide expansion of activities on elder abuse, the INPEA was formed in 1997, with representation from all six inhabited continents. INPEA presented a number of country reports regarding their progress toward formulating and implementing policies and programs on aging and elder abuse (INPEA, 2009). One example is Austria's 2004 parliamentary law to ban age discrimination against the elderly. Israel is another example, as it has established specialized units within welfare departments in 20 local municipalities that address elder abuse. It has employed protocols to identify and report elder abuse and neglect within the health system. The Israeli Ministry of Welfare also issued special regulations for detecting and intervening against elder abuse in residential settings. In addition, Germany has implemented a 3-year governmental program called Secure Life in Old Age (2008–2011), which focuses on specific problems facing elderly for which preventive actions seem necessary. Portugal has established a free counseling service for older adults who feel victimized, mistreated, and neglected in any way. There is a training program for health professionals, including physicians, nurses, psychologists, and social assistants, who work in facilities for continuing care. Running a national project, the University of Helsinki/Palmenia Centre for Continuing Education in Finland is trying to include protection of elderly in the security plans of municipalities. They pay special attention to domestic violence, with a particular attention to elderly women who may be experiencing this form of abuse. In Spain, the Centre Reina Sofia in Spain works to increase the visibility of elder abuse in the country, and in 2008, it has completed the first nationwide research on the ill treatment of elders within the family.

Efforts have also been made to increase the level of surveillance and the level of knowledge among health care providers regarding elder abuse. In 2001, an advisory group to WHO and several national representatives determined basic strategies for developing a global response against elder abuse (WHO & INPEA, 2001). This included taking global inventory of "best practices" regarding the health care response to elder abuse, conducting additional training about elder abuse for HCPs, developing and evaluating screening tools for HCPs to use in developing countries, and promoting further policy changes within countries. The group also stressed the importance of mobilizing civil society against elder abuse by raising awareness and decreasing stigma surrounding the issue. It also committed to ensuring the dissemination of any research findings on the topic area through peer-reviewed, scientific journals.

A PUBLIC HEALTH NURSING APPROACH

From a public health nursing approach, family violence may be addressed at the primary, secondary, or tertiary level of prevention.

Primary Prevention

To prevent family violence, it is necessary to take a community approach. Because family violence is a reflection of the normative acceptance of aggression in a given society (Vandello & Cohen, 2003), primary prevention is needed in order to revise this norm within communities. Through public education programs, nurses can teach communities that family violence causes harm not only to the victims and perpetrators but also to the community as a whole. Through media campaigns against family violence, nurses can also help communities to challenge social norms that condone the use of violence against family members. Nurses can maximize their efforts to raise public awareness by participating in global primary prevention activities. For example, they can participate in the World Elder Abuse Awareness Day, which is organized by INPEA. On June 15th every year, groups and organizations from all over the world contribute to raising awareness about elder abuse. Nurses can use this forum to disseminate messages of elder abuse prevention to large audiences with minimal costs.

As clinicians, nurses must be aware that while public education and campaigns may raise awareness and may even bring about social attitudinal change, in some instances, tolerance of family violence may be so entrenched in the social norms that the survivors are still blamed and the perpetrators are still absolved of wrongdoing. For example, in Palestinian society, women as well as men believe that wife beating is justified in certain circumstances (Haj-Yahia, 1998). Similar views have also been found in Arab (Haj-Yahia, 2005; Khawaja, 2004, Oweis, Gharaibeh, Al-Natour, & Froelicher, 2009) and Asian communities (Bhuyan, Mell, Senturia, Sullivan, & Shiu-Thornton, 2005; Chan, 2006; Shiu-Thornton, Senturia, & Sullivan, 2005).

Such erroneous beliefs are not just confined to IPV. Worldwide, corporal punishment is still commonly used to discipline children (Donnelly & Straus, 2005) despite the clear

---

EXHIBIT 16.1 | *Prevention of Family Violence*

- Primary prevention: Stop family violence before it happens through public education, community sanctions against violence, provision of support to at-risk families, and regulation and legislation.
- Secondary prevention: Reduce or end family violence through early detection and by providing timely interventions.
- Tertiary prevention: For those experiencing family violence, provide therapeutic interventions including referrals.

link between the corporal punishment of children and child maltreatment (Burns, 1993) and despite The United Nations Convention on the Rights of the Child (1989), which specifically noted the deleterious effects of such punishment. In addition, victims of elder abuse may falsely believe that they are to be blamed for the abuse (Kosberg, 1988). Prevention of elder abuse is further delayed in Asian communities because many falsely believe that the Confucian ethic of filial piety prevents its occurrence (Doe et al., 2009).

When developing strategies, health professionals also need to pay closer attention to families in greatest need of services, including those with low birth weight and preterm infants; children with chronic illness and disabilities; low-income, unmarried teenage mothers; and those with a history of substance misuse. Needed services include early interventions in pregnancy that continue to at least the second year of a child's life or even to 5 years of age. These services need to be flexible so that the duration and frequency of visits and the types of assistance provided can be adjusted to a family's need and level of risk. Such early childhood programs should (a) actively promote positive physical- and mental health-related behaviors and specific qualities of infant caregiving; (b) reduce stress within the family by enhancing social and physical environments; (c) have HCPs teach child management skills, so that each newly learnt skill would form the basis for the next skill; and (d) adequately identify and report problematic behaviors at home.

Nurses should be aware of prevailing beliefs about family violence and take the lead to challenge and correct unfounded or misguided assumptions where needed. An example is the use of strict discipline for childrearing in many societies, a common practice that is influenced by the principles of filial piety and obedience. Nurses can, through their contact with parents, challenge the long-held societal beliefs about the use of corporal punishment as an effective childrearing method, provide evidence on the vulnerability of young children to physical and psychological abuse, and educate parents on how to raise children without resorting to shame and/or violence. One example of a nurse-led project to decrease child abuse is a community-based project using UNICEF's Child Friendly Family framework that has been instituted in a socially impoverished community in Hong Kong. Its goals include (1) eliminating corporal punishment of children in the home; (2) promoting the use of positive parenting skills; and (3) sustaining communitywide participation in "Child Friendly Families" through a collaboration of professionals, parents, and volunteers (Tiwari et al., 2008). This low-cost project provides an example of what can be done to change public perception about child abuse and empower parents to provide a child friendly environment for their children.

Addressing the roots of the issue of child abuse is fundamental to eliminating injustice against children. Reducing poverty, improving standards and levels of education, creating more employment opportunities, as well as increasing the availability of resources and quality of childcare at the national and global levels can both prevent and reduce child maltreatment. WHO (2006a) outlined strategies for preventing child maltreatment and reducing the underlying causes and risk factors, as well as strengthening the protective factors, in the hope of preventing the occurrence of new instances of maltreatment at the individual and community levels. These strategies included providing early childhood education and care and offering universal primary and secondary education about child abuse. In addition, strategies aimed at community-level factors included reducing unemployment and implementing good social protection systems that include the provision of benefits for people living with disabilities, health insurance, child care, income or food supplements, and unemployment benefits.

Because nurses are educated to seek understanding of the contextual influences on a person's health, they can work with families to develop healthy and effective coping mechanisms to use when they encounter stressful life events. This strategy can also be considered a primary preventive measure of family violence. For example, while becoming a parent may bring many rewards including a sense of achievement and family life enhancement (Feeney, Hohaus, Noller, & Alexander, 2001), caring for a new infant can be very demanding for the parents (Petch & Halford, 2008). The many changes associated with new parenthood can further strain the couple's relationship (Shapiro, Gottman, & Carere, 2000) and may even lead to marital conflict (Brown, 1994). It is important for nurses who work with expectant couples and new parents to offer support during this time because marital distress can have a negative impact on the infant as well as the couple (Bond & McMahon 1984; Krishnakmuar & Buehler, 2000). Through antenatal education, nurses can help couples prepare for parenthood, teaching them how to care for their infant (such as feeding, diapering, and soothing a crying baby) and the acceptable ways to discipline children. In addition, components of marital communication, fondness and admiration, and conflict management (Shapiro & Gottman, 2005) can be incorporated in antenatal education to enhance marital quality and reduce couple conflict. When deciding which of the antenatal education programs may be appropriate for supporting expectant couples, nurses must ensure that the selected program is evidence-based (Gagnon & Sandall, 2008) and culturally appropriate for the target group. The latter criterion is particularly important when programs developed in one culture are applied to another culture. Nurses should, for instance, consult recommendations on cultural adaptation when adopting Western couple education programs for Asian couples (Huang, 2005).

Primary prevention of family violence may also take place at a macro, societal level through the development of regulation and legislation designed to prevent or respond to abusive situations. Nurses can play an important role at this level by (a) lobbying their elected officials to make nonviolence in families a priority, (b) canvassing for ratification of international conventions (such as the United Nations Convention on the Rights of the Child), and (c) ensuring that an adequate knowledge of family violence and reporting laws is included in nurses' education.

Secondary Prevention

Once family violence has occurred, early identification and timely intervention are needed to reduce or end the violence and prevent further violence-related complications. One US-based study showed that, of the women who were killed by their intimate partners, 41% had utilized the health care system in the year before their murder (Sharps, et al., 2001). This finding suggests that nurses are in an ideal position to detect family violence, partly because they routinely conduct client/patient assessments. Therefore, screening for family violence could easily be incorporated in nursing assessments.

In addition, because of nurses' experience in making highly personal and sensitive inquiries, they should be able to help survivors of family violence recount their abusive experiences. Although people from different cultures may vary in their willingness to disclose sensitive issues such as family violence, some of the principles of good practices for screening are nevertheless applicable across cultures. These include the need to conduct the assessment in private and in the absence of the perpetrator, to ensure confidentiality, and to adopt a caring and empathetic approach.

In addition, nurses should be sensitive to how culture and traditions influence the disclosure of family violence. For example, some ethnic groups may believe that the use of violence against women in intimate relationships can be justified under certain circumstances (Haj-Yahia, 1998; Legerwood, 1990; Yick & Agbayani-Siewert, 1997; Yoshioka, DiNoia, & Ullah, 2001). Among Russian women, disclosure of IPV may be viewed as "airing dirty laundry" (Crandall, Senturia, Sullivan, & Sihiu-Thorntom, 2005). Similar views may also be shared by other ethnic groups due to a "felt-need" to preserve the face and honor of the family, maintain harmony, and sacrifice the self for the greater good of the family/community (Ho, 1990; Lee, 2002; Shiu-Thornton et al., 2005; Yamashiro & Matsuoka, 1997).

This custom does not absolve nurses from asking the much-needed questions because even in societies that emphasize close family ties and saving family face, abused women are prepared to disclose their abuse to an "outsider" if the assessment is conducted by trained professionals in a culturally sensitive manner (Tiwari et al., 2005; Tiwari, Chan et al., 2007). Thus, when explaining the need for screening to those thought unwilling to report family violence, nurses should emphasize that disclosure is the first step to restoring harmony and is essential in preventing the breakup of family ties. Furthermore, nurses should recognize that different forms of family violence may not be perceived in the same way across different cultures. For example, neglect may be viewed as a serious form of elder abuse in Turkey (Yalcinkaya, Mandiracioglu, & Turan, 2006) but only as a mild or moderate form of abuse in Russia (Rinsky & Malley-Morrison, 2006), Greece (Daskalopoulos, Kakouros, & Stathopoulou, 2006), and Italy (Daskalopoulos & Borrelli, 2006). Knowing how the same construct may be interpreted differently in different cultures (Krahe, Bieneck, & Moller, 2005), nurses can use questions that are meaningful to the respondents when eliciting the history of family violence. As an example, in cultures where sexual chastisement is accepted as part of a husband's marital prerogative, asking a woman if she has been sexually abused by her intimate partner may not elicit the true picture. In these cases, behavior-specific questions that describe inappropriate sexual demands are preferred, as they do not require women to interpret whether their experience is abusive or not.

In addition, nurses should use screening tools that are appropriate for the target population. An example is the Abuse Assessment Screen (AAS) used to screen Chinese women for IPV. Although the AAS has been used extensively in North America, modification was required to ensure that it accurately detects the psychological abuse that predominates in Chinese abusive intimate relationships (Tiwari, Fong et al., 2007).

Providing timely interventions once the abuse has been detected is also important. On a community level, nurses can form collaborative relationships with community agencies to target both the persons who have been mistreated and the perpetrators. Health service-based interventions may also be provided in the health care setting. Regardless of the setting, secondary preventive interventions should be theory-led, evidence-based, and protocol-driven. In particular, theory-led interventions can help nurses decide whether such interventions are appropriate to address the problem. For instance, as coercive tactics are often used by the perpetrators of IPV, nurses may select the Empowerment Intervention (Parker, McFarlane, Soeken, Silva, & Reel, 1999), which is based on an empowerment model (Dutton, 1992) and designed to increase the survivor's independence and control. However, since the perception of family violence is much influenced by the beliefs and values of a given society, interventions that are consistent with the subscribed norms of the recipients are more likely to be accepted and yield positive results. Tiwari et al. (2005) found this was the case when the Empowerment Intervention (Parker et al., 1999) was adopted for use in a study of abused pregnant Chinese women. In the shame-oriented Chinese society, many of the women participants were too afraid to reveal their shameful feelings especially if they had been ridiculed previously for doing so. The researchers concluded that, in addition to the original key components of the intervention, an empathetic understanding component (Rogers, 1951) was also required. The modified intervention succeeded in reducing IPV and improving the psychological health of the women (Tiwari et al., 2005).

Nurses offering secondary preventive measures might suggest certain services and assistance for those identified as susceptible to perpetration, in order to reduce levels of stress before an act of maltreatment occurs. These could include, for example, periods of respite care or attendance at a support group for caregivers of older adults (Penhale, 2008). Even in cultures that are thought to protect their elders, economic burden, multi-generational households, fragile support systems for the elderly, and a lack of preparation for old age may seriously strain the older adult–caregiver relationship and give rise to the risk of elder abuse (Dong & Simon, 2008; Oh, Kim, Martins, & Kim, 2005). Nurses should identify those in need of protection and provide timely intervention. In addition, nurses could help those at risk to utilize factors that are known to offer protection from family violence, such as increased social support. In the case of elder abuse, for example, good family relationships can be an important modifying factor in reducing the stress arising from a dependent older person and a stressed caregiver (Reis & Nahmiash, 1998).

Tertiary Prevention

Ensuring the safety of an abused person should be paramount in a nurse's mind, particularly at the tertiary prevention level. Relevant interventions may include developing a safety plan with the client and making timely and appropriate referrals. In the United States, for instance, nurses are mandated reporters of child abuse, and if such a case is even suspected, the nurse has the responsibility to call the necessary agencies to file a report (see chapter 10 for further discussion.) However, national, regional, and local mandates related to IPV and elder abuse vary; thus, it is incumbent upon each nurse to know those legal requirements in order to adhere to necessary standards of practice.

As previously mentioned, referral is an important component of intervening with family violence at the tertiary level. Not only should nurses know about community resources for survivors and perpetrators of family violence, they should also be sensitive to their client's needs. Failure to match the identified needs with the appropriate help could result in a refusal to accept help—a result that is all too often observed in abused or neglected older adults (Spencer, 2005). It is important to recognize older adults' concerns about privacy and independence and that they may be reluctant to relinquish what little control they still have. In response, a harm reduction approach (Spencer, 2005) may be a helpful way of dealing with elder abuse. With a focus on reducing the negative consequences of abuse for the abused older adult, the harm reduction model allows the elder to decide what is important to address (rather than having to make hard choices such as giving up contact with the perpetrator, as is the case in the traditional models of care).

Nurses may have already used some aspects of harm reduction in their care of abused older adults. They can further propagate the principles of harm reduction so that older persons can still live with dignity, even in complex abusive and neglectful situations. Although the idea of harm reduction originates in Canada, it may also be an acceptable model in Asian communities in which making compromises in order to maintain family harmony is often preferred, especially by the older generation.

Social support has generally been shown to enhance abused women's coping (Kocot & Goodman, 2003; Nurius, Furrey, & Berliner, 1992). However, nurses should be aware that the perceived benefits of social support may not be universal. For instance, Asian people may not perceive social support as beneficial because of cultural (e.g., seeking outside help threatens family reputation and harmony) and language (e.g., immigrants unable to understand the language) barriers (Yoshihama, 1999; Yoshioka, Dang, Shewmangal, Chan, & Tan, 2000). Therefore, nurses should not assume that all clients will be keen to seek help or accept assistance from social services or other agencies. Instead, time and effort may need to be spent to help them resolve their own attitudes, understand their dilemma of wanting to end the abuse and yet keeping their family together, and accept that they may still feel trapped in the abusive relationship despite the social support.

Nurses can work to empower the family in abusive situations by recognizing and capitalizing on the family's strengths. Families can often generate solutions that are more culturally appropriate and individualized than those proposed by others. An example is the adoption of a coping strategy known as fatalistic voluntarism that is used by many Chinese (Lee, 1995). Believing that life events are determined not only by human self-determination and effort but also by external forces beyond human control, some Chinese people facing life's adversities will do all that is humanly possible but "leave the rest to heaven." Tiwari, Wong, and Ip (2001) found that Chinese women used the concepts of fatalistic voluntarism (*ren* and *yuan*) at different stages of their abusive relationship. Specifically, while they were still in the abusive relationship, they would use *ren* (patience and forbearance) in order to wait for the right moment and not to take a hasty action. Once they had left their abusive partners, they would use *yuan* (relationships are predetermined by external, invisible forces) to provide ready answers about life's vicissitudes, to help them avoid guilty feelings and hostility, and to give them hope for a better future. Although no study has explored the phenomenon of fatalistic voluntarism in elder abuse, in view of the pervasiveness of this coping orientation in some Chinese people, it is likely that such a belief is also endorsed by abused older adults. Given the positive and activistic orientation of the fatalistic voluntarism belief, nurses can empower Chinese abuse survivors by affirming their coping behaviors and supporting them in developing their own resources.

Learning about other cultural practices and philosophies, either similar to or different from these examples, would help nurses to provide culturally sensitive care to abused individuals. Nurses must also be aware of their own culturally bound perceptions and how these may affect their approach to the client. Furthermore, nurses can better meet the therapeutic needs of survivors of family violence by being sensitive to how the survivors perceive the health impact of the abuse. As well, nurses should recognize that the survivors' health beliefs often influence their perception of illness and the manifestation of symptoms arising from the abuse. For example, under the influence of traditional Chinese health beliefs, Chinese people may not see a clear distinction between physical and mental disorders; they may view internal organs as the centers for combined physiological and psychological functions (Lin, 1982). As a result, Chinese clients may use vital organs (such as heart and lungs) in colloquial expressions of feelings. Instead of expressing emotional states associated with the mental health condition (e.g., depressive symptoms), they may present symptoms of the related bodily function (e.g., headache and back pain). Without an understanding of the health concepts influencing Chinese patients' expressions of symptoms, it is easy to dismiss patients as lacking psychological awareness or having a tendency toward somatization. Thus, when making health assessments of Chinese survivors of family violence, nurses should inquire about emotional as well as somatic symptoms and acknowledge the survivors' expressed physical health problems.

SUMMARY

Family violence is a global problem facing most societies. Nurses, who interact with clients in various health care settings, are well positioned to make a positive impact on the prevention of violence and to mitigate the long-term health consequences of violence that has already occurred. Being aware of the prevalence and risk factors for violence in cross-cultural settings enables nurses to promote their clients' health in sensitive and proactive ways.

EXHIBIT 16.2
Useful Links

GENERAL RESOURCES

United Nations Convention on the Elimination of All Forms of Discrimination against Women, General Assembly resolution 34/180. (1981). Available from http://www. childinfo.org/files/childmarriage_cedaw.pdf

Civil and political rights, including questions of disappearances and summary executions: Report of the special rapporteur, Ms. Asma Jahangir. Submitted Pursuant to Commission on Human Rights Resolution 1999/35 (E/CN.4/2000/3). New York, NY: United Nations, Commission on Human Rights. Available from http://www.unhchr.ch/huridocda/huridoca.nsf/AllSymbols/B72F2CFE9AA28E58802568AB003C572E/$File/G0010389.pdf?OpenElement

United Nations & Pinheiro, P. S. (2006). *Report of the independent expert for the United Nations study on violence against children:* Pursuant to GeneralAssembly resolution 57/90 of 2002. Available from http://www.violencestudy.org/IMG/pdf/English-2-2.pdf

United Nations Children's Fund (UNICEF) (2006). *Child marriage.* Available from http://www.childinfo.org/marriage.html

United Nations Population Fund (UNFPA). (2000). Chapter 3: Ending violence against women and girls. In, *State of the world population.* Available from http://www.unfpa.org/swp/2000/english/ch03.html

World Health Organization (WHO) (2002). *World report on violence and health.* Available from http://www.who.int/violence_injury_prevention/violence/world_report/en/

Preventing violence: A guide to implementing the recommendations of the World Report on Violence and Health. Available from http://www.who.int/violence_injury_prevention/media/news/08_09_2004/en/index.html

---

Continued

EXHIBIT 16.2 *Continued*

Child Maltreatment. (2008). Available from http://www.who.int/topics/child_abuse/en/

Global school-based student health survey (GSHS). (2008). Available from http://www.who.int/chp/gshs/en/

Missing voices: The views of older persons on elder abuse. (2001). Available from http://www.who.int/ageing/projects/elder_abuse/missing_voices/en/

Guidelines for conducting community surveys on injuries and violence (2004). Available from http://www.who.int/violence_injury_prevention/publications/surveillance/06_09_2004/en/index.html

---

Elder Abuse Foundation
http://www.elder-abuse-foundation.com/index.html

International Network for the Prevention of Elder Abuse
http://www.inpea.net/home.html

HelpAge International
http://www.helpage.org/Home

International Association of Gerontology and Geriatrics
http://www.iagg.com.br/webforms/index.aspx

World Health Organisation Ageing Programme
http://www.who.int/ageing/en/

Help the Aged, Canada
http://helptheaged.ca/index.htm

International Longevity Centre—UK
http://www.ilcuk.org.uk/

United Nations Programme on Ageing
http://www.un.org/esa/socdev/ageing/index.html

International Society for Prevention of Child Abuse and Neglect (ISPCAN)
http://www.ispcan.org/

Child Abuse and Neglect in Eastern Europe
http://www.canee.net/links

American Professional Society on the Abuse of Children
www.APSAC.org

Association for Treatment of Sexual Abusers
www.ATSA.com

Center on Child Abuse and Neglect. University of Oklahoma Health Sciences Center
http://w3.ouhsc.edu/ccan/

Center on Sex Offender Management
www.csom.org

Child Physical and Sexual Abuse: Guidelines for Treatment. National Crime Victims Research and Treatment Center
www.musc.edu/cvc/

Childtrafficking.com. Terre des hommes Foundation, Lausanne, (Tdh)
http://www.childtrafficking.com

Child Trauma Academy. "Incubated in Terror: Neurodevelopmental Factors in the 'Cycle of Violence'"
http://www.childtrauma.org/CTAMATERIALS/incubated.asp

Child Welfare League of America
http://www.cwla.org/advocacy/

Children's Defense Fund
www.childrensdefense.org

The Future of Children—Domestic Violence and Children http://www.
futureofchildren.org/pubs-info2825/pubs-info.htm?doc_id=70473

The Greenbook Initiative
http://www.thegreenbook.info/

HandsOnScotland
http://www.handsonscotland.co.uk/

"In Harm's Way: Domestic Violence and Child Maltreatment."
http://www.calib.com/nccanch/pubs/otherpubs/harmsway.cfm

Kempe Children's Center
http://www.kempecenter.org

Minnesota Center Against Violence and Abuse
http://www.mincava.umn.edu/hart/risks&r.htm

National Center on the Sexual Behavior of Youth
www.NCSBY.org

National Child Protection Clearinghouse
http://www.aifs.org.au/nch/issues2.html

National Children's Alliance
http://www.nca-online.org/statutes.html

National Clearinghouse on Child Abuse and Neglect
http://nccanch.acf.hhs.gov

National Crime Victims Research and Treatment Center
http://www.musc.edu/cvc/

National Exchange Center
http://www.preventchildabuse.com

National Parent Information Network
http://www.npin.org

Office for Victims of Crime
http://www.ojp.usdoj.gov/ovc/

Prevent Child Abuse America
http://www.preventchildabuse.org

Profile of Child Trafficking in Nigeria
http://www.ispcan.org/documents/ChildTraffickingNigeriaOutline.pdf

Continued

EXHIBIT 16.2 *Continued*

Violence Against Women Online Resources
http://www.vaw.umn.edu/library/ccp/

Additional Resources on Violence Against Women

Minnesota Center Against Violence and Abuse
http://www.mincava.umn.edu/hart/risks&r.htm

Violence Against Women Online Resources
Available from http://www.vaw.umn.edu/library/ccp/

Interagency Gender Working Group
Available from http://www.igwg.org/pubstools/systemaletizing/system-gbv.htm

---

REFERENCES

Abraham, M. (1999). Sexual abuse in South Asian immigrant marriages. *Violence Against Women, 5,* 591–618.

Abraham, M. (2000). Isolation as a form of marital violence: The South Asian immigrant experience. *Journal of Social Distress and the Homeless, 9,* 221–236.

Abraham, M. (2002). *Speaking the unspeakable. Marital violence among South Asian immigrants in the United States.* New Brunswick, NJ: Rutgers University Press.

Adinkrah, M. (2003). Men who kill their own children: Paternal filicide incidents in contemporary Fiji. *Child Abuse &Neglect, 27,* 557–568.

African Network for the Prevention and Protection against Child Abuse and Neglect (ANPPCAN). (2002). *Awareness and views regarding child abuse and child rights in selected communities in Kenya.* Nairobi, Kenya.

Agnew, V. (1998). *In search of a safe place: Abused women and culturally sensitive services.* Toronto, Ontario, Canada: University of Toronto Press.

Ajdukovic, M., Ogresta, J., & Rusac, S. (2009). Family violence and health among elderly in Croatia. *Journal of Aggression, Maltreatment & Trauma, 18,* 261–279.

Aldridge, M. L., & Browne, K. D. (2003). Perpetrators of spousal homicide: A review. *Trauma, Violence & Abuse, 4,* 265–276.

Alyahri, A., & Goodman, R. (2008). Harsh corporal punishment of Yemeni children: Occurrence, type and associations. *Child Abuse & Neglect, 32,* 766–773.

Amodeo, M., Griffin, M. L., Fassler, I. R., Clay, C. M., & Ellis, M. A. (2006). Childhood sexual abuse among black women and white women from two-parent families. *Child Maltreatment, 11,* 237–247.

Antonopoulou, C. (1999). Domestic violence in Greece. *American Psychologist, 54*(1), 63–64.

Arai, M. (2006). Elder abuse in Japan. *Educational Gerontology, 32*(1), 13–23.

Bagley, C., & Ramsay, R. (1986). Sexual abuse in childhood: Psychosocial outcomes and implications for social work practice. *Journal of Social Work and Human Sexuality, 4,* 33–47.

Bardi, M., & Borgognini-Tari, S. M. (2001). A survey of parent–child conflict resolution: Intrafamily violence in Italy. *Child Abuse & Neglect, 25,* 839–853.

Barnett, O.W., & Fagan, R.W. (1993). Alcohol use in male spouse abusers and their female partners. *Journal of Family Violence, 8,* 1–25.

Barnett, O., Miller, M., Perrin, C., & Perrin, R. (1997). *Family violence across the lifespan.* Thousand Oaks, CA: Sage.

Barnett, O. W., Miller-Perrin, C. L., & Perrin, R. D. (2005). Child abuse. In *Family violence across the lifespan.* Thousand Oaks, CA: Sage.

Barrata, P. C., McNally, M. J., Sales, I. M., & Stewart, D. E. (2005). Portuguese immigrant women's perspectives on wife abuse: A cross-generational comparison. *Journal of Interpersonal Violence, 20,* 1132–1150.

Bawah, A. A., Akweongo, P., Simmons, R., & Philips, J. F. (1999). Women's fears and men's anxieties: The impact of family planning on gender relations in Northern Ghana. *Studies in Family Planning, 30*(1), 54–66.

Bezerra-Flanders, W., & Clark, J. C. (2006). Perspectives on elder abuse and neglect in Brazil. *Educational Gerontology, 32*(1), 63–72.

Bhuyan, R., Mell, M., Senturia, K., Sullivan, M., & Shiu-Thornton, S. (2005). "Women must endure according to their karma": Cambodian immigrant women talk about domestic violence. *Journal of Interpersonal Violence, 20*, 902–921.

Biggs, S., Manthorpe, J., Tinker, A., Doyle, M., & Erens, B. (2009). Mistreatment of older people in the United Kingdom: Findings from the first national prevalence study. *Journal of Elder Abuse & Neglect, 21*, 1–14.

Black, D. A., et al. (1999). *Partner, child abuse risk factor literature review: National network of family resiliency*. Retrieved from http://www.nnh.org/risk.

Bond, C. R., & McMahon, R. J. (1984). Relationship between marital distress and child behavior problems, marital personal adjustment, maternal personality, and maternal parenting behavior. *Journal of Abnormal Psychology, 93*, 348–351.

Brown, M. (1994). Marital discord during pregnancy: A family systems approach. *Family System Medicine, 12*, 221–234.

Browne, K. et al. (2002). *Child abuse and neglect in Romanian families: A national prevalence study 2000*. Copenhagen, Denmark: WHO Regional Office for Europe.

Brownridge, D. A., & Halli, S. S. (2002). Culture variation in male partner violence against women. *Violence Against Women, 8*, 87–115.

Bui, H. N., & Morash, M. (1999). Domestic violence in the Vietnamese immigrant community: An exploratory study. *Violence Against Women, 5*, 769–795.

Burns, N. M. (1993). *Literature review of issues related to the use of corrective force against children* (Department of Justice Canada, Working Document WD1993-6e).

Byrne, C. A., et al. (1999). The socioeconomic impact of interpersonal violence on women. *Journal of Consulting and Clinical Psychology, 67*, 362–366.

Canadian Centre for Justice Statistics. (2000). *Family violence in Canada: A statistical profile 2000*. Retrieved from http://www.statcan.gc.ca/pub/85-224-x/85-224-x000000-eng.pdf.

Cavanagh, K., Dobash, R. E., & Dobash, R. P. (2007). The murder of children by fathers in the context of child abuse. *Child Abuse & Neglect, 31*, 731–746.

Chan, K. L. (2006). The Chinese concept of face and violence against women. *International Social Work, 49*, 65–73.

Chen, J. Q., Dunne, M. P., & Han, P. (2004). Child sexual abuse in China: A study of adolescents in four provinces. *Child Abuse & Neglect, 28*, 1171–1186.

Children's Bureau. (2009). *Child maltreatment 2007*. Washington, DC: U.S. Department of Health and Human Services. Retrieved from http://www.acf.hhs.gov/programs/cb/stats_research/ index.htm#can.

Cohen, M., Levin, S. H., Gagin, R., & Friedman, G. (2007). Elder abuse: Disparities between older people's disclosure of abuse, evident abuse, and high risk of abuse. *Journal of American Geriatrics Society, 55*, 1224–1230.

Comijs, H. C., Pot, A. M., Smit, J. H., Bouter, L. M., & Jonker, C. (1998). Elder abuse in the community: Prevalence and consequences. *Journal of the American Geriatric Society, 46*, 885–888.

Cox, C. E., Kotch, J. B., & Everson, M. D. (2003). A longitudinal study of modifying influences in the relationship between domestic violence and child maltreatment. *Journal of Family Violence, 18*, 5–17.

Crandall, M., Senturia, K., Sullivan, M., & Shiu-Thornton, S. (2005). "No way out": Russian-speaking women's experiences with domestic violence. *Journal of Interpersonal Violence, 20*, 941–958.

Daichman, L. S. (2005). Elder abuse in developing countries. In M. Johnson, V. L. Bengtson, P. G. Coleman, & T. B. L. Kirkwood (Eds.), *The Cambridge handbook of age and ageing* (pp. 323–331). Cambridge, UK: Cambridge University Press.

Daskalopoulos, M. D., & Borrelli, S. E. (2006). Definitions of elder abuse in an Italian sample. *Journal of Elder Abuse & Neglect, 18*, 67–85.

Daskalopoulos, M. D., Kakouros, A., & Stathopoulou, G. (2006). Perspectives on elder abuse in Greece. *Journal of Elder Abuse & Neglect, 18*, 87–104.

deAlwis, M. (2004). The "purity" of displacement and the reterritorialization of longing. In W. Giles & J. Hyndman (Eds.), *Sites of violence: Feminist politics in conflict zones.* Berkeley, CA: University of California Press.

Doe, S. S. (2000). Cultural factors in child maltreatment and domestic violence in Korea. *Children and Youth Services Review, 22*, 231–236.

Doe, S. S., Han, H. K., & McCaslin, R. (2009). Cultural and ethical issues in Korea's recent elder abuse reporting system. *Journal of Elder Abuse & Neglect, 21*, 170–185.

Dong, X. Q., & Simon, M. A. (2008). Is greater social support a protective factor against elder maltreatment? *Gerontology, 54*, 381–388.

Dong, X. Q., Simon, M. A., & Gorbein, M. J. (2007). Elder abuse and neglect in an urban Chinese population. *Journal of Elder Abuse & Neglect, 19*, 79–96.

Dong, X. Q., Simon, M. A., Gorbein, M. J., Percak, B. A., & Golden, R. (2007). Loneliness in older Chinese adults: A risk factor for elder mistreatment. *Journal of the American Geriatrics Society, 55*, 1832–1835.

Donnelly, M., & Straus, M. A. (2005). *Corporal punishment of children in theoretical perspective.* New Haven, CT: Yale University Press.

Dubowitz, H., & Bennett, S. (2007). Physical abuse and neglect of children. *The Lancet, 369*, 1891–1900.

Dunne, M. P., Purdie, D., Cook, M., Boyle, F. M., & Najman, J. M. (2003). Is child sexual abuse declining? Evidence from a population-based survey of men and women in Australia. *Child Abuse & Neglect, 27*, 141–152.

Dutton, M. (1992). *Empowering and healing the battered women.* New York: Springer.

Ellsberg, M. C., Pena, R., Herrera, A., Liljestrand, J., & Winkvist, A. (2000). Candies in hell: Women's experiences of violence in Nicaragua. *Social Science & Medicine, 51*, 1595–1610.

Eriksson, H. (2001). *Våld mot äldre kvinnor och män–en omfångsstudie* [Violence against elderly women and men: A prevalence study]. Umeå: rottsoffermyndigheten.

Estroff, S. E. (1997). A cultural perspective of experiences of illness, disability, and deviance. In G. E. Henderson, et al. (Eds.), *The social medicine reader* (pp. 6–11). Durham, NC: Duke University Press.

Facchin, P., Barbieri, E., Boin, F., et al, (1998). *European strategies on child protection: Preliminary report.* Padua, Italy: University of Padua, Epidemiology and Community Medicine Unit.

Fanslow, J. L. & Robinson, E. (2004). Violence against women in New Zealand: Prevalence and health consequences. *The New Zealand Medical Journal, 117*, 1–12.

Feeney, J. A., Hohaus, L. H., Noller, P., & Allexander, R. A. (2001). *Becoming parents: Exploring the bonds between mothers, fathers, and their infants.* New York: Cambridge University Press.

Finkelhor, D., Hotaling, G., Lewis, I. A., & Smith, C. (1990). Sexual abuse in a national survey of adult men and women: Prevalence, characteristics, and risk factors. *Child Abuse & Neglect, 14*, 19–28.

Fong, J. (2000). Silent no more: How women experienced wife abuse in the local Chinese community. Unpublished doctoral dissertation, York University, Toronto, Canada.

Ford-Gilboe, M., Wuest, J., & Merrit-Gray, M. (2005). Strengthening capacity to limit intrusion: Theorizing family health promotion in the aftermath of woman abuse. *Qualitative Health Research, 15*, 477–501.

Fox, J. A. & Zawitz, M. W. (2006). *Homicide trends in the United States.* Washington, DC: Department of Justice. Retrieved from http://www.ojp.usdoj.gov/bjs/homicide/homtrnd.htm.

Gagnon, A., & Sandall, J. (2008). *Individual or group antenatal education for childbirth or parenthood, or both.* The Cochrane Library.

Garcia-Moreno, C. (2000). Violence against women: International perspectives. *American Journal of Preventative Medicine, 19*, 330–333.

Garcia-Moreno, C., et al. (2006). *WHO Multi-Country Study on Women's Health and Domestic Violence against Women.* Geneva, Switzerland: World Health Organization.

Global Initiative. (2006). *Global summary of the legal status of corporal punishment of children.* Retrieved June 28, 2006, from http://www.violencestudy.org/IMG/pdf/140705-02.pdf.

Glodava, M., & Onizuko, R. (1994). Mail-order brides: Women for sale. Fort Collins, CO: Alaken.

Gonzales-de Olarte, E., & Gavilano, L. P. (1999). Does poverty cause domestic violence? Some answers from Lima. In A. R. Morrison & M. L. Biehl (Eds.), *Too close to home: Domestic violence in the Americas* (pp. 35–49). Washington, DC: Inter-American Development Bank.

Department of Justice, Canada, Government of Canada. (2009). *Abuse of older adults: Department of Justice Canada overview paper.* Retrieved from http://canada.justice.gc.ca/eng/pi/fv-vf/facts-info/old-age/index.html.

Gunaratne, S. (2002). *State and community responses to domestic violence in Sri Lanka.* Center for Women's Research.

Guruge, S. (2007). *The influence of gender, racial, social, and economic inequalities on the production of and responses to intimate partner violence in the post- migration context.* Doctoral dissertation, University of Toronto, Toronto, Canada.

Guruge, S., & Humphreys, J. (2009). Barriers that affect abused immigrant women's access to and use of formal social supports. *Canadian Journal of Nursing Research, 41,* 64–84.

Guruge, S., Khanlou, N., & Gastaldo, D. (2010). The production of intimate male partner violence in the migration process: Intersections of gender, race, and class. Journal of Advanced Nursing, *66*(1): 103–113.

Hahm, H. C., & Guterman, N. B. (2001). The emerging problems of physical child abuse in South Korea. *Child Maltreatment, 6,* 169–179.

Haj-Yahia, M.M. (1998). A patriarchal perspective of beliefs about wife beating among Palestinian men from the West Bank and the Gaza Strip. *Journal of Family Issues, 19,* 595–621.

Haj-Yahia, M.M. (2005). Can people's patriarchal ideology predict their beliefs about wife abuse?: The case of Jordanian men. *Journal of Community Psychology, 33,* 545–567.

Haj-Yahia, M. M., & Abdo-Kaloti, R. (2003). The rates and correlates of the exposure of Palestinian adolescents to family violence: Toward an integrative-holistic approach. *Child Abuse & Neglect, 27,* 781–806.

Haj-Yahia, M. M., & Tamish, S. (2001). The rates of child sexual abuse and its psychological consequences as revealed by a study among Palestinian university students. *Child Abuse & Neglect, 25,* 1303–1327.

Health Canada. (1999). *Women's health strategy.* Retrieved from http://www/hc-gc.ca/women/english/womenstrat.htm.

Heise, L. L. (1998). Violence against women: An integrated, ecological framework. *Violence Against Women, 4,* 262–290.

Heise, L. L., Pitanguy, J., & Germain, A. (1994). *Violence against women: The hidden health burden.* Washington, DC: World Bank.

Ho, C. K. (1990). An analysis of domestic violence in Asian American communities: A multicultural approach to counselling. *Women & Therapy, 9,* 129–150.

Hoffman, K. L., Demo, D. H., & Edwards, J. H. (1994). Physical wife abuse in a non-western society: An integrated theoretical approach. *Journal of Marriage and the Family, 56,* 131–146.

Huang, W. J. (2005). An Asian perspective on relationship and marriage education. *Family Process, 44,* 161–173.

Hyman, I., Guruge, S., & Mason, R. (2008). The impact of post-migration changes on marital relationships: A study of Ethiopian immigrant couples in Toronto. *Journal of Comparative Family Studies, 39,* 149–164.

Hyman, I., Guruge, S., Mason, R., Mekonned, G., Stuckless, N., Tang, T., et al. (2006). *Post migration changes in gender relations in the Ethiopian community in Toronto: Phase II.* Toronto, Ontario, Canada: Centre of Excellence for Research on Immigration and Settlement. Retrieved from http://ceris.metropolis.net/Virtual%20Library/RFPReports/Hyman_PhaseII2004.pdf.

Hyman, I., Guruge, S, Mason, R., Stuckless, N., Gould, J., Tang, T., et al. (2004). Post migration changes in gender relations among Ethiopian immigrant couples in Toronto. *Canadian Journal of Nursing Research, 36,* 74–89.

INPEA. (2009). *Reports on elder abuse prevention from around the world.* Retrieved from http://sites.google.com/a/nicenet.ca /weaad2009/inspiration-stories.

International Society for the Prevention of Child Abuse and Neglect (ISPCAN). (2006). *World perspectives on child abuse* (6th ed.). Retrieved from http://www.ispcan.org/wp/ISPCANWorldPerspectives2006.pdf.

ISPCAN (2008). *World perspectives on child abuse.* Retrieved from http://www.ispcan.org/wp/images/Executive_Summary_2008.pdf.

Jewkes, R., Penn-Kekana, L., Levin, J., Ratsaka, M., & Schrieber, M. (2001). Prevalence of emotional, physical and sexual abuse of women in three South African provinces. *South African Medical Journal, 91,* 421–428.

Keskinoglu, P., Picakciefe, M., Bilgic, N., Giray, H., Karakus, N., & Ucku, R. (2008). Home accidents in the community-dwelling elderly in Izmir, Turkey: How do prevalence and risk factors differ between high and low socioeconomic districts? *Journal of Aging and Health, 20,* 824–836.

Ketsela, T., & Kebede, D. (1997). Physical punishment of elementary school children in urban and rural communities in Ethiopia. *Ethiopian Medical Journal, 35,* 23–33.

Khan, M. E., Townsend, J. W., Sinha, R., & Lakhanpal, S. (1996). *Sexual violence within marriage*. New Delhi, India: Population Council.

Khawaja, M. (2004). Domestic violence in refugee camps in Jordan. *International Journal of Gynaecology & Obstetrics, 86*, 67–69.

Kirschner, R. H., & Wilson H. (2001). Pathology of fatal child abuse. In R. M. Reece & S. Ludwig (Eds.), *Child abuse: Medical diagnosis and management* (2nd ed., pp. 467–516). Philadelphia, PA: Lippincott Williams & Wilkins.

Kocot, T., & Goodman, L. (2003). The roles of coping and social support in battered women's mental health. *Violence Against Women, 9*, 323–346.

König, J., & Leembruggen-Kallberg, E. (2006). Perspectives on elder abuse in Germany. *Educational Gerontology, 32*(1), 25–35.

Kosberg, J. I. (1988). Preventing elder abuse: Identification of high risk factors prior to placement decisions. *The Gerontologist, 28*, 43–50.

Koss, M. P., Goodman, L. A., Browne, A., Fitzgerald, L. F., Keita, G. P., & Russo, N. F. (1994). *No safe haven: Male violence against women at home, at work, and in the community*. Washington, DC: American Psychological Association.

Krahe, B., Bieneck, S., & Moller, I. (2005). Understanding gender and intimate partner violence from an international perspective. *Sex Roles, 52*, 807–827.

Krishnakmuar, A., & Buehler, C. (2000). Inter-parental conflict and parenting behaviors: A meta analytic review. *Family Relations, 49*, 25–44.

Krug, E. G., Dahlberg, L. L., Mercy, J. A., Zwi, A. B., & Lozano, R. (2002). World report on violence and health. Geneva, Switzerland: World Health Organization.

Kurrle, S., & Naughtin, G. (2008). An overview of elder abuse and neglect in Australia. *Journal of Elder, 20*(2), 108–125.

Lalor, K. (2004). Child sexual abuse in Tanzania and Kenya. *Child Abuse & Neglect, 28*, 833–844.

Larrain, S. H. (1994). *Violencia puertas adentro: La mujer golpeada. [Violence behind closed doors: The battered women]*. Santiago, Chile: Editorial Universitaria.

Lee, M. (2002). Asian battered women: Assessment and treatment. In A. R. Roberts (Ed.), *Handbook of domestic violence intervention strategies* (pp. 472–482). New York: Oxford University Press.

Lee, R. (1995). Cultural tradition and stress management in modern society: Learning from the Hong Kong experience. In T. Y. Lin, W. S. Tseng, & E. K. Yeh (Eds.), *Chinese societies and mental health* (pp. 40–56). Hong Kong, China: Oxford University Press.

Legerwood, J. (1990). Changing Khmer conception of gender: Women, stories, and the social order. *Dissertation Abstracts International*. Ann Arbor, MI: University Microfilms.

Leibrich, J., Paulin, J., & Ransom, R. (1995). *Hitting home. Men speak about abuse of women partners*. Wellington: New Zealand Department of Justice.

Levesque, R. J. R. (2002). *Culture and family violence: Fostering change through human rights law*. Washington, DC: American Psychological Association.

Lin, K. M. (1982). Traditional Chinese medical health beliefs and their relevance for mental illness and psychiatry. In A. Kleinman & T. Lin (Eds.), *Normal and abnormal behavior in Chinese culture* (pp. 95–111). London, UK: Reidel.

Lowenstein, A., Eisikovits, Z., Band-Winterstein, T., & Enosh, G. (2009). Is elder abuse and neglect a social phenomenon?: Data from the first national prevalence survey in Israel. *Journal of Elder Abuse & Neglect, 21*, 253–277.

Maclean, H., & Sicchia, S. R. (2004). *Gender, globalization and health*: Excerpts from the background paper prepared for the CIHR–IGH. Retrieved from http://www.womensresearch.ca/PDF/Stonehouse-Abridged.pdf.

MacMillan, H. I., Fleming, J. E., Trocme, N., Boyle, M. H., Wong, M., Racine, Y. A., et al. (1997). Prevalence of child physical and sexual abuse in the community: Results from the Ontario Health Supplement. *Journal of the American Medical Association, 278*, 131–135.

Madhu, S. N., & Peltzer, K. (2000). Risk factors and child sexual abuse among secondary school students in the Northern Province (South Africa). *Child Abuse & Neglect, 24*(2), 259–268.

Madu, S. N., & Peltzer, K. (2000). Risk factors and child sexual abuse among secondary students in the Northern Province (South Africa). *Child Abuse & Neglect, 24*, 259–268.

Malley-Morrison, K., Nolido, N. E., & Chawla, S. (2006). International perspectives on elder abuse: Five case studies. *Educational Gerontology, 32*(1), 1–11.

Manoochechri, H., Ghorbi, B., Hosseini, M., Nasiri Oskuyee, N., & Karbakhsh, M. (2009). Degree and types of domestic abuse in the elderly in Tehran [Farsi]. *SBMU Faculty of Nursing & Midwifery Quarterly, 18*(63).

Martin, S., Tsui, A., Maitra, K., & Marinshaw, R. (1999). Domestic violence in northern India. *American Journal of Epidemiology, 150*(4), 417.

Mathews, S., Abrahams, N., Jewkes, R., Martin, L., Lombard, C., & Vetten, L. (2008). Intimate femicide-suicide in South Africa: a cross-sectional study. *Bulletin of the World Health Organization, 86*, 542–558.

May-Chahal, C., & Cawson, P. (2005). Measuring child maltreatment in the United Kingdom: A study of the prevalence of child abuse and neglect. *Child Abuse & Neglect, 29*, 969–984.

Mehotra, M. (1999). The social construction of wife abuse: Experiences of Asian Indian women in the United States. *Violence Against Women, 5*, 619–640.

Ministry of Women and Child Development, Government of India. (2007). *Study on child abuse: India 2007*. Retrieved from http://wcd.nic.in/childabuse.pdf.

Mirrlees-Black, C. (1999). Domestic violence: *Findings from a new British crime survey self-completion questionnaire* (Home Office Research Study No. 191). Retrieved from http://www.homeoffice.gov.uk/rds/pdfs/hors191.pdf.

Moreno, M. F. (1999). La violencia en la pareja [Intimate partner violence]. *Revista Panamericana de Salud Pu´ blica, 5*, 245–258.

Morrison, L., Guruge, S., & Snarr, K. A. (1999). Sri Lankan Tamil immigrants in Toronto: Gender, marriage patterns, and sexuality. In G. A. Kelson & D. L. DeLaet (Eds.), *Gender and immigration* (pp. 144–161). New York: New York University Press.

Mulroney, J. (2003). *Australian statistics on domestic violence*. Retrieved from http://www.austdvclearinghouse.unsw.edu.au/topics/topics_pdf_files /Statistics_final.pdf.

Nelson, E., & Zimmerman, C. (1996). *Household survey on domestic violence in Cambodia*. Phnom Penh, Vietnam: Ministry of Women's Affairs and Project Against Domestic Violence.

Nurius, P.S., Furrey, J., & Berliner, L. (1992). Coping capacity among women with abusive partners. *Violence and Victims, 7*, 229–243.

Ogg, J., & Bennett, G. C. J. (1992). Elder abuse in Britain, *British Medical Journal, 305*, 998–999.

Oh, J., Kim, H. S., Martin, D., & Kim, H. (2005). A study of elder abuse in Korea. *International Journal of Nursing Studies, 43*, 203–214.

Oh, J., Kim, H., Martins, D., & Kim, H. (2006). A study of elder abuse in Korea. *International Journal of Nursing Studies, 43*(2), 203–214.

Older Persons Programme (2009). *Active Ageing Programme Calendar (2009)*. Retrieved from http://olderpersonsprogramme.co.za/oppcal.html.

Oweis, A., Gharaibeh, M., Al-Natour, A., & Froelicher, E. (2009). Violence against women: Unveiling the suffering of women with a low income in Jordan. *Journal of Transcultural Nursing, 20*, 69–76.

Pan American Health Organization. (n.d.). *Abuse (mistreatment) and neglect (abandonment): Diagnostic and management guide I*. Retrieved from http://www.imsersomayores.csic.es/documentos/documentos/paho-manualen-01.pdf

Parker, B., McFarlane, J., Soeken, K., Silva, C., & Reel, S. (1999). Testing an intervention to prevent further abuse to pregnant women. *Research in Nursing and Health, 22*, 59–66.

Patterson, M., & Malley-Morrison, K. (2006). A cognitive-ecological approach to elder abuse in five cultures: Human rights and education. *Educational Gerontology, 32*(1), 73–82.

Penhale, B. (2008). Elder abuse in the United Kingdom. *Journal of Elder Abuse & Neglect, 20*, 151–168.

Petch, J., & Halford, W. K. (2008). Psycho-education to enhance couples' transition to parenthood. *Clinical Psychology Review, 28*, 1125–1137.

Podnieks, E. (1992). National survey on abuse of the elderly in Canada. *Journal of Elder Abuse & Neglect, 4*, 5–58.

Rabi, K. (2006). Israeli perspectives on elder abuse. *Educational Gerontology, 32*(1), 49–62.

Raj, A., & Silverman, J. (2002). Violence against immigrant women. *Violence Against Women, 8*, 367–398.

Reece, R. M., & Krous, H. F. (2001). Fatal child abuse and sudden infant death syndrome. In R. M. Reece & S. Ludwig (Eds.), *Child abuse: Medical diagnosis and management* (2nd ed., pp. 517–543). Philadelphia, PA: Lippincott Williams & Wilkins.

Reis, M., & Nahmiash, D. (1998). Validation of the indicators of abuse (IOA) screen. *Gerontology, 38*, 5–30.

Rinsky, K., & Malley-Morrison, K. (2006). Russian perspectives on elder abuse: An exploratory study. *Journal of Elder Abuse & Neglect, 18*, 123–139.

Rogers, C. (1951). *Client-centered therapy, its current practice, implications and theory.* Boston, MA: Houghton Mifflin.

Rodgers, K. (1994). Wife assault: The findings of a national survey. *Juristat Service Bulletin, 14*, 1–22.

Rosales, J., et al (1999). *Encuesta Nicaraguense de demografiay salud, 1998 [1998 Nicaraguan demographic and health survey].* Managua, Nicaragua: Instituto Nacional de Estadisticas y Censos.

Shapiro A. F, Gottman J. M, & Carrére S. (2000). The baby and the marriage: Identifying factors that buffer against decline in marital satisfaction after the first baby arrives. *Journal of Family Psychology,14*, 59–70.

Shapiro, A. F., & Gottman, J. M. (2005). Effects on marriage of a psycho-communicative-educational intervention with couples undergoing the transition to parenthood: Evaluation at 1-year post intervention. *The Journal of Family Communication, 5*, 1–24.

Sharps, P. W., Koziol-McLain, J., Campbell, J., McFarlane, J., Sachs, C., & Xu, X. (2001). Health care providers' missed opportunities for preventing femicide. *Preventive Medicine, 33*, 373–380.

Sherman, C. W., Rosenblatt, D. E., & Antonucci, T. C. (2008). Elder abuse and mistreatment: A life span and cultural context. *Indian Journal of Gerontology, 22*, 319–339.

Shiu-Thornton, S., Senturia, K., & Sullivan, M. (2005). "Like a bird in a cage": Vietnamese women survivors talk about domestic violence. *Journal of Interpersonal Violence, 20*, 959–976.

Shumba, A. (2001). Epidemiology and etiology of reported cases of child physical abuse in Zimbabwean primary schools. *Child Abuse & Neglect, 25*, 265–277.

Spencer, C. (2005, October 26). *Harm reduction and abuse in later life.* Paper presented at World Conference on Family Violence, Banff, Canada.

Stathopoulou, G. (2004). Greece. In K. Malley-Morrison (Ed.), *International perspectives on family violence and abuse* (pp. 131–149). Florence, KY: Routledge.

Stephenson, R., Sheikhattari, P., Assasi, N., Eftekhar, H., Zamani, Q., Maleki, B., et al. (2006). Child maltreatment among school children in the Kurdistan province, Iran. *Child Abuse & Neglect, 30*, 231–245.

Straus, M., et al. (1986). Societal change and change in family violence from 1975 to 1985 as revealed by two national surveys. *Journal of Marriage and the Family, 48*, 465–479.

Straus, M. A., & Hamby, S. L. (1997). Measuring physical and psychological maltreatment of children with the Conflict Tactics Scales. In K. Kantor, et al. (Eds), *Out of the darkness: Contemporary perspectives on family violence* (pp. 119–135). Thousand Oaks, CA: Sage.

Straus, M. A., Hamby, S. L., Finkelhor, D., Moore, D., & Runyan, D. (1998). Identification of child maltreatment with the Parent–Child Conflict Tactics Scales: Development and psychometric data for a national sample of American parents. *Child Abuse & Neglect, 22*, 249–270.

Tang, C. S. (2002). Childhood experience of sexual abuse among Hong Kong Chinese college students. *Child Abuse & Neglect, 26*, 23–37.

Tang, C. S. (2006). Corporal punishment and physical maltreatment against children: A community study of Chinese parents in Hong Kong. *Child Abuse & Neglect, 30*, 893–907.

Tang, C. S, & Yan, E. C. (2004). Intention to participate in child sexual abuse prevention programs: A study of Chinese adults in Hong Kong. *Child Abuse & Neglect, 28*, 1187–1197.

Tauriac, J., & Scruggs, N. (2006). Elder abuse among African Americans. *Educational Gerontology, 32*(1), 37–48.

Tiwari, A., Chan, K. L., Fong, D. Y. T., Leung, W. C., Brownridge, D. A., Lam, H., et al. (2007). A territory-wide survey on intimate partner violence among pregnant women in Hong Kong. *Hong Kong Journal of Gynaecology, Obstetrics and Midwifery, 7*, 7–15.

Tiwari, A., Fong, D. Y. T., Chan, K. L., Leung, W. C., Parker, B., & Ho, P. C. (2007). Identifying intimate partner violence: Comparing the Chinese Abuse Assessment Screen with the Chinese Revised Conflict Tactics Scale. *British Journal of Obstetrics & Gynaecology, 114*, 1065–1071.

Tiwari, A., Leung, W. C., Leung, T. W., Humphreys, J., Parker, B., & Ho, P. C. (2005). A randomised controlled trial of empowerment training for Chinese abused pregnant women in Hong Kong. *British Journal of Obstetrics & Gynaecology, 112*, 1249–1256.

Tiwari, A., Wong, M., & Ip, H. (2001). Ren and Yuan: A cultural interpretation of Chinese women's responses to battering. *Canadian Journal of Nursing Research, 33*, 63–80.

Tiwari, A., Yuk, H., Pang, P., Yuen, F., Fong, D. Y. T., & Chan, K. L. (2008). *Building partnership to promote health in the community: Collaboration of parents, volunteers and professionals for better parenting.* Hong Kong, China: The University of Hong Kong, Department of Nursing Studies.

Tjaden, P., & Thonnes, N. (2000). *Full report on the prevalence, incidence and consequences of intimate partner violence against women: Findings from the National Violence against Women Survey.* Washington, DC: National Institute of Justice and the Centers for Disease Control and Prevention.

Troeme, N. H., & Wolfe, D. (2001). *Child maltreatment in Canada: Selected results from the Canadian Incidence Study of Reported Child Abuse and Neglect.* Ottawa, Ontario, Canada: Minister of Public Works and Government Services Canada.

Tyler, K. A. (2002). Social and emotional outcomes of childhood sexual abuse: A review of recent research. *Aggression and Violent Behavior, 7,* 567–589.

United Nations. (1981). *Convention on the Elimination of All Forms of Discrimination against Women: General Assembly resolution 34/180.* Retrieved from http://www.childinfo.org/files/childmarriage_cedaw.pdf.

United Nations. (1991). *Vienna International Plan of Action on Ageing.* Retrieved from http://www.un.org/esa/socdev/ageing/vienna_intlplanofaction.html.

United Nations. (2002). *Elder abuse widespread and unreported, says new report by secretary-general.* Retrieved from http://www.globalaging.org/waa2/articles/elderabuse.htm.

United Nations. (2004). *World population prospects: The 2004 revision highlights.* Retrieved from http://www.un.org/esa/population/publications/WPP2004/2004Highlights_finalrevised.pdf.

United Nations & Pinheiro, P. S. (2006). *Report of the independent expert for the United Nations study on violence against children: Pursuant to General Assembly resolution 57/90 of 2002.* Retrieved from http://www.violencestudy.org/IMG/pdf/English-2-2.pdf.

United Nations Children's Fund (UNICEF). (2003). *The state of the world children 2003.* Retrieved from http://www.unicef.org/sowc03/.

UNICEF. (2006). *Child marriage.* Retrieved from http://www.childinfo.org/marriage.html.

United Nations Population Fund (2000). Chapter 3: Ending violence against women and girls. In *State of the world population.* Retrieved from http://www.unfpa.org/swp/2000/english/ch03.html.

Vandello, & Cohen, D. (2003). Male honor and female fidelity: Implicit cultural scripts that perpetuate domestic violence. *Journal of Personal and Social Psychology, 84,* 887–1010.

Varcoe, C., & Irwin, L. (2004). "If I killed you, I'd get the kids": Women's survival and protection work with child custody and access in the context of woman abuse. *Qualitative Sociology, 27*(1), 77–99.

Wijeyatilake, K. (2003). *Harsh realities: A pilot study on gender based violence in the plantation sector.* UNFPA.

Winton, M. A., & Mara, B. A. (2001). *Child abuse and neglect: Multidisciplinary approaches.* Boston, MA: Allyn and Bacon.

Wong, W. C. W., Chen, W. Q., Goggins, W. B., Tang, C. S., & Leung, P. W. (2009). Individual, familial and community determinants of child physical abuse among high school students in China. *Social Science & Medicine, 68,* 1819–1825.

Wood, K., & Jewkes, R. (1997). Violence, rape and sexual coercion: Everyday love in South Africa. *Gender and Development, 5*(2), 23–30.

World Health organization (WHO). (2002a). *Child abuse and neglect by parents and other caregivers.* Geneva, Switzerland: WHO.

WHO. (2002b). Child abuse and neglect by parents and other caregivers. In, *World report on violence and health.* Geneva, Switzerland: WHO. Retrieved from http://www.who.int/violence_injury_prevention/violence/global_campaign/en/chap3.pdf.

WHO. (2002c). *Active aging: A policy framework.* Retrieved from http://www.alter-migration.ch/data/5/WHOactiveageing.pdf.

WHO. (2002d). Violence by intimate partners. In *World report on violence and health.* Geneva, Switzerland: WHO. Retrieved from http://www.who.int/violence_injury_prevention/violence/.../chap4.pdf.

WHO. (2002e). *Intimate partner violence and alcohol fact sheet.* Geneva, Switzerland: WHO. Retrieved from http://www.who.int/violence_injury.../world .../factsheets/ft_intimate.pdf.

WHO. (2006a). *Preventing child maltreatment: A guide to taking action and generating evidence.* Geneva, Switzerland: WHO.

WHO. (2006b). *Multi-country study on women's health and domestic violence against women: Summary report. Initial results on prevalence, health outcomes and women's responses.* Geneva, Switzerland: WHO.

WHO. (2008a). *A global response to elder abuse and neglect: Building primary health care capacity to deal with the problem worldwide. Main report.* Geneva, Switzerland: WHO.

WHO. (2008b). *Discussing screening for elder abuse at primary health care level.* Geneva, Switzerland: WHO.

WHO. (2008c). *Child maltreatment.* Retrieved from http://www.who.int/topics/child_abuse/en/.

WHO and International Network for the Prevention of Elder Abuse. (2001). *Missing voices: The views of older persons on elder abuse*. Geneva, Switzerland: Author.

Wuest, J., Ford-Gilboe, M., & Merrit-Gray, M. (2005). Regenerating family: Strengthening the emotional health of mothers and children in the context of intimate partner violence. *Advances in Nursing Science, 27*, 257–274.

Yalcinkaya, A., Mandiracioglu A., & Turan, F. (2006). Turkey: A pilot study of elder mistreatment in a convenient sample. *Journal of Elder Abuse & Neglect, 18*, 105–121.

Yamashiro, G. Y., & Matsuoka, J. K. (1997). Help-seeking among Asian and Pacific Americans: A multiperspective analysis. *Social Work, 42*, 176–186.

Yen, C. F., Yang, M. S., Yang, M. J., Su, Y. C., Wang, M. H., & Lan, C. M. (2008). Childhood physical and sexual abuse: Prevalence and correlates among adolescents living in rural Taiwan. *Child Abuse & Neglect, 32*, 429–438.

Yick, A. G., & Agbayani-Siewert, P. (1997). Perception of domestic violence in a Chinese American community. *Journal of Interpersonal Violence, 12*, 832–846.

Yoshihama, M., & Sorenson, S. B. (1994). Physical, Sexual, and Emotional Abuse by Male Intimates: Experiences of Women in Japan. *Violence and Victims, 9*, 63–77.

Yoshihama, M. (1999). Domestic violence against women of Japanese decent in Los Angeles: Two methods of estimating prevalence. *Violence Against Women, 5*, 869–897.

Yoshioka, M. R., DiNoia, J., & Ullah, K. (2001). Attitudes toward marital violence: An examination of four Asian communities. *Violence Against Women, 7*, 900–926.

Yoshioka, M., Dang, Q., Shewmangal, N., Chan, C., & Tan, C. (2000). Asian family violence report: A study of the Cambodian, Chinese, Korean, South Asian and Vietnamese communities in Massachusetts. *Boston: Asian Task Force Against Domestic Violence, Inc. Retrieved January, 10*, 2008.

Youssef, R. M., Attia, M. S., & Kamel, M. I. (1998). Children experiencing violence: Parental use of corporal punishment. *Child Abuse & Neglect, 22*, 959–973.

Zeira, A., Astor, R., & Benbenishty, R. (2002). Sexual harassment in Jewish and Arab public schools in Israel. *Child Abuse & Neglect, 26*, 149–166.

APPENDIX A

Abuse Assessment Screen

1. Have you ever been emotionally or physically abused by your partner or someone important to you? _____
2. Within the last year, have you been hit, slapped, kicked, pushed or shoved, or otherwise physically hurt by your partner or ex-partner?
   If yes, by whom _____
   Number of times _____
3. Does your partner ever force you into sex? _____
4. Are you afraid of your partner or ex-partner? _____

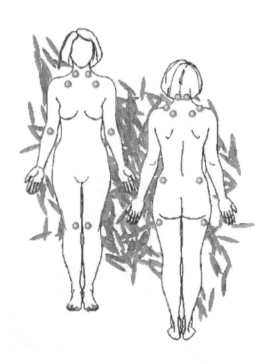

Mark the area of any injury on body map.
(Helton & McFarlane, 1986)

APPENDIX B

Danger Assessment

Jacquelyn C. Campbell, PhD, RN, FAAN

Several risk factors have been associated with increased risk of homicides (murders) of women and men in violent relationships. We cannot predict what will happen in your case, but we would like you to be aware of the danger of homicide in situations of abuse and for you to see how many of the risk factors apply to your situation.

Using the calendar, please mark the approximate dates during the past year when you were abused by your partner or ex-partner. Write on that date how bad the incident was according to the following scale:

1. Slapping, pushing; no injuries and/or lasting pain
2. Punching, kicking; bruises, cuts, and/or continuing pain
3. "Beating up"; severe contusions, burns, broken bones
4. Threat to use weapon; head injury, internal injury, permanent injury, choking, miscarriage
5. Use of weapon; wounds from weapon

(If **any** of the descriptions for the higher number apply, use the higher number.)

Mark **Yes** or **No** for each of the following.

("He" refers to your husband, partner, ex-husband, ex-partner, or whoever is currently physically hurting you.)

Yes	No		
_____	_____	1.	Has the physical violence increased in severity or frequency over the past year?
_____	_____	2.	Does he own a gun?
_____	_____	3.	Have you left him after living together during the past year?
			3a. (If you have *never* lived with him, check here___)
_____	_____	4.	Is he unemployed?
_____	_____	5.	Has he ever used a weapon against you or threatened you with a lethal weapon?
			(If yes, was the weapon a gun?____)
_____	_____	6.	Does he threaten to kill you?
_____	_____	7.	Has he avoided being arrested for domestic violence?
_____	_____	8.	Do you have a child that is not his?
_____	_____	9.	Has he ever forced you to have sex when you did not wish to do so?
_____	_____	10.	Does he ever try to choke you?

_____ _____ 11. Does he use illegal drugs? By drugs, I mean "uppers" or amphetamines, "meth," speed, angel dust, cocaine, "crack," street drugs, or mixtures.

_____ _____ 12. Is he an alcoholic or problem drinker?

_____ _____ 13. Does he control most or all of your daily activities? (For instance: does he tell you who you can be friends with, when you can see your family, how much money you can use, or when you can take the car)?
(If he tries, but you do not let him, check here: _____)

_____ _____ 14. Is he violently and constantly jealous of you?
(For instance, does he say "If I can't have you, no one can.")

_____ _____ 15. Have you ever been beaten by him while you were pregnant?
(If you have never been pregnant by him, check here: _____)

_____ _____ 16. Has he ever threatened or tried to commit suicide?

_____ _____ 17. Does he threaten to harm your children?

_____ _____ 18. Do you believe he is capable of killing you?

_____ _____ 19. Does he follow or spy on you, leave threatening notes or messages, destroy your property, or call you when you do not want him to?

_____ _____ 20. Have you ever threatened or tried to commit suicide?

_____ Total "Yes" Answers

Thank you. Please talk to your nurse, advocate, or counselor about what the Danger Assessment means in terms of your situation.

APPENDIX C

Safer and Stronger Abuse Measure Questions

1. In the last year, has anyone you know made you feel unsafe?
2. In the last year, has anyone you know yelled at you over and over again or hurt your feelings on purpose?
3. In the last year, has anyone you know refused or forgotten to help you with an important personal need such as: toileting or going to the bathroom, bathing, helping you move, getting dressed, getting food or water?
4. In the last year, has anyone you know broken or kept you from using important things such as a: phone, wheelchair, cane, walker, respirator, communication device, service animal, other assistive devices?
5. In the last year, has anyone you know: kept you from taking your medication? Give you too much or too little medication?
6. In the last year, has anyone you know: stolen your money, important items or equipment, signed your checks to take money from you, used your credit or debit card without your OK?
7. In the last year, has anyone you know made you afraid they would hit, kick, slap or shove you?
8. In the last year, has anyone you know actually hit, kicked, slapped or shoved you?
9. In the last year, has anyone you know handled you roughly?
10. In the last year, has anyone you know held or tied you down or made you stay someplace when you did not want to?
11. In the last year, has anyone you know physically hurt you in anyway?
12. In the last year, has anyone you know made you afraid they were going to touch you in a sexual way that you did not want?
13. In the last year, has anyone you know actually touched you in a sexual way that you did not want? In the last year, has anyone you know taken advantage of you in sexual ways you did not want?
14. In the last year, has anyone made you look at or taken sexual pictures of you?
15. In the last year, has anyone been naked in front of you or made you be naked?
16. In the last year, has anyone asked about your sex life?
17. In the last year, has anyone made you feel bad about your body?

Safer and Stronger Perpetrator Risk Characteristics

1. Is the person someone you depend on for personal care (like dressing, bathing, or using the toilet?)
2. Is the person someone who drinks too much or abuses drugs?
3. Is the person someone who controls whether you get the services and health care you need?
4. Is the person someone who controls most of your daily activities?
5. Is the person someone who gets jealous or has severe fits of anger?
6. Is the person someone who decides whether or not you see your family or friends?
7. Is the person someone who makes you afraid they would or actually has hurt your pet, children, or someone else important to you?
8. Is the person someone who has hurt other people?
9. As time goes by, is the abuse getting worse or happening more often?
10. Has the person ever tried to choke you?
11. Has the person ever used a weapon against you or threatened you with a lethal weapon?
12. If "yes," was the weapon a gun?

Index